Bioelectromagnetism

Bioelectromagnetism

■ ■ ■ ■ ■ ■

Principles and Applications
of Bioelectric
and Biomagnetic Fields

JAAKKO MALMIVUO
Ragnar Granit Institute
Tampere University of Technology
Tampere, Finland

ROBERT PLONSEY
Department of Biomedical Engineering
Duke University
Durham, North Carolina

New York   Oxford
OXFORD UNIVERSITY PRESS
1995

Oxford University Press

Oxford New York Toronto
Delhi Bombay Calcutta Madras Karachi
Kuala Lumpur Singapore Hong Kong Tokyo
Nairobi Dar es Salaam Cape Town
Melbourne Auckland Madrid

and associated companies in
Berlin Ibadan

Published by Oxford University Press, Inc.,
200 Madison Avenue, New York, New York 10016

Oxford is a registered trademark of Oxford University Press

Library of Congress Cataloging-in-Publication Data
Malmivuo, Jaakko.
Bioelectromagnetism : principles and applications of bioelectric
and biomagnetic fields / Jaakko Malmivuo, Robert Plonsey.
p. cm. Includes bibliographical references and index.
ISBN-13 978-0-19-505823-9

1. Electrophysiology. 2. Biomagnetism.
I. Plonsey, Robert.
II. Title.
QP341.M235 1995
612'.01442—dc20 93-42971

5 7 9 8 6 4

Printed in the United States of America
on acid-free paper

The authors dedicate this book to

Ragnar Granit

(1900–1991)

*the Finnish-born pioneer of bioelectromagnetism
and Nobel Prize winner*

Preface

Bioelectric phenomena have been a part of medicine throughout its history. The first written document on bioelectric events is an ancient Egyptian hieroglyph of 4000 B.C. describing the electric sheatfish. Bioelectromagnetism is, of course, based strongly on the general theory of electromagnetism. In fact, until the middle of the nineteenth century the history of electromagnetism was also the history of bioelectromagnetism. From the viewpoint of modern science, bioelectric phenomena have had scientific value for the past 200 years. Many of the fundamental contributions to the theory of bioelectromagnetism were made in the nineteenth century. Only in the past 100 years has bioelectromagnetism had real diagnostic or therapeutic value. As we know, this is actually the case for most of medicine as well.

During the past few decades, advances in the theory and technology of modern electronics have led to improvements in medical diagnostic and therapeutic methods and, as a result, bioelectric and biomagnetic phenomena have become increasingly important. Today it is impossible to imagine a hospital without electrocardiography and electroencephalography. The development of microelectronics has made such equipment portable and has increased their diagnostic power. Implantable cardiac pacemakers have allowed millions of people to return to normal life. The development of superconducting technology has made it possible to detect the weak biomagnetic fields induced by bioelectric currents. The latest advances in the measurement of electric currents flowing through a single ion channel of the cell membrane with the patch clamp have opened up completely new applications for bioelectromagnetism. With the patch clamp, bioelectromagnetism can also be applied to molecular biology, for instance, in developing new pharmaceuticals. These examples illustrate that bioelectromagnetism is a vital part of our everyday life.

This book first provides a short introduction to the anatomy and physiology of excitable tissues, and then introduces the theory and associated equations of bioelectric and biomagnetic phenomena; this theory underlies all practical methods. The book then describes current measurement methods and research results and provides an account of their historical development.

The chapters dealing with the anatomy and physiology of various organs are necessarily elementary as comprehensive texts are available in these disciplines. Nevertheless, we wanted to include introductory descriptions of the anatomy and physiology of neural and cardiac tissues in particular so that readers would have a review of the structures and functions upon which electrophysiological models are based. We have also introduced readers to the relevant vocabulary and to important general references.

The theory of bioelectromagnetism deals mainly with electrophysiological models of bioelectric generators, excitability of tissues, and the behavior of bioelectric and biomagnetic fields in and around the volume conductors formed by the body. Because of the nature of the bioelectric sources and the volume conductors, the theory and the analytic methods of bioelectromagnetism are very different from those of general electromagnetism. The theoretical methods are presented as a logical structure. As part of this theory the lead field theoretical approach has been emphasized. Besides the obvious benefits of this approach, it is also true that lead field theory has not been discussed widely in other didactic publications. The lead field theory ties together the sensitivity distribution of the measurement of bioelectric sources, the distribution of stimulation energy, and the sensitivity distribution of impedance measurements, in both electric and magnetic applications. Moreover, lead field theory clearly explains the similarities and differences between the electric and the corresponding magnetic methods, which are tightly related by Maxwell's equations. Thus, all the subfields of bioelectromagnetism are closely related.

We have aimed to present bioelectromagnetism as a theoretical discipline and, in later chapters, to provide much practical material so that the book can also serve as a reference. These chapters also provide an opportunity to introduce some relevant history. In particular, we wanted to present the theory and applications of bioelectricity in parallel with those of biomagnetism to show that in principle they form an inseparable pair. This gave us an opportunity to introduce some relevant history so that readers may recognize how modern research is grounded in older theory and how the fundamentals of many contemporary methods were actually developed years ago.

Our scope in the later chapters is necessarily limited, and thus readers will find only an overview of the topics (applications). Despite their brevity, these applications should help clarify

and strengthen the reader's understanding of basic principles. While better measurement methods than those existing today will undoubtedly be developed in the future, they will necessarily be based on the same theory and mathematical equations given in this book; hence, we believe that its underlying ''truth'' will remain relevant.

This book is intended for readers with a background in physics, mathematics, and/or engineering (at roughly the second- or third-year university level). Readers will find that some chapters require a solid background in physics and mathematics in order to be fully understood but that most can be understood with only an elementary grounding in these subjects.

The initiative for writing this book came from Dr. Jaakko Malmivuo. It is for the most part based on lectures he has given at the Ragnar Granit Institute (formerly Institute of Biomedical Engineering) of Tampere University of Technology and at Helsinki University of Technology in Finland. He has also lectured on bioelectromagnetism as a visiting professor at the Technical University of Berlin, at Dalhousie University in Halifax, and at Sophia University in Tokyo, and has conducted various international tutorial courses. All the illustrations were drawn by Dr. Malmivuo with a microcomputer using the graphics program Corel-DRAW!. The calculations of the curves and the fields were made with MathCad and the data were accurately transferred to the illustrations.

The manuscript was read and carefully critiqued by Dr. Milan Horáček at Dalhousie University and Dr. David Geselowitz of Pennsylvania State University. Their valuable comments are acknowledged with gratitude. Sir Alan Hodgkin and Sir Andrew Huxley read Chapter 4. We are grateful for their detailed comments and the support they gave our illustration of the Hodgkin-Huxley membrane model. We are grateful also to the staff of Oxford University Press, especially Jeffrey House, Dolores Oetting, Edith Barry, Rosalind Corman, and Alasdair Ritchie. Dr. Ritchie carefully read several chapters and made detailed suggestions for improvement. We also thank the anonymous reviewer provided by Oxford University Press for many valuable comments. Ms. Tarja Erälaukko and Ms. Soile Lönnqvist, at

Ragnar Granit Institute, provided editorial assistance in the preparation of the manuscript and the illustrations. We also appreciate the work of the many students and colleagues who critiqued earlier versions of the manuscript. The encouragement and support of our wives, Kirsti and Vivian, are also gratefully acknowledged.

Financial support from the Academy of Finland and Ministry of Education in Finland is greatly appreciated.

We hope that this book will raise our readers' interest in bioelectromagnetism and provide the background that will allow them to delve into research and practical applications in the field. We also hope that the book will facilitate the development of medical diagnosis and therapy.

Tampere, Finland   J.M.
Durham, North Carolina   R.P.

Contents

Symbols and Units

$\alpha_h, \alpha_m, \alpha_n$	transfer rate coefficients (Hodgkin-Huxley model)
$\beta_h, \beta_m, \beta_n$	transfer rate coefficients (Hodgkin-Huxley model)
δ_s, δ_v	two-dimensional $[m^{-2}]$ and three-dimensional $[m^{-3}]$ Dirac delta functions
ϵ	permittivity [F/m]
$\mathscr{E}$	electromotive force (emf) [V]
Θ	conduction velocity (of wave) [m/s]
λ	membrane length constant [cm] $(\approx \sqrt{(r_m/r_i)} = \sqrt{(R_m a/2\rho_i)})$
μ	magnetic permeability of the medium [H/m = Vs/Am]
μ, μ_0	electrochemical potential of the ion in general and in the reference state [J/mol]
ν	nodal width $[\mu m]$
ρ	resistivity $[\Omega m]$, charge density $[C/m^3]$
ρ_i^b, ρ_o^b	intracellular and interstitial bidomain resistivities $[k\Omega \cdot cm]$
ρ_m^b	bidomain membrane resistivity $[k\Omega \cdot cm]$
ρ_t^b	bidomain total tissue impedance $[k\Omega \cdot cm]$
ρ_i, ρ_o	intracellular and interstitial resistivities $[k\Omega \cdot cm]$
σ	conductivity [S/m]
σ_i^b, σ_o^b	intracellular and interstitial bidomain conductivities [mS/cm]
σ_i, σ_o	intracellular and interstitial conductivities [mS/cm]
τ	membrane time constant [ms] $(= r_m c_m$ in one-dimensional problem, $= R_m C_m$ in two-dimensional problem)
ϕ, Θ	longitude (azimuth), coltitude, angles in spherical polar coordinates
Φ	potential [V]
Φ_i, Φ_o	potential inside and outside the membrane [mV]

Φ_{LE}	reciprocal electric scalar potential field of electric lead due to unit reciprocal current [V/A]
Φ_{LM}	reciprocal magnetic scalar potential field of magnetic lead due to reciprocal current of unit time derivative [Vs/A]
Φ, ψ	two scalar functions (in Green's theorem)
χ	surface-to-volume ratio of a cell [1/cm]
ω	radial frequency [rad] ($= 2\pi f$)
Ω	solid angle [sr (steradian) $= m^2/m^2$]
a	radius [m], fiber radius [μm]
$\bar{a}$	unit vector
A	azimuth angle in spherical coordinates [°]
A	cross-sectional area [m^2]
$\bar{A}$	magnetic vector potential [Wb/m $=$ Vs/m]
$\bar{B}$	magnetic induction (magnetic field density) [Wb/m^2 $=$ Vs/m^2]
$\bar{B}_{LM}$	reciprocal magnetic induction of a magnetic lead due to reciprocal current of unit time derivative [Wb·s/Am^2 $=$ Vs^2/Am^2]
c	particle concentration [mol/m^3]
$\bar{c}$	lead vector
c_i, c_o	intracellular and extracellular ion concentrations (monovalent ion) [mol/m^3]
c^k	ion concentration of the kth permeable ion [mol/m^3]
c_m	membrane capacitance per unit length [μF/cm fiber length]
C	electric charge [C (Coulomb) $=$ As]
C_m	membrane capacitance per unit area (specific capacitance) [μF/cm^2]
d	double layer thickness, diameter [μm]
d_i, d_o	fiber internal and external myelin diameters [μm]
$d\bar{S}$	outward surface normal
D	Fick's constant (diffusion constant) [cm^2/s $=$ cm^3/(cm·s)]
D	electric displacement [C/m^2]
E	elevation angle in spherical coordinates [°]
$\bar{E}$	electric field [V/m]
$\bar{E}_{LE}$	reciprocal electric field of electric lead due to unit reciprocal current [V/Am]
$\bar{E}_{LM}$	reciprocal electric field of magnetic lead due to reciprocal current of unit time derivative [Vs/Am]
F	Faraday's constant [9.649·10^4 C/mol]
F	magnetic flux [Wb $=$ Vs]
g_K, g_{Na}, g_L	membrane conductances per unit length for potassium, sodium, and chloride (leakage) [mS/cm fiber length]
G_K, G_{Na}, G_L	membrane conductances per unit area for potassium, sodium, and chloride (leakage) [mS/cm^2]
G_{Kmax}, G_{Namax}	maximum values of potassium and sodium conductances per unit area [mS/cm^2]
G_m	membrane conductance per unit area [mS/cm^2]

h	distance (height) [m]
h	membrane thickness [μm]
h,m,n	gating variables (Hodgkin-Huxley model)
Hct	hematocrit [%]
$\overline{H}$	magnetic field [A/m]
$\overline{H}_{LM}$	reciprocal magnetic field of a magnetic lead due to reciprocal current of unit time derivative [s/m]
i_m	membrane current per unit length [μA/cm fiber length] ($= 2\pi a I_m$)
i_r	reciprocal current through a differential source element [A]
I	electric current [A]
I_a	applied steady-state (or stimulus) current [μA]
I_i, I_o	axial currents [μA] and axial currents per unit area [μA/cm^2] inside and outside the cell
i_K, i_{Na}, i_L	membrane current carried by potassium, sodium, and chloride (leakage) ions per unit length [μA/cm fiber length]
I_K, I_{Na}, I_L	membrane current carried by potassium, sodium, and chloride (leakage) ions per unit area [μA/cm^2]
I_L	lead current in general [A]
I_m	membrane current per unit area [μA/cm^2] ($= I_{mC} + I_mR$), bidomain membrane current per unit volume [μA/cm^3]
i_{mC}, i_{mI}, i_{mR}	capacitive, ionic, and resistive components of the membrane current per unit length [μA/cm fiber length] ($= 2\pi a I_{mC}, = 2\pi a I_{mI}, = 2\pi a I_{mR}$)
I_{mC}, I_{mI}, I_{mR}	capacitive, ionic, and resistive components of the membrane current per unit area [μA/cm^2]
I_r	total reciprocal current [A]
I_{rh}	rheobasic current per unit area [μA/cm^2]
I_s	stimulus current per unit area [μA/cm^2]
j, j_k	ionic flux, ionix flux due to the kth ion [mol/(cm^2·s)]
j_D, j_e	ionic flux due to diffusion, due to electric field [mol/(cm^2·s)]
$\overline{J}$	electric current density [A/m^2]
$\overline{J} dv$	source element
$\overline{J}^i$	impressed current density [μA/cm^2], impressed dipole moment per unit volume [μA·cm/cm^3]
$\overline{J}_i, \overline{J}_o$	intracellular and interstitial current densities [μA/cm^2]
$\overline{J}_F^i, \overline{J}_V^i$	flow (flux) and vortex source components of the impressed current density [μA/cm^2]
$\overline{J}_r^i, \overline{J}_t^i$	radial and tangential components of the impressed current density [μA/cm^2]
$\overline{J}_L$	lead field in general [A/m^2]
$\overline{J}_{LE}$	electric lead field due to unit reciprocal current [1/m^2]
$\overline{J}_{LI}$	lead field of current feeding electrodes for a unit current [1/m^2] (in impedance measurement)
$\overline{J}_{LM}$	magnetic lead field due to reciprocal current of unit time derivative [s/m^2]

K	constant
$K(k), E(k)$	complete elliptic integrals
$\overline{K}_j$	secondary current source for electric fields [μA/cm^2]
l	length [m], internodal spacing [μm]
ℓ	liter
L	inductance [H = Wb/A = Vs/A]
$\overline{m}$	magnetic dipole moment of a volume source [Am^2]
M	vector magnitude in spherical coordinates
M_1, M_2, M_3	peak vector magnitudes during the initial, mid, and terminal phases of the QRS-complex in ECG [mV] and MCG [pT]
n	number of moles
$\overline{n}$	surface normal (unit length)
$\overline{n}_j$	surface normal of surface S_j directed from the primed region to the double-primed one
p	electric dipole moment per unit area [Am/m^2 = A/m]
$\overline{p}$	electric dipole moment of a volume source [Am]
P	pressure [N/m^2]
P_{Cl}, P_K, P_{Na}	membrane permeabilities of chloride, potassium, and sodium ions [m/s]
r	radius, distance [m], vector magnitude in spherical polar coordinates
r	correlation coefficient
$\overline{r}$	radius vector
r_i, r_o	axial intracellular and interstitial resistances per unit length [kΩ/cm fiber length] ($r_i = 1/\sigma_i \pi a^2$)
r_m	membrane resistance times unit length [k$\Omega\cdot$cm fiber length] (= $R_m/2\pi a$)
R	gas constant [8.314 J/(mol·K)]
R_i, R_o	axial resistances of the intracellular and interstitial media [kΩ]
R_m	membrane resistance times unit area (specific resistance) [k$\Omega\cdot$cm^2]
R_s	series resistance [MΩ]
S_{Cl}, S_K, S_{Na}	electric current densities due to chloride, potassium, and sodium ion fluxes [μA/cm^2]
t	time [s]
T	temperature [°C], absolute temperature [K]
u	ionic mobility [cm^2/(V·s)]
v	velocity [m/s]
v	volume [m^3]
V	voltage [V]
V'	deviation of the membrane voltage from the resting state [mV] (= $V_m - V_r$)
V_c	clamp voltage [mV]
V_L	lead voltage in general [V]
V_{LE}	lead voltage of electric lead due to unit reciprocal current [V]

V_{LM}	lead voltage of magnetic lead due to reciprocal current of unit time derivative [V]
V_K, V_{Na}, V_L	Nernst voltages for potassium, sodium, and chloride (leakage) ions [mV]
V_m	membrane voltage [mV] ($= \Phi_i - \Phi_o$)
V_r, V_{th}	resting and threshold voltages of membrane [mV]
V_R	reversal voltage [mV]
V_Z	measured voltage (in impedance measurement) [V]
W	work [J/mol]
X,Y,Z	rectangular coordinates
z	valence of the ions
Z	impedance [Ω]

The *List of Symbols and Units* includes the main symbols existing in the book. Symbols, which appear only in one connection or are obvious extensions of those in the list, are not necessarily included. They are defined in the text as they are introduced.

The dimensions for *general variables* follow the SI system.

The dimensions for *variables used in electrophysiological measurements* follow, for practical reasons, usually the tradition in this discipline. Lower case symbols are used in the one-dimensional problem, where they are defined "per unit length." Upper case symbols are used in the two-dimensional problem, where they are defined "per unit area." Upper case symbols may also represent a variable defined "for the total area." (As usual in the bioelectric literature, the symbol "I" is used for membrane currents also in the two-dimensional problem, though in physics current density is represented with the symbol "J.")

Abbreviations

ac	alternating current
AV	atrioventricular
CO	cardiac output
DC	direct current
ECG,MCG	electrocardiogram, magnetocardiogram
EDR	electrodermal response
EEG,MEG	electroencephalogram, magnetoencephalogram
EHV,MHV	electric heart vector, magnetic heart vector
emf	electromotive force
EMG,MMG	electromyogram, magnetomyogram
ENG,MNG	electronystagmogram, magnetonystagmogram
EOG,MOG	electro-oculogram, magneto-oculogram
EPSP,IPSP	excitatory and inhibitory post-synaptic potentials
ERG,MRG	electroretinogram, magnetoretinogram
ERP	early receptor potential
ESR	electric skin resistance
F,V	flow, vortex
FN,FP	false negative, false positive
GSR	galvanic skin reflex
HR	heart rate
IPL	inner plexiform layer
LA,RA,LL	left arm, right arm, left leg
LBBB,RBBB	left bundle-branch block, right bundle-branch block

LVED	left ventricular end-diastolic
LVH,RVH	left ventricular hypertrophy, right ventricular hypertrophy
LRP	late receptor potential
MFV	magnetic field vector
MI	myocardial infarction
MSPG	magnetic susceptibility plethysmography
OPL	outer plexiform layer
PAT	paroxysmal atrial tachycardia
PCG	phonocardiogram
PGR	psychogalvanic reflex
REM	rapid eye movements
rf	radio-frequency
rms	root mean square
RPE	retinal pigment epithelium
SA	sinoatrial
SQUID	Superconducting QUantum Interference Device
SV	stroke volume
TEA	tetraethylammonium
TN,TP	true negative, true positive
TTS	transverse tubular system
TTX	tetrodotoxin
V	ECG lead (V_F, V_L, V_R, aV_F, aV_L, aV_R, $V_1, \ldots, V_6$)
VCG	vectorcardiography
VECG,VMCG	vector electrocardiography, vector magnetocardiography
WPW	Wolff-Parkinson-White (syndrome)

Physical Constants

Quantity	Symbol	Value	Dimension
Absolute temperature	T	T[°C] − 273.16	(kelvin)
Avogadro's number	N	6.022×10^{23}	1/mol
Electric permittivity for free space	ϵ_0	8.854	C/(V·m)
		1.602×10^{-19}	
Elementary charge	e	9.648×10^4	C
Faraday's constant	F	1.987	C/mol
Gas constant (in energy units)	R	8.315	cal/(K·mol) J/(K·mol)
Joule	J	1	kg·m^2/s^2
		1	V·C = W·s
		0.2389	cal
Magnetic permeability for free space	μ	$4\pi \cdot 10^{-7}$	H/m

Bioelectromagnetism

1

Introduction

1.1 THE CONCEPT OF BIOELECTROMAGNETISM

Bioelectromagnetism is a discipline that examines the electric, electromagnetic, and magnetic phenomena which arise in biological tissues. These phenomena include:

The behavior of excitable tissue (the sources)

The electric currents and potentials in the volume conductor

The magnetic field at and beyond the body

The response of excitable cells to electric and magnetic field stimulation

The intrinsic electric and magnetic properties of the tissue

It is important to separate the concept of bioelectromagnetism from the concept of *medical electronics;* the former involves bioelectric, bioelectromagnetic, and biomagnetic *phenomena* and measurement and stimulation *methodology,* whereas the latter refers to the actual *devices* used for these purposes.

By definition, bioelectromagnetism is interdisciplinary since it involves the association of the life sciences with the physical and engineering sciences. Consequently, we have a special interest in those disciplines that combine engineering and physics with biology and medicine. These disciplines are briefly defined as follows:

Biophysics: The science that is concerned with the solution of biological problems in terms of the concepts of physics.

Bioengineering: The application of engineering to the development of health care devices, analysis of biological systems, and manufacturing of products based on advances in this technology. This term is also frequently used to encompass both biomedical engineering and biochemical engineering (biotechnology).

Biotechnology: The study of microbiological process technology. The main fields of application of biotechnology are agriculture, and food and drug production.

Medical electronics: A division of biomedical engineering concerned with electronic devices and methods in medicine.

Medical physics: A science based upon physical problems in clinical medicine.

Biomedical engineering: An engineering discipline concerned with the application of science and technology (devices and methods) to biology and medicine.

3

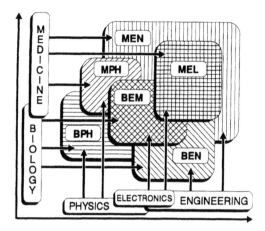

Fig. 1.1 Currently recognized interdisciplinary fields that associate physics and engineering with medicine and biology: BEN = bioengineering; BPH = biophysics; BEM = bioelectromagnetism; MPH = medical physics; MEN = medical engineering; MEL = medical electronics.

Figure 1.1 illustrates the relationships between these disciplines. The coordinate origin represents the more theoretical sciences, such as biology and physics. As one moves away from the origin, the sciences become increasingly applied. Combining a pair of sciences from medical and technical fields yields interdisciplinary sciences such as medical engineering. It must be understood that the disciplines are actually *multi*dimensional, and thus their *two*-dimensional description is only suggestive.

1.2 SUBDIVISIONS OF BIOELECTROMAGNETISM

1.2.1 Division on a Theoretical Basis

The discipline of bioelectromagnetism may be subdivided in many different ways. One such classification divides the field on theoretical grounds according to two universal principles: *Maxwell's equations* (the electromagnetic connection) and the *principle of reciprocity.* This philosophy is illustrated in Figure 1.2 and is discussed in greater detail below.

Maxwell's Equations

Maxwell's equations, that is, the electromagnetic connection, connect time-varying electric

and magnetic fields so that when there are *bioelectric* fields there always are also *biomagnetic* fields, and vice versa (Maxwell, 1865). Depending on whether we discuss electric, electromagnetic, or magnetic phenomena, bioelectromagnetism may be divided along one conceptual dimension (horizontally in Fig. 1.2) into three subdivisions, namely

(A) Bioelectricity,
(B) Bioelectromagnetism (biomagnetism), and
(C) Biomagnetism.

Subdivision B has historically been called "biomagnetism" which unfortunately can be confused with our Subdivision C. Therefore, in this book, for Subdivision B we also use the conventional name "biomagnetism" but, where appropriate, we emphasize that the more precise term is "bioelectromagnetism." (The reader experienced in electromagnetic theory will note the omission of a logical fourth subdivision: measurement of the electric field induced by variation in the magnetic field arising from magnetic material in tissue. However, because this field is not easily detected and does not have any known value, we have omitted it from our discussion).

Reciprocity

Owing to the principle of reciprocity, the sensitivity distribution in the detection of bioelectric signals, the energy distribution in electric stimulation, and the sensitivity distribution of electric impedance measurements are the same. This is also true for the corresponding bioelectromagnetic and biomagnetic methods, respectively. Depending on whether we discuss the measurement of the field, of stimulation/magnetization, or the measurement of intrinsic properties of tissue, bioelectromagnetism may be divided within this framework (vertically in Fig. 1.2) as follows:

(I) Measurement of an electric or a magnetic field from a bioelectric source or (the magnetic field from) magnetic material
(II) Electric stimulation with an electric or a magnetic field or the magnetization of materials (with a magnetic field)
(III) Measurement of the intrinsic electric or magnetic properties of tissue.

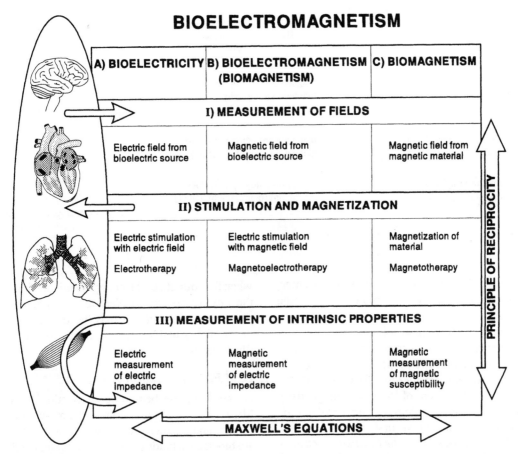

Fig. 1.2 Organization of bioelectromagnetism into its subdivisions. It is first divided horizontally: A) bioelectricity; B) bioelectromagnetism (biomagnetism); and C) biomagnetism. Then the division is made vertically: I) measurement of fields; II) stimulation and magnetization; and III) measurement of intrinsic electric and magnetic properties of tissue. The horizontal divisions are tied together by Maxwell's equations and the vertical divisions by the principle of reciprocity.

Description of the Subdivisions

The aforementioned taxonomy is illustrated in Figure 1.2 and a detailed description of its elements is given in this section.

(I) *Measurement of an electric or a magnetic field* refers, essentially, to the electric or magnetic signals produced by the activity of living tissues. In this subdivision of bioelectromagnetism, the active tissues produce electromagnetic energy, which is measured either electrically or magnetically within or outside the organism in which the source lies. This subdivision includes also the magnetic field produced by magnetic material in the tissue. Examples of these fields in the three horizontal subdivisions are shown in Table 1.1.

(II) *Electric stimulation with an electric or a magnetic field or the magnetization of materials* includes the effects of applied electric and magnetic fields on tissue. In this subdivision of bioelectromagnetism, electric or magnetic energy is generated with an electronic device outside biological tissues. When this electric or magnetic energy is applied to *excitable tissue* in order to activate it, it is called *electric stimulation* or *magnetic stimulation,* respectively. When the magnetic energy is applied to tissue containing ferromagnetic material, the material is *magnetized.* (To be accurate, an insulated human body may also be charged to a high electric potential. This kind of experiment, called *electrifying,* were made already during the early development of bio-

Table 1.1   I) Measurements of fields

(A) Bioelectricity	(B) Bioelectromagnetism (Biomagnetism)	(C) Biomagnetism
Neural cells		
electroencephalography (EEG)	magnetoencephalography (MEG)	
electroneurography (ENG)	magnetoneurography (MNG)	
electroretinography (ERG)	magnetoretinography (MRG)	
Muscle cells		
electrocardiography (ECG)	magnetocardiography (MCG)	
electromyography (EMG)	magnetomyography (MMG)	
Other tissue		
electro-oculography (EOG)	magneto-oculography (MOG)	
electronystagmography (ENG)	magnetonystagmography (MNG)	
		magnetopneumogram
		magnetohepatogram

electricity but their value is only in the entertainment.) Similarly the nonlinear membrane properties may be defined with both subthreshold and transthreshold stimuli. Subthreshold electric or magnetic energy may also be applied for other therapeutic purposes, called *electrotherapy* or *magnetotherapy*. Examples of this second subdivision of bioelectromagnetism, also called *electrobiology* and *magnetobiology*, respectively, are shown in Table 1.2.

(III) *Measurement of the intrinsic electric or magnetic properties of tissue* is included in bioelectromagnetism as a third subdivision. As in Subdivision II, electric or magnetic energy is generated by an electronic device outside the biological tissue and applied to it. However,

when the strength of the energy is *sub*threshold, the *passive (intrinsic) electric and magnetic properties of the tissue* may be obtained by performing suitable measurements. Table 1.3 illustrates this subdivision.

Lead Field Theoretical Approach

As noted in the beginning of Section 1.2.1, Maxwell's equations connect time-varying electric and magnetic fields, so that when there are bioelectric fields there are also biomagnetic fields, and vice versa. This electromagnetic connection is the universal principle unifying the three subdivisions—A, B, and C—of bioelectromagnetism in the horizontal direction in Figure 1.2. As noted in the beginning of this

Table 1.2   II) Stimulation and magnetization

(A) Bioelectricity	(B) Bioelectromagnetism (Biomagnetism)	(C) Biomagnetism
Stimulation		
patch clamp, voltage clamp		
electric stimulation of the central nervous system or of motor nerve/muscle	magnetic stimulation of the central nervous system or of motor nerve/muscle	
electric cardiac pacing	magnetic cardiac pacing	
electric cardiac defibrillation	magnetic cardiac defibrillation	
Therapeutic applications		
electrotherapy	electromagnetotherapy	magnetotherapy
electrosurgery (surgical diathermy)		
Magnetization		
		magnetization of ferromagnetic material

Table 1.3 III) Measurement of intrinsic properties

(A) Bioelectricity	(B) Bioelectromagnetism (Biomagnetism)	(C) Biomagnetism
electric measurement of electric impedance	magnetic measurement of electric impedance	measurement of magnetic susceptibility
impedance cardiography		magnetic susceptibility plethysmography
impedance pneumography		magnetic remanence measurement
impedance tomography	impedance tomography	magnetic resonance imaging (MRI)
electrodermal response (EDR)		

section, the sensitivity distribution in the detection of bioelectric signals, the energy distribution in electric stimulation, and the sensitivity distribution of the electric impedance measurement are the same. All of this is true also for the corresponding bioelectromagnetic and biomagnetic methods, respectively. The universal principle that ties together the three subdivisions I, II, and III and unifies the discipline of bioelectromagnetism in the vertical direction in Figure 1.2 is the principle of reciprocity.

These fundamental principles are further illustrated in Figure 1.3, which is drawn in the same format as Figure 1.2 but also includes a description of the applied methods and the *lead fields* that characterize their sensitivity/energy distributions. Before finishing this book, the reader may have difficulty understanding Figure 1.3 in depth. However, we wanted to introduce this figure early, because it illustrates the fundamental principles governing the entire discipline of bioelectromagnetism, which will be amplified later on.

1.2.2 Division on an Anatomical Basis

Bioelectromagnetism can be classified also along anatomical lines. This division is appropriate especially when one is discussing clinical applications. In this case, bioelectromagnetism is subdivided according to the applicable tissue. For example, one might consider

(a) neurophysiological bioelectromagnetism;
(b) cardiological bioelectromagnetism; and
(c) bioelectromagnetism of other organs or tissues.

1.2.3 Organization of This Book

Because it is inappropriate from a didactic perspective to use only one of the aforementioned divisional schemes (i.e., division on a theoretical or an anatomical basis), both of them are utilized in this book. This book includes 28 chapters which are arranged into nine parts. Table 1.4 illustrates how these chapters fit into the scheme whereby bioelectromagnetism is divided on a theoretical basis, as introduced in Figure 1.2.

Part I discusses the anatomical and physiological basis of bioelectromagnetism. From the anatomical perspective, for example, Part I considers bioelectric phenomena first on a cellular level (i.e., involving nerve and muscle cells) and then on an organ level (involving the nervous system (brain) and the heart).

Part II introduces the concepts of the *volume source* and *volume conductor* and the concept of modeling. It also introduces the concept of *impressed current source* and discusses general theoretical concepts of *source-field models* and the *bidomain* volume conductor. These discussions consider only electric concepts.

Part III explores theoretical methods and thus anatomical features are excluded from discussion. For practical (and historical) reasons, this discussion is first presented from an electric perspective in Chapter 11. Chapter 12 then relates most of these theoretical methods to magnetism and especially considers the difference between concepts in electricity and magnetism.

The rest of the book (i.e., Parts IV–IX) explores clinical applications. For this reason, bioelectromagnetism is first classified on an anatomical basis into bioelectric and

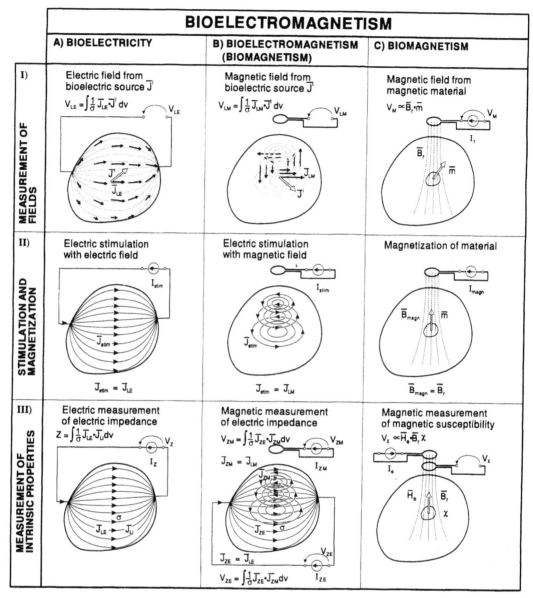

Fig. 1.3 Lead field theoretical approach to describe the subdivisions of bioelectromagnetism. The sensitivity distribution in the detection of bioelectric signals, the energy distribution in electric stimulation, and the distribution of measurement sensitivity of electric impedance are the same, owing to the principle of reciprocity. This is true also for the corresponding bioelectromagnetic and biomagnetic methods. Maxwell's equations tie time-varying electric and magnetic fields together so that when there are bioelectric fields there are also bioelectromagnetic fields, and vice versa.

bio(electro)magnetic constituents to point out the parallelism between them. Part IV describes electric and magnetic measurements of bioelectric sources of the nervous system, and Part V those of the heart.

In Part VI, Chapters 21 and 22 discuss electric and magnetic stimulation of neural and Part VII, Chapters 23 and 24, that of cardiac tissue. These subfields are also referred to as *electrobiology* and *magnetobiology*.

Part VIII focuses on Subdivision III of bioelectromagnetism—that is, the measurement of

Table 1.4 Organization of this book (by chapter number) according to the division of bioelectromagnetism on a theoretical basis

(A) Bioelectricity	(B) Bioelectromagnetism (Biomagnetism)	(C) Biomagnetism
(I) Measurement of fields		
Electric field from bioelectric source	Magnetic field from bioelectric source	Magnetic field from magnetic material
04 Active behavior of the membrane		Not discussed
05 Physiology of the synapse and brain		
06 Bioelectric behavior of the heart		
07 Volume source and volume conductor		
08 Source-field models		
09 Bidomain model		
11 Theoretical methods	12 Theory of biomagnetic measurements	
13 Electroencephalography	14 Magnetoencephalography	
15 12-lead ECG	20 Magnetocardiography	
16 Vectorcardiography		
17 Other ECG systems		
18 Distortion in ECG		
19 ECG diagnosis		
28 Electric signals of the eye		
(II) Stimulation and magnetization		
Electric stimulation with electric field	Electric stimulation with magnetic field	Magnetization of material
03 Subthreshold membrane phenomena		Not discussed
21 Functional electric stimulation	22 Magnetic stimulation	
23 Cardiac pacing		
24 Cardiac defibrillation		
(III) Measurement of intrinsic properties		
Electric measurement of electric impedance	Magnetic measurement of electric impedance	Magnetic measurement of magnetic susceptibility
25 Impedance plethysmography		Not discussed
26 Impedance tomography	26 Magnetic measurement of electric impedance tomography	
27 Electrodermal response		

the intrinsic electric properties of biological tissue. Chapters 25 and 26 examine the measurement and imaging of tissue impedance, and Chapter 27 the measurement of the electrodermal response.

In Part IX, Chapter 28 introduces the reader to a bioelectric signal that is not generated by excitable tissue: the electro-oculogram (EOG). The electroretinogram (ERG) also is discussed in this connection for anatomical reasons, al-though the signal is due to an excitable tissue, namely the retina.

The discussion of the effects of an electromagnetic field on tissue, which is part of Subdivision II, includes topics on cellular physiology and pathology rather than electromagnetic theory. Therefore this book does not include this subject. The reader may get an overview of this for instance from Gandhi (1990) or Reilly (1992).

Because discussion of Subdivision C would require the introduction of additional fundamentals, we have chosen not to include it in this volume. As mentioned earlier, Subdivision C entails measurement of the magnetic field from magnetic material, magnetization of material, and measurement of magnetic susceptibility. The reader interested in these topics should consult Maniewski et al. (1988) and other sources. At the present time, interest in the Subdivision C topic is limited.

1.3 IMPORTANCE OF BIOELECTROMAGNETISM

Why should we consider the study of electric and magnetic phenomena in living tissues as a separate discipline? The main reason is that bioelectric phenomena of the cell membrane are vital functions of the living organism. The cell uses the membrane potential in several ways. With rapid opening of the channels for sodium ions, the membrane potential is altered radically within a thousandth of a second. Cells in the nervous system communicate with one another by means of such electric signals that rapidly travel along the nerve processes. In fact, life itself begins with a change in membrane potential. As the sperm merges with the egg cell at the instant of fertilization, ion channels in the egg are activated. The resultant change in the membrane potential prevents access of other sperm cells.

Electric phenomena are easily measured, and therefore, this approach is direct and feasible. In the investigation of other modalities, such as biochemical and biophysical events, special transducers must be used to convert the phenomenon of interest into a measurable electric signal. In contrast electric phenomena can easily be directly measured with simple electrodes; alternatively, the magnetic field they produce can be detected with a magnetometer.

In contrast to all other biological variables, bioelectric and biomagnetic phenomena can be detected in real time by noninvasive methods because the information obtained from them is manifested immediately throughout and around the volume conductor formed by the body. Their source may be investigated by applying the modern theory of volume sources and volume conductors, utilizing the computing capability of modern computers. (The concepts of volume sources and volume conductors denote three-dimensional sources and conductors, respectively, having large dimensions relative to the distance of the measurement. These are discussed in detail later.) Conversely, it is possible to introduce temporally and spatially controlled electric stimuli to activate paralyzed regions of the neural or muscular systems of the body.

The electric nature of biological tissues permits the transmission of signals for information and for control and is therefore of vital importance for life. The first category includes such examples as vision, audition, and tactile sensation; in these cases a peripheral transducer (the eye, the ear, etc.) initiates afferent signals to the brain. Efferent signals originating in the brain can result in voluntary contraction of muscles to effect the movement of limbs, for example. And finally, homeostasis involves closed-loop regulation mediated, at least in part, by electric signals that affect vital physiologic functions such as heart rate, strength of cardiac contraction, humoral release, and so on.

As a result of the rapid development of electronic instrumentation and computer science, diagnostic instruments, which are based on bioelectric phenomena, have developed very quickly. Today it is impossible to imagine any hospital or doctor's office without electrocardiography and electroencephalography. The development of microelectronics has made such equipment portable and strengthened their diagnostic power. Implantable cardiac pacemakers have allowed millions of people with heart problems to return to normal life. Biomagnetic applications are likewise being rapidly developed and will, in the future, supplement bioelectric methods in medical diagnosis and therapy. These examples illustrate that bioelectromagnetism is a vital part of our everyday life.

Bioelectromagnetism makes it possible to investigate the behavior of living tissue on both cellular and organic levels. Furthermore, the latest scientific achievements now allow scientists to do research at the subcellular level by measuring the electric current flowing through a single ion channel of the cell membrane with the patch-clamp method. With the latter approach, bioelectromagnetism can be applied to molecular biology and to the development of new pharmaceuticals. Thus bioelectromagnetism offers new and important opportunities for the development of diagnostic and therapeutic methods.

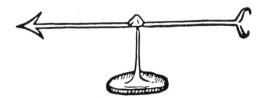

Fig. 1.4 The first instrument to detect electricity was the electroscope invented by William Gilbert (Gilbert 1600).

1.4 SHORT HISTORY OF BIOELECTROMAGNETISM

1.4.1 The First Written Documents and First Experiments in Bioelectromagnetism

The first written document on bioelectric events is in an ancient Egyptian hieroglyph of 4000 B.C. The hieroglyph describes the electric sheatfish (catfish) as a fish that "releases the troops." Evidently, when the catch included such a fish, the fish generated electric shocks with an amplitude of more than 450 V, which forced the fishermen to release all of the fish. The sheatfish is also illustrated in an Egyptian sepulcher fresco (Morgan, 1868).

The Greek philosophers Aristotle (384–322 B.C.) and Thales (c.625–547 B.C.) experimented with amber and recognized its power to attract light substances (Smith, 1931). The first written document on the medical application of electricity is from the year A.D. 46, when Scribonius Largus recommended the use of torpedo fish for curing headaches and gouty arthritis (Kellaway, 1946). The electric fish remained the only means of producing electricity for electrotherapeutic experiments until the seventeenth century.

William Gilbert (1544–1603), physician to Queen Elizabeth I of England, was the first to subject the attractive power of amber to planned experiment. Gilbert constructed the first instrument to measure this power. This *electroscope* was a light metal needle pivoted on a pin so that it would turn toward the substances of attracting power (see Fig. 1.4). Gilbert called the substances possessing this power of attraction *electricks,* from the Greek name

for amber (ηλεκτρον). Thus he coined the term that eventually became the new science of electricity. Gilbert published his experiments in 1600 in a book entitled *De Magnete* (Gilbert, 1600). (The reader may refer to Fig. 1.20 at the end of this chapter. It presents a chronology of important historical events in bioelectromagnetism from the year 1600 until today.)

The first carefully documented scientific experiments in neuromuscular physiology were conducted by Jan Swammerdam (Dutch; 1637–80). At that time it was believed that contraction of a muscle was caused by the flow of "animal spirits" or "nervous fluid" along the nerve to the muscle. In 1664, Swammerdam conducted experiments to study the muscle volume changes during contraction (see Fig. 1.5). Swammerdam placed a frog muscle (b) into a glass vessel (a). When contraction of the muscle was initiated by stimulation of its motor nerve, a water droplet (e) in a narrow tube, projecting from the vessel, did not move, indicating that the muscle did not expand. Thus, the contraction could not be a consequence of inflow of nervous fluid.

In many similar experiments, Swammerdam stimulated the motor nerve by pinching it. In fact, in this experiment stimulation was achieved by pulling the nerve with a wire (c) made of silver (filium argenteum) against a loop (d) made of copper (filium aeneum). According to the principles of electrochemistry, the dissimilar metals in this experiment, which are embedded in the electrolyte provided by the tissue, are the origin of an *electromotive force (emf)* and an associated *electric current.* The latter flows through the metals and the tissue, and is responsible for the stimulation (*activation*) of the nerve in this tissue preparation.

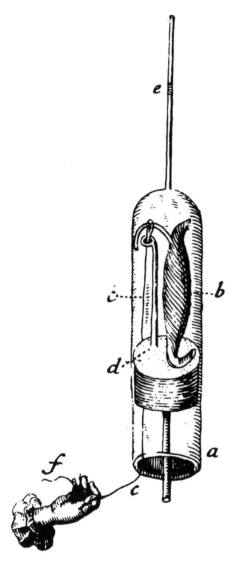

Fig. 1.5 Stimulation experiment of Jan Swammerdam in 1664. Touching the motoric nerve of a frog muscle (b) in a glass vessel (a) with silver wire (c) and a copper loop (d) produces stimulation of the nerve, which elicits a muscular contraction; however, it is uncertain as to whether the stimulation was produced as a result of electricity from the two dissimilar metals or from the mechanical pinching. See also text (Swammerdam, 1738).

The nerve, once activated, initiates a flow of current of its own. These are of biological origin, driven from sources that lie in the nerve and muscle membranes, and are distinct from the aforementioned stimulating currents. The active region of excitation propagates from the nerve to the muscle and is the immediate cause of the muscle contraction. The electric behavior of nerve and muscle forms the subject matter of ''bioelectricity,'' and is one central topic in this book.

It is believed that this was the first documented experiment of motor nerve stimulation resulting from an emf generated at a bimetallic junction (Brazier, 1959). Swammerdam probably did not understand that neuromuscular excitation is an electric phenomenon. On the other hand, some authors interpret the aforementioned stimulation to have resulted actually from the mechanical stretching of the nerve. The results of this experiment were published posthumously in 1738 (Swammerdam, 1738b).

The first *electric machine* was constructed by Otto von Guericke (German; 1602–1686). It was a sphere of sulfur (''the size of an infant's head'') with an iron axle mounted in a wooden framework, as illustrated in Figure 1.6. When the sphere was rotated and rubbed, it generated static electricity (von Guericke, 1672). The second electric machine was invented in 1704 by Francis Hauksbee the Elder (British; 1666–1713). It was a sphere of glass rotated by a wheel (see Fig. 1.7). When the rotating glass was rubbed, it produced electricity continuously (Hauksbee, 1709). It is worth mentioning that Hauksbee also experimented with evacuating the glass with an air pump and was able to generate brilliant light, thus anticipating the discovery of *cathode rays, x-rays,* and the *electron.*

At that time the main use of electricity was for entertainment and medicine. One of the earliest statements concerning the use of electricity was made in 1743 by Johann Gottlob Krüger of the University of Halle: ''All things must have a usefulness; that is certain. Since electricity must have a usefulness, and we have seen that it cannot be looked for either in theology or in jurisprudence, there is obviously nothing left but medicine'' (Licht, 1967).

1.4.2 Electric and Magnetic Stimulation

Systematic application of electromedical equipment for therapeutic use started in the 1700s. One can identify four different historical pe-

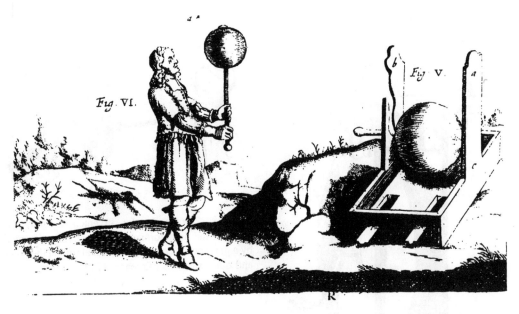

Fig. 1.6 Otto von Guericke constructed the first electric machine which included a sphere of sulfur with an iron axle. When the sphere was rotated and rubbed it generated static electricity (Guericke, 1672).

riods of electromagnetic stimulation, each based on a specific type or origin of electricity. These periods are named after Benjamin Franklin (American; 1706–1790), Luigi Galvani (Italian; 1737–1798), Michael Faraday (British; 1791–1867), and Jacques Arsène d'Arsonval (French; 1851–1940), as explained in Table 1.5. These men were the discoverers or promoters of different kinds of electricity: static electricity, direct current, induction coil shocks, and radiofrequency current, respectively (Geddes, 1984a).

The essential invention necessary for the application of a stimulating electric current was the *Leyden jar,* invented on the 11th of October, 1745, by the German inventor Ewald Georg von Kleist (c. 1700–1748) (Krueger, 1746). It was also invented independently by a Dutch scientist, Pieter van Musschenbroek (1692–1761) of the University of Leyden in The Netherlands in 1746, whose university affiliation explains the origin of the name. The Leyden jar is a capacitor formed by a glass bottle covered with metal foil on the inner and outer surfaces, as illustrated in Figure 1.8. The first practical *electrostatic generator* was invented by Jesse Ramsden (British; 1735–1800) in 1768 (Mottelay, 1975).

Benjamin Franklin deduced the concept of *positive and negative electricity* in 1747 during his experiments with the Leyden jar. He also studied *atmospheric electricity* with his famous kite experiment in 1752.

Soon after the Leyden jar was invented, it was applied to muscular stimulation and treatment of paralysis. As early as 1747, Jean Jallabert (Italian; 1712–1768), professor of mathematics in Genova, applied electric stimulation to a patient whose hand was paralyzed. The treatment lasted three months and was successful. This experiment, which was carefully documented (Jallabert, 1748), represents the beginning of *therapeutic stimulation of muscles by electricity.*

The most famous experiments in neuromuscular stimulation were performed by Luigi Galvani, professor of anatomy at the University of Bologna. His first important finding is dated January 26, 1781. A dissected and prepared frog was lying on the same table as an electric machine. When his assistant touched with a scalpel the femoral nerve of the frog sparks were simultaneously discharged in the nearby electric machine, and violent muscular contractions occurred (Galvani, 1791; Rowbottom and Susskind, 1984, p. 35). (It has been suggested that

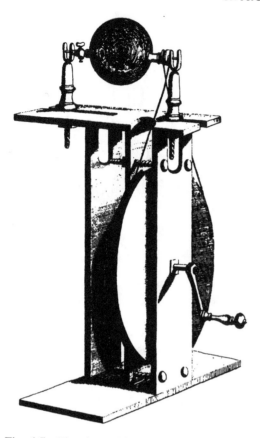

Fig. 1.7 Electric machine invented by Hauksbee in 1704. It had a sphere of glass rotated by a wheel. When the glass was rotated and rubbed it produced electricity continuously. If the glass was evacuated with an air pump it generated brilliant light (Hauksbee, 1709).

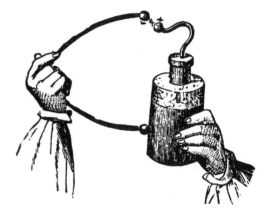

Fig. 1.8 The Leyden Jar, invented in 1745, was used for the first storage of electricity. It is formed by a glass bottle covered with metal foil on the inner and outer surfaces (Krueger, 1746).

the assistant was Galvani's wife Lucia, who is known to have helped him with his experiments.) This is cited as the first documented experiment in *neuromuscular electric stimulation.*

Galvani continued the stimulation studies

Table 1.5 Different historical eras of electric and electromagnetic stimulation

Scientist	Lifetime	Historical era
Benjamin Franklin	1706–1790	static electricity
Luigi Galvani	1737–1798	direct current
Michael Faraday	1791–1867	induction coil shocks
Jacques d'Arsonval	1851–1940	radiofrequency current

with atmospheric electricity on a prepared frog leg. He connected an electric conductor between the side of the house and the nerve of the frog leg. Then he grounded the muscle with another conductor in an adjacent well. Contractions were obtained when lightning flashed. In September 1786, Galvani was trying to obtain contractions from atmospheric electricity during calm weather. He suspended frog preparations from an iron railing in his garden by brass hooks inserted through the spinal cord. Galvani happened to press the hook against the railing when the leg was also in contact with it. Observing frequent contractions, he repeated the experiment in a closed room. He placed the frog leg on an iron plate and pressed the brass hook against the plate, and muscular contractions occurred.

Continuing these experiments systematically, Galvani found that when the nerve and the muscle of a frog were simultaneously touched with a *bimetallic arch of copper and zinc,* a contraction of the muscle was produced. This is illustrated in Figure 1.9 (Galvani, 1791). This experiment is often cited as the classic study to demonstrate the *existence of bioelectricity* (Rowbottom and Susskind, 1984 p. 39), although, as mentioned previously, it is possible that Jan Swammerdam had already conducted similar experiments in 1664. It is well known that Galvani did not understand the mechanism of the stimulation with the bimetallic arch. His

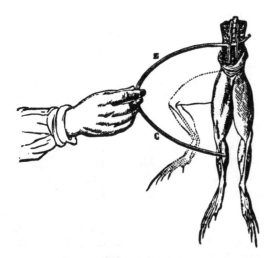

Fig. 1.9 Stimulation experiment of Luigi Galvani. The electrochemical behavior of two dissimilar metals [(zinc (Z) and copper (C)] in a bimetallic arch, in contact with the electrolytes of tissue, produces an electric stimulating current that elicits muscular contraction.

tion of the *Voltaic pile*, a battery that could produce continuous electric current (Volta, 1800). Giovanni (Joannis) Aldini (Italian; 1762–1834), a nephew of Galvani, applied stimulating current from Voltaic piles to patients (Aldini, 1804). For electrodes he used water-filled vessels in which the patient's hands were placed. He also used this method in an attempt to resuscitate people who were almost dead.

In 1872, T. Green described *cardiorespiratory resuscitation*, a method used to resuscitate surgical patients who were anesthetized with chloroform, an anesthetic with the side effect of depressing respiration and the cardiac pulse. Using a battery of up to 200 cells generating about 300 volts, he applied this voltage to the patient between the neck and the lower ribs on the left side. It is documented that T. Green used this method successfully on five or seven patients who suffered sudden respiratory arrest and were without a pulse (Green, 1872).

Michael Faraday's invention of the *induction coil* in 1831 initiated the faradic era of electromedicine (Faraday, 1834). However, it was Emil Heinrich du Bois-Reymond (German; 1818–96), who in 1846 introduced the induction coil to medical applications (du Bois-Reymond, 1849). This was called the *Faraday stimulation*. An induction coil with hammer break is shown in Figure 1.10. An early experiment of Faraday stimulation of the cerebral

explanation for this phenomenon was that the bimetallic arch was discharging the "animal electricity" existing in the body.

Alessandro Volta (Italian; 1745–1827), professor of physics in Pavia, continued the experiments on *galvanic stimulation*. He understood better the mechanism by which electricity is produced from two dissimilar metals and an electrolyte. His work led in 1800 to the inven-

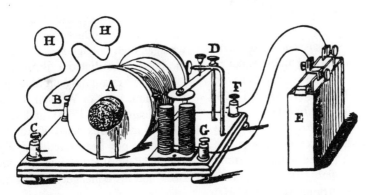

Fig. 1.10 Induction coil with hammer break. Electric current from the battery (E) is fed to the primary circuit of the induction coil (A). This current pulls the hammer with the magnetic field of the solenoid (close to G) and breaks the circuit with the contactor (D). Through the vibration of the hammer this breaking is continuous and it induces a high voltage alternating current in the secondary circuit in (A). This current is applied to the patient with electrodes (H).

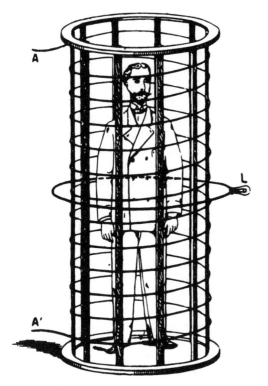

Fig. 1.11 d'Arsonval's great solenoid (d'Arsonval, 1893).

cortex was made in 1874 by Dr. Robert Bartholow, a professor of medicine in Cincinnati (Bartholow, 1881). Robert Bartholow stimulated the exposed cerebral cortex with faradic currents and observed that they would elicit movements of the limbs of the opposite side and also the turning of the head to that side (York, 1987).

In the late 1800s, Jacques Arsène d'Arsonval heated living tissue by applying high-frequency electric current either with an electrode or with a large coil (see Fig. 1.11) (d'Arsonval, 1893). This was the beginning of *diathermy*.

Jacques d'Arsonval (1896) reported on a flickering visual sensation perceived when an individual's head was placed within a strong time-varying magnetic field. This was generated with a large coil carrying 32 A at 42 Hz. He called this phenomenon *"magnetophosphenes."* It was caused by the stimulating effect of the magnetic field to the retina, which is known to be very sensitive to it. This was the first experiment on magnetic stimulation of the nervous system. The first *transcranial magnetic*

stimulation of the motor cortex was achieved in 1985 (Barker, Jalinous, and Freeston, 1985).

The first scientist to report *direct cardiac pacing* was F. Steiner (1871), who demonstrated this method in a dog anesthetized with an overdose of chloroform. In 1882, Hugo Wilhelm von Ziemssen (German; 1829–1902) applied this technique to a human (Ziemssen, 1882). It was only in 1932, when cardiac pacing was reported by Albert Salisbury Hyman (American; 1893–1972), that this method was applied clinically to atrial pacing (Hyman, 1932).

The modern era of cardiac pacing started in August 1952, when Paul Maurice Zoll (American; 1911–) performed cardiac pacing for a duration of 20 min (Zoll, 1952). In 1958, Furman and Schwedel succeeded in supporting a patient for 96 days with cardiac pacing (Furman and Schwedel, 1959).

The first implantation of a cardiac pacemaker, a milestone in the history of bioelectromagnetism, was accomplished in Stockholm by the surgeon Åke Senning (1915–). On October 8, 1958, at the Karolinska Institute, he implanted the *pacemaker* made by engineer Rune Elmqvist. The development of the implantable pacemaker was made possible by the invention of the *transistor* by Bardeen and Brattain in 1948.

The first report on *cardiac defibrillation,* in 1899, is that by Jean Louis Prevost (Swiss; 1838–1927) and Frédéric Battelli (Italian; 1867–1941) (Prevost and Battelli, 1899). They found, in animal experiments, that low-voltage electric shocks induced ventricular fibrillation whereas high-voltage shocks did not. Instead, the latter defibrillated a fibrillating heart.

Modern ventricular defibrillation started with the famous work of William B. Kouwenhoven (American; 1886–1975) and his colleagues who, in the 1930s, used 60 Hz current to defibrillate a dog heart (Geddes, 1976). The first human defibrillation was accomplished by Beck and his colleagues in 1947.

1.4.3 Detection
of Bioelectric Activity

The *connection between electricity and magnetism* was discovered in 1819 by Hans Christian Örsted (Danish; 1777–1851). Örsted conducted

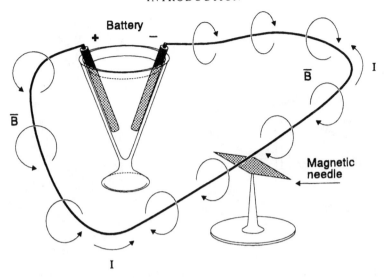

Fig. 1.12 Reconstruction of the first demonstration of the electromagnetic connection by Hans Christian Örsted in 1819. The battery generates an electric current I to flow in the circuit formed by a metal wire. This current induces a magnetic induction $\bar{B}$ around the wire. The magnetic needle under the wire turns parallel to the direction of the magnetic induction demonstrating its existence (Örsted, 1820a,b,c).

his first experiment during his lecture at the University of Copenhagen. Passing an electric current through a wire above a magnetic needle, he forced the needle to move to the direction normal to the wire (see Fig. 1.12) (Örsted, 1820a–c). By reversing the direction of the electric current, he reversed the direction of the needle deflection. (The magnetic needle (i.e., the compass) was invented in China about A.D. 100 and is the first detector of a magnetic field.)

After this discovery, it was possible to devise a *galvanometer,* an instrument detecting weak electric currents. Invented by Johann Salemo Christopf Schweigger (German; 1779–1875) in 1821, it is based on the deflection of a magnetized needle in the magnetic field inside a coil, into which the current to be measured is introduced. Because he increased the magnetic field by using multiple loops of wire forming the coil, Schweigger called his instrument *multiplikator* (Schweigger, 1821). In 1825, Leopold Nobili (Italian; 1784–1835), a professor of physics in Florence, invented the *astatic galvanometer* (Nobili, 1825). In its construction, Nobili employed a double coil of 72 turns wound in a figure eight (see Fig. 1.13A). One magnetic needle was located in each of the two openings. The needles were connected on the same suspension. They were parallel, but of

opposite polarity. Since the current flowed in opposite direction in the two coils, both needles moved in the same direction. Because of their opposite direction, the needles did not respond to Earth's magnetic field. Another version of the astatic galvanometer is illustrated in Figure 1.13B. This construction includes only one coil around one of the two magnetic needles. The other needle (identical but opposite in direction), provided with a scale, serves also as an indicator.

Carlo Matteucci (Italian; 1811–65) was the first to measure a bioelectric current. Using the astatic galvanometer, he made his first measurement of *muscle impulse* in frog muscle in 1838 (Matteucci, 1838), although the report did not appear in print until 1842.

In 1841, the German physiologist Emil du Bois-Reymond had received a copy of Matteucci's short essay on animal electricity, and thus was aware of the experiments of Matteucci. He repeated the studies with improved instrumentation. Besides detecting the bioelectric current from frog muscle, du Bois-Reymond, in 1842 (shortly before Matteucci's paper was published), measured the current arising from a frog *nerve impulse* (du Bois-Reymond, 1843). One of his experiments is shown in Figure 1.14.

The English school of neurophysiology be-

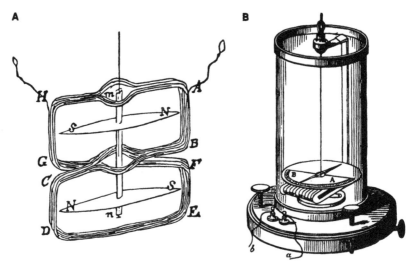

Fig. 1.13 (A) Astatic galvanometer invented by Nobili in 1825. He compensated for the effect of the Earth's magnetic field by placing two identical magnetic needles connected on the same suspension in opposite directions in the openings of a coil wound in the form of figure eight (Nobili, 1825). (B) A technically more advanced version of the astatic galvanometer. Only one of the two identical (but opposite) needles is surrounded by a coil. The other needle serves as an indicator.

gan when Richard Caton (British; 1842–1926) became interested in the recording technique of du Bois-Reymond and applied it to the measurement of the electric activity of the brains of rabbits and monkeys. The first report of his experiments, published in 1875 (Caton, 1875), is believed to constitute the discovery of the *electroencephalogram* (EEG). In 1888, a young Polish scientist Adolf Beck (1863–1942), working for the great physiologist Napoleon Nicodemus Cybulski (1854–1919) at the University of Krakow, succeeded in demon-

strating that the electric impulse propagated along a nerve fiber without attenuation (Beck, 1888). Without knowledge of the work of Caton, Beck studied the electric activity of the brain in animal experiments and independently arrived at many of Caton's conclusions (Beck, 1891). The German psychiatrist Hans Berger (1873–1941), made the first recording of the EEG on a human in 1924, and identified the two major rhythms, α and β (Berger, 1929). Berger's recordings on EEG are illustrated in Figure 1.15.

The tracings of the electric activity of the human heart, the *electrocardiogram* (ECG), was first measured in 1887 by Augustus Waller (British; 1856–1922) using *capillary electrometer* (Waller, 1887; see Fig. 1.16). In a capillary electrometer a moving photographic film is exposed along a glass capillary tube filled with sulfuric acid and mercury. Their interface moves in response to an electric field. The sensitivity of the capillary electrometer is about 1 mV, but its time response is very poor. The capillary electrometer was invented in 1873 by Gabriel Lippman (1873), and the photographic technique by which the signal was recorded by E. J. Marey and G. J. Lippman (1876).

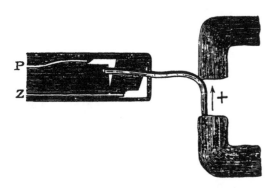

Fig. 1.14 Du Bois-Reymond's apparatus for studying effect of continuous current on nerve.

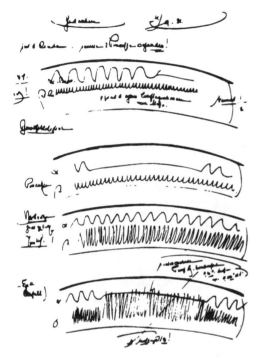

Fig. 1.15 A page from Berger's notebook illustrating early recordings of the human EEG.

Waller found that the cardiac electric generator has a *dipolar nature* (Fig. 1.17) and suggested that the ECG should be measured between the five measurement points formed by the hands, legs, and mouth (a total of 10 bipolar leads). He was also the first to record a set of three nearly orthogonal leads, including mouth-to-left arm, mouth-to-left leg, and back-to-front.

A pioneer in modern electrocardiography was Willem Einthoven (Dutch; 1860–1927) who, at the beginning of this century, developed the first high-quality ECG recorder based on the *string galvanometer* (Einthoven, 1908). Though Einthoven is often credited with inventing the string galvanometer, that honor actually belongs to Clément Ader (1897). However, Einthoven undoubtedly made important improvements in this device such that it was possible to apply it to clinical electrocardiography. Einthoven summarized his fundamental results in ECG research in 1908 and 1913 (Einthoven, 1908; Einthoven et al., 1913), and received the Nobel Prize for his work in 1924.

Horatio Williams, who was the first to construct a sequence of instantaneous vectors (Williams, 1914), is usually considered to be the inventor of *vectorcardiography*. Hubert Mann made further studies in vectorcardiography to develop it as a clinical tool. He published his first two-dimensional vectorcardiogram based on Einthoven's triangle in 1916 (see Fig. 1.18) and called this construction the *"monocardiogram"* (Mann, 1920). After J. B. Johnson (1921) of the Western Electric Company invented the low-voltage cathode ray tube, it became possible to display bioelectric signals in

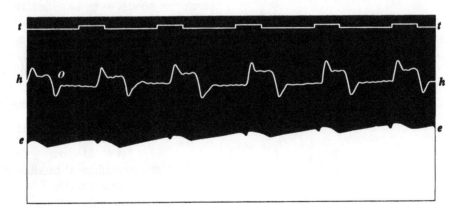

Fig. 1.16 The first recording of the human electrocardiogram by Augustus Waller (1887). The recording was made with a capillary electrometer. The ECG recording (e) is the borderline between the black and white areas. The other curve (h) is the *apexcardiogram*, a recording of the mechanical movement of the apex of the heart.

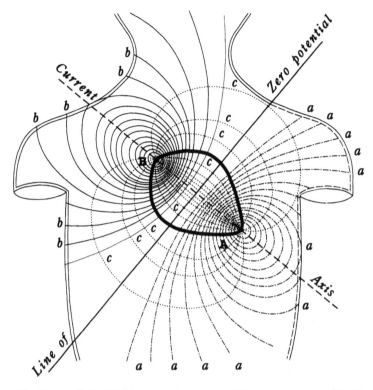

Fig. 1.17 Electric field of the heart on the surface of the thorax, recorded by Augustus Waller (1887). The curves (a) and (b) represent the recorded positive and negative isopotential lines, respectively. These indicate that the heart is a dipolar source having the positive and negative poles at (A) and (B), respectively. The curves (c) represent the assumed current flow lines.

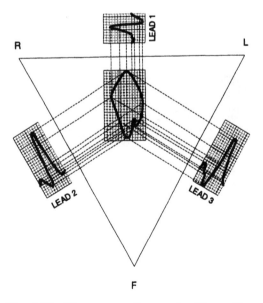

Fig. 1.18 The monocardiogram by Mann. (Redrawn from Mann, 1920.)

vector form in real time. This invention allowed vectorcardiography to be used as a clinical tool.

The invention of the *electron tube* by Lee de Forest (American; 1873–1961) in 1906 allowed bioelectric signals to be amplified, revolutionizing measurement technology. Finally, the invention of the transistor by John Bardeen and Walter Brattain in 1948 marked the beginning of the semiconductor era. It also allowed the instrumentation of bioelectromagnetism to be miniaturized, made portable and implantable, and more reliable.

1.4.4 Modern Electrophysiological Studies of Neural Cells

The term *neuron* was first applied to the neural cell in 1891 by Heinrich Wilhelm Gottfried Waldeyer (German; 1837–1921). Basic research into the study of neurons was undertaken at the end of the nineteenth century by August Forel (Swiss; 1848–1931), Wilhelm His, Sr. (Swiss; 1831–1904), and Santiago Ramón y Cajal (Spanish; 1852–1934). According to their theory, it is the neural cell that is the functional unit in the nervous system. (In 1871, Santiago Ramón y Cajal also discovered that neurons could be selectively stained with a special silver preparation.)

Sir Charles Scott Sherrington (British; 1856–1952) introduced the concept of the *synapse* (Sherrington, 1897). He also contributed the concept of the *reflex arc*. Lord Edgar Douglas Adrian (British; 1889–1977) formulated the *all-or-nothing law* of the neural cell in 1912 (Adrian and Lucas, 1912; Adrian, 1914) and measured the electric impulse of a single nerve 1926. Adrian and Sherrington won the Nobel Prize in 1932.

The founder of membrane theory was Julius Bernstein (German; 1839–1917), a pupil of Hermann von Helmholtz. Bernstein stated that the potential difference across the membrane was maintained by the difference in concentration of potassium ions on opposite sides of the membrane. The membrane, which is selectively permeable to all ions, has a particularly high permeability to potassium. This formed the basis for an evaluation of the transmembrane voltage as proportional to the logarithm of the concentration ratio of the potassium ions, as expressed by the *Nernst equation*.

Herbert Spencer Gasser (American; 1888–1963) and Joseph Erlanger (American; 1874–1965) studied nerve impulses with the aid of a cathode ray tube. Because they could not get a *cathode-ray oscilloscope* from the Western Electric Company, which had recently invented it, they built such a device themselves from a distillation flask. Linking the device to an amplifier, they could record the time course of nerve impulses for the first time (Gasser and Erlanger, 1922). With their experiments they were also able to confirm the hypothesis that axons of large diameter within a nerve bundle transmit nerve impulses more quickly than do thin axons. For their studies Gasser and Erlanger received the Nobel Prize in 1944.

Sir Alan Lloyd Hodgkin (English; 1914–) and Sir Andrew Fielding Huxley (English; 1914–) investigated the behavior of the cell membrane in great detail and developed a very accurate mathematical model of the activation process (Hodgkin and Huxley, 1952). Sir John Eccles (Australian; 1903–) investigated synaptic transmission in Canberra, Australia, in the 1950s. Eccles, Hodgkin, and Huxley won the Nobel Prize in 1963.

Ragnar Arthur Granit (Finnish; 1900–1991) undertook fundamental research in the bioelectric phenomena of the retina and the nervous system in the 1930s and 1940s. In 1935 he could show experimentally that inhibitory synapses are found in the retina. Hermann von Helmholtz had proposed that the human ability to discriminate a spectrum of colors could be explained if it could be proven that the eye contains receptors sensitive to different wavelengths of light. Granit's first experiments in color vision, performed in 1937, employed the electroretinogram (ERG) to confirm the extent of spectral differentiation. In 1939, Granit developed a microelectrode, a device that permits the measurement of electric potentials inside a cell. With this technique Granit further studied the color vision and established the spectral sensitivities of the three types of cone cells—blue, green, and red. Ragnar Granit shared the 1967 Nobel Prize with H. Keffer Hartline and George Wald ''for their discoveries concerning the primary physiological and chemical visual processes in the eye'' (Granit, 1955).

The behavior of ion channels in the biological membrane has been described in greater detail through the invention of the *patch clamp* technique by Erwin Neher (German; 1944–) and Bert Sakmann (German; 1942–) (Neher and Sakmann, 1976). With the patch clamp method it is possible to measure the electric current from a single ionic channel. This extends the origins of bioelectromagnetism to molecular biology so that this technique can also be used, for instance, in developing new pharmaceuticals. Neher and Sakmann won the Nobel Prize in 1991.

1.4.5 Bioelectromagnetism

As mentioned in Section 1.4.3, the connection between electricity and magnetism was experimentally discovered in 1819 by Hans Christian Örsted. French scientists Jean Baptiste Biot

(1774–1862) and Félix Savart (1791–1841) proved that the force between a current-carrying helical wire and a magnet pole is inversely proportional to the distance between them (Biot, 1820). André Marie Ampère (French; 1775–1836) showed that a current-carrying helical wire, which he called the *solenoid*, behaved magnetically as a permanent magnet (Ampère, 1820), hence linking the electric current to the production of a magnetic field. Ampère also developed the mathematical theory of electrodynamics (Ampère, 1827). The electromagnetic connection was theoretically formulated in 1864 by James Clerk Maxwell (British; 1831–79), who developed equations that link time-varying electricity and magnetism (Maxwell, 1865). Since Örsted's discovery, electromagnetic interdependence has been widely utilized in a large variety of devices. Examples of these include those used for the measurement of electric current (galvanometers and ammeters), electric generators, electric motors, and various radiofrequency devices. However, biomagnetic signals were not detected for a long time because of their extremely low amplitude.

The first biomagnetic signal, the *magnetocardiogram* (MCG), was detected by Gerhard M. Baule and Richard McFee in 1963 with an induction coil magnetometer (Baule and McFee, 1963). The magnetometer was made by winding two million turns of copper wire around a ferrite core. In addition to the detector coil, which was placed in front of the heart, another identical coil was connected in series and placed alongside. The two coils had opposite senses and thereby canceled the distributing common magnetic fields arising from distant external sources (see Fig. 1.19). A remarkable increase in the sensitivity of biomagnetic measurements was obtained with the introduction of the *Superconducting QUantum Interference Device* (SQUID), working at the temperature of liquid helium (−269°C) (Zimmerman, Thiene, and Hardings, 1970; Cohen, 1972).

Although David Cohen succeeded to measure the magnetic alpha rhythm with an induction coil magnetometer (Cohen, 1968), the magnetic signal generated by the electric activ-

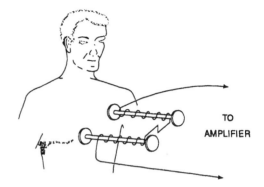

Fig. 1.19 Detection of the first biomagnetic signal, the magnetocardiogram (MCG), by Baule and McFee. (Redrawn from Baule and McFee, 1963.)

ity of the brain, measured in the *magnetoencephalogram* (MEG), is so low that in practice its detection is possible only by using the SQUID. With such a device the MEG was first detected by David Cohen in 1970 (Cohen, 1972). John Wikswo and his co-workers were first to measure the magnetic field of a frog nerve bundle in 1980 (Wikswo, Barach, and Freeman, 1980).

In this connection we want to draw the readers' attention to the fact that the difference between the measurement principles in the first measurements of the bioelectric and biomagnetic signals is surprisingly small:

In the first measurement of the *bioelectric signal*, Matteucci (1838) used a magnetized needle as the detector. (The bioelectric field is, of course, far too low to deflect the needle of an electroscope.) The biomagnetic field, produced by the bioelectric currents flowing in the frog leg, was too small to deflect the magnetic needle directly. It was therefore multiplied by feeding the bioelectric current to a coil of multiple turns and with placement of the needle inside the coil, an application of the invention of Schweigger (1821). The effect of the Earth's magnetic field was compensated by winding the coil in the form of a figure eight, placing two identical magnetic needles on the same suspension and oriented in opposite directions in the two openings of the coil. This formed an astatic galvanometer, as described earlier.

In the first measurement of a *biomagnetic signal* (the *magnetocardiogram*), the magnetic field produced by the bioelectric currents circulating in the human body was measured with a coil (Baule and McFee, 1963). Because of the low amplitude of this biomagnetic field, multiple turns of wire had to be wound around the core of the coil. To compensate for the effect of the magnetic field of the Earth and other sources of "noise", two identical coils wound in opposite directions were used (Fig. 1.19).

Thus, in terms of measurement technology, the first measurements of bioelectric and biomagnetic signals can be discriminated on the basis of whether the primary loop of the conversion of the bioelectric current to a magnetic field takes place outside or within the body, respectively. Since the invention of the capillary electrometer by G. J. Lippman (1873) and especially after the invention of electronic amplifiers, electric measurements have not directly utilized induced magnetic fields, and therefore the techniques of bioelectric and biomagnetic measurements have been driven apart.

In terms of measurement theory, the first measurements of bioelectric signals were measurements of the *flow source*, and thus truly electric. The first measurement of the biomagnetic signal by Richard McFee was the measurement of the *vortex source*, and thus truly magnetic. It will be shown later that with magnetic detectors it is possible to make a measurement which resembles the detection of the flow source. However, such a measurement does not give new information about the source compared to the electric measurement.

This example should draw our readers' attention to the fact that from a *theoretical point of view*, the essential difference between the bioelectric and biomagnetic measurements lies in the *sensitivity distributions* of these methods. Another difference stems from the diverse *technical properties* of these instrumentations, which impart to either method specific advantages in certain applications.

1.4.6   Theoretical Contributions to Bioelectromagnetism

The German scientist and philosopher Hermann Ludwig Ferdinand von Helmholtz (1821–1894) made the earliest significant contributions of the theory of bioelectromagnetism. A physician by education and, in 1849, appointed professor of physiology at Königsberg, he moved to the chair of physiology at Bonn in 1855. In 1871 he was awarded the chair of physics at the University of Berlin, and in 1888 was also appointed the first director of Physikalisch-Technische Bundesanstalt in Berlin.

Helmholtz's fundamental experimental and theoretical scientific contributions in the field of bioelectromagnetism include the following topics, which are included in this book:

1. The demonstration that *axons are processes of nerve cell bodies* (1842)
2. The establishment of the law of *conservation of energy* (the *First Law of Thermodynamics*) (1847)
3. The invention of the *myograph* and the first measurement of the *conduction velocity* of a motor nerve axon (1850)
4. The concept of *double layer source* (1853)
5. The *solid angle theorem* for electric potentials
6. The *principle of superposition* (1853)
7. The *reciprocity theorem* (1853)
8. The insolvability of the *inverse problem* (1853)
9. Helmholtz's theorem concerning the *independence of flow and vortex sources*
10. The *Helmholtz coils* (applied in biomagnetic instrumentation)

Besides these, the contributions of Helmholtz to other fields of science include fundamental works in physiology, acoustics, optics, electrodynamics, thermodynamics, and meteorology. He is the author of the *theory of hearing* (1863) from which all modern theories of resonance are derived. He also invented, in 1851, the *ophthalmoscope*, which is used to investigate the retina of a living eye.

Until the end of the nineteenth century, the physics of electricity was not fully understood. It was known, however, that neither pure water nor dry salts could by themselves transmit an electric current, whereas in aqueous solution salts could. Svante August Arrhenius (Swedish; 1859–1927) hypothesized in his 1884 doctoral thesis that molecules of some substances *dissociate*, or split, into two or more particles *(ions)* when they are dissolved in a liquid. Although each intact molecule is electrically balanced, the particles carry an electric charge, either positive or negative depending on the nature of the particle. These charged bodies form only in solution and permit the passage of electricity. This theory is fundamental for understanding the nature of the bioelectric current, because it flows in solutions and is carried by ions. Svante Arrhenius won the Nobel Prize in Chemistry in 1903.

At the end of the nineteenth century, Walther Hermann Nernst (German; 1864–1941) did fundamental work in thermochemistry, investigating the behavior of electrolytes in the presence of electric currents. In 1889, he developed a fundamental law, known as the *Nernst equation*. Nernst also developed many other fundamental laws, including the Third Law of Thermodynamics. He was awarded the Nobel Prize in Chemistry in 1920.

Dutch scientists Hermann Carel Burger (1893–1965) and Johan Bernhard van Milaan (1886–1965) introduced the concept of the *lead vector* in 1946 (Burger and van Milaan, 1946). They also extended this to the concept of the *image surface*. In 1953, Richard McFee and Franklin D. Johnston introduced the important concept of the *lead field*, which is based on the reciprocity theorem of Helmholtz (McFee and Johnston, 1953, 1954ab). The invention of the electromagnetic connection in 1819 by Örsted tied bioelectric and biomagnetic fields together. The invention of the reciprocity theorem in 1853 by Helmholtz showed that the sensitivity distribution of a lead for measuring bioelectric sources is the same as the distribution of stimulation current introduced into the same lead. Furthermore, this is the same as the sensitivity distribution of a tissue impedance measurement with the same lead. All this is true for corresponding magnetic methods as well. These principles are easily illustrated with the concept of lead field.

Dennis Gabor (British; 1900–1979) and Clifford V. Nelson published the *Gabor-Nelson theorem* in 1954 (Gabor and Nelson, 1954). This theorem explains how an equivalent dipole of a volume source and its location may be calculated from measurements on the surface of a homogeneous volume conductor.

1.4.7 Summary of the History of Bioelectromagnetism

The history of bioelectromagnetism is summarized chronologically in Figure 1.20. The historical events are divided into four groups: theory, instrumentation, stimulation, and measurements. This figure should serve as a useful overview for our readers and help them recognize how one contribution follows from an earlier one and how the development of an entire discipline thereby takes place. From this figure we may summarize the following thoughts.

1. Up to the middle of the nineteenth century, the *history of electromagnetism* has actually also been the *history of bioelectromagnetism*. The first electric machines and the Leyden jar were constructed to produce static electricity for a specific purpose: to "electrify" and to stimulate humans. The Voltaic pile was developed with the idea of galvanic stimulation. The universal principles of reciprocity and superposition were introduced in connection with their application to bioelectromagnetism. Bioelectric and biomagnetic measurements have also been the incentive for the development of sensitive measurement instruments. The latter include not only the astatic galvanometer, capillary electrometer, and string galvanometer of the nineteenth century but also the low-voltage cathode ray tube and the SQUID in the twentieth century. An understanding of the function of nerve cells and brain and their simulation with electronic models has led to the development of a new generation of computers: the neurocomputer. These events emphasize the importance of bioelectromagnetism.

2. In the seventeenth and early eighteenth centuries, it is surprising how quickly a new invention in the field of bioelectromagnetism became the basis for still further applications and new inventions, even in different countries, although travel and communication were limited to the horse. As examples one may mention the invention of the Leyden jar in Germany and the Netherlands in 1745 and 1746, respectively, and its systematic application to human functional electric stimulation in Italy in 1747. Another example is the invention of the electromagnetic connection in 1819 in Denmark and

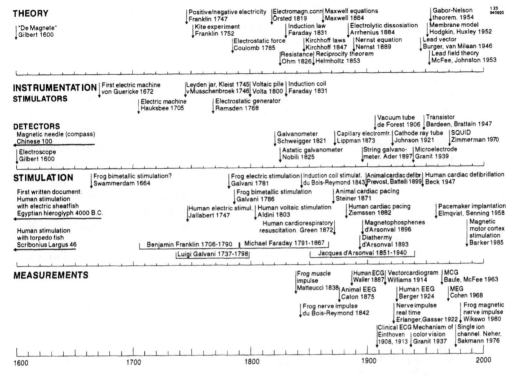

Fig. 1.20 Chronology of the history of bioelectromagnetism. The historical events are divided into four groups: theory, instrumentation, stimulation, and measurements.

the development of the galvanometer in 1821 in Germany and the astatic galvanometer in 1825 in Italy.

3. On the other hand, some inventions have been rediscovered, having been "forgotten" for about 100 years. Exactly 100 years elapsed following the publication of the reciprocity theorem before the lead field theory was introduced. The magnetic stimulation of the motor cortex was developed almost 100 years after the observation of magnetophosphenes. The time span from the first bioelectric measurements to the first corresponding biomagnetic measurements has been, on average, 100 years—quite a long time!

4. Several fundamental techniques used today in bioelectromagnetic instrumentation date back to the earliest instruments. The astatic galvanometer of 1825 included an ingenious method of compensation for the magnetic noise field. This principle was applied to the first measurement of MCG in 1963. Actually the planar gradiometers, applied in the multichannel

MEG-instruments using SQUID, are constructed exactly according to the same principle as the astatic galvanometer coil was more than 150 years ago. The basic clinical ECG leads— the limb leads—were invented 100 years ago by Waller. Similarly, Waller also introduced the dipole model to ECG, and it still has a strong role in electro- and magnetocardiology.

A more detailed review of the history of bioelectromagnetism can be found in the following references: Brazier (1988), Geddes (1984ab), McNeal (1977), Mottelay (1975), Rautaharju (1987, 1988), Rowbottom and Susskind (1984), and Wasson (1987).

1.5 NOBEL PRIZES
IN BIOELECTROMAGNETISM

The discipline of bioelectromagnetism is strongly reflected in the work of many Nobel laureates. It should be noted that 16 Nobel

Table 1.6 Nobel prizes awarded to bioelectromagnetism and closely related subject areas

Year	Name of recipient	Nationality	Subject of research
1901	Jacobus van't Hoff*	Neth.	laws of chemical dynamics and osmotic pressure
1903	Svante Arrhenius*	Sweden	theory of electrolytic dissociation
1906	Camillo Golgi Santiago Ramón y Cajal	Italy Spain	work on the structure of nervous system
1920	Walther Nernst*	Germany	work in thermochemistry
1924	Willem Einthoven	Neth.	discovery of electrocardiogram mechanism
1932	Edgar Douglas Adrian Sir Charles Sherrington	Britain Britain	discoveries regarding function of neurons
1936	Sir Henry Hallet Dale Otto Loewi	Britain Germany	work on chemical transmission of nerve impulses
1944	Joseph Erlanger Herbert Spencer Gasser	U.S. U.S.	researches on differentiated functions of nerve fibers
1949	Walter Rudolf Hess	Switz.	discovery of function of middle brain
1961	Georg von Békésy	U.S.	discoveries of the physical mechanism of the inner ear
1963	Sir John Eccles Alan Lloyd Hodgkin Andrew Fielding Huxley	Austr. Britain Britain	study of the transmission of nerve impulses along a nerve fiber
1967	Ragnar Arthur Granit Haldan Keffer Hartline George Wald	Finland U.S. U.S.	discoveries about chemical and physiological visual processes in the eye
1968	Lars Onsager*	U.S.	work on theory of thermodynamics of irreversible processes
1970	Julius Axelrod Sir Bernard Katz Ulf von Euler	U.S. Britain Sweden	discoveries concerning the chemistry of nerve transmission
1981	David Hunter Hubel Torsten Nils Wiesel	U.S. Sweden	discoveries concerning information processing in the visual system
1991	Erwin Neher Bert Sakmann	Germany Germany	discoveries concerning the function of single ion channels in cells

*Nobel Prize in chemistry. All other prizes were received in physiology or medicine.

prizes have been given for contributions to the discipline of bioelectromagnetism and closely related subjects. Of these prizes, 12 were in physiology or medicine; four were in chemistry. Although some perhaps do not directly concern bioelectromagnetism, they are very closely related. Since several individuals may have shared an award, the actual number of Nobel laureates is 28. The large number of these Nobel laureates shows that bioelectromagnetism is recognized as a very important discipline. Nobel laureates associated with bioelectromagnetism are listed in Table 1.6.

One should probably add to this list the names of Gabriel Jonas Lippman and Dennis Gabor, although they did not receive their Nobel Prize for their work in bioelectromagnetism.

Gabriel Lippman received the Nobel Prize in physics in 1908 for his photographic reproduction of colors. But he was also the inventor of the capillary electrometer (Lippman, 1873). The capillary electrometer was a more sensitive measuring instrument than the astatic galvanometer and was an important contribution to the technology by which bioelectric events were recorded.

Dennis Gabor received the Nobel Prize in physics in 1971 for the invention of holography. He was also the senior author of the Gabor-Nelson theorem, which is used to ascertain the equivalent dipole of a volume source by measurements of the electric potential on the surface of the volume conductor (Gabor and Nelson, 1954).

One should also note that Georg von Békésy received the Nobel prize for his discoveries of the *physical* mechanism of stimulation within the cochlea. His discoveries have, however, contributed most significantly to the analysis of the relation between the mechanical and the electric phenomena in the receptors involved in the transformation of sound into nerve impulses. Therefore, von Békésy's name is included in this list.

REFERENCES

Ader C (1897): Sur un nouvel appareil enregistreur pour cables sousmarins. *Compt. rend. Acad. Sci. (Paris)* 124: 1440–2.

Adrian ED (1914): The all-or-none principle in nerve. *J. Physiol. (Lond.)* 47: 460–74.

Adrian ED, Lucas K (1912): On the summation of propagated disturbances in nerve and muscle. *J. Physiol. (Lond.)* 44: 68–124.

Aldini G (1804): *Essai Théorique et Expérimental sur le Galvanisme,* Vol. 2, Fournier, Paris.

Ampère AM (1820): Du mémoire sur l'action mutuelle entre deux courans électriques, entre un courant électrique et un aimant ou le globe terrestre, et entre deux aimants. *Ann. Chim. Phys.* 15: 170–218.

Ampère AM (1827): Mémoire sur la théorie mathématique des phénomènes électro-dynamiques uniquemant déduit de l'éxperience. *Mém. de l'Institut* 6: 175–386.

Barker AT, Jalinous R, Freeston IL (1985): Noninvasive magnetic stimulation of human motor cortex. *Lancet* 1:(8437) 1106–7.

Bartholow R (1881): *Electro-Therapeutics,* Philadelphia.

Baule GM, McFee R (1963): Detection of the magnetic field of the heart. *Am. Heart J.* 55:(7) 95–6.

Beck A (1888): O pobudiwosci róznych miejsc tego samego nerwu. *Rozpr. Wydz. mat.-przyr. polsk. Akad. Um.* 15: 165–95. (On the excitability of the various parts of the same nerve).

Beck A (1891): The determination of localization in the brain and spinal cord by means of electrical phenomena. *Polska Akademija Umiejetnosci,* Series 2, pp. 187–232. (thesis)

Berger H (1929): Über das Elektroenkephalogram des Menschen. *Arch. f. Psychiat.* 87: 527–70.

Biot JB (1820): Note sur le magnétisme de la pile de Volta. *Ann. Chim. Phys.* 15: 222–4.

du Bois-Reymond EH (1843): Vorläufiger Abriss einer Untersuchung ueber den sogenannten Froschstrom und ueber die elektromotorischen Fische. *Ann. Physik und Chemie* 58: 1–30.

du Bois-Reymond EH (1848): *Untersuchungen ueber thierische Elektricität,* Vol. 1, 56+743 pp. G Reimer, Berlin.

du Bois-Reymond EH (1849): *Untersuchungen ueber thierische Elektricität,* Vol. 2, pp. 393–4. G. Reimer, Berlin.

Brazier MAB (1959): The historical development of neurophysiology. In *Handbook of Physiology. Section I: Neurophysiology,* Vol. I, ed. IJ Field, HW Magoun, VE Hall, pp. 1–58, American Physiological Society, Washington.

Burger HC, van Milaan JB (1946): Heart vector and leads—I. *Br. Heart J.* 8:(3) 157–61.

Caton R (1875): The electric currents of the brain. *Br. Med. J.* 2: 278.

Cohen D (1968): Magnetoencephalography, evidence of magnetic fields produced by alpharhythm currents. *Science* 161: 784–6.

Cohen D (1972): Magnetoencephalography: Detection of brain's electric activity with a superconducting magnetometer. *Science* 175:(4022) 664–6.

Cohen D, Edelsack EA, Zimmerman JE (1970): Magnetocardiograms taken inside a shielded room with a superconducting point-contact magnetometer. *Appl. Phys. Letters* 16: 178–280.

d'Arsonval J (1893): Action physiologique de courants alternatifs à grande frequence. *Arch. Physiol. Norm. et Pathol.* 5: 401–8, 780–90.

d'Arsonval JA (1896): Dispositifs pour la mésure des courants alternatifs de toutes fréquences. *C. R. Soc. Biol. (Paris)* 2: 450–1.

Einthoven W (1908): Weiteres über das Elektrokardiogram. *Pflüger Arch. ges. Physiol.* 122: 517–48.

Einthoven W, Fahr G, de Waart A (1913): Über die Richtung und die Manifeste Grösse der Potentialschwankungen im mennschlichen Herzen und über den Einfluss der Herzlage auf die form des Elektrokardiogramms. *Pflüger Arch. ges. Physiol.* 150: 275–315.

Faraday M (1834): Experimental researches on electricity, 7th series. *Phil. Trans. R. Soc. (Lond.)* 124: 77–122.

Furman S, Schwedel JB (1959): An intracardiac pacemaker for Stokes-Adams seizures. *N. Engl. J. Med.* 261:(5 Nov) 943–8.

Gabor D, Nelson CV (1954): Determination of the

resultant dipole of the heart from measurements on the body surface. *J. Appl. Phys.* 25:(4) 413–6.

Galvani L (1791): De viribus electricitatis in motu musculari. Commentarius. *De Bononiesi Scientarium et Ertium Instituto atque Academia Commentarii* 7: 363–418. (Commentary on the effects of electricity on muscular motion. Burndy Library edition, 1953, Norwalk, Conn.).

Gasser HS, Erlanger J (1922): A study of the action currents of the nerve with the cathode ray oscillograph. *Am. J. Physiol.* 62: 496–524.

Geddes LA (1976): Kouwenhoven WB. *Med. Instrum.* 10:(2) 141–3.

Gilbert W (1600): *De Magnete, Magneticisque Corporibus, et de Magno Magnete Tellure; Physiologica Nova Plumiris et Argumentis et Experimentis Demonstrata,* Peter Short, London. (Transl. SP Thompson, London: The Gilbert Club, 1900: facsimile ed. New York: Basic Books, 1958: transl. PF Mottelay, 1893, facsimile ed.: Dover, New York, 1958.)

Granit R (1955): *Receptors and Sensory Perception,* 369 pp. Yale University Press, New Haven.

Green T (1872): On death from chloroform: Its prevention by a galvanism. *Br. Med. J.* 1:(May 25) 551–3.

von Guericke O (1672): *Experimenta Nova (Ut Vocantur) Magdeburgica,* Amsterdam.

Hauksbee F (1709): *Physico-Mechanical Experiments,* 1st ed., London.

Helmholtz HLF (1842): De fabrica systematis nervosi evertebratorum. *Berlin,* Thesis, (Structure of the nervous system in invertebrates.) (Dr. Phil. thesis)

Helmholtz HLF (1847): *Über die Erlangung der Kraft,* Berlin. (On the conservation of energy)

Helmholtz HLF (1850): Über die Fortpflanzungsgeschwindigkeit der Nervenreizung. *Arch. anat. physiol. wiss. Med.* : 71–3. (On the speed of propagation of nerve stimulation).

Helmholtz HLF (1853): Ueber einige Gesetze der Vertheilung elektrischer Ströme in körperlichen Leitern mit Anwendung auf die thierisch-elektrischen Versuche. *Ann. Physik und Chemie* 89: 211–33, 354–77.

Helmholtz HLF (1863): *Die Lehre von den Tonempfindungen als Physiologische Grundlage für die Theorie der Musik,* Braunschweig. (On the sensations of tone)

Hodgkin AL, Huxley AF (1952): A quantitative description of membrane current and its application to conduction and excitation in nerve. *J. Physiol. (Lond.)* 117: 500–44.

Hyman S (1932): Resuscitation in stopped heart. *Arch. Int. Med.* 50: 283–305.

Jallabert J (1748): *Expériences Sur L'électricité Avec Quelques Conjectures Sur La Cause De Ses Effets,* Geneva.

Johnson JB (1921): A low voltage cathode ray oscillograph. *Physical Rev.* 17: 420–1.

Kellaway P (1946): *Bull. Hist. Med.* 20: 112–37.

Krueger J (1746): *Beschichte der Erde,* Lubetvatbischen Buchhandlung, Helmstädt.

Licht S (1967): *Therapeutic Electricity and Ultraviolet Radiation,* Baltimore.

Lippman GJ (1873): Beziehungen zwischen der Capillaren und elektrischen Erscheinungen. *Ann. Physik und Chemie* (Series 2) 149: 546–61.

Maniewski R, Katila T, Poutanen T, Siltanen P, Varpula T, Wikswo JP (1988): Magnetic measurement of cardiac mechanical activity. *IEEE Trans. Biomed. Eng.* 35:(9) 662–70.

Mann H (1920): A method for analyzing the electrocardiogram. *Arch. Int. Med.* 25: 283–94.

Marey EJ, Lippman GJ (1876): Inscription photographique des indications de l'électromètre de Lippman. *Compt. rend. Acad. Sci. (Paris)* 83: 278–80.

Matteucci C (1838): Sur le courant électrique où propre de la grenouille. Second memoire sur l'électricité animale, faisant suite à celui sur la torpille. *Ann. Chim. Phys.* (2ème serie), 67: 93–106.

Matteucci C (1842): Deuxième mémoire sur le courant électrique propre de la grenouille et sur celui des animaux à sang chaud (1). *Ann. Chim. Phys.* (3ème serie), 6: 301–39.

Maxwell J (1865): A dynamical theory of the electromagnetic field. *Phil. Trans. R. Soc. (Lond.)* 155: 459–512.

McFee R, Johnston FD (1953): Electrocardiographic leads I. Introduction. *Circulation* 8:(10) 554–68.

McFee R, Johnston FD (1954a): Electrocardiographic leads II. Analysis. *Circulation* 9:(2) 255–66.

McFee R, Johnston FD (1954b): Electrocardiographic leads III. Synthesis. *Circulation* 9:(6) 868–80.

Morgan CE (1868): *Electro-Physiology and Therapeutics,* Williams, Wood, New York.

Neher E, Sakmann B (1976): Single-channel currents recorded from membrane of denervated frog muscle fibers. *Nature* 260: 799–802.

Nobili L (1825): Ueber einen neuen Galvanometer. *J. Chem. und Physik* 45: 249–54.

Örsted HC (1820a): Experimenta circa effectum conflictus electrici in acum magneticam. *J. F. Chem. Phys.* 29: 275–81.

Örsted HC (1820b): Galvanic magnetsim. *Phil. Mag.* 56: 394.

Örsted HC (1820c): Neuere elektro-magnetische Versuche. *J. Chem. und Physik* 29: 364–9.

Polson MJ, Barker AT, Freeston IL (1982): Stimulation of nerve trunks with time-varying magnetic fields. *Med. & Biol. Eng. & Comput.* 20:(2) 243–4.

Prevost JL, Battelli F (1899): On some effects of electric discharges on the heart of mammals. *Compt. rend. Acad. Sci. (Paris)* 129: 943–8.

de la Rive A (1853): *A Treatise on Electricity*, London.

Schweigger JSC (1821): Elektromagnetischer Multiplikator. *J. Chem. und Physik* 31: 35–41.

Sherrington CS (1897): The central nervous system. In *A Textbook of Physiology*, Vol. 3, ed. M Forster, Macmillan, London.

Smith JA, (Transl.) (1931): De anima. In *The Works of Aristotle*, Vol. 3, ed. WD Ross, p. 405, Oxford University Press, Oxford.

Steiner F (1871): Über die Elektropunctur des Herzens als Wiederbelebungsmittel in der Chloroformsyncope. *Archiv. f. klin. Chir.* 12: 748–80.

Swammerdam J (1738a): *Biblia Naturae*, Vol. 2, ed. H. Boerhaave, Leyden.

Swammerdam J (1738b): *Biblia Naturae*, Vol. 2, ed. H. Boerhaave, pp. 839–50. Leyden.

Volta A (1800): On the electricity excited by the mere contact of conducting substances of different kinds. *Phil. Trans. R. Soc. (Lond.)* 90: 403–31. (In French.).

Waller AD (1887): A demonstration on man of electromotive changes accompanying the heart's beat. *J. Physiol. (Lond.)* 8: 229–34.

Wikswo JP, Barach JP, Freeman JA (1980): Magnetic field of a nerve impulse: First measurements. *Science* 208: 53–5.

Williams HB (1914): On the cause of the phase difference frequently observed between homonymous peaks of the electrocardiogram. *Am. J. Physiol.* 35: 292–300.

York DH (1987): Review of descending motor pathways involved with transcranial stimulation. *Neurosurg.* 20:(1) 70–3.

Ziemssen H (1882): Studien über die Bewegungsvorgange am menschlichen Herzen. *Deuts. Archiv f. klin. Med.* 30: 270–303.

Zimmerman JE, Thiene P, Hardings J (1970): Design and operation of stable r-f biased superconducting point-contact quantum devices. *J. Appl. Phys.* 41: 1572.

Zoll PM (1952): Excitation of the heart in ventricular standstill by external electric stimulation. *N. Engl. J. Med.* 247: 768–71.

REVIEW ARTICLES

Brazier MAB (1959): The historical development of neurophysiology. In *Handbook of Physiology. Section I: Neurophysiology*, Vol. I, ed. IJ Field, HW Magoun, VE Hall, pp. 1–58, American Physiological Society, Washington.

Brazier MA (1988): *A History of Neurophysiology in the 19th Century*, 265 pp. Raven Press, New York.

Gandhi OP (ed.) (1990): *Biological Effects and Medical Applications of Electromagnetic Energy*, (Series ed, A Nordgraaf: Biophysics and Bioengineering Series.) 573 pp. Prentice Hall, Englewood Cliffs, N.J.

Geddes LA (1984a): The beginnings of electromedicine. *IEEE Eng. Med. Biol. Mag.* 3:(4) 8–23.

Geddes LA (1984b): A short history of the electrical stimulation of excitable tissue: Including electrotherapeutic applications. *Physiologist* 27(Suppl.):(1) 15–265.

McNeal DR (1977): 2000 years of electrical stimulation. In *Functional Electrical Stimulation. Applications in Neural Prostheses. Biomedical Engineering and Instrumentation Series*, Vol. 3, ed. FT Hambrecht, JB Reswick, pp. 3–35, Marcel Dekker, New York and Basel.

Mottelay PF (1975): *Bibliographical History of Electricity and Magnetism*, 673 pp. Charles Griffin, New York.

Rautaharju PM (1987): A hundred years of progress in electrocardiography, 1: Early contributions from Waller to Wilson. *Can. J. Cardiol.* 3:(8) 362–74.

Rautaharju PM (1988): A hundred years of progress in electrocardiography, 2: The rise and decline of vectorcardiography. *Can. J. Cardiol.* 4:(2) 60–71.

Reilly JP (1992): *Electrical Stimulation & Electropathology*, 504 pp. Cambridge University Press, Cambridge.

Rowbottom M, Susskind C (1984): *Electricity and Medicine. History of Their Interaction*, 303 pp. San Francisco Press, San Francisco.

Wasson T (ed.) (1987): *Nobel Prize Winners*, 1165 pp. H. W. Wilson, New York.

I

Anatomical and Physiological Basis of Bioelectromagnetism

The purpose of Part I is to introduce the anatomy and physiology of excitable tissues and the mechanism of bioelectric phenomena.

Chapter 2 begins on a cellular level, with a discussion of the anatomy and physiology of nerve and muscle cells. A discussion of cellular electrophysiology on a *qualitative* basis follows in this chapter and then on a *quantitative* basis in Chapter 3. This chapter explores the bioelectric behavior of the cell membrane under the firing threshold, and Chapter 4 the activation mechanism. Biomagnetic phenomena are not yet discussed in Part I.

Next the anatomy and physiology of excitable tissues at the organ level is briefly reviewed first in Chapter 5 on neural tissue and then in Chapter 6 on cardiac tissue. Our purpose is to introduce the necessary vocabulary and to provide an overview of the source of bioelectric phenomena.

2

Nerve and
Muscle Cells

2.1 INTRODUCTION

In this chapter we consider the structure of nerve and muscle tissue and in particular their membranes, which are excitable. A *qualitative* description of the activation process follows. Many new terms and concepts are mentioned only briefly in this chapter but in more detail in the next two chapters, where the same material is dealt with from a quantitative rather than a qualitative point of view.

The first documented reference to the nervous system is found in ancient Egyptian records. The Edwin Smith Surgical Papyrus, a copy (dated 1700 B.C.) of a manuscript composed about 3500 B.C., contains the first use of the word "brain," along with a description of the coverings of the brain which was likened to the film and corrugations that are seen on the surface of molten copper as it cooled (Elsberg, 1931; Kandel and Schwartz, 1985).

The basic unit of living tissue is the cell. Cells are specialized in their anatomy and physiology to perform different tasks. All cells exhibit a voltage difference across the cell membrane. Nerve cells and muscle cells are excitable. Their cell membrane can produce electrochemical impulses and conduct them along the membrane. In muscle cells, this electric phenomenon is also associated with the contraction of the cell. In other cells, such as gland cells and ciliated cells, it is believed that the membrane voltage is important to the execution of cell function.

The origin of the membrane voltage is the same in nerve cells as in muscle cells. In both cell types, the membrane generates an impulse as a consequence of excitation. This impulse propagates in both cell types in the same manner. What follows is a short introduction to the anatomy and physiology of nerve cells. The reader can find more detailed information about these questions in other sources such as Berne and Levy (1988), Ganong (1991), Guyton (1992), Patton et al. (1989) and Ruch and Patton (1982).

2.2 NERVE CELL

2.2.1 The Main Parts of the Nerve Cell

The nerve cell may be divided on the basis of its structure and function into three main parts:

(1) the *cell body,* also called the *soma;*
(2) numerous short processes of the soma, called the *dendrites;* and,
(3) the single long nerve fiber, the *axon.* These are described in Figure 2.1.

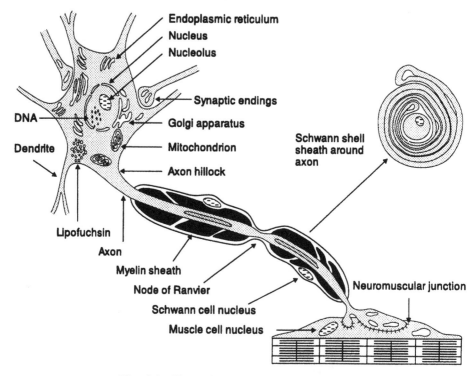

Fig. 2.1 The major components of a neuron.

The body of a nerve cell (see also Schadé and Ford, 1973) is similar to that of all other cells. The cell body generally includes the nucleus, mitochondria, endoplasmic reticulum, ribosomes, and other organelles. Since these are not unique to the nerve cell, they are not discussed further here. Nerve cells are about 70–80% water; the dry material is about 80% protein and 20% lipid. The cell volume varies between 600 and 70,000 μm^3 (Shadé and Ford, 1973).

The short processes of the cell body, the dendrites, receive impulses from other cells and transfer them to the cell body *(afferent signals).* The effect of these impulses may be *excitatory* or *inhibitory.* A *cortical neuron* (shown in Fig. 2.2) may receive impulses from tens or even hundreds of thousands of neurons (Nunez, 1981).

The long nerve fiber, the *axon,* transfers the signal from the cell body to another nerve or to a muscle cell. Mammalian axons are usually about 1–20 μm in diameter. Some axons in larger animals may be several meters in length. The axon may be covered with an insulating layer called the *myelin sheath,* which is formed by *Schwann cells* (named for the German phys-

iologist Theodor Schwann, 1810–1882, who first observed the myelin sheath in 1838). The myelin sheath is not continuous but divided into sections, separated at regular intervals by the *nodes of Ranvier* (named for the French anatomist Louis Antoine Ranvier, 1834–1922, who observed them in 1878).

2.2.2 The Cell Membrane

The cell is enclosed by a cell membrane whose thickness is about 7.5–10.0 nm. Its structure and composition resemble a soap-bubble film (Thompson, 1985), since one of its major constituents, *fatty acids,* has that appearance. The fatty acids that constitute most of the cell membrane are called *phosphoglycerides.* A phosphoglyceride consists of phosphoric acid and fatty acids called *glycerides* (see Fig. 2.3). The head of this molecule, the phosphoglyceride, is *hydrophilic* (attracted to water). The fatty acids have *tails* consisting of hydrocarbon chains which are *hydrophobic* (repelled by water).

If fatty acid molecules are placed in water, they form little clumps, with the acid heads that are attracted to water on the outside, and the

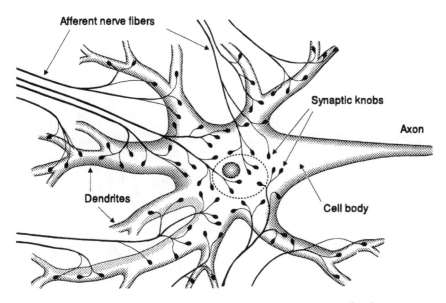

Fig. 2.2 Cortical nerve cell and nerve endings connected to it.

hydrocarbon tails that are repelled by water on the inside. If these molecules are very carefully placed on a water surface, they orient themselves so that all acid heads are in the water and all hydrocarbon tails protrude from it. If another layer of molecules were added and more water put on top, the hydrocarbon tails would line up with those from the first layer, to form a double (two molecules thick) layer. The acid heads would protrude into the water

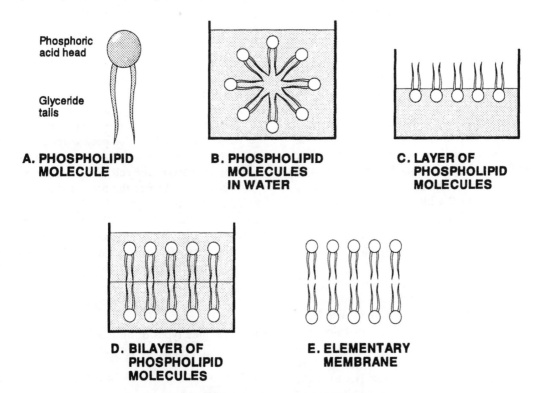

Fig. 2.3 A sketch illustrating how the phosphoglyceride (or phospholipid) molecules behave in water. See text for discussion.

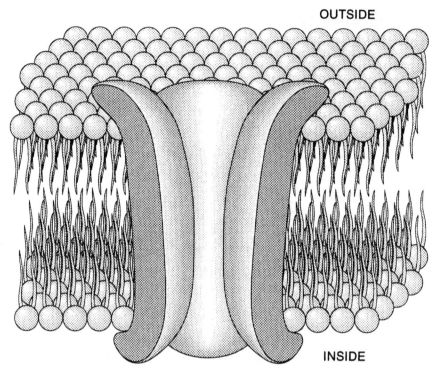

Fig. 2.4 The construction of a cell membrane. The main constituents are two lipid layers, with the hydrophobic tails pointing inside the membrane (away from the aqueous intracellular and interstitial mediums). The macromolecular pores in the cell membrane form the ionic channels through which sodium, potassium, and chloride molecules flow through the membrane and generate the bioelectric phenomena.

on each side and the hydrocarbons would fill the space between. This bilayer is the basic structure of the cell membrane.

From the bioelectric viewpoint, the *ionic channels* constitute an important part of the cell membrane. These are macromolecular pores through which sodium, potassium, and chloride ions flow through the membrane. The flow of these ions forms the basis of bioelectric phenomena. Figure 2.4 illustrates the construction of a cell membrane.

2.2.3 The Synapse

The junction between an axon and the next cell with which it communicates is called the *synapse*. Information proceeds from the cell body unidirectionally over the synapse, first along the axon and then across the synapse to the next nerve or muscle cell. The part of the synapse that is on the side of the axon is called the *presynaptic terminal;* that part on the side of

the adjacent cell is called the *postsynaptic terminal.* Between these terminals, there exists a gap, the *synaptic cleft,* with a thickness of 10–50 nm. The fact that the impulse transfers across the synapse only in one direction, from the presynaptic terminal to the postsynaptic terminal, is due to the release of a chemical transmitter by the presynaptic cell. This transmitter, when released, activates the postsynaptic terminal, as shown in Figure 2.5. The synapse between a motor nerve and the muscle it innervates is called *the neuromuscular junction.* Information transfer in the synapse is discussed in more detail in Chapter 5.

2.3 MUSCLE CELL

There are three types of muscles in the body:

smooth muscle,

striated muscle (skeletal muscle), and

cardiac muscle.

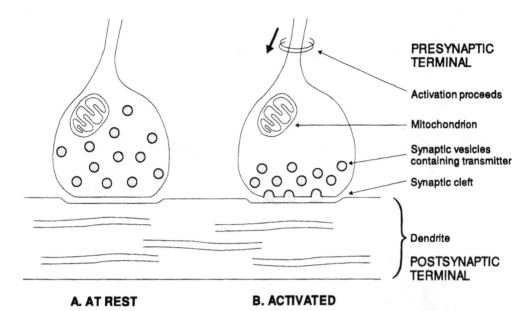

PRESYNAPTIC TERMINAL

Activation proceeds

Mitochondrion

Synaptic vesicles containing transmitter

Synaptic cleft

Dendrite

POSTSYNAPTIC TERMINAL

A. AT REST   **B. ACTIVATED**

Fig. 2.5 Simplified illustration of the anatomy of the synapse. (A) The synaptic vesicles contain a chemical transmitter. (B) When the activation reaches the presynaptic terminal the transmitter is released and it diffuses across the synaptic cleft to activate the postsynaptic membrane.

Smooth muscles are *involuntary* (i.e., they cannot be controlled voluntarily). Their cells have a variable length but are in the order of 0.1 mm. Smooth muscles exist, for example, in the digestive tract, in the wall of the trachea, uterus, and bladder. The contraction of smooth muscle is controlled from the brain through the autonomic nervous system.

Striated muscles, are also called *skeletal muscles* because of their anatomical location, are formed from a large number of muscle fibers, that range in length from 1 to 40 mm and in diameter from 0.01 to 0.1 mm. Each fiber forms a (muscle) cell and is distinguished by the presence of alternating dark and light bands. This is the origin of the description "striated," as an alternate terminology of skeletal muscle (see Fig. 2.6).

The striated muscle fiber corresponds to an (unmyelinated) nerve fiber but is distinguished electrophysiologically from nerve by the presence of a periodic *transverse tubular system* (TTS), a complex structure that, in effect, continues the surface membrane into the interior of the muscle. Propagation of the impulse over the surface membrane continues radially into the fiber via the TTS, and forms the trigger of myofibrillar contraction. The presence of the TTS affects conduction of the muscle fiber so that it differs (although only slightly) from propagation on an (unmyelinated) nerve fiber. Striated muscles are connected to the bones via tendons. Such muscles are voluntary and form an essential part of the organ of support and motion.

Cardiac muscle is also striated, but differs in other ways from skeletal muscle: Not only is it involuntary, but also when excited, it generates a much longer electric impulse than does skeletal muscle, lasting about 300 ms. Correspondingly, the mechanical contraction also lasts longer. Furthermore, cardiac muscle has a special property: The electric activity of one muscle cell spreads to all other surrounding muscle cells, owing to an elaborate system of *intercellular* junctions.

2.4 BIOELECTRIC FUNCTION OF THE NERVE CELL

The *membrane voltage (transmembrane voltage)* (V_m) of an excitable cell is defined as the potential at the inner surface (Φ_i) relative to that at the outer (Φ_o) surface of the membrane, i.e., $V_m = \Phi_i - \Phi_o$. This definition is indepen-

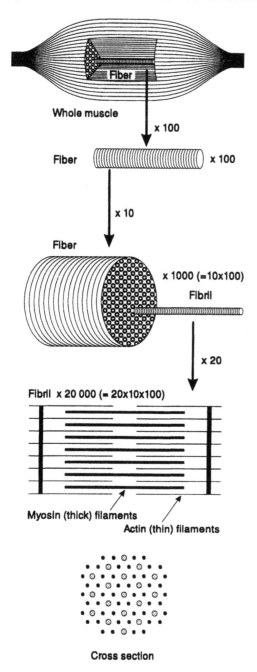

Fig. 2.6 Anatomy of striated muscle. The fundamental physiological unit is the fiber.

dent of the cause of the potential, and whether the membrane voltage is constant, periodic, or nonperiodic in behavior. Fluctuations in the membrane potential may be classified according to their character in many different ways. Figure 2.7 shows the classification for nerve cells developed by Theodore Holmes Bullock (1959). According to Bullock, these transmem-

brane potentials may be resolved into a resting potential and potential changes due to activity. The latter may be classified into three different types:

1. *Pacemaker potentials:* the intrinsic activity of the cell which occurs without external excitation.
2. *Transducer potentials* across the membrane, due to external events. These include *generator potentials* caused by receptors or *synaptic potential* changes arising at synapses. Both subtypes can be inhibitory or excitatory.
3. As a consequence of transducer potentials, further response will arise. If the magnitude does not exceed the threshold, the response will be *nonpropagating (electrotonic).* If the response is great enough, a *nerve impulse (action potential impulse) will be produced which obeys the all-or-nothing law (see below) and proceeds unattenuated along the axon or fiber.*

2.5 EXCITABILITY OF NERVE CELL

If a nerve cell is stimulated, the transmembrane voltage necessarily changes. The stimulation may be

excitatory (i.e., *depolarizing;* characterized by a change of the potential inside the cell relative to the outside in the *positive* direction, and hence by a *decrease* in the normally negative resting voltage), or

inhibitory (i.e., *hyperpolarizing,* characterized by a change in the potential inside the cell relative to the outside in the *negative* direction, and hence by an *increase* in the magnitude of the membrane voltage).

After stimulation the membrane voltage returns to its original resting value.

If the membrane stimulus is insufficient to cause the transmembrane potential to reach the threshold, then the membrane will not activate. The response of the membrane to this kind of stimulus is essentially passive. Notable research on membrane behavior under *subthreshold* conditions has been performed by Lorente de Nó (1947) and Davis and Lorente de Nó (1947).

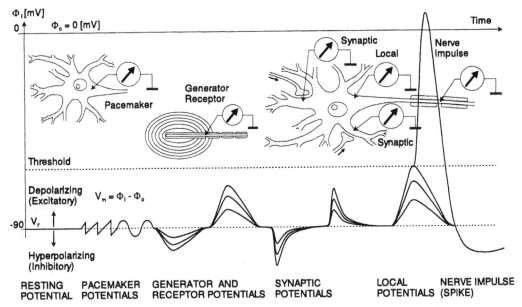

Fig. 2.7 Transmembrane potentials according to Theodore H. Bullock.

If the excitatory stimulus is strong enough, the transmembrane potential reaches the threshold, and the membrane produces a characteristic electric impulse, the *nerve impulse*. This potential response follows a characteristic form regardless of the strength of the transthreshold stimulus. It is said that the *action impulse* of an activated membrane follows an *all-or-nothing law*. An inhibitory stimulus increases the amount of concurrent excitatory stimulus necessary for achieving the threshold (see Fig. 2.8). (The electric recording of the nerve impulse is called the *action potential*. If the nerve impulse is recorded magnetically, it may be called an *action current*. The terminology is further explicated in Section 2.8 and in Fig. 2.11, below.)

2.6 THE GENERATION OF THE ACTIVATION

The mechanism of the activation is discussed in detail in Chapter 4 in connection with the Hodgkin-Huxley membrane model. Here the generation of the activation is discussed only in general terms.

The concentration of sodium ions (Na^+) is about 10 times higher outside the membrane than inside, whereas the concentration of the potassium (K^+) ions is about 30 times higher

inside as compared to outside. When the membrane is stimulated so that the transmembrane potential rises about 20 mV and reaches the threshold—that is, when the membrane voltage changes from -70 mV to about -50 mV (these are illustrative and common numerical values)—the sodium and potassium ionic permeabilities of the membrane change. The sodium ion permeability increases very rapidly at first, allowing sodium ions to flow from outside to inside, making the inside more positive. The inside reaches a potential of about $+20$ mV. After that, the more slowly increasing potassium ion permeability allows potassium ions to flow from inside to outside, thus returning the intracellular potential to its resting value. The maximum excursion of the membrane voltage during activation is about 100 mV; the duration of the nerve impulse is around 1 ms, as illustrated in Figure 2.9. While at rest, following activation, the Na-K pump restores the ion concentrations inside and outside the membrane to their original values.

2.7 CONCEPTS ASSOCIATED WITH THE ACTIVATION PROCESS

Some basic concepts associated with the activation process are briefly defined in this section.

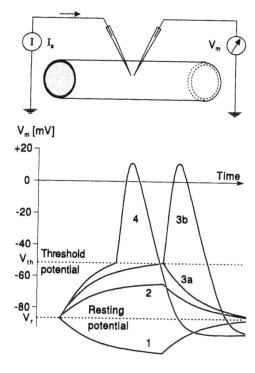

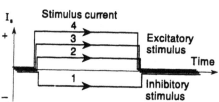

Fig. 2.8 The response of the membrane potential to inhibitory (1) and excitatory (2, 3, 4) stimuli. The current stimulus (2), while excitatory is, however, subthreshold, and only a passive response is seen. For the excitatory level (3), threshold is marginally reached; the membrane is sometimes activated (3b), whereas at other times only a local response (3a) is seen. For a stimulus (4), which is clearly trans-threshold, a nerve impulse is invariably initiated.

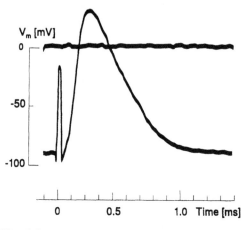

Fig. 2.9 Nerve impulse recorded from a cat motoneuron following a transthreshold stimulus. The stimulus artifact may be seen at $t = 0$.

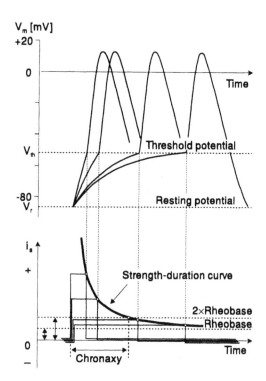

Fig. 2.10 The response of the membrane to various stimuli of changing strength, the strength-duration curve. The level of current strength which will just elicit activation after a very long stimulus is called *rheobase*. The minimum time required for a stimulus pulse twice the rheobase in strength to trigger activation is called *chronaxy*. (For simplicity, threshold is shown here to be independent of stimulus duration.)

Whether an excitatory cell is activated depends largely on the strength and duration of the stimulus. The membrane potential may reach the threshold by a short, strong stimulus or a longer, weaker stimulus. The curve illustrating this dependence is called the *strength-duration curve;* a typical relationship between these variables is illustrated in Figure 2.10. The smallest current adequate to initiate activation is called the *rheobasic current* or *rheobase*. Theoretically, the rheobasic current needs an infinite duration to trigger activation. The time needed to excite the cell with twice rheobase current is called *chronaxy.*

Accommodation and *habituation* denote the adaptation of the cell to a continuing or repetitive stimulus. This is characterized by a rise in the excitation threshold. *Facilitation* denotes an increase in the excitability of the cell; correspondingly, there is a decrease in the threshold. *Latency* denotes the delay between two events. In the present context, it refers to the time between application of a stimulus pulse and the beginning of the activation. Once activation has been initiated, the membrane is insensitive to new stimuli, no matter how large the magnitude. This phase is called the *absolute refractory period.* Near the end of the activation impulse, the cell may be activated, but only with a stimulus stronger than normal. This phase is called the *relative refractory period.*

The activation process encompasses certain specifics such as currents, potentials, conductivities, concentrations, ion flows, and so on. The term *action impulse* describes the whole process. When activation occurs in a nerve cell, it is called a *nerve impulse;* correspondingly, in a muscle cell, it is called a *muscle impulse.* The *bioelectric* measurements focus on the *electric potential* difference across the membrane; thus the electric measurement of the action impulse is called the *action potential* that describes the behavior of the *membrane potential* during the activation. Consequently, we speak, for instance, of *excitatory postsynaptic potentials* (EPSP) and *inhibitory postsynaptic potentials* (IPSP). In *biomagnetic* measurements, it is the electric *current* that is the source of the magnetic field. Therefore, it is logical to use the term *action current* to refer to the source of the biomagnetic signal during the action impulse. These terms are further illustrated in Figure 2.11.

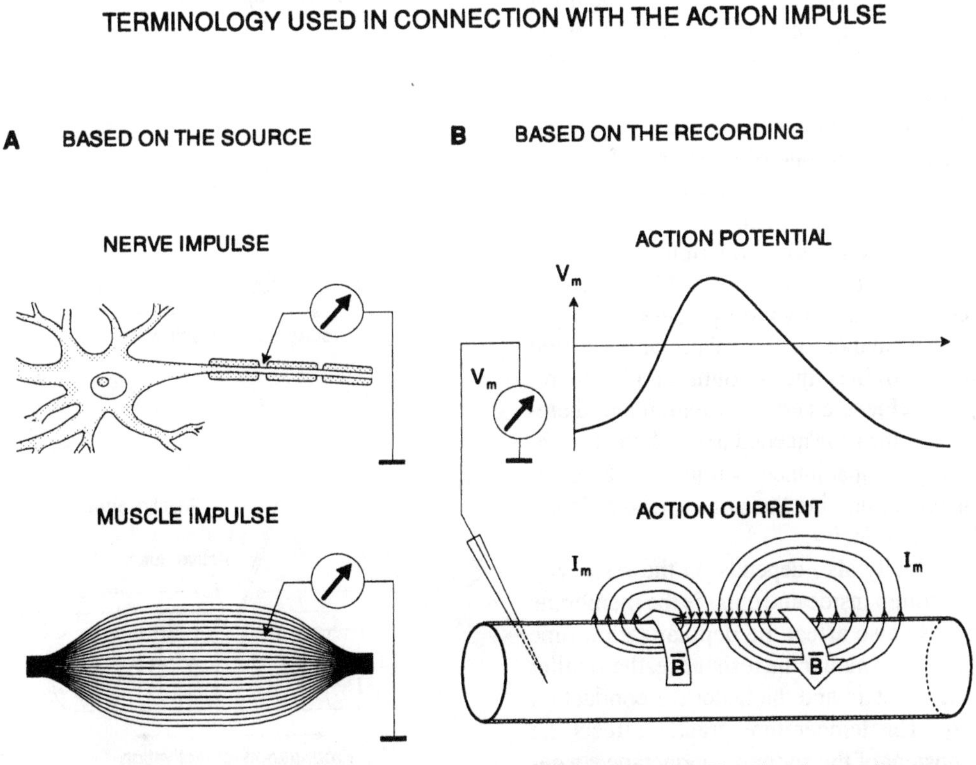

TERMINOLOGY USED IN CONNECTION WITH THE ACTION IMPULSE

A   BASED ON THE SOURCE   **B   BASED ON THE RECORDING**

Fig. 2.11 Clarification of the terminology used in connection with the action impulse. (A) The source of the action impulse may be nerve or muscle cell. Correspondingly, it is called a nerve impulse or a muscle impulse. (B) The electric quantity measured from the action impulse may be potential or current. Correspondingly, the recording is called an action potential or an action current.

2.8 CONDUCTION OF THE NERVE IMPULSE IN AN AXON

Ludvig Hermann (1872, 1905) correctly proposed that the activation propagates in an axon as an unattenuated nerve impulse. He suggested that the potential difference between excited and unexcited regions of an axon would cause small currents, now called *local circuit currents*, to flow between them in such a direction that they stimulate the unexcited region.

Although excitatory inputs may be seen in the dendrites and/or soma, activation originates normally only in the soma. Activation in the form of the nerve impulse (action potential) is first seen in the *root* of the axon—the initial segment of the axon, often called the *axon hillock*. From there it propagates along the axon. If excitation is initiated artificially somewhere along the axon, propagation then takes place in *both* directions from the stimulus site. The conduction velocity depends on the electric properties and the geometry of the axon.

An important physical property of the membrane is the change in sodium conductance due to activation. The higher the maximum value achieved by the sodium conductance, the higher the maximum value of the sodium ion current and the higher the rate of change in the membrane voltage. The result is a higher gradient of voltage, increased local currents, faster excitation, and increased conduction velocity. The decrease in the threshold potential facilitates the triggering of the activation process.

The capacitance of the membrane per unit length determines the amount of charge required to achieve a certain potential and therefore affects the time needed to reach the threshold. Large capacitance values, with other parameters remaining the same, mean a slower conduction velocity.

The velocity also depends on the resistivity of the medium inside and outside the membrane since these also affect the depolarization time constant. The smaller the resistance, the smaller the time constant and the faster the conduction velocity. The temperature greatly affects the time constant of the sodium conductance; a decrease in temperature decreases the conduction velocity.

The above effects are reflected in an expression derived by Müler and Markin (1978) using an idealized nonlinear ionic current function. For the velocity of the propagating nerve impulse in unmyelinated axon, they obtained

$$v = \sqrt{\frac{i_{Namax}}{r_i c_m^2 V_{th}}} \qquad (2.1)$$

where

v = velocity of the nerve impulse [m/s]
$i_{Na\ max}$ = maximum sodium current per unit length [A/m]
V_{th} = threshold voltage [V]
r_i = axial resistance per unit length [Ω/m]
c_m = membrane capacitance per unit length [F/m]

A myelinated axon (surrounded by the myelin sheath) can produce a nerve impulse only at the nodes of Ranvier. In these axons the nerve impulse propagates from one node to another, as illustrated in Figure 2.12. Such a propagation is called *saltatory conduction* (*saltare*, "to dance" in Latin).

The membrane capacitance per unit length

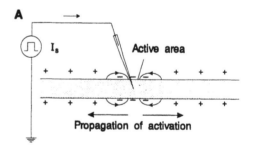

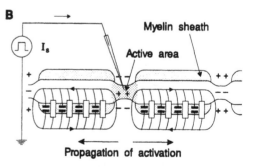

Fig. 2.12 Conduction of a nerve impulse in a nerve axon. (A) Continuous conduction in an unmyelinated axon; (B) saltatory conduction in a myelinated axon.

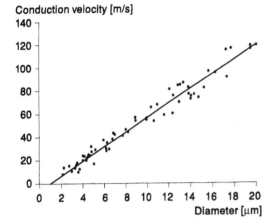

Fig. 2.13 Experimentally determined conduction velocity of a nerve impulse in a mammalian myelinated axon as a function of the diameter. (Adapted from Ruch and Patton, 1982.)

of a myelinated axon is much smaller than in an unmyelinated axon. Therefore, the myelin sheath increases the conduction velocity. The resistance of the axoplasm per unit length is inversely proportional to the cross-sectional area of the axon and thus to the square of the diameter. The membrane capacitance per unit length is directly proportional to the diameter. Because the time constant formed from the product controls the nodal transmembrane potential, it is reasonable to suppose that the velocity would be inversely proportional to the time constant. On this basis the conduction velocity of the myelinated axon should be directly proportional to the diameter of the axon. This is confirmed in Figure 2.13, which shows the conduction velocity in mammalian myelinated axons as linearly dependent on the diameter. The conduction velocity in myelinated axon has the approximate value shown:

$$v \approx 6d \qquad (2.2)$$

where

v = velocity [m/s]
d = axon diameter [μm]

REFERENCES

Berne RM, Levy MN (1993): *Physiology,* 3rd ed., 1091 pp. C. V. Mosby, St. Louis.

Bullock TH (1959): Neuron doctrine and electrophysiology. *Science* 129:(3355) 997–1002.

Davis LJ, Lorente de Nó R (1947): Contributions to the mathematical theory of the electrotonus. *Stud. Rockefeller Inst. Med. Res.* 131: 442–96.

Elsberg CA (1931): The Edwin Smith surgical papyrus. *Ann. Med. Hist.* 3: 271–9.

Ganong WF (1991): *Review of Medical Physiology,* 15th ed., Appleton & Lange, Norwalk, Conn.

Guyton AC (1992): *Human Physiology and Mechanisms of Disease,* 5th ed., 690 pp. Saunders, Philadelphia.

Hermann L (1872): *Grundriss der Physiologie,* 4th ed., (Quoted in L Hermann (1899): Zur Theorie der Erregungsleitung und der elektrischen Erregung. Pflüger Arch. ges. Physiol. 75: 574–90.)

Hermann L (1905): *Lehrbuch der Physiologie,* 13th ed., 762 pp. August Hirschwald, Berlin.

Kandel ER, Schwartz JH (1985): *Principles of Neural Science,* Elsevier Publishing, New York.

Lorente de Nó R (1947): *A Study of Nerve Physiology,* 293 pp. Rockefeller Institute for Medical Research, New York.

Müler AL, Markin VS (1978): Electrical properties of anisotropic nerve-muscle syncytia—II. Spread of flat front of excitation. *Biophys.* 22: 536–41.

Nunez PL (1981): *Electric Fields of the Brain: The Neurophysics of EEG,* 484 pp. Oxford University Press, New York.

Patton HD, Fuchs AF, Hille B, Scher AM, Steiner R (eds.) (1989): *Textbook of Physiology,* 21st ed., 1596 pp. W. B. Saunders, Philadelphia.

Ruch TC, Patton HD (eds.) (1982): *Physiology and Biophysics,* 20th ed., 1242 pp. W. B. Saunders, Philadelphia.

Schadé JP, Ford DH (1973): *Basic Neurology,* 2nd ed., 269 pp. Elsevier Scientific Publishing, Amsterdam.

Thompson CF (1985): *The Brain—An Introduction to Neuroscience,* 363 pp. W. H. Freeman, New York.

3

Subthreshold Membrane Phenomena

3.1 INTRODUCTION

In the previous chapter the subthreshold behavior of the nerve cell was discussed qualitatively. This chapter describes the physiological basis of the resting voltage and the subthreshold response of an axon to electric stimuli from a *quantitative* perspective.

The membrane plays an important role in establishing the resting and active electric properties of an excitable cell, through its regulation of the movement of *ions* between the extracellular and intracellular spaces. The word *ion* (Greek for "that which goes") was introduced by Faraday (1834). The ease with which an ion crosses the membrane, namely the *membrane permeability*, differs among ion species; this *selective permeability* will be seen to have important physiological consequences. Activation of a cell affects its behavior by altering these permeabilities. Another important consideration for transmembrane ion movement is the fact that the ionic composition inside the cell differs greatly from that outside the cell. Consequently, concentration gradients exist for all permeable ions that contribute to the net ion movement or flux. The principle whereby ions flow from regions of high to low concentration is called *diffusion*.

One consequence of this ion flow is the tendency for ions to accumulate at the inner and outer membrane surfaces, a process by which an electric field is established within the membrane. This field exerts forces on the ions crossing the membrane since the latter carry an electric charge. Thus to describe membrane ion movements, electric-field forces as well as diffusional forces should be considered. *Equilibrium* is attained when the diffusional force balances the electric field force for all permeable ions.

For a membrane that is permeable to only one type of ion, equilibrium requires that the force due to the electric field be equal and opposite to the force due to diffusion. In the next section we shall explore the *Nernst equation*, which expresses the equilibrium voltage associated with a given concentration ratio. Equilibrium can also be defined by equating the electrochemical potential on both sides of the membrane.

The Nernst equation is derived from two basic concepts involving ionic flow—those resulting from an electric field force and those resulting from a diffusional force. A more rigorous thermodynamic treatment is available, and the interested reader should consult references such as van Rysselbergh (1963) and Katchalsky and Curran (1965).

We shall also derive the Goldman-Hodgkin-

Katz equation, which gives the steady-state value of the membrane voltage when there are several types of ions in the intracellular and extracellular media, and when the membrane is permeable to all of them. As will be seen, the Goldman-Hodgkin-Katz equation is a straightforward extension of the Nernst equation.

A more detailed discussion of physical chemistry, which contributes to many topics in this chapter, can be found in standard textbooks such as Edsall and Wyman (1958) and Moore (1972).

3.2 NERNST EQUATION

3.2.1 Electric Potential and Electric Field

In electrostatics the electric potential Φ at point P is defined as the work required to move a unit positive charge from a reference position O to position P. If the reference potential is Φ_O and the potential at point P designated Φ_P, then the work W_e, required to move a quantity of charge Q from point O to point P is simply

$$W_e = Q(\Phi_P - \Phi_O) \qquad (3.1)$$

where

W_e = work [J/mol]
Q = charge [C] (coulombs)
Φ = potential [V]

In electrophysiological problems the quantity of ions is usually expressed in *moles*. (One mole equals the molecular weight in grams—hence 6.0225×10^{23}, *Avogadro's number* of molecules.) If *one mole* of an ion is transferred from a reference point O at potential Φ_O to an arbitrary point P at potential Φ_P, then from Equation 3.1 the required work is

$$W_e = zF(\Phi_P - \Phi_O) \qquad (3.2)$$

where

W_e = work [J/mol]
z = valence of the ions
F = Faraday's constant [9.649×10^4 C/mol]
Φ = potential [V]

Faraday's constant converts quantity of moles to quantity of charge for a univalent ion.

The factor z, called *valence*, takes into account multivalent ions and also introduces the sign. Note that if $\Phi_P - \Phi_O$ and z are both positive (i.e., the case where a positive charge is moved from a lower to higher potential), then work must be done, and W_e is positive as expected.

The *electric field* is defined by the *force that it exerts on a unit charge*. If a unit positive charge is moved from reference point O to a nearby point P, where the corresponding vector displacement is $d\bar{s}$, then the work done *against* the electric field force $\bar{E}$, according to the basic laws of mechanics, is the work dW given by

$$dW = -\bar{E} \cdot d\bar{s} \qquad (3.3)$$

Applying Equation 3.1 to Equation 3.3 (replacing Q by unity) gives:

$$\Phi_P - \Phi_O = dW = -\bar{E} \cdot d\bar{s} \qquad (3.4)$$

The Taylor series expansion of the scalar field Φ about the point O and along the path s is:

$$\Phi_P = \Phi_O + d\Phi/ds + \cdots \qquad (3.5)$$

Since P is very close to O, the remaining higher terms may be neglected in Equation 3.5. The second term on the right-hand side of Equation 3.5 is known as the directional derivative of Φ in the direction s. The latter, by the vector-analytic properties of the gradient, is given by $\nabla\Phi \cdot d\bar{s}$. Consequently, Equation 3.5 may be written as

$$\Phi_P - \Phi_O = \nabla\Phi \cdot d\bar{s} \qquad (3.6)$$

From Equations 3.4 and 3.6 we deduce that

$$\bar{E} = -\nabla\Phi \qquad (3.7)$$

This relationship is valid not only for electrostatics but also for electrophysiological problems since *quasistatic conditions* are known to apply to the latter (see Section 8.2.2).

According to Ohm's law, current density $\bar{J}$ and electric field $\bar{E}$ are related by

$$\bar{J} = \sigma\bar{E} = -\sigma \nabla\Phi \qquad (3.8)$$

where σ is the conductivity of the medium. This current, for obvious reasons, is called a *conduction current*.

We are interested mainly in those charged particles that arise from ionization in an electrolyte and, in particular, in those ions present in the intracellular and extracellular spaces in electrically excitable tissues. Because of their charges, these ions are subject to the electric field forces summarized above. The *flux* (i.e., flow per unit area per unit time) that results from the presence of an electric field depends on the electric resistance, which, in turn, is a function of the *ionic mobility* of the ionic species. The latter is defined by u_k, the velocity that would be achieved by the kth ion in a unit electric field. Then the ionic flux is given by

$$\bar{j}_{ke} = -u_k \frac{z_k}{|z_k|} c_k \nabla\Phi \qquad (3.9)$$

where

$\bar{j}_{ke}$ = ionic flux (due to electric field) [mol/(cm²·s)]
u_k = ionic mobility [cm²/(V·s)]
z_k = valence of the ion
c_k = ionic concentration [mol/cm³]

and further:

$\dfrac{z_k}{|z_k|}$ = the sign of the force (positive for cations and negative for anions)

$-u_k\dfrac{z_k}{|z_k|}$ = the mean velocity achieved by these ions in a unit electric field (according to the definition of u_k) the subscript k denotes the kth ion.

Multiplying ionic concentration c_k by velocity gives the ionic flux. A comparison of Equation 3.8 with Equation 3.9 shows that the mobility is proportional to the conductivity of the kth ion in the electrolyte. The ionic mobility depends on the viscosity of the solvent and the size and charge of the ion.

3.2.2   Diffusion

If a particular ionic concentration is not uniform in a compartment, redistribution occurs that ultimately results in a uniform concentration. To accomplish this, flow must necessarily take place from high- to low-density regions. This process is called *diffusion,* and its quantitative description is expressed by *Fick's law* (Fick, 1855). For the kth ion species, this is expressed as

$$\bar{j}_{kD} = -D_k \nabla c_k \qquad (3.10)$$

where

$\bar{j}_{kD}$ = ionic flux (due to diffusion) [mol/(cm²·s)]
D_k = Fick's constant (diffusion constant) [cm²/s]
c_k = ion concentration [mol/cm³]

This equation describes flux in the direction of *decreasing* concentration (accounting for the minus sign), as expected.

Fick's constant relates the "force" due to diffusion (i.e., $-\nabla c_k$) to the consequent flux of the kth substance. In a similar way the mobility couples the electric field force ($-\nabla\Phi$) to the resulting ionic flux. Since in each case the flux is limited by the same factors (collision with solvent molecules), a connection between u_k and D_k should exist. This relationship was worked out by Nernst (1889) and Einstein (1905) and is

$$D_k = \frac{u_k RT}{|z_k|F} \qquad (3.11)$$

where

T = absolute temperature [K]
R = gas constant [8.314 J/(mol·K)]

3.2.3   Nernst-Planck Equation

The total ionic flux for the kth ion, $\bar{j}_k$, is given by the sum of ionic fluxes due to diffusion and electric field of Equations 3.10 and 3.9. Using the Einstein relationship of Equation 3.11, it can be expressed as

$$\bar{j}_k = \bar{j}_{kD} + \bar{j}_{ke} = -D_k \left(\nabla c_k + \frac{c_k z_k F}{RT} \nabla\Phi \right) \qquad (3.12)$$

Equation 3.12 is known as the *Nernst-Planck* equation (after Nernst, 1888, 1889; Planck, 1890ab). It describes the flux of the kth ion under the influence of both a concentration gradient and an electric field. Its dimension depends on those used to express the ionic concentration and the velocity. Normally the units are expressed as [mol/(cm²·s)].

The ionic flux $\bar{j}$ can be converted into an electric current density $\bar{J}$ by multiplying the former by zF, the number of charges carried by each mole (expressed in coulombs, [C]). The result is, for the kth ion,

$$\bar{J}_k = -D_k z_k F \left(\nabla c_k + \frac{c_k z_k F}{RT} \nabla\Phi \right) \qquad (3.13)$$

where

$\bar{J}_k$ = electric current density due to the kth ion
$[C/(s \cdot cm^2)] = [A/cm^2]$

Using Equation 3.11, Equation 3.13 may be rewritten as

$$\bar{J}_k = - \left(u_k RT \frac{z_k}{|z_k|} \nabla c_k + u_k c_k |z_k| F \nabla \Phi \right)$$

(3.14)

3.2.4 Nernst Potential

Figure 3.1 depicts a small portion of a cell membrane of an excitable cell (i.e., a nerve or muscle cell). The membrane element shown is described as a *patch*. The significant ions are potassium (K^+), sodium (Na^+), and chloride (Cl^-), but we shall assume that the membrane is permeable only to one of them (potassium) which we denote as the kth ion, to allow later generalization. The ion concentrations on each side of the membrane are also illustrated schematically in Figure 3.1. At the sides of the figure, the sizes of the symbols are given in proportion to the corresponding ion concentrations. The ions are shown to cross the membrane through channels, as noted above. The number of ions flowing through an open channel may be more than 10^6 per second.

It turns out that this is a reasonable approximation to actual conditions at rest. The concentration of potassium is normally around 30–50 times greater in the intracellular space compared to the extracellular. As a consequence, potassium ions diffuse outward across the cell membrane, leaving behind an equal number of negative ions (mainly chloride). Because of the strong electrostatic attraction, as the potassium efflux takes place, the potassium ions accumulate on the outside of the membrane. Simultaneously, (an equal number of) chloride ions (left behind from the KCl) accumulate on the inside of the membrane. In effect, the membrane capacitance is in the process of charging, and an electric field directed inward increasingly develops in proportion to the net potassium efflux.

The process described above does not continue indefinitely because the increasing electric field forms a force on the permeable po-

INTRACELLULAR MEDIUM

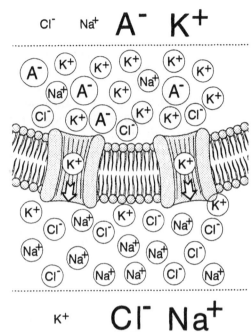

Fig. 3.1 A patch of membrane of an excitable cell at rest with part of the surrounding intracellular and extracellular media. The main ions capable of transmembrane flow are potassium (K^+), sodium (Na^+), and chloride (Cl^-). The intracellular ionic composition and extracellular ionic composition are unequal. At the sides of the figure, the sizes of the symbols reflect the proportions of the corresponding ion concentration. The intracellular anion (A^-) is important to the achievement of electroneutrality; however, A^- is derived from large immobile and impermeable molecules (KA), and thus A^- does not contribute to ionic flow. At rest, the membrane behaves as if it were permeable only to potassium. The ratio of intracellular to extracellular potassium concentration is in the range 30–50:1.

tassium ion that is directed inward and, hence, opposite to the diffusional force. An equilibrium is reached when the two forces are equal in magnitude. The number of the potassium ions required to cross the membrane to bring this about is ordinarily *extremely small* compared to the number available. Therefore, in the above process for all practical purposes we may consider the intracellular and extracellular concentrations of the potassium ion as unchanging throughout the transient. The transmembrane potential achieved at equilibrium is simply the *equilibrium potential.*

A quantitative relationship between the potassium ion concentrations and the aforementioned equilibrium potential can be derived from the Nernst-Planck equation. To generalize the result, we denote the potassium ion as the kth ion. Applying Equation 3.13 to the membrane at equilibrium we must satisfy a condition of zero current so that

$$\bar{J}_k = 0 = -D_k z_k F \left(\nabla c_k + \frac{c_k z_k F}{RT} \nabla \Phi \right) \quad (3.15)$$

where the subscript k refers to an arbitrary k^{th} ion. Transposing terms in Equation 3.15 gives

$$\nabla c_k = -\frac{c_k z_k F}{RT} \nabla \Phi \quad (3.16)$$

Since the membrane is extremely thin, we can consider any small patch as planar and describe variations across it as one-dimensional (along a normal to the membrane). If we call this direction x, we may write out Equation 3.16 as

$$\frac{dc_k}{dx} = -\frac{c_k z_k F}{RT} \frac{d\Phi}{dx} \quad (3.17)$$

Equation 3.17 can be rearranged to give

$$\frac{dc_k}{c_k} = -\frac{z_k F}{RT} d\Phi \quad (3.18)$$

Equation 3.18 may now be integrated from the intracellular space (i) to the extracellular space (o); that is:

$$\int_i^o \frac{dc_k}{c_k} = -\frac{z_k F}{RT} \int_i^o d\Phi \quad (3.19)$$

Carrying out the integrations in Equation 3.19 gives

$$\ln \frac{c_{o,k}}{c_{i,k}} = -\frac{z_k F}{RT} (\Phi_o - \Phi_i) \quad (3.20)$$

where $c_{i,k}$ and $c_{o,k}$ denote the intracellular and extracellular concentrations of the kth ion, respectively. The equilibrium voltage across the membrane for the kth ion is, by convention, the intracellular minus the extracellular potential ($V_k = \Phi_i - \Phi_o$), hence:

$$V_k = -\frac{RT}{z_k F} \ln \frac{c_{i,k}}{c_{o,k}} \quad \textbf{(3.21)}$$

where

V_k = equilibrium voltage for the kth ion across the membrane ($\Phi_i - \Phi_o$) i.e., the Nernst voltage [V]

R = gas constant [8.314 J/(mol × K)]

T = absolute temperature [K]

z_k = valence of the kth ion

F = Faraday's constant [9.649 × 10^4 C/mol]

$c_{i,k}$ = intracellular concentration of the kth ion

$c_{o,k}$ = extracellular concentration of the kth ion

Equation 3.21 is the famous *Nernst equation* derived by Walther Hermann Nernst in 1888 (Nernst, 1888). By substituting 37°C, which gives $T = 273 + 37$ and +1 for the valence, and by replacing the natural logarithm (the Napier logarithm) with the decadic logarithm (the Briggs logarithm), one may write the Nernst equation for a monovalent cation as:

$$V = -61 \times \log_{10} \frac{c_i}{c_o} \text{ [mV]} \quad (3.22)$$

At room temperature (20°C), the coefficient in Equation 3.22 has the value of 58; at the temperature of seawater (6°C), it is 55. The latter is important when considering the squid axon.

Example

We discuss the subject of equilibrium further by means of the example described in Figure 3.2, depicting an axon lying in a cylindrical experimental chamber. The potential inside the axon may be changed with three interchangeable batteries (A, B, and C) which may be placed between the intracellular and extracellular spaces. We assume that the intracellular and the extracellular spaces can be considered *isopotential* so that the transmembrane voltage V_m (difference of potential across the membrane) is the same everywhere. (This technique is called *voltage clamp,* and explained in more detail in Section 4.2.) Furthermore, the membrane is assumed to be permeable only to potassium ions. The intracellular and extracellular concentrations of potassium are $c_{i,K}$ and $c_{o,K}$, respectively. In the resting state, the membrane voltage V_m (= $\Phi_i - \Phi_o$) equals V_K, the Nernst voltage for K^+ ions according to Equation 3.21.

In Figure 3.2 the vertical axis indicates the potential Φ, and the horizontal axis the radial distance r measured from the center of the axon.

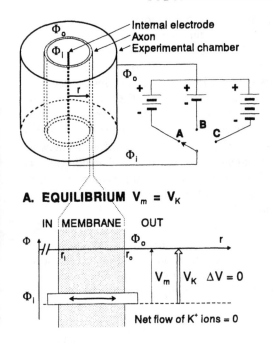

A. EQUILIBRIUM $V_m = V_K$

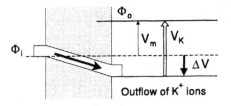

B. DEPOLARIZED $|V_m| < |V_K|$

C. HYPERPOLARIZED $|V_m| > |V_K|$

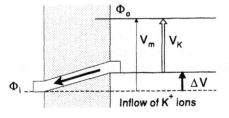

Transmembrane voltage: $V_m = \Phi_i - \Phi_o$

Nernst voltage for K$^+$ ions: $V_K = -\dfrac{RT}{zF} \ln \dfrac{c_{i,K}}{c_{o,K}}$

Force moving K$^+$ ions: $\Delta V = V_m - V_K$

Fig. 3.2 An example illustrating the Nernst equation and ion flow through the membrane in (A) equilibrium at rest, (B) depolarized membrane, and (C) hyperpolarized membrane. The diffusional force arising from the concentration gradient is equal and opposite to the equilibrium electric field V_K which, in turn, is calculated from the Nernst potential (see

The membrane is located between the radial distance values r_i and r_o. The length of the arrows indicates the magnitude of the voltage (inside potential minus outside potential). Their direction indicates the polarity so that upward arrows represent negative, and downward arrows positive voltages (because all the potential differences in this example are measured from negative potentials). Therefore, when ΔV is positive (downward), the transmembrane current (for a positive ion) is also positive (i.e., outward).

A. Suppose that the electromotive force *emf* of the battery A equals V_K. In this case $V_m = V_K$ and the condition corresponds precisely to the one where equilibrium between diffusion and electric field forces is achieved. Under this condition no net flow of potassium ions exists through the membrane (see Figure 3.2A). (The flow through the membrane consists only of diffusional flow in both directions.)

B. Suppose, now, that the voltage of battery B is smaller than V_K ($|V_m| < |V_K|$). Then the potential inside the membrane becomes less negative, a condition known as *depolarization* of the membrane. Now the electric field is no longer adequate to equilibrate the diffusional forces. This imbalance is $\Delta V = V_m - V_K$ and an outflow of potassium (from a higher electrochemical potential to a lower one) results. This condition is illustrated in Figure 3.2B.

C. If, on the other hand, battery C is selected so that the potential inside the membrane becomes more negative than in the resting state ($|V_m| > |V_K|$), then the membrane is said to be *hyperpolarized*. In this case ions will flow inward (again from the higher electrochemical potential to the lower one). This condition is described in Figure 3.2C.

Equation 3.21). The Nernst electric field force V_K is described by the open arrow. The thin arrow describes the actual electric field V_m across the membrane that is imposed when the battery performs a voltage clamp (see Section 4.2 for the description of voltage clamp). The bold arrow is the net electric field driving force ΔV in the membrane resulting from the difference between the actual electric field (thin arrow) and the equilibrium electric field (open arrow).

3.3 ORIGIN
OF THE RESTING VOLTAGE

The resting voltage of a nerve cell denotes the value of the membrane voltage (difference between the potential inside and outside the membrane) when the neuron is in the resting state in its natural, physiological environment. It should be emphasized that the resting state is not a passive state but a stable active state that needs metabolic energy to be maintained. Julius Bernstein, the founder of membrane theory, proposed a very simple hypothesis on the origin of the resting voltage, depicted in Figure 3.3 (Bernstein, 1902, 1912). His hypothesis is based on experiments performed on the axon of a squid, in which the intracellular ion concentrations are, for potassium, $c_{i,K} = 400$ mol/m^3; and, for sodium, $c_{i,Na} = 50$ mol/m^3. It is *presumed* that the membrane is permeable to potassium ions but fully *im*permeable to sodium ions.

The axon is first placed in a solution whose ion concentrations are the same as inside the axon. In such a case the presence of the membrane does not lead to the development of a difference of potential between the inside and outside of the cell, and thus the membrane voltage is zero.

The axon is then moved to seawater, where the potassium ion concentration is $c_{o,K} = 20$ mol/m^3 and the sodium ion concentration is $c_{o,Na} = 440$ mol/m^3. Now a concentration gradient exists for both types of ions, causing them to move from the region of higher concentration to the region of lower concentration. However, because the membrane is assumed to be im-

permeable to sodium ions, despite the concentration gradient, they cannot move through the membrane. The potassium ions, on the other hand, flow from inside to outside. Since they carry a positive charge, the inside becomes more negative relative to the outside. The flow continues until the membrane voltage reaches the corresponding potassium Nernst voltage— that is, when the electric and diffusion gradients are equal (and opposite) and equilibrium is achieved. At equilibrium the membrane voltage is calculated from the Nernst equation (Equation 3.21).

The hypothesis of Bernstein is, however, incomplete, because the membrane is *not* fully impermeable to sodium ions. Instead, particularly as a result of the high electrochemical gradient, some sodium ions flow to the inside of the membrane. Correspondingly, potassium ions flow, as described previously, to the outside of the membrane. Because the potassium and sodium Nernst voltages are unequal, there is *no* membrane voltage that will equilibrate both ion fluxes. Consequently, the membrane voltage at rest is merely the value for which a steady-state is achieved (i.e., where the sodium influx and potassium efflux are equal). The steady resting sodium influx and potassium efflux would eventually modify the resting intracellular concentrations and affect the homeostatic conditions; however, the Na-K pump, mentioned before, transfers the sodium ions back outside the membrane and potassium ions back inside the membrane, thus keeping the ionic concentrations stable. The pump obtains its energy from the metabolism of the cell.

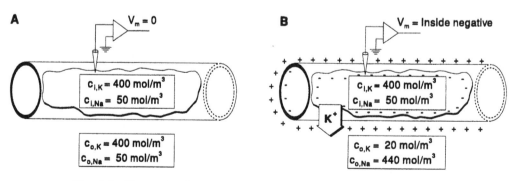

Fig. 3.3 The origin of the resting voltage according to Julius Bernstein.

3.4 MEMBRANE WITH MULTI-ION PERMEABILITY

3.4.1 Donnan Equilibrium

The assumption that biological membranes are permeable to a single ion only is not valid, and even low permeabilities may have an important effect. We shall assume that when several permeable ions are present, the flux of each is independent of the others (an assumption known as the *independence principle* and formulated by Hodgkin and Huxley (1952)). This assumption is supported by many experiments.

The biological membrane patch can be represented by the model drawn in Figure 3.4, which takes into account the primary ions potassium, sodium, and chloride. If the membrane potential is V_m, and since V_k is the equilibrium potential for the kth ion, then $(V_m - V_k)$ evaluates the net driving force on the kth ion. Considering potassium (K), for example, the net driving force is given by $(V_m - V_K)$; here we can recognize that V_m represents the electric force and V_K the diffusional force (in electric

terms) on potassium. When $V_m = V_K$, the net force is zero and there is no flux since the potential is the same as the potassium equilibrium potential. The reader should recall, that V_K is negative; thus if $V_m - V_K$ is positive, the electric field force is less than the diffusional force, and a potassium efflux (a positive transmembrane current) results, as explained in the example given in Section 3.2.4.

The unequal intracellular and extracellular composition arises from active transport (Na-K pump) which maintains this imbalance (and about which more will be said later). We shall see that despite the membrane ion flux, the pump will always act to restore normal ionic composition. Nevertheless, it is of some interest to consider the end result if the pump is disabled (a consequence of ischemia, perhaps). In this case, very large ion movements will ultimately take place, resulting in changed ionic concentrations. When equilibrium is reached, every ion is at its Nernst potential which, of course, is also the common transmembrane potential. In fact, in view of this common potential, the required equilibrium concentration ratios must satisfy Equation 3.23 (derived from Equation 3.21)

$$\frac{c_{o,K}}{c_{i,K}} = \frac{c_{o,Na}}{c_{i,Na}} = \frac{c_{i,Cl}}{c_{o,Cl}} \tag{3.23}$$

Note that Equation 3.23 reflects the fact that all ions are univalent and that chloride is negative. The condition represented by Equation 3.23 is that *all* ions are in equilibrium; it is referred to as the *Donnan equilibrium*.

3.4.2 The Value of the Resting Voltage, Goldman-Hodgkin-Katz Equation

The relationship between membrane voltage and ionic flux is of great importance. Research on this relationship makes several assumptions: first, that the biological membrane is homogeneous and neutral (like very thin glass); and second, that the intracellular and extracellular regions are completely uniform and unchanging. Such a model is described as an *electrodiffusion model*. Among these models is that by Goldman-Hodgkin-Katz which is described in this section.

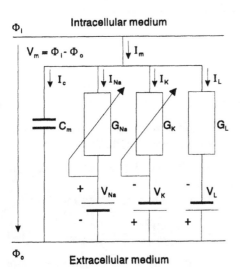

Fig. 3.4 An electric circuit representation of a membrane patch. In this diagram, V_{Na}, V_K, and V_L represent the absolute values of the respective emf's and the signs indicate their directions when the extracellular medium has a normal composition (high Na and Cl, and low K, concentrations).

In view of the very small thickness of a biological membrane as compared to its lateral extent, we may treat any element of membrane under consideration as *planar*. The Goldman-Hodgkin-Katz model assumes, in fact, that the membrane is *uniform, planar,* and *infinite* in its lateral extent. If the x-axis is chosen normal to the membrane with its origin at the interface of the membrane with the extracellular region, and if the membrane thickness is h, then $x = h$ defines the interface of the membrane with the intracellular space. Because of the assumed lateral uniformity, variations of the potential field Φ and ionic concentration c within the membrane are functions of x only. The basic assumption underlying the Goldman-Hodgkin-Katz model is that the field within the membrane is constant; hence

$$\frac{d\Phi}{dx} = \frac{\Phi_h - \Phi_0}{h} = \frac{V_m}{h} \qquad (3.24)$$

where

Φ_0 = potential at the outer membrane surface
Φ_h = potential at the inner membrane surface
V_m = transmembrane voltage
h = membrane thickness

This approximation was originally introduced by David Goldman (1943).

The Nernst equation evaluates the equilibrium value of the membrane voltage when the membrane is permeable to only one kind of ion or when all permeable ions have reached a Donnan equilibrium. Under physiological conditions, such an equilibrium is not achieved as can be verified with examples such as Table 3.1. To determine the membrane voltage when there are several types of ions in the intra- and extracellular media, to which the membrane may be permeable, an extended version of the Nernst equation must be used. This is the particular application of the Goldman-Hodgkin-Katz equation whose derivation we will now describe.

For the membrane introduced above, in view of its one dimensionality, we have $\nabla\Phi \equiv d\Phi/dx$, $\nabla c_k \equiv dc_k/dx$, and, using Equation 3.12, we get

$$j_k = -D_k \left(\frac{dc_k}{dx} + \frac{c_k z_k F}{RT} \frac{d\Phi}{dx} \right) \qquad (3.25)$$

for the kth ion flux. If we now insert the constant field approximation of Equation 3.24 ($d\Phi/dx = V_m/h$) the result is

$$\frac{dc_k}{dx} = -\frac{j_k}{D_k} - \frac{V_m z_k F}{RTh} c_k \qquad (3.26)$$

(To differentiate ionic concentration within the membrane from that outside the membrane (i.e., inside versus outside the membrane), we use the symbol c^m in the following where *intra*membrane concentrations are indicated.) Rearranging Equation 3.26 gives the following differential equation:

$$\frac{dc_k^m}{-\dfrac{j_k}{D_k} - \dfrac{V_m z_k F c_k^m}{RTh}} = dx \qquad (3.27)$$

We now integrate Equation 3.27 *within* the membrane from the left-hand edge ($x = 0$) to the right-hand edge ($x = h$). We assume the existence of resting conditions; hence each ion flux must be in steady state and therefore uniform with respect to x. Furthermore, for V_m to remain constant, the total transmembrane electric current must be zero. From the first condition we require that $j_k(x)$ be a constant; hence on the left-hand side of Equation 3.27, only $c_k^m(x)$ is a function of x. The result of the integration is then

$$-\frac{RTh}{V_m z_k F} \ln \left[\frac{\dfrac{V_m z_k F}{RTh} c_k^h + \dfrac{j_k}{D_k}}{\dfrac{V_m z_k F}{RTh} c_k^0 + \dfrac{j_k}{D_k}} \right] = h \qquad (3.28)$$

where

c_k^h = concentration of the kth ion at $x = h$
c_k^0 = concentration of the kth ion at $x = 0$

Both variables are defined within the membrane.

Equation 3.28 can be solved for j_k, giving

$$j_k = -\frac{D_k V_m z_k F}{RTh} \cdot \frac{c_k^h - c_k^0 e^{-V_m z_k F/RT}}{1 - e^{-V_m z_k F/RT}} \qquad (3.29)$$

The concentrations of the kth ion in Equation 3.29 are those within the membrane. However, the known concentrations are those in the intracellular and extracellular (bulk) spaces. Now the concentration ratio from just outside to just inside the membrane is described by a *partition coefficient*, β. These are assumed to be the same at both the intracellular and extracellular interface. Consequently, since $x = 0$ is at the extracellular surface and $x = h$ the intracellular interface, we have

$$c_k^h = \beta_k c_i \qquad (3.30)$$
$$c_k^0 = \beta_k c_o$$

where

β = partition coefficient
c_i = measurable intracellular ionic concentration
c_o = measurable extracellular ionic concentration

The electric current density J_k can be obtained by multiplying the ionic flux j_k from Equation 3.29 by Faraday's constant and valence. If, in addition, the permeability P_k is defined as

$$P_k = \frac{D_k \beta_k}{h} \qquad (3.31)$$

then

$$J_k = -\frac{P_k V_m z_k^2 F^2}{RT} \cdot \frac{c_i - c_o e^{-V_m z_k F/RT}}{1 - e^{-V_m z_k F/RT}} \qquad (3.32)$$

When considering the ion flux through the membrane at the resting state, the sum of all currents through the membrane is necessarily zero, as noted above. The main contributors to the electric current are potassium, sodium, and chloride ions. So we may write

$$J_K + J_{Na} + J_{Cl} = 0 \qquad (3.33)$$

By substituting Equation 3.32 into Equation 3.33, appending the appropriate indices, and noting that for potassium and sodium the valence $z = +1$ whereas for chloride $z = -1$, and canceling the constant $z_k^2 F^2/RT$, we obtain:

$$-P_K \frac{c_{i,K} - c_{o,K} e^{-V_m F/RT}}{1 - e^{-V_m F/RT}}$$
$$- P_{Na} \frac{c_{i,Na} - c_{o,Na} e^{-V_m F/RT}}{1 - e^{-V_m F/RT}}$$
$$-P_{Cl} \frac{c_{i,Cl} - c_{o,Cl} e^{+V_m F/RT}}{1 - e^{+V_m F/RT}} = 0 \qquad (3.34)$$

In Equation 3.34 the expression for sodium ion current is seen to be similar to that for potassium (except for exchanging Na for K); however, the expression for chloride requires, in addition, a change in sign in the exponential term, a reflection of the negative valence.

The denominator can be eliminated from Equation 3.34 by first multiplying the numerator and denominator of the last term by factor $-e^{-FV_m/RT}$ and then multiplying term by term by $1 - e^{-FV_m/RT}$. Thus we obtain

$$P_K(c_{i,K} - c_{o,K} e^{-V_m F/RT})$$
$$+ P_{Na}(c_{i,Na} - c_{o,Na} e^{-V_m F/RT})$$
$$+ P_{Cl}(c_{o,Cl} - c_{i,Cl} e^{-V_m F/RT}) = 0 \qquad (3.35)$$

Multiplying through by the permeabilities and collecting terms gives:

$$P_K c_{i,K} + P_{Na} c_{i,Na} + P_{Cl} c_{o,Cl}$$
$$= e^{-V_m F/RT}(P_K c_{o,K} + P_{Na} c_{o,Na} + P_{Cl} c_{i,Cl}) \qquad (3.36)$$

From this equation, it is possible to solve for the potential difference V_m across the membrane, as follows:

$$V_m = -\frac{RT}{F} \ln \frac{P_K c_{i,K} + P_{Na} c_{i,Na} + P_{Cl} c_{o,Cl}}{P_K c_{o,K} + P_{Na} c_{o,Na} + P_{Cl} c_{i,Cl}} \qquad \mathbf{(3.37)}$$

where V_m evaluates the intracellular minus extracellular potential (i.e., transmembrane voltage). This equation is called the *Goldman-Hodgkin-Katz equation*. Its derivation is based on the works of David Goldman (1943) and Hodgkin and Katz (1949). One notes in Equation 3.37 that the relative contribution of each ion species to the resting voltage is weighted by that ion's permeability. For the squid axon, we noted (Section 3.5.2) that $P_{Na}/P_K = 0.04$, which explains why its resting voltage is relatively close to V_K and quite different from V_{Na}.

By substituting 37°C for the temperature and the Briggs logarithm (with base 10) for the Napier logarithm (to the base e), Equation 3.37 may be written as:

$$V_m =$$
$$-61 \log_{10} \frac{P_K c_{i,K} + P_{Na} c_{i,Na} + P_{Cl} c_{o,Cl}}{P_K c_{o,K} + P_{Na} c_{o,Na} + P_{Cl} c_{i,Cl}} \text{ [mV]} \qquad (3.38)$$

Example

It is easy to demonstrate that the Goldman-Hodgkin-Katz equation (Equation 3.37) reduces to the Nernst equation (Equation 3.21). Suppose that the chloride concentration both inside and outside the membrane were zero (i.e., $c_{o,Cl} = c_{i,Cl} = 0$). Then the third terms in the numerator and denominator of Equation 3.37 would be absent. Suppose further that the permeability to sodium (normally very small) could be taken to be exactly zero (i.e., $P_{Na} = 0$). Under these conditions the Goldman-Hodgkin-Katz equation reduces to the form of the Nernst equation (note that the absolute value of the valence of the ions in question $|z| = 1$). This demonstrates again that the Nernst equation expresses the equilibrium potential difference across an ion permeable membrane for systems containing only a single permeable ion.

3.4.3 The Reversal Voltage

The membrane potential at which the (net) membrane current is zero is called the *reversal voltage* (V_R). This designation derives from the fact that when the membrane voltage is increased or decreased, it is at this potential that the membrane current reverses its sign. When the membrane is permeable for two types of ions, A^+ and B^+, and the permeability ratio for these ions is P_A/P_B, the reversal voltage is defined by the equation:

$$V_R = \frac{RT}{zF} \ln \frac{(P_A/P_B)A_o + B_o}{(P_A/P_B)A_i + B_i} \qquad (3.39)$$

This equation resembles the Nernst equation (Equation 3.21), but it includes *two* types of ions. It is the simplest form of the Goldman-Hodgkin-Katz equation (Equation 3.37).

3.5 ION FLOW THROUGH THE MEMBRANE

3.5.1 Factors Affecting Ion Transport Through the Membrane

This section explores the flow of various ions through the membrane under normal resting conditions.

The flow of ions through the cell membrane depends mainly on three factors:

1. the ratio of ion concentrations on both sides of the membrane,
2. the voltage across the membrane, and
3. the membrane permeability.

The effects of concentration differences and membrane voltages on the flow of ions may be made commensurable if, instead of the concentration ratio, the corresponding Nernst voltage is considered. The force affecting the ions is then proportional to the difference between the membrane voltage and the Nernst voltage.

Regarding membrane permeability, we note that if the biological membrane consisted solely of a lipid bilayer, as described earlier, all ionic flow would be greatly impeded. However, specialized proteins are also present which cross the membrane and contain aqueous channels. Such channels are specific for certain ions; they also include gates which are sensitive to membrane voltage. The net result is that membrane permeability is different for different ions, and it may be affected by changes in the transmembrane voltage, and/or by certain ligands.

As mentioned in Section 3.4.1, Hodgkin and Huxley (1952) formulated a quantitative relation called the *independence principle*. According to this principle the flow of ions through the membrane does not depend on the presence of other ions. Thus, the flow of each type of ion through the membrane can be considered independent of other types of ions. The total membrane current is then, by superposition, the sum of the currents due to each type of ions.

3.5.2 Membrane Ion Flow in a Cat Motoneuron

We discuss the behavior of membrane ion flow with an example. For the cat motoneuron the following ion concentrations have been measured (see Table 3.1). For each ion, the following equilibrium voltages may be *calculated* from the Nernst equation:

$$V_{Na} = -61 \, \log_{10}(15/150) = +61 \text{ mV}$$
$$V_K = -61 \, \log_{10}(150/5.5) = -88 \text{ mV}$$
$$V_{Cl} = +61 \, \log_{10}(9/125) = -70 \text{ mV}$$

Table 3.1 Ion concentrations measured from cat motoneuron

	Outside the membrane [mol/m^3]	Inside the membrane [mol/m^3]
Na$^+$	150	15
K$^+$	5.5	150
Cl$^-$	125	9

The resting voltage of the cell was *measured* to be −70 mV.

When Hodgkin and Huxley described the electric properties of an axon in the beginning of the 1950s (see Chapter 4), they believed that two to three different types of ionic channels (Na^+, K^+, and Cl^-) were adequate for characterizing the excitable membrane behavior. The number of different channel types is, however, much larger. In 1984, Bertil Hille (Hille, 1984/1992) summarized what was known at that time about ion channels. He considered that about four to five different channel types were present in a cell and that the genome may code for a total number of 50 different channel types. Now it is believed that each cell has at least 50 different channel types and that the number of different channel proteins reaches one thousand.

We now examine the behavior of the different constituent ions in more detail.

Chloride Ions

In this example the equilibrium potential of the chloride ion is the same as the resting potential of the cell. While this is not generally the case, it is true that the chloride Nernst potential does approach the resting potential. This condition arises because chloride ion permeability is relatively high, and even a small movement into or out of the cell will make large changes in the concentration ratios as a result of the very low intracellular concentration. Consequently the concentration ratio, hence the Nernst potential, tends to move toward equilibrium with the resting potential.

Potassium Ions

In the example described by Table 3.1, the equilibrium voltage of potassium is 19 mV more negative than the resting voltage of the cell. In a subsequent section we shall explain that this is a typical result and that the resting potential always exceeds (algebraically) the potassium Nernst potential. Consequently, we must always expect a net flow of potassium ions from the inside to the outside of a cell under resting conditions. To compensate for this flux, and thereby maintain normal ionic composition, the potassium ion must also be transported into the cell. Such a movement, however, is in the direction of increasing potential and consequently requires the expenditure of energy. This is provided by the Na-K pump, that functions to transport potassium at the expense of energy.

Sodium Ions

The equilibrium potential of sodium is +61 mV, which is given by the concentration ratio (see Table 3.1). Consequently, the sodium ion is 131 mV from equilibrium, and a sodium influx (due to both diffusion and electric field forces) will take place at rest. Clearly neither sodium nor potassium is in equilibrium, but the resting condition requires only a steady state. In particular, the *total* membrane current has to be zero. For sodium and potassium, this also means that the total efflux and total influx must be equal in magnitude. Since the driving force for sodium is 6.5 times greater than that for potassium, the potassium permeability must be 6.5 times greater than for sodium. Because of its low resting permeability, the contribution of the sodium ion to the resting transmembrane potential is sometimes ignored, as an approximation.

In the above example, the ionic concentrations and permeabilities were selected for a cat motoneuron. In the squid axon, the ratio of the resting permeabilities of potassium, sodium and chloride ions has been found to be $P_K:P_{Na}:P_{Cl}$ = 1:0.04:0.45.

3.5.3 Na-K Pump

The long-term ionic composition of the intracellular and extracellular space is maintained by the Na-K pump. As noted above, in the steady state, the total passive flow of electric current is zero, and the potassium efflux and sodium influx are equal and opposite (when these are the only contributing ions). When the Na-K pump was believed to exchange 1 mol potassium for 1 mol sodium, no net electric current was expected. However recent evidence is that for 2 mol potassium pumped in, 3 mol sodium is pumped out. Such a pump is said to be *electrogenic* and must be taken into account in any quantitative model of the membrane currents (Junge, 1992).

3.5.4 Graphical Illustration of the Membrane Ion Flow

The flow of potassium and sodium ions through the cell membrane (shaded) and the electrochemical gradient causing this flow are illustrated in Figure 3.5. For each ion the clear stripe represents the ion flux; the width of the stripe, the amount of the flux; and the inclination (i.e., the slope), the strength of the electrochemical gradient.

As in Figure 3.2, the vertical axis indicates the potential, and the horizontal axis distance normal to the membrane. Again, when ΔV is positive (downward), the transmembrane current (for a positive ion) is also positive (i.e., outward). For a negative ion (Cl^-), it would be inward.

3.6 CABLE EQUATION OF THE AXON

Ludvig Hermann (1905) was the first to suggest that under subthreshold conditions the cell membrane can be described by a uniformly distributed leakage resistance and parallel capacitance. Consequently, the response to an arbitrary current stimulus can be evaluated from an elaboration of circuit theory. In this section, we describe this approach in a cell that is circularly cylindrical in shape and in which the length greatly exceeds the radius. (Such a model applies to an unmyelinated nerve axon.)

3.6.1 Cable Model of the Axon

Suppose that an axon is immersed in an electrolyte of finite extent (representing its extracellular medium) and an excitatory electric impulse is introduced via two electrodes—one located just outside the axon in the extracellular medium and the other inside the axon, as illustrated in Figure 3.6. The total stimulus current (I_i), which flows axially inside the axon, diminishes with distance since part of it continually crosses the membrane to return as a current (I_o) outside the axon. Note that the definition of the direction of positive current is to the right for both I_i and I_o, in which case conservation of current requires that $I_o = -I_i$. Suppose also that both inside and outside of the

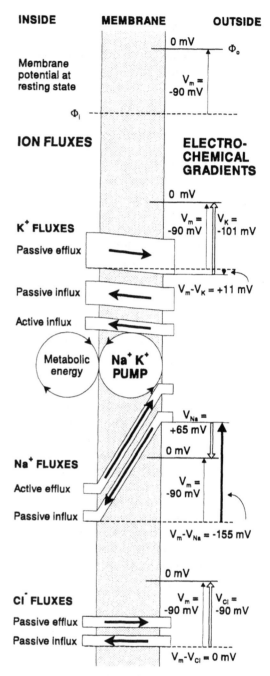

Fig. 3.5   A model illustrating the transmembrane ion flux. (After Eccles, 1968.) Note that K^+ and Cl^- passive flux due to diffusion and electric field are shown separately.

axon, the potential is uniform within any cross-section (i.e., independent of the radial direction) and the system exhibits axial symmetry. These approximations are based on the cross-sectional dimensions being very small compared to the

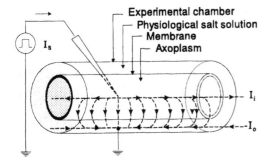

Fig. 3.6 The experimental arrangement for deriving the cable equation of the axon.

length of the active region of the axon. Suppose also that the length of the axon is so great that it can be assumed to be infinite.

Under these assumptions the equivalent circuit of Figure 3.7 is a valid description for the axon. One should particularly note that the limited extracellular space in Figure 3.6 confines current to the axial direction and thus serves to justify assigning an axial resistance R_o to represent the interstitial fluid. In the model, each section, representing an axial element of the axon along with its bounding extracellular fluid, is chosen to be short in relation to the total axon length. Note, in particular, that the subthreshold membrane is modeled as a distributed resistance and capacitance in parallel. The resistive component takes into account the ionic membrane current i_{mI}; the capacitance reflects the fact that the membrane is a poor conductor but a good dielectric, and consequently, a membrane capacitive current i_{mC} must be included

as a component of the total membrane current. The axial intracellular and extracellular paths are entirely resistive, reflecting experimental evidence regarding nerve axons.

The components of the equivalent circuit described in Figure 3.7 include the following: Note that instead of the MKS units, the dimensions are given in units traditionally used in this connection. Note also that quantities that denote ''per unit length'' are written with lower-case symbols.

r_i = intracellular axial resistance of the axoplasma per unit length of axon [$k\Omega$/cm axon length]

r_o = extracellular axial resistance of the (bounding) extracellular medium per unit length of axon [$k\Omega$/cm axon length]

r_m = membrane resistance times unit length of axon [$k\Omega \cdot$cm axon length] (note that this is in the radial direction, which accounts for its dimensions)

c_m = membrane capacitance per unit length of axon [μF/cm axon length]

We further define the currents and voltages of the circuit as follows (see Figs. 3.6 and 3.7):

I_i = total longitudinal intracellular current [μA]

I_o = total longitudinal extracellular current [μA]

i_m = total transmembrane current per unit length of axon [μA/cm axon length] (in radial direction)

i_{mC} = capacitive component of the transmembrane current per unit length of axon [μA/cm axon length]

i_{mI} = ionic component of the transmembrane current per unit length of axon [μA/cm axon length]

Φ_i = potential inside the membrane [mV]

Φ_o = potential outside the membrane [mV]

$V_m = \Phi_i - \Phi_o$ = membrane voltage [mV]

V_r = membrane voltage in the resting state [mV]

$V' = V_m - V_r$ = deviation of the membrane voltage from the resting state [mV]

A graphical sketch defining of various potentials and voltages in the axon is given in Figure 3.8.

We note once again that the direction of positive current is defined as the direction of the positive x-axis both inside and outside the axon. Therefore, for all values of x, conservation of current requires that $I_i + I_o = 0$ provided that x does not lie between stimulating electrodes.

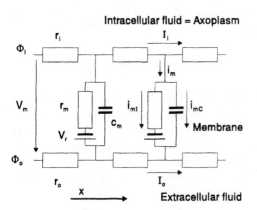

Fig. 3.7 The equivalent circuit model of an axon. An explanation of the component elements is given in the text.

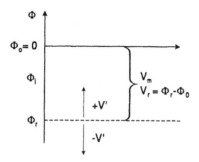

Fig. 3.8 A graphical sketch depicting various potentials and voltages in the axon used in this book.

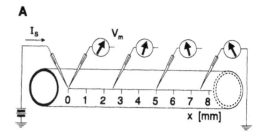

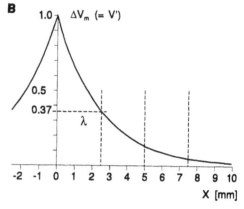

Fig. 3.9 (A) Stimulation of a nerve with current step. (B) Variation of the membrane voltage as a function of distance.

For a region lying between the stimulating electrodes, $I_i + I_o$ must equal the net applied current.

In the special case when there are no stimulating currents (i.e., when $I_i = I_o = I_m = 0$), then $V_m = V_r$ and $V' = 0$. However, once activation has been initiated we shall see that it is possible for $I_i + I_o = 0$ everywhere and $V' \neq 0$ in certain regions.

Since V_r, the membrane resting voltage, is the same everywhere, it is clear that

$$\frac{\partial V'}{\partial x} = \frac{\partial V_m}{\partial x} \quad \text{and} \quad \frac{\partial V'}{\partial t} = \frac{\partial V_m}{\partial t} \quad (3.40)$$

based on the definition of V' given above.

3.6.2   The Steady-State Response

We first consider the stationary case (i.e., $\partial/\partial t = 0$) which is the steady-state condition achieved following the application of current step. This corresponds to the limit $t \to \infty$. The steady-state response is illustrated in Figure 3.9. It follows from Ohm's law that

$$\frac{\partial \Phi_i}{\partial x} = -I_i r_i, \qquad \frac{\partial \Phi_o}{\partial x} = -I_o r_o \quad (3.41)$$

From the current conservation laws, it follows also that the transmembrane current per unit length, i_m, must be related to the loss of I_i or to the gain of I_o as follows:

$$i_m = -\frac{\partial I_i}{\partial x} = \frac{\partial I_o}{\partial x} \quad (3.42)$$

Note that this expression is consistent with $I_i + I_o = 0$. The selection of the signs in Equation 3.42 is based on outward-flowing current being defined as positive. From these definitions and

Equations 3.40 and 3.41 (and recalling that $V' = \Phi_i - \Phi_o - V_r$), it follows that

$$\frac{\partial V'}{\partial x} = \frac{\partial \Phi_i}{\partial x} - \frac{\partial \Phi_o}{\partial x} = -I_i r_i + I_o r_o \quad (3.43)$$

Furthermore, by differentiating with respect to x, we obtain:

$$\frac{\partial^2 V'}{\partial x^2} = -r_i \frac{\partial I_i}{\partial x} + r_o \frac{\partial I_o}{\partial x} \quad (3.44)$$

Substituting Equation 3.42 into Equation 3.44 gives:

$$\frac{\partial^2 V'}{\partial x^2} = (r_i + r_o)i_m \quad \mathbf{(3.45)}$$

which is called the *general cable equation*.

Under stationary and subthreshold conditions the capacitive current $c_m \, dV'/dt = 0$; so that the membrane current per unit length is simply $i_m = V'/r_m$; according to Ohm's law. Consequently, Equation 3.45 can be written in the form

$$\frac{\partial^2 V'}{\partial x^2} = V' \frac{r_i + r_o}{r_m} \quad (3.46)$$

whose solution is

$$V' = Ae^{-x/\lambda} + Be^{x/\lambda} \qquad (3.47)$$

The constant λ in Equation 3.47 has the dimension of length and is called the *characteristic length* or *length constant* of the axon. It is called also the *space constant*. The characteristic length λ is related to the parameters of the axon by Equation 3.46, and is given by:

$$\lambda = \sqrt{\frac{r_m}{r_i + r_o}} \approx \sqrt{\frac{r_m}{r_i}} \qquad (3.48)$$

The latter form of Equation 3.48 may be written because the extracellular axial resistance r_o is frequently negligible when compared to the intracellular axial resistance r_i.

With the boundary conditions:

$$V'_{x=0} = V'(0) \quad \text{and} \quad V'_{x=\infty} = 0$$

the constants A and B take on the values A = $V'(0)$ and B = 0, and from Equation 3.47 we obtain the solution:

$$V' = V'(0)e^{-x/\lambda} \qquad (3.49)$$

This expression indicates that V' decreases exponentially along the axon beginning at the point of stimulation ($x = 0$), as shown in Figure 3.9B. At $x = \lambda$ the amplitude has diminished to 36.8% of the value at the origin. Thus λ is a measure of the distance from the site of stimulation over which a significant response is obtained. For example at $x = 2\lambda$ the response has diminished to 13.5%, whereas at $x = 5\lambda$ it is only 0.7% of the value at the origin.

3.6.3 Stimulation with a Step-Current Impulse

In this section we consider the transient (rather than steady-state) response of the axon to a subthreshold current-step input. In this case the membrane current is composed of both resistive and capacitive components reflecting the parallel *RC* nature of the membrane:

$$i_m = i_{mR} + i_{mC} \qquad (3.50)$$

where

i_m = the total membrane current per unit length [μA/cm axon length]

i_{mR} = the resistive component of the membrane current per unit length [μA/cm axon length]

i_{mC} = the capacitive component of the membrane current per unit length [μA/cm axon length]

Under transient conditions Equation 3.50 substituted into Equation 3.45 may be written:

$$\frac{1}{r_i + r_o} \frac{\partial^2 V'}{\partial x^2} = \frac{V'}{r_m} + c_m \frac{\partial V'}{\partial t} \qquad (3.51)$$

The left side of Equation 3.51 evaluates the total membrane current i_m, whereas on the right side the first term represents the resistive component (formed by the ionic currents), and the second term the capacitive current which must now be included since $\partial/\partial t \neq 0$. Equation 3.51 may also be written in the form:

$$\frac{r_m}{r_i + r_o} \frac{\partial^2 V'}{\partial x^2} = V' + r_m c_m \frac{\partial V'}{\partial t} \qquad (3.52)$$

which can be easily expressed as

$$-\lambda^2 \frac{\partial^2 V'}{\partial x^2} + \tau \frac{\partial V'}{\partial t} + V' = 0 \qquad \textbf{(3.53)}$$

where $\tau = r_m c_m$ is the *time constant* of the membrane and λ is the *space constant* as defined in Equation 3.48.

Here the time constant was derived for a long, thin axon corresponding to a *one-dimensional problem*. The time constant may be derived with a similar method also for the surface of a membrane as a *two-dimensional problem*. In such case instead of the variables defined "times unit length" and "per unit length," variables defined "times unit area" and "per unit area" are used. Then we obtain for the time constant $\tau = R_m C_m$.

The temporal and spatial responses of the membrane voltage for several characteristic values of x and t are illustrated in Figure 3.10. One should note that the behavior of V' as a function of x is nearly exponential for all values of t, but the response as a function of t for large values of x differs greatly from an exponential behavior (becoming S-shaped). These curves illustrate the interpretation of λ, the space constant, as a measure of the spatial extent of the response to the stimulating current. For values of x/λ less than around 2, τ is essentially a measure of the time to reach steady state. However, for large x/λ this interpretation becomes poor because the temporal curve deviates greatly from exponential. In Figure 3.10, where

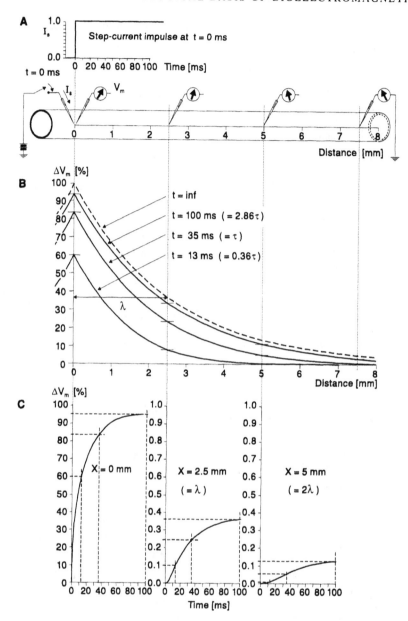

Fig. 3.10   The response of the axon to a step-current impulse. (A) The physical setup, including the waveform of the applied current and the placement of stimulating and recording electrodes. (B) The spatial response at t = 13, 35, 100 ms; and $t = \infty$. The latter curve is the steady-state response and corresponds to Equation 3.49. (C) The temporal response of three axial sites at x = 0, 2.5, 5 mm.

λ = 2.5 mm, the electrode at x = 5 mm is at 2λ, and the amplitude, after an interval τ, has reached only 37% of steady state. Were we to examine x = 25 mm (corresponding to 5λ), only 0.8% of steady state would be reached after the interval τ.

While a closed-form solution to Equation 3.53 can be described, we have chosen to omit it from this text because of its complexity. One can find a derivation in Davis and Lorente de Nó (1947). Rather than include this analytical material, we have chosen instead to illustrate

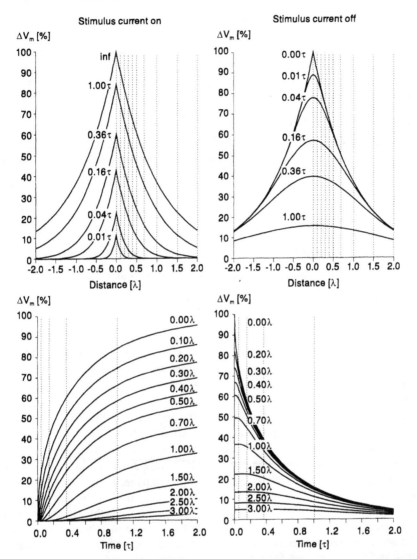

Fig. 3.11   Subthreshold transmembrane voltage response to a step current of very long duration at different instants of time (upper graphs) and at different distances from the sites of stimulation (lower graphs). The responses when the current is turned on and off are shown in the left and right sides of the figure, respectively.

the temporal and spatial response of the transmembrane voltage to a current step for a range of values of λ and τ. This is provided in Figure 3.11.

Specifically, Figure 3.11 describes the subthreshold transmembrane voltage response to a current step of very long duration introduced extracellularly at the center of a cable of infinite length. The response, when the current is turned on, is shown in the left-hand side of the figure, whereas the response, when the current is sub-

sequently turned off, is on the right. The transmembrane voltage is described as a function of time for given positions of the fiber. The transmembrane voltage is also described as a function of position at given times following the application of the current or its termination. The figure is drawn from a recalculation of its quantities from the original publication of Hodgkin and Rushton (1946).

Note that distance is shown normalized to the space constant λ, whereas time is normal-

Table 3.2   Cable constants for unmyelinated axons of different species

Quantity	Dimension	Species Squid	Lobster	Crayfish
diameter	[μm]	500	75	30
characteristic length λ	[cm]	0.5	0.25	0.25
time constant τ	[ms]	0.7	2.0	5.0
specific resistance of the membrane*	[kΩ·cm^2]	0.7	2.0	5.0
specific capacitance of the membrane*	[μF/cm^2]	1	1	1

*The specific resistance and specific capacitance of the membrane can be calculated from values of resistance and capacitance per unit length by use of the following:

$$R_m = 2\pi a r_m \qquad (3.54)$$

$$C_m = c_m/(2\pi a) \qquad (3.55)$$

where

R_m = specific resistance of the membrane (membrane resistance times unit area) [kΩ·cm^2]
r_m = membrane resistance times unit length [kΩ·cm axon length]
C_m = specific capacitance of the membrane (membrane capacitance per unit area) [μF/cm^2]
c_m = membrane capacitance per unit length [μF/cm axon length]
a = fiber radius [cm]

ized to the time constant τ. Normalization, such as this, results in "universal" curves that can be adapted to any actual value of λ and τ. Note also that the points on a particular voltage versus distance curve drawn at some values of t in the upper graph can also be found at the same values of t in the lower graph for the particular distance values, and vice versa. The fact that the upper and lower curves show the same phenomenon but in different dimensions is emphasized by the dotted vertical lines which indicate the corresponding location of points in the two sets of curves.

Table 3.2 lists measured values of characteristic lengths and time constants for several axons for several different species. A significant variation from species to species is seen.

3.7   STRENGTH-DURATION RELATION

When an excitable membrane is depolarized by a stimulating current whose magnitude is gradually increased, a current level will be reached, termed the *threshold*, when the membrane undergoes an action impulse. The latter is characterized by a rapid and phasic change in membrane permeabilities, and associated transmembrane voltage. An illustration of this process was given in Figure 2.8, where the response to

stimulus level 2 is *sub*threshold, whereas stimulus 3 appears just *at* threshold (since sometimes an action potential (3B) results whereas at other times a passive response (3A) is observed). An action potential is also clearly elicited for the *trans*threshold stimulus of 4.

Under active conditions the membrane can no longer be characterized as linear, and the RC model described in the previous section is not applicable. In the next chapter, we present a detailed study of the active membrane.

A link between this chapter, which is limited to the passive membrane, and the next, which includes the nonlinear membrane, lies in the modeling of conditions that lead to excitation. Although it is only an approximation, one can consider the membrane just up to the point of activation as linear (i.e., passive). Consequently, membrane behavior within this limit can be analyzed using ordinary electric circuits. In particular, if threshold values are known, it then becomes possible to elucidate conditions under which activation will just be achieved. Since activation is affected not only by the strength of a stimulating current but also its duration, the result is the evaluation of *strength-duration* curves that describe the minimum combinations of strength and duration just needed to produce the activation (Arvanitaki, 1938), as was illustrated in Figure 2.10.

A simple example of these ideas is furnished

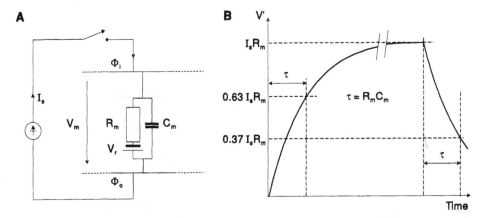

Fig. 3.12 The derivation of the strength-duration curve. (A) An approximate lumped-parameter RC-network which replaces the actual distributed parameter structure. (B) The response of the network to a current pulse of magnitude I_s is exponential and is shown for a pulse of very long duration.

by a cell that is somewhat spherical in shape and in which one stimulating electrode is placed intracellularly and the other extracellularly. One can show that for cells of such shape, both the intracellular and extracellular space is isopotential at all times. Thus, if a current is passed between the electrodes, it passes uniformly across the membrane so that all membrane elements behave similarly. As a consequence, the corresponding electric circuit is a lumped R_m and C_m in parallel. The value of R_m is the membrane resistance times unit area, whereas C_m is the membrane capacitance per unit area.

If I_s is the stimulus current per unit area then from elementary circuit theory applied to this parallel RC circuit, we have

$$V' = I_s R_m (1 - e^{-t/\tau}) \qquad (3.56)$$

where

V' = change in the membrane voltage [mV]
I_s = stimulus current per unit area [μA/cm^2]
R_m = membrane resistance times unit area [kΩ·cm^2]
t = stimulus time [ms]
τ = membrane time constant = $R_m C_m$ [ms]
C_m = membrane capacitance per unit surface [μF/cm^2]

Unfortunately, this simple analysis cannot be applied to cells with other shapes (e.g., the fiberlike shape of excitable cells), where the re-

sponse to a stimulating current follows that governed by Equation 3.53 and described in Figure 3.11. However, Equation 3.56 could still be viewed as a first-order approximation based on a lumped-parameter representation of what is actually a distributed-parameter structure. Following this argument, in Figure 3.12 we have assumed that a long fiber can be approximated by just a single (lumped) section, hence leading to an equation of the type described in Equation 3.56. A characteristic response based on Equation 3.56 is also shown in Figure 3.12.

The membrane is assumed to be activated if its voltage reaches the threshold value. We consider this condition if we substitute $V' = \Delta V_{th}$ into Equation 3.56, where ΔV_{th} is the change in the resting voltage needed just to reach the threshold voltage. Equation 3.56 may now be written in the form:

$$I_s = \frac{\Delta V_{th}}{R_m(1 - e^{-t/\tau})} \qquad (3.57)$$

The smallest current that is required for the transmembrane voltage to reach threshold is called the *rheobasic current*. With this stimulus current, the required stimulus duration is infinite. Because the rheobasic current is given by $I_{rh} = \Delta V_{th}/R_m$, the strength-duration curve takes on the form:

$$I_s = \frac{I_{rh}}{1 - e^{-t/\tau}} \qquad (3.58)$$

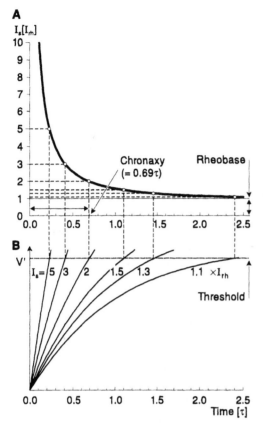

Fig. 3.13 (A) Strength-duration curve. The units are relative. (B) The subthreshold transient response prior to excitation.

If the stimulus current is twice rheobasic current, then $I_s = 2(\Delta V_{th}/R_m)$, and we obtain for chronaxy:

$$t = \tau \ln 2 = 0.693\tau \qquad (3.62)$$

The analytical results above are approximate for several reasons. First, the excitable tissue cannot normally be well approximated by a lumped R since such elements are actually distributed. (In a space clamp stimulation the membrane can be more accurately represented with a lumped model.) Also the use of a linear model is satisfactory up to perhaps 80% of the threshold, but beyond this the membrane behaves nonlinearly. Another approximation is the idea of a fixed threshold; in a subsequent chapter, we describe *accommodation*, which implies a threshold rising with time.

In a particular situation, a strength-duration curve can be found experimentally. In this case, rheobase and chronaxy are more realistic measures of the stimulus-response behavior. This type of data for chronaxy is given in Table 3.3, which lists chronaxies measured for various nerve and muscle tissues. Note that, in general, the faster the expected response from the phys-

The strength-duration curve is illustrated in Figure 3.13. Here the stimulus current is normalized so that the rheobasic current has the strength of unity. (Note again, that this result is derived for a space clamp situation.)

The time needed to reach the threshold voltage with twice the rheobasic stimulus current is called *chronaxy*. For the relation between chronaxy and the membrane time constant, Equation 3.57 can be written as:

$$1 - e^{-t/\tau} = \frac{\Delta V_{th}}{I_s R_m} \qquad (3.59)$$

$$e^{t/\tau} = \frac{1}{1 - \frac{\Delta V_{th}}{I_s R_m}} \qquad (3.60)$$

$$t = \tau \ln \frac{1}{1 - \frac{\Delta V_{th}}{I_s R_m}} \qquad (3.61)$$

Table 3.3 Chronaxy values for excitable tissues

Tissue	Time [ms]
Skeletal muscle	
Frog (gastrocnemius)	0.2–0.3
Frog (sartorius)	0.3
Turtle (leg flexors and extensors)	1–2
Man (arm flexors)	0.08–0.1
Man (arm extensors)	0.16–0.3
Man (thigh muscles)	0.10–0.7
Man (facial muscles)	0.24–0.7
Cardiac muscle	
Frog (ventricle)	3
Turtle (ventricle)	2
Dog (ventricle)	2
Man (ventricle)	2
Smooth muscle	
Frog (stomach)	100
Nerve	
Frog (sciatic)	0.3
Man (A fibers)	0.2
Man (vestibular)	14–22
Receptors	
Man (tongue)	1.4–1.8
Man (retinal rods)	1.2–1.8
Man (retinal cones)	2.1–3.0

iological system, the shorter the chronaxy value.

REFERENCES

Arvanitaki A (1938): *Les Variations Graduées De La Polarisation Des Systèmes Excitables*, Hermann, Paris.

Bernstein J (1902): Untersuchungen zur Termodynamik der bioelektrischen Ströme. *Pflüger Arch. ges. Physiol.* 9: 521–62.

Bernstein J (1912): *Elektrobiologie*, 215 pp. Viewag, Braunschweig.

Davis LJ, Lorente de Nó R (1947): Contributions to the mathematical theory of the electrotonus. *Stud. Rockefeller Inst. Med. Res.* 131: 442–96.

Eccles JC (1968): *The Physiology of Nerve Cells*, 270 pp. The Johns Hopkins Press, Baltimore.

Einstein A (1905): Über die von der molekularkinetischen Theorie die wärme Gefordertebewegung von in ruhenden flüssigkeiten suspendierten Teilchen. *Ann. Physik* 17: 549–60.

Faraday M (1834): Experimental researches on electricity, 7th series. *Phil. Trans. R. Soc. (Lond.)* 124: 77–122.

Fick M (1855): Über Diffusion. *Ann. Physik und Chemie* 94: 59–86.

Goldman DE (1943): Potential, impedance, and rectification in membranes. *J. Gen. Physiol.* 27: 37–60.

Hermann L (1905): Beiträge zur Physiologie und Physik des Nerven. *Pflüger Arch. ges. Physiol.* 109: 95–144.

Hille B (1992): *Ionic Channels of Excitable Membranes*, 2nd ed., 607 pp. Sinauer Assoc., Sunderland, Mass. (1st ed., 1984)

Hodgkin AL, Huxley AF (1952): A quantitative description of membrane current and its application to conduction and excitation in nerve. *J. Physiol. (Lond.)* 117: 500–44.

Hodgkin AL, Huxley AF, Katz B (1952): Measurement of current-voltage relations in the membrane of the giant axon of Loligo. *J. Physiol. (Lond.)* 116: 424–48.

Hodgkin AL, Katz B (1949): The effect of sodium ions on the electrical activity of the giant axon of the squid. *J. Physiol. (Lond.)* 108: 37–77.

Hodgkin AL, Rushton WA (1946): The electrical constants of a crustacean nerve fiber. *Proc. R. Soc. (Biol.)* B133: 444–79.

Junge, D (1992): *Nerve and Muscle Excitation*, 3rd ed., 263 pp. Sinauer Assoc., Sunderland, Mass.

Katchalsky A, Curran PF (1965): *Nonequilibrium Thermodynamics in Biophysics*, 248 pp. Harvard University Press, Cambridge, Mass.

Kortum G (1965): *Treatise on Electrochemistry*, 2nd ed., 637 pp. Elsevier, New York.

Nernst WH (1888): Zur Kinetik der Lösung befindlichen Körper: Theorie der Diffusion. *Z. Phys. Chem.* 3: 613–37.

Nernst WH (1889): Die elektromotorische Wirksamkeit der Ionen. *Z. Phys. Chem.* 4: 129–81.

Planck M (1890a): Über die Erregung von Elektricität und Wärme in Elektrolyten. *Ann. Physik und Chemie, Neue Folge* 39: 161–86.

Planck M (1890b): Über die Potentialdifferenz zwischen zwei verdünnten Lösungen binärer Elektrolyte. *Ann. Physik und Chemie, Neue Folge* 40: 561–76.

Ruch TC, Patton HD (eds.) (1982): *Physiology and Biophysics*, 20th ed., 1242 pp. W. B. Saunders, Philadelphia.

van Rysselberghe P (1963): *Thermodynamics of Irreversible Processes*, 165 pp. Hermann, Paris, and Blaisedell, New York.

FURTHER READING

Edsall JT, Wyman J (1958): *Biophysical Chemistry*, Vol. 1, 699 pp. Academic Press, New York.

Moore WJ (1972): *Physical Chemistry*, 4th ed., 977 pp. Prentice-Hall, Englewood Cliffs, N.J.

4

Active Behavior
of the Membrane

4.1 INTRODUCTION

When a stimulus current pulse is arranged to depolarize the resting membrane of a cell to or beyond the threshold voltage, then the membrane will respond with an *action impulse*. An example of this is seen in Figure 2.8 in the action potential responses 3b and 4 to the trans-threshold stimuli 3 and 4, respectively. The response is characterized by an initially rapidly rising transmembrane potential, which reaches a positive peak and then more slowly recovers to the resting voltage. This phasic behavior typifies what is meant by an action impulse.

A quantitative analysis of the action impulse was successfully undertaken by Alan L. Hodgkin and Andrew F. Huxley and colleagues in Cambridge (Hodgkin and Huxley, 1952a–d). Their work was made possible because of two important factors. The first was the selection of the giant axon of the squid, a nerve fiber whose diameter is around 0.5 mm, and consequently large enough to permit the insertion of the necessary two electrodes into the intracellular space. (Credit for discovering the applicability of the squid axon to electrophysiological studies is given to J. Z. Young (1936).) The second was the development of a feedback control device called the *voltage clamp*, capable

of holding the transmembrane voltage at any prescribed value.

This chapter describes the voltage clamp device, the experiments of Hodgkin and Huxley, the mathematical model into which their data were fitted, and the resulting simulation of a wide variety of recognized electrophysiological phenomena (activation, propagation, etc.). The voltage clamp procedure was developed in 1949 separately by K. S. Cole (1949) and G. Marmont (1949). Because of its importance, we first discuss the principle of the voltage clamp method in detail. The Hodgkin and Huxley work is important not only for its ability to describe *quantitatively* both the active and the passive membrane, but for its contribution to a deeper understanding of the membrane mechanisms that underlie its electrophysiological behavior.

A remarkable improvement in the research of membrane electrophysiology was made by Erwin Neher and Bert Sakmann, who in 1976 published a method for the measurement of ionic currents in a single ionic channel (Neher and Sakmann, 1976). This method, called *patch clamp*, is a further development of the voltage clamp technique. The patch clamp technique allows the researcher to investigate the operation of single ion channels and receptors and

66

has a wide application, for instance, in the pharmaceutical research. By measuring the capacitance of the plasma membrane with the patch clamp technique, the researcher may also investigate the regulation of exocytosis of the cell.

The electric behavior of the axon membrane is, of course, described by the net ion flow through a great number of ion channels. The ion channels seem to behave "digitally" (as seen in the measurement result of the patch clamp experiment); however, because of the large number of ion channels, the electric currents of a large area of the axon membrane exhibit "analog" behavior, as seen in the measurement result obtained in a voltage clamp experiment.

Logically, discussion of the electric behavior of the membrane should begin by examining the behavior of single ion channels and then proceed to explain the electric behavior of the membrane as the summation of the behavior of a large number of its constituent ionic channels. For historical reasons, however, membrane behavior and the voltage clamp method are discussed here first, before ionic channel behavior and the patch clamp method are explored.

4.2   VOLTAGE CLAMP METHOD

4.2.1   Goal of the Voltage Clamp Measurement

In order to describe the activation mechanism *quantitatively*, one must be able to *measure selectively the flow of each constituent ion of the total membrane current*. In this section, we describe how this is accomplished by the voltage clamp measurement procedure.

The following current components arise when the axon is stimulated at one end and the membrane voltage as well as current of a propagating nerve impulse are measured distally:

1. The axial (longitudinal) currents due to propagation of the nerve impulse:
   a. I_o = total axial current outside the axon
   b. I_i = total axial current inside the axon
   Note that $I_o = -I_i$.

2. The transmembrane current i_m per unit length arising from intrinsic membrane properties and enumerated by the following:
   a. Capacitive current component i_{mC} per unit length
   b. Ionic current component i_{mI} per unit length including:
      (1) Sodium current i_{Na} per unit length
      (2) Potassium current i_K per unit length
      (3) Chloride (or leakage) current i_L per unit length.

Our particular goal is to measure selectively each individual ionic current, especially the sodium and potassium currents. Note that because we examine the ionic currents during the propagating nerve impulse, the membrane resistance (r_m) is not constant; hence it is represented by a symbol indicating a variable resistance. Any measurement of membrane current with a propagating nerve impulse, however, will yield the sum of these currents.

The total membrane current (as illustrated in Fig. 4.1) satisfies Equation 3.48, which can be rewritten in the form:

$$i_m = i_{mI} + c_m \frac{\partial V_m}{\partial t} = \frac{1}{r_i + r_o} \frac{\partial^2 V_m}{\partial x^2} \quad (4.1)$$

where

i_m = total transmembrane current per unit length [μA/cm axon length]

i_{mI} = ionic component of the transmembrane current per unit length [μA/cm axon length]

c_m = membrane capacitance per unit length [μF/cm axon length]

V_m = membrane voltage [mV]

t = time [ms]

r_i = intracellular axial resistance per unit length of axon [kΩ/cm axon length]

r_o = interstitial resistance per unit length [kΩ/cm axon length]

x = distance [cm]

By measuring $V_m(t)$ and the propagation velocity Θ, we could obtain $V_m (t - x/\Theta)$ and hence i_m from Equation 4.1. Although the determination of i_m is straightforward, the accuracy depends on the uniformity of the preparation as well as knowledge of the parameters r_i, rc_o, and Θ. A more satisfactory procedure is based on the elimination of the axial currents.

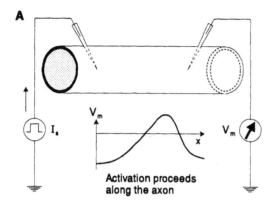

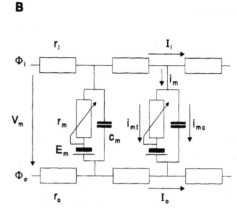

Fig. 4.1 The principle of membrane current measurement with a propagating nerve impulse. (A) It is assumed that a propagating wave is initiated at the left and has a uniform velocity at the site where the voltage is measured. To obtain the transmembrane current, Equation 4.1 can be used; implementation will require the measurement of the velocity of propagation so that $\partial^2 V_m/\partial x^2 = (1/\Theta^2)\partial^2 V_m/\partial t^2$ can be evaluated. (B) A portion of the linear core conductor model (assuming the extracellular medium to be bounded) which reflects the physical model above. (Note that because we examine the ionic currents during the propagating nerve impulse, the membrane resistance r_m is not constant; hence it is represented by a symbol indicating a variable resistance. To the extent that the ion concentrations may change with time, then E_m can also be time-varying.) The symbols are explained in the text.

By convention V_m, the transmembrane voltage, is taken as the intracellular potential, Φ_i, relative to the extracellular potential, Φ_o. That is, $V_m = \Phi_i - \Phi_o$. Further, the positive direction of transmembrane current is chosen as outward (from the intracellular to the extracellular space). These conventions were adopted in the mid-1950s so that in reading earlier papers one should be alert to encountering an opposite choice. The aforementioned conventions are reflected in Equation 4.1. Also, to maintain consistency with the tradition of drawing electronic circuits, in the equivalent circuits of the cell membrane, the reference terminal, that is the outside of the cell, is selected to be at the bottom, and the terminal representing the measured signal, that is the inside of the cell, is at the top. In those figures, where it is appropriate to illustrate the membrane in the vertical direction, the inside of the membrane is located on the left-hand side and the outside on the right-hand side of the membrane.

4.2.2 Space Clamp

With appropriate instrumentation, it is possible to stimulate the axon simultaneously throughout the entire length of the preparation. Then the membrane voltage at each instant of time is identical over the entire length of the axon. This situation can be brought about by inserting a thin stimulation electrode along the axis of the entire length of the dissected axon, whereas the other electrode, a concentric metal cylinder of the same length, is outside the axon. As a result, there is complete longitudinal uniformity of potential along the axon. This means that the potential can vary only with respect to the radius from the axis, and only radial currents can arise. Furthermore, all membrane elements behave synchronously, so the entire axon membrane behaves as whole. (Hodgkin and Huxley further designed a compartment to eliminate any fringing effects at the ends.) Consequently, between the concentric electrodes, a membrane current will be measured that obeys the equation:

$$i_m = i_I + c_m \frac{\partial V_m}{\partial t} \qquad (4.2)$$

where

i_m = the total current per unit length [μA/cm axon length]

i_{mI} = the ionic current per unit length [μA/cm axon length]

c_m = the capacitance of the preparation per unit length [μF/cm axon length]

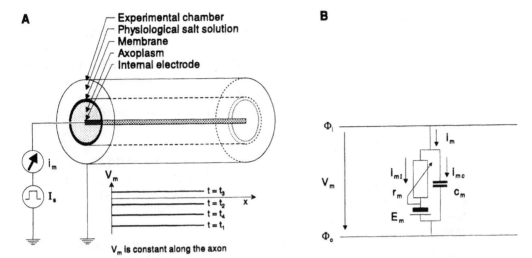

A
- Experimental chamber
- Physiological salt solution
- Membrane
- Axoplasm
- Internal electrode

V_m is constant along the axon

B

Fig. 4.2 Simplified principle and electric model of the space clamp measurement procedure. (A) The physical structure of the device that ensures axial uniformity, hence current flow that is in the radial direction only. The problem is thus reduced to one dimension. (B) The total current (i_m), through the membrane (per unit length), consisting of the components of ionic current i_{mI} and capacitive current i_{mC}.

Because the apparatus ensures axial uniformity, it is described as *space clamped*. The electric model of the space clamped measurement is illustrated in Figure 4.2.

4.2.3 Voltage Clamp

In the space clamp procedure, the membrane current includes the capacitive component as a confounding source. The capacitive component can be eliminated by keeping the membrane voltage constant during the measurement. Such a procedure is called *voltage clamp*. Because the capacitive current, the first term on the right side of Equation 4.2, is proportional to the time derivative of the voltage, the capacitive current is zero if the derivative of voltage is zero. In this case the equation representing the membrane current reduces to:

$$i_m = i_{mI} \qquad (4.3)$$

and the membrane current is composed solely of ionic currents. (In the moment following the onset of the voltage step, a very brief current pulse arises owing to the capacitance of the membrane. It disappears quickly and does not affect the measurement of the ensuing activation currents.)

The voltage clamp procedure is illustrated in the space clamp device shown in Figure 4.3. A desired voltage step is switched between the

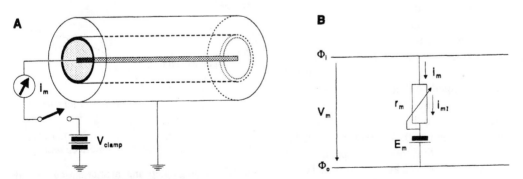

Fig. 4.3 Voltage clamp experiment. (A) The simplified principle of the experiment. (B) Electric model of the axon membrane in voltage clamp experiment.

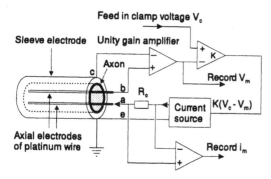

Fig. 4.4 Realistic voltage clamp measurement circuit. Current is applied through electrodes (a) and (e), while the transmembrane voltage, V_m, is measured with electrodes (b) and (c). The current source is controlled to maintain the membrane voltage at some preselected value V_c.

inner and outer electrodes, and the current flowing between these electrodes (i.e., the transmembrane current) is measured.

The actual voltage clamp measurement circuit is somewhat more complicated than the one described above and is shown in Figure 4.4. Separate electrodes are used for current application (a, e) and voltage sensing (b, c) to avoid voltage errors due to the electrode-electrolyte interface and the resistance of the thin current electrode wires. Figure 4.4 illustrates the principle of the measurement circuit used by Hodgkin, Huxley, and Katz (1952). The circuit includes a unity gain amplifier (having high input impedance), which detects the membrane voltage V_m between a wire inside the axon (b) and outside the axon (c). The output is sent to an *adder*, where the difference between the clamp voltage (V_c) and the measured membrane voltage (V_m) is detected and amplified. This output, $K(V_c - V_m)$, drives the current generator. The current generator feeds the current to the electrode system (a, e) and hence across the membrane. The current is detected through measurement of the voltage across a calibrated resistance, R_c. The direction of the controlled current is arranged so that V_m is caused to approach V_c, whereupon the feedback signal is reduced toward zero. If K is large, equilibrium will be established with V_m essentially equal to V_c and held at that value. The principle is that of negative feedback and proportional control.

The measurements were performed with the giant axon of a squid. The thickness of the diameter of this axon—approximately 0.5 mm— makes it possible to insert the two internal electrodes described in Figure 4.4 into the axon. (These were actually fabricated as interleaved helices on an insulating mandrel.)

4.3 EXAMPLES OF RESULTS OBTAINED WITH THE VOLTAGE CLAMP METHOD

4.3.1 Voltage Clamp to Sodium Nernst Voltage

Figure 4.5 illustrates a typical transmembrane current obtained with the voltage clamp method. The potential inside the membrane is changed abruptly from the resting potential of −65 mV to +20 mV with an 85 mV step. As a result, an ionic current starts to flow which is inward at first but which, after about 2 ms, turns outward, asymptotically approaching the value 2 mA/cm^2.

Let us examine the membrane current arising

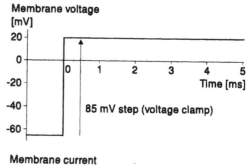

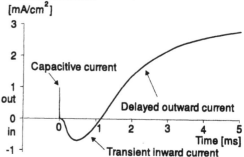

Fig. 4.5 Voltage step and membrane current in voltage clamp experiment.

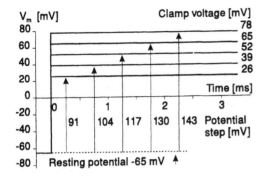

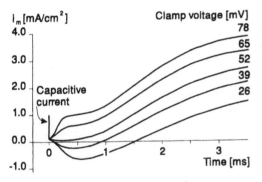

Fig. 4.6 A series of voltage clamp steps.

with different voltage steps. Figure 4.6 presents the results from experiments comprising five measurements at the voltage steps of 91–143 mV. In the series of curves, it may be noted that the membrane current is again composed of two components—an early and a late behavior as was the case in Figure 4.5.

The early current is directed inward for the smaller voltage steps. As the voltage step increases, the amplitude of the inward component decreases, and it disappears entirely with the voltage step of 117 mV. With higher voltage steps, the early current is directed outward and increases proportionally to the voltage step. The late component of the membrane current on the other hand is always outward and increases monotonically, approaching an asymptotic limit. This limit grows as a function of the size of the voltage step.

Assuming a resting membrane voltage of −65 mV, a 117 mV voltage step results in a membrane voltage of +52 mV. Based on the sodium concentration inside and outside the membrane, the Nernst equation evaluates an

equilibrium voltage of +50 mV. (Note the example in Section 3.1.3.) Hence one can conclude that the early component of the membrane current is carried by sodium ions since it reduces to zero precisely at the sodium equilibrium voltage and is inward when V_m is less than the sodium Nernst voltage and outward when V_m exceeds the sodium Nernst voltage. The outward (late) component must therefore be due to potassium ion flow. Because chloride tends to be near equilibrium, for the axon at rest while the chloride permeability does not increase during an action potential the chloride current tends to be small relative to that of sodium and potassium and can be ignored.

4.3.2 Altering the Ion Concentrations

An approach to the selective measurement of the potassium ion flow alone is available by utilizing a voltage clamp step corresponding to the sodium Nernst potential. This maneuver effectively eliminates sodium flow. By systematically altering the sodium concentration outside the axon, and then choosing the voltage clamp step at the respective sodium Nernst voltage, we can study the behavior of K^+ alone. And if we return to the current measurement under normal conditions (with both sodium and potassium), subtracting the potassium current leaves the sodium current alone.

This procedure is illustrated in Figure 4.7. This figure shows results from a voltage clamp experiment that was first done in normal seawater with a 56 mV step. Figure 4.7.A illustrates the Nernst potentials for different ions and the clamp voltage. The curve in (B) represents the measured total membrane current consisting of sodium and potassium components. Curve (C) is the membrane current measured after the extracellular sodium ions were reduced so that the 56 mV step reached the (new) sodium Nernst voltage. This curve, consequently, represents only potassium current. By subtracting curve (C) from curve (B), we obtain curve (D), which is the membrane current due to sodium ions in the original (unmodified sodium) situation. Thus curves (C) and (D) are the desired components of (B). Note that Hodgkin and Huxley assumed that the potassium current is unaf-

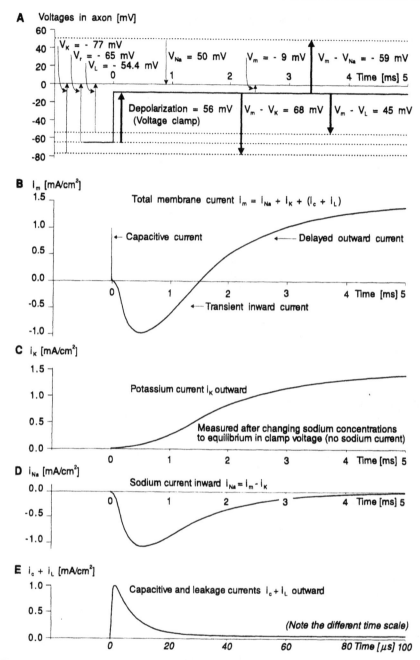

A Voltages in axon [mV]

$V_K = -77$ mV
$V_r = -65$ mV
$V_L = -54.4$ mV
$V_{Na} = 50$ mV
$V_m = -9$ mV
$V_m - V_{Na} = -59$ mV

Depolarization = 56 mV
(Voltage clamp)
$V_m - V_K = 68$ mV
$V_m - V_L = 45$ mV

B i_m [mA/cm^2]

Total membrane current $i_m = i_{Na} + i_K + (i_c + i_L)$

← Capacitive current   ← Delayed outward current

← Transient inward current

C i_K [mA/cm^2]

Potassium current i_K outward

Measured after changing sodium concentrations
to equilibrium in clamp voltage (no sodium current)

D i_{Na} [mA/cm^2]

Sodium current inward $i_{Na} = i_m - i_K$

E $i_c + i_L$ [mA/cm^2]

Capacitive and leakage currents $i_c + i_L$ outward

(Note the different time scale)

Fig. 4.7 Selective measurement of sodium and potassium current: The extracellular
sodium ions are replaced with an inactive cation to reduce the sodium Nernst potential
so that it corresponds to the clamp voltage value.

fected by changes in extracellular sodium so
that (C) is the same in both normal and reduced-
sodium seawater.

A very clever technique was also developed
by Baker, Hodgkin, and Shaw (1962) which

enabled a change to be made in the internal
ionic composition as well. Figure 4.8 illustrates
how to do the preparation of the axon for the
type of experiment conducted by Hodgkin and
Huxley. For this experiment, it is first necessary

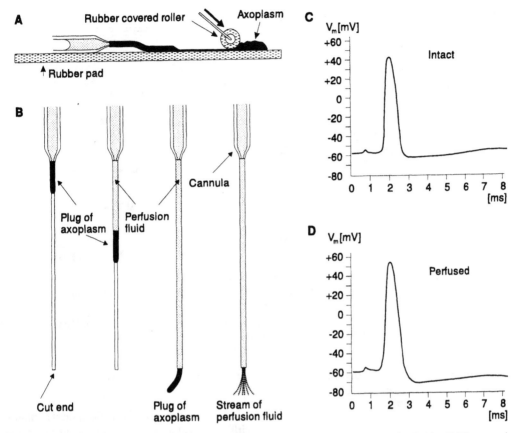

Fig. 4.8 Preparation of the squid axon for a voltage clamp experiment, where the internal ionic concentrations of the axon are changed. (A) The axoplasm is first squeezed out with a roller. (B) The axon is filled with perfusion fluid. (C) The axon impulse is measured before perfusion. (D) The axon impulse after perfusion.

to squeeze out the normal axoplasm; this is accomplished using a roller (A). Then the axon is filled with perfusion fluid (B). The membrane voltage is measured during action impulse before (C) and after (D) the procedures. Measurements following restoration of initial conditions are also performed to ensure that the electric behavior of the axon membrane has not changed.

4.3.3 Blocking of Ionic Channels with Pharmacological Agents

The sodium and potassium currents may also be separated by applying certain pharmacological agents that selectively block the sodium and potassium channels. Narahashi, Moore, and their colleagues showed that *tetrodotoxin*

(TTX) selectively blocks the flow of sodium across the membrane (Narahashi, Moore, and Scott, 1964; Moore et al., 1967). Armstrong and Hille (1972) showed that *tetraethylammonium* (TEA) blocks the flow of potassium ions. (It may be interesting to know that tetrodotoxin is the poisonous chemical that exists in the viscera of the Japanese fugu fish. The fugu fish is considered as an exotic dish. Before it can be used in a meal, it must be carefully prepared by first removing the poisonous parts.)

Figure 4.9 shows a series of voltage clamp experiments, which begin with normal conditions. Then the sodium channels are blocked with tetrodotoxin, and the measurement represents only the potassium current. Thereafter, the tetrodotoxin is flushed away, and a control measurement is made. After this, the potassium

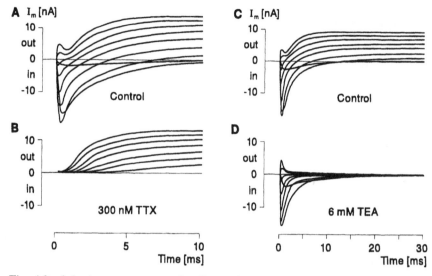

Fig. 4.9 Selective measurement of sodium and potassium currents by selective blocking of the sodium and potassium channels with pharmacological agents. (A) Control measurement without pharmacological agents. (B) Measurement after application of tetrodotoxin (TTX). (C) Control measurement without pharmacological agents. (D) Measurement after application of tetraethylammonium (TEA).

channels are blocked with tetraethylammonium which allows selective measurement of the sodium current (Hille, 1970).

4.4 HODGKIN-HUXLEY MEMBRANE MODEL

4.4.1 Introduction

In the following, membrane kinetics is discussed in detail, based on the model by A. L. Hodgkin and A. F. Huxley (1952d). Hodgkin's and Huxley's model is based on the results of their voltage clamp experiments on giant axons of the squid. The model is not formulated from fundamental principles but, rather is a combination of theoretical insight and curve fitting. Hodgkin and Huxley described their work by saying:

Our object here is to find equations which describe the conductances with reasonable accuracy and are sufficiently simple for theoretical calculation of the action potential and refractory period. For sake of illustration we shall try to provide a physical basis for the equations, but must emphasize that the interpretation given is unlikely to provide a correct

picture of the membrane. (Hodgkin and Huxley, 1952d, p. 506)

In spite of its simple form, the model explains with remarkable accuracy many nerve membrane properties. It was the first model to describe the ionic basis of excitation correctly. For their work, Hodgkin and Huxley received the Nobel Prize in 1963. Although we now know many specific imperfections in the Hodgkin-Huxley model, it is nevertheless essential to discuss it in detail to understand subsequent work on the behavior of voltage-sensitive ionic channels.

The reader should be aware that the original Hodgkin and Huxley papers were written at a time when the definition of V_m was chosen opposite to the convention adopted in the mid-1950s. In the work described here, we have used the present convention: V_m equals the intracellular minus extracellular potential.

4.4.2 Total Membrane Current and Its Components

Hodgkin and Huxley considered the electric current flowing across the cell membrane dur-

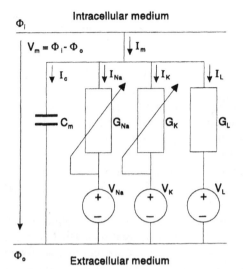

Intracellular medium

Φ_i

$V_m = \Phi_i - \Phi_o$ I_m

I_c I_{Na} I_K I_L

C_m G_{Na} G_K G_L

V_{Na} V_K V_L

Φ_o Extracellular medium

Fig. 4.10 The equivalent circuit of the Hodgkin-Huxley model. The voltage sources show the polarity of the positive value. The calculated Nernst voltages of sodium, potassium, and chloride designate the value of each corresponding voltage source. With the normal extracellular medium, V_{Na} has a positive value (Equation 4.7) while V_K and V_L have negative values (Equations 4.8 and 4.9). During an action impulse, G_{Na} and G_K vary as a function of transmembrane voltage and time.

ing activation to be described by what we now call the *parallel conductance model* (called also the *chord conductance model*) (Junge, 1992), which for the first time separated several ion-conducting branches. This model is illustrated in Figure 4.10. It consists of four current components:

1. Current carried by sodium ions
2. Current carried by potassium ions
3. Current carried by other ions (designated leakage current, constituted mainly from chloride ions)
4. Capacitive (displacement) current

In this model, each of these four current components is assumed to utilize its own (i.e., independent) path or channel. To follow the modern sign notation, the *positive* direction of membrane current and Nernst voltage is chosen to be from *inside to outside*.

The model is constructed by using the basic electric circuit components of voltage source,

resistance, and capacitance as shown in Figure 4.10. The ion permeability of the membrane for sodium, potassium, and other ions (introduced in Equation 3.34) is taken into account through the specification of a sodium, potassium, and leakage conductance per unit area (based on Ohm's law) as follows:

$$G_{Na} = \frac{I_{Na}}{V_m - V_{Na}} \tag{4.4}$$

$$G_K = \frac{I_K}{V_m - V_K} \tag{4.5}$$

$$G_L = \frac{I_L}{V_m - V_L} \tag{4.6}$$

where

G_{Na}, G_K, G_L = membrane conductance per unit area for sodium, potassium, and other ions—referred to as the *leakage* conductance [S/cm^2]

I_{Na}, I_K, I_L = the electric current carried by sodium, potassium and other ions *(leakage current)* per unit area [mA/cm^2]

V_{Na}, V_K, V_L = Nernst voltage for sodium, potassium, and other ions *(leakage voltage)* [mV]

V_m = membrane voltage [mV]

The above-mentioned Nernst voltages are defined by the Nernst equation, Equation 3.21, namely:

$$V_{Na} = -\frac{RT}{zF} \ln \frac{c_i^{Na}}{c_o^{Na}} \tag{4.7}$$

$$V_K = -\frac{RT}{zF} \ln \frac{c_i^K}{c_o^K} \tag{4.8}$$

$$V_L = -\frac{RT}{zF} \ln \frac{c_i^{Cl}}{c_o^{Cl}} \tag{4.9}$$

where the subscripts "i" and "o" denote the ion concentrations inside and outside the cell membrane, respectively. Other symbols are the same as in Equation 3.21 and $z = 1$ for Na and K but $z = -1$ for Cl.

In Figure 4.10 the polarities of the voltage sources are shown as having the same polarity which corresponds to the positive value. We may now insert the Nernst voltages of sodium, potassium, and chloride, calculated from Equations 4.7 to 4.9 to the corresponding voltage sources so that a calculated positive Nernst voltage is directed in the direction of the voltage source polarity and a calculated negative Nernst voltage is directed in the opposite direction. With the sodium, potassium, and chloride concentration ratios existing in nerve and muscle cells, the voltage sources of Figure 4.10 in practice achieve the polarities of those shown in Figure 3.4.

Because the internal concentration of chloride is very low, small movements of chloride ion have a large effect on the chloride concentration ratio. As a result, a small chloride ion flux brings it into equilibrium and chloride does not play an important role in the evaluation of membrane potential (Hodgkin and Horowicz, 1959). Consequently, Equation 4.9 was generalized to include not only chloride ion flux but that due to any non-specific ion. The latter flux arises under experimental conditions since, in preparing an axon for study, small branches are cut leaving small membrane holes through which small amounts of ion diffusion can take place. The conductance G_L was assumed constant while V_L was chosen so that the sum of all ion currents adds to zero at the resting membrane potential.

When $V_m = V_{Na}$, the sodium ion is in equilibrium and there is no sodium current. Consequently, the deviation of V_m from V_{Na} (i.e., $V_m - V_{Na}$) is a measure of the driving voltage causing sodium current. The coefficient that relates the driving force ($V_m - V_{Na}$) to the sodium current density I_{Na} is the sodium conductance, G_{Na}—that is, $I_{Na} = G_{Na}(V_m - V_{Na})$, consistent with Ohm's law. A rearrangement leads to Equation 4.4. Equations 4.5 and 4.6 can be justified in the same way.

Now the four currents discussed above can be evaluated for a particular membrane voltage, V_m. The corresponding circuits are formed by:

1. Sodium Nernst voltage and the membrane conductance for sodium ions
2. Potassium Nernst voltage and the membrane conductance for potassium ions
3. Leakage voltage (at which the leakage current is zero due to chloride and other ions) and membrane leakage conductance
4. Membrane capacitance

(Regarding these circuit elements, Hodgkin and Huxley had experimental justification for assuming linearly ohmic conductances in series with each of the emf's. They observed that the current changed linearly with voltage when a sudden change of membrane voltage was imposed. These conductances are, however, not included in the equivalent circuit in Figure 4.10 (Huxley, 1993).)

On the basis of their voltage clamp studies, Hodgkin and Huxley determined that the membrane conductance for sodium and potassium are functions of *transmembrane voltage and time*. In contrast, the leakage conductance is constant. Under subthreshold stimulation, the membrane resistance and capacitance may also be considered constant.

One should recall that when the sodium and potassium conductances are evaluated during a particular voltage clamp, their dependence on voltage is eliminated because the voltage during the measurement is *constant*. The voltage nevertheless *is* a parameter, as may be seen when one compares the behavior at different voltages. For a voltage clamp measurement the only variable in the measurement is *time*. Note also that the capacitive current is zero, because $dV/dt = 0$.

For the Hodgkin-Huxley model, the expression for the total transmembrane current density is the sum of the capacitive and ionic components. The latter consist of sodium, potassium, and leakage terms and are given by rearranging Equations 4.4 through 4.6. Thus

$$I_m = C_m \frac{dV_m}{dt} + (V_m - V_{Na})G_{Na} + (V_m - V_K)G_K + (V_m - V_L)G_L \quad (4.10)$$

where

$$\begin{aligned} I_m &= \text{membrane current per unit area} \\ &\quad [\text{mA/cm}^2] \\ C_m &= \text{membrane capacitance per unit} \\ &\quad \text{area } [\text{F/cm}^2] \\ V_m &= \text{membrane voltage } [\text{mV}] \\ V_{Na}, V_K, V_L &= \text{Nernst voltage for sodium,} \\ &\quad \text{potassium and leakage ions } [\text{mV}] \end{aligned}$$

G_{Na}, G_K, G_L = sodium, potassium, and leakage conductance per unit area [S/cm^2]

As noted before, in Figure 4.10 the polarities of the voltage sources are shown in a universal and mathematically correct way to reflect the Hodgkin-Huxley equation (Equation 4.10). With the sodium, potassium, and chloride concentration ratios existing in nerve and muscle cells the voltage sources of Figure 4.10 in practice achieve the polarities of those shown in Figure 3.4.

Note that in Equation 4.10, the sum of the current components for the *space clamp action impulse* is necessarily zero, since the axon is stimulated simultaneously along the whole length and since after the stimulus the circuit is open. There can be no *axial* current since there is no potential gradient in the axial direction at any instant of time. On the other hand, there can be no *radial* current (i.e., $I_m = 0$) because in this direction there is an open circuit. In the *voltage clamp experiment* the membrane current in Equation 4.10 is not zero because the voltage clamp circuit permits a current flow (necessary to maintain the clamp voltage).

4.4.3 Potassium Conductance

Because the behavior of the potassium conductance during the voltage clamp experiment is simpler than that of the sodium conductance, it will be discussed first.

Hodgkin and Huxley speculated on the ion conductance mechanism by saying that

[it] *depends on the distribution of charged particles which do not act as carriers in the usual sense, but which allow the ions to pass through the membrane when they occupy particular sites in the membrane.* On this view the rate of movement of the activating particles determines the rate at which the sodium and potassium conductances approach their maximum but has little effect on the (maximum) magnitude of the conductance. (italics ours; Hodgkin and Huxley, 1952d, p. 502)

Hodgkin and Huxley did not make any assumptions regarding the nature of these particles in chemical or anatomical terms. Because the only role of the particles is to identify the fraction of channels in the open state, this could

be accomplished by introducing corresponding abstract random variables that are measures of the probabilities that the configurations are open ones. In this section, however, we describe the Hodgkin-Huxley model and thus follow their original idea of charged particles moving in the membrane and controlling the conductance. (These are summarized later in Fig. 4.13.)

The time course of the potassium conductance (G_K) associated with a voltage clamp is described in Figure 4.11 and is seen to be continuous and monotonic. (The curves in Fig. 4.11 are actually calculated from the Hodgkin-Huxley equations. For each curve the individual values of the coefficients, listed in table 1 of Hodgkin and Huxley (1952d), are used; therefore, they follow closely the measured data.) Hodgkin and Huxley noted that this variation could be fitted by a first-order equation toward the end of the record, but required a third- or fourth-order equation in the beginning. This character is, in fact, demonstrated by its sigmoidal shape, which can be achieved by supposing G_K to be proportional to the fourth power of a variable, which in turn satisfies a first-order equation. Hodgkin and Huxley gave this mathematical description a physical basis with the following assumptions.

As is known, the potassium ions cross the membrane only through channels that are specific for potassium. Hodgkin and Huxley supposed that the opening and closing of these channels are controlled by electrically charged particles called n-particles. These may stay in a *permissive* (i.e., open) position (for instance inside the membrane) or in a *nonpermissive* (i.e., closed) position (for instance outside the membrane), and they move between these states (or positions) with first-order kinetics. The probability of an n-particle being in the open position is described by the parameter n, and in the closed position by $(1 - n)$, where $0 \le n \le 1$. Thus, when the membrane potential is changed, the changing distribution of the n-particles is described by the probability of n relaxing exponentially toward a new value.

In mathematical form, the voltage- and time-dependent transitions of the n-particles between the open and closed positions are described by the changes in the parameter n with the voltage-dependent transfer rate coefficients α_n and β_n.

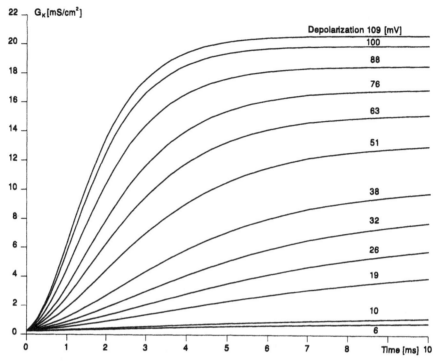

Fig. 4.11 Behavior of potassium conductance as a function of time in a voltage clamp experiment. The displacement of transmembrane voltage from the resting value [in mV] is shown (all are depolarizations). These theoretical curves correspond closely to the measured values.

This follows a first-order reaction given by:

$$n \underset{\beta_n}{\overset{\alpha_n}{\rightleftharpoons}} (1 - n) \qquad (4.11)$$

where

α_n = the transfer rate coefficient for n-particles from closed to open state [1/s]

β_n = the transfer rate coefficient for n-particles from open to closed state [1/s]

n = the fraction of n-particles in the open state

$1 - n$ = the fraction of n-particles in the closed state

If the initial value of the probability n is known, subsequent values can be calculated by solving the differential equation

$$\frac{dn}{dt} = \alpha_n(1 - n) - \beta_n n \qquad (4.12)$$

Thus, the rate of increase in the fraction of n-particles in the open state dn/dt depends on their fraction in the closed state $(1 - n)$, and their fraction in the open state n, and on the transfer rate coefficients α_n and β_n. Because the n-particles are electrically charged, the transfer rate coefficients are voltage-dependent (but do not depend on time). Figure 4.12A shows the variations of the transfer rate coefficients with membrane voltage. Expressions for determining their numerical values are given at the end of this section.

Furthermore Hodgkin and Huxley supposed that the potassium channel will be open only if *four* n-particles exist in the permissive position (inside the membrane) within a certain region. It is assumed that the probability of any one of the four n-particles being in the permissive position does not depend on the positions of the other three. Then the probability of the channel being open equals the joint probability of these four n-particles being at such a site and, hence, proportional to n^4. (These ideas appear to be well supported by studies on the acetylcholine receptor, which consists

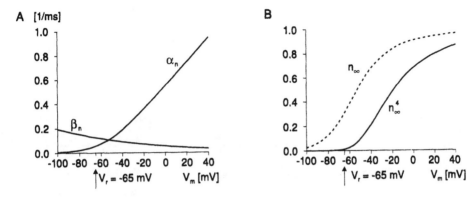

Fig. 4.12 (A) Variation of transfer rate coefficients α_n and β_n as functions of membrane voltage. (B) Variation of n_∞ and n_∞^4 as functions of membrane voltage ($G_K \propto n^4$).

of five particles surrounding an aqueous channel, and where a small cooperative movement of all particles can literally close or open the channel (Unwin and Zampighi, 1980).)

The potassium conductance per unit area is then the conductance of a single channel times the number of open channels. Alternatively, if $G_{K\,max}$ is the conductance per unit area when all channels are open (i.e., its maximum value), then if only the fraction n^4 are open, we require that

$$G_K = G_{K\,max}n^4 \qquad (4.13)$$

where $G_{K\,max}$ = maximum value of potassium conductance [mS/cm^2], and n obeys Equation 4.12.

Equations 4.12 and 4.13 are among the basic expressions in the Hodgkin and Huxley formulation.

Equation for n at Voltage Clamp

For a voltage step (voltage clamp), the transfer rate coefficients α_n and β_n change immediately to new (but constant) values. Since at a constant voltage, the transfer rate coefficients in Equation 4.12 are constant, the differential equation can be readily solved for n, giving

$$n(t) = n_\infty - (n_\infty - n_0)e^{-t/\tau_n} \qquad (4.14)$$

where

$$n_\infty = \frac{\alpha_n}{\alpha_n + \beta_n} = \text{steady-state value of } n$$

$$\tau_n = \frac{1}{\alpha_n + \beta_n} = \text{time constant [s]}$$

We see that the voltage step initiates an exponential change in n from its initial value of n_0 (the value of n at $t = 0$) toward the steady-state value of n_∞ (the value of n at $t = \infty$). Figure 4.12B shows the variation of n_∞ and n_∞^4 with membrane voltage.

Summary of the Hodgkin-Huxley Model for Potassium Conductance

Figure 4.13 presents an interpretation of the ideas of the Hodgkin-Huxley model for potassium conductance though representing the authors' interpretation. In Figure 4.13A the response of the n-particles to a sudden depolarization is shown before and at two successive instants of time during the depolarization. Initially, the fraction of n-particles in the permissive position (inside the membrane), n, is small since α_n is small and β_n is large. Therefore, the potassium channels (of which two are illustrated) are closed. Depolarization increases α_n and decreases β_n so that n rises exponentially (following first-order kinetics) toward a maximum value of n_∞. When four n-particles occupy the site around the channel inside the membrane, the channel opens; therefore, the potassium conductance G_K is proportional to n^4, as shown in Equation 4.13. Figure 4.13A illustrates this phenomenon first at one channel and then at two channels. The magnitude of α_n and β_n is shown in Figures 4.13A by the thickness of the arrows and in 4.13B by the curves. In Figure 4.13C, the response of n and n^4 to

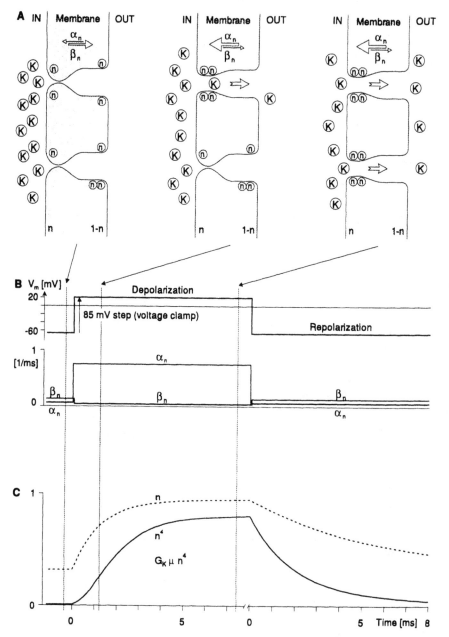

Fig. 4.13 In the Hodgkin-Huxley model, the process determining the variation of potassium conductance with depolarization and repolarization with voltage clamp. (A) Movement of n-particles as a response to sudden depolarization. Initially, α_n is small and β_n is large, as indicated by the thickness of the arrows. Therefore, the fraction n of n-particles in the permissive state (inside the membrane) is small. Depolarization increases α_n and decreases β_n. Thus n rises exponentially to a larger value. When four n-particles occupy the site around the channel inside the membrane, the channel opens. (B) The response of the transfer rate coefficients α_n and β_n to sudden depolarization and repolarization. (C) The response of n and n^4 to a sudden depolarization and repolarization ($G_K \propto n^4$).

a sudden depolarization and repolarization is shown.

The reader may verify that the potassium conductance really is proportional to n^4, by comparing this curve and the curve in Figure 4.11 representing the potassium conductance at 88 mV depolarization (which is the value closest to 85 mV used in Figure 4.13). These curves are very similar in form.

4.4.4 Sodium Conductance

The results that Hodgkin and Huxley obtained for sodium conductance in their voltage clamp experiments are shown in Figure 4.14 (Hodgkin and Huxley, 1952d). The curves in Figure 4.14 are again calculated from the Hodgkin-Huxley equations and fit closely to the measured data.

The behavior of sodium conductance is initially similar to that of potassium conductance, except that the speed of the conductance increase during depolarization is about 10 times

faster. The rise in sodium conductance occurs well before the rise in potassium conductance becomes appreciable. Hodgkin and Huxley assumed again that at the sodium channels certain electrically charged particles called *m-particles* exist whose position control the opening of the channel. Thus they have two states, open (permissive) and closed (nonpermissive); the proportion m expresses the fraction of these particles in the open state (for instance inside the membrane) and $(1 - m)$ the fraction in the closed state (for instance outside the membrane), where $0 \leq m \leq 1$.

The mathematical form for the voltage- and time-dependent transitions of the m-particles between the open and closed positions is similar to that for potassium. We identify these with a subscript "m"; thus the voltage-dependent transfer rate coefficients are α_m and β_m. These follow a first-order process given by

$$m \underset{\beta_m}{\overset{\alpha_m}{\rightleftharpoons}} (1 - m) \qquad (4.15)$$

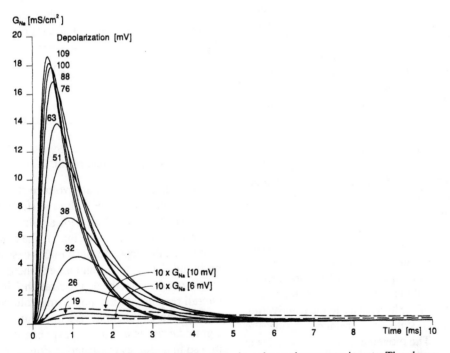

Fig. 4.14 Behavior of sodium conductance in voltage clamp experiments. The clamp voltage is expressed as a change from the resting value (in [mV]). Note that the change in sodium conductance is small for subthreshold depolarizations but increases greatly for transthreshold depolarization ($\geq \Delta V_m = 26$ mV).

where

α_m = the transfer rate coefficient for m-particles from closed to open state [1/s]

β_m = the transfer rate coefficient for m-particles from open to closed state [1/s]

m = the fraction of m-particles in the open state

$1 - m$ = the fraction of m-particles in the closed state

An equation for the behavior of sodium activation may be written in the same manner as for the potassium, namely that m satisfies a first-order process:

$$\frac{dm}{dt} = \alpha_m(1 - m) - \beta_m m \qquad (4.16)$$

The transfer rate coefficients α_m and β_m are voltage-dependent but do not depend on time.

On the basis of the behavior of the early part of the sodium conductance curve, Hodgkin and Huxley supposed that the sodium channel is open only if *three* m-particles are in the permissive position (inside the membrane). Then the probability of the channel being open equals the joint probability that three m-particles in the permissive position; hence the initial increase of sodium conductance is proportional to m^3.

The main difference between the behavior of sodium and potassium conductance is that the rise in sodium conductance, produced by membrane depolarization, is not maintained. Hodgkin and Huxley described the falling conductance to result from an inactivation process and included it by introducing an inactivating *h-particle*. The parameter h represents the probability that an h-particle is in the non-inactivating (i.e., open) state—for instance, outside the membrane. Thus $(1 - h)$ represents the number of the h-particles in the inactivating (i.e., closed) state—for instance, inside the membrane. The movement of these particles is also governed by first-order kinetics:

$$(1 - h) \underset{\beta_h}{\overset{\alpha_h}{\rightleftharpoons}} h \qquad (4.17)$$

where

α_h = the transfer rate coefficient for h-particles from inactivating to non-inactivating state [1/s]

β_h = the transfer rate coefficient for h-particles from non-inactivating to inactivating state [1/s]

h = the fraction of h-particles in the non-inactivating state

$1 - h$ = the fraction of h-particles in the inactivating state

and satisfies a similar equation to that obeyed by m and n, namely:

$$\frac{dh}{dt} = \alpha_h(1 - h) - \beta_h h \qquad (4.18)$$

Again, because the h-particles are electrically charged, the transfer rate coefficients α_h and β_h are voltage-dependent but do not depend on time.

The sodium conductance is assumed to be proportional to the number of sites inside the membrane that are occupied simultaneously by three activating m-particles and not blocked by an inactivating h-particle. Consequently, the behavior of sodium conductance is proportional to m^3h, and

$$G_{Na} = G_{Na\,max}m^3h \qquad \textbf{(4.19)}$$

where

$G_{Na\,max}$ = maximum value of sodium conductance [mS/cm^2], and

m = obeys Equation (4.16), and

h = obeys Equation (4.18).

Following a depolarizing voltage step (voltage clamp), m will rise with time (from m_0 to m_∞) according to an expression similar to Equation 4.14 (but with m replacing n). The behavior of h is just the opposite since in this case it will be found that $h_0 \gg h_\infty$ and an exponential decrease results from the depolarization. Thus the overall response to a depolarizing voltage step includes an exponential rise in m (and thus a sigmoidal rise in m^3) and an exponential decay in h so that G_{Na}, as evaluated in Equation 4.19, will first increase and then decrease. This behavior is just exactly that needed to fit the data described in Figure 4.14. In addition, it turns out that the normal resting values of m are close

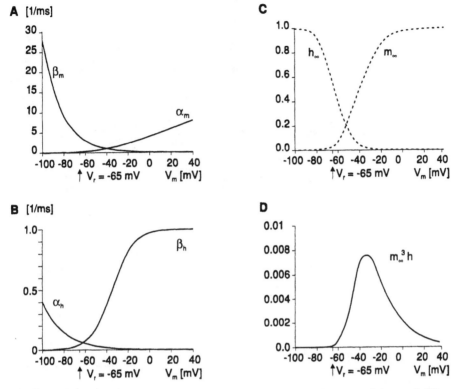

Fig. 4.15 Variation in (A) α_m and β_m, (B) α_h and β_h, (C) m_∞ and h_∞, and (D) $m_\infty^3 h_\infty$ as a function of membrane voltage. Note that the value of $m_\infty^3 h_\infty$ is so small that the steady-state sodium conductance is practically zero.

to zero, whereas h is around 0.6. For an initial hyperpolarization, the effect is to decrease m; however, since it is already very small, little additional diminution can occur. As for h, its value can be increased to unity, and the effect on a subsequent depolarization can be quite marked. This effect fits experimental observations closely. The time constant for changes in h is considerably longer than for m and n, a fact that can lead to such phenomena as "anode break," discussed later in this chapter. Figure 4.15A shows variations in the transfer rate coefficients α_m, β_m, α_h, and β_h with membrane voltage. Figure 4.15B shows the variations in m_∞, h_∞, and $m_\infty^3 h_\infty$ with membrane voltage.

Summary
of the Hodgkin-Huxley Model
for Sodium Conductance

Similar to Figure 4.13, Figure 4.16 summarizes the voltage clamp behavior of the Hodgkin-

Huxley model but for sodium conductance. Figure 4.16A shows the response of the m- and h-particles to a sudden depolarization at rest and at two successive moments during depolarization. (Because the h-particles have inactivating behavior, they are drawn with negative color (i.e., a white letter on a filled circle).) Initially, the fraction of m-particles in the permissive position (inside the membrane), m, is small since α_m is small and β_m is large. Therefore, the sodium channels (of which two are illustrated) are not open. Initially, the fraction of h-particles in the non-inactivating (open-channel) position (outside the membrane), h, is large since α_h is large and β_h is small. Depolarization increases α_m and β_h, and decreases β_m and α_h, as shown in Figure 4.16A by the thickness of the arrows and in 4.16B by the curves.

Because the time constant τ_m is much shorter than τ_h, m rises faster toward a maximum value of unity than h decays toward zero. Both pa-

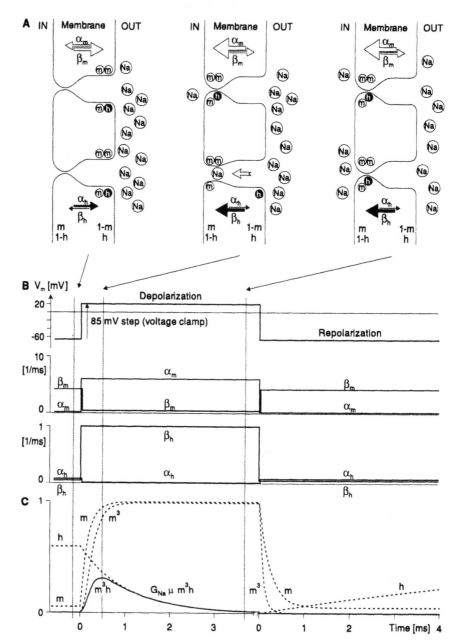

Fig. 4.16 The process, in the Hodgkin-Huxley model, determining the variation of sodium conductance with depolarization and repolarization with voltage clamp. (A) Movement of m- and h-particles as a response to sudden depolarization. Initially, α_m is small and β_m is large, as indicated by the thickness of the arrows. Therefore, the fraction of particles of type m in the permissive state (inside the membrane) is small. Initially also the value of α_h is large and β_h is small. Thus the h-particles are in the non-inactivating position, outside the membrane. Depolarization increases α_m and β_h and decreases β_m and α_h. Thus the number of m-particles inside the membrane, m, rises exponentially toward unity, and the number of h-particles outside the membrane, h, decreases exponentially toward zero. (B) The response of transfer rate coefficients α_m, β_m, α_h, and β_h to sudden depolarization and repolarization. (C) The response of m, h, m^3, and m^3h to a sudden depolarization and repolarization. Note that according to Equation 4.20, G_{Na} is proportional to m^3h.

rameters behave exponentially (following first-order kinetics) as seen from Figure 4.16C. When three m-particles occupy the site around the channel inside the membrane and one h-particle occupies a site outside the membrane, the channel opens. Therefore, the initial increase of sodium conductance G_{Na} is proportional to m^3 (since initially h is large and the non-inactivating h-particles occupy the open-channel site outside the membrane). In figure 4.16A, the short time constant τ_m is indicated by the almost simultaneous opening of two sodium channels. Later on, because of the longer time constant τ_h, the inactivating h-particles move to the inside of the membrane, blocking the sodium channels. Consequently, as shown in Equation 4.19, the overall behavior of the sodium conductance G_{Na} is proportional to m^3h.

The reader may again verify that the sodium conductance is proportional to m^3h by comparing this curve and the curve in Figure 4.14, representing the sodium conductance at 88 mV depolarization (which is the value closest to 85mV used in Figure 4.16).

4.4.5 Hodgkin-Huxley Equations

Transfer Rate Coefficients

The transfer rate coefficients α and β of the gating variables n, m, and h are determined from Equations 4.20 through 4.25. These equations were developed by Hodgkin and Huxley and, when substituted into Equations 4.12, 4.14 (and similar ones for m and h), 4.16, and 4.18, lead to the curves plotted in Figures 4.11 and 4.13. This compares well to measurements on the entire range of voltage clamp values. The dimension is [1/ms] for the transfer rate coefficients α and β.

$$\alpha_n = \frac{0.1 - 0.01V'}{e^{(1-0.1V')} - 1} \qquad (4.20)$$

$$\beta_n = \frac{0.125}{e^{0.0125V'}} \qquad (4.21)$$

$$\alpha_m = \frac{2.5 - 0.1V'}{e^{(2.5-0.1V')} - 1} \qquad (4.22)$$

$$\beta_m = \frac{4}{e^{(V'/18)}} \qquad (4.23)$$

$$\alpha_h = \frac{0.07}{e^{0.05V'}} \qquad (4.24)$$

$$\beta_h = \frac{1}{e^{(3-0.1V')} + 1} \qquad (4.25)$$

In these equations $V' = V_m - V_r$, where V_r is the resting voltage. All voltages are given in millivolts. Therefore, V' is the deviation of the membrane voltage from the resting voltage in millivolts, and it is positive if the potential inside the membrane changes in the positive direction (relative to the outside). The equations hold for the giant axon of the squid at a temperature of 6.3°C.

Please note again that in the voltage clamp experiment the α and β are constants because the membrane voltage is kept constant during the entire procedure. During an unclamped activation, where the transmembrane voltage is continually changing, the transfer rate coefficients will undergo change according to the above equations.

Constants

In addition to the variables discussed above, the constants of the Hodgkin-Huxley model are given here. The voltages are described in relation to the resting voltage (as shown):

C_m	=	1	μF/cm^2
$V_r - V_{Na}$	=	-115	mV
$V_r - V_K$	=	$+12$	mV
$V_r - V_L$	=	-10.613	mV
$G_{Na\,max}$	=	120	mS/cm^2
$G_{K\,max}$	=	36	mS/cm^2
G_L	=	0.3	mS/cm^2

Note that the value of V_L is not measured experimentally, but is calculated so that the current is zero when the membrane voltage is equal to the resting voltage. The voltages in the axon are illustrated in Figure 4.17 in graphical form.

In Table 4.1 we summarize the entire set of Hodgkin-Huxley equations that describe the Hodgkin-Huxley model.

4.4.6 Propagating Nerve Impulse

When analyzing the propagating nerve impulse instead of the nonpropagating activation (i.e., when the membrane voltage is in the space clamp condition), we must consider the axial currents in addition to the transmembrane currents. Let us examine Figure 4.18 (Plonsey, 1969).

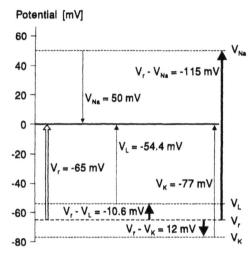

Fig. 4.17 An illustration of the voltages in the squid axon.

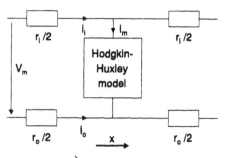

Fig. 4.18 Application of the Hodgkin-Huxley model to a propagating nerve impulse.

describing the behavior of the membrane, is a Hodgkin-Huxley model. For the circuit in this figure, Equation 3.42 was derived in the previous chapter for the total membrane current, and it applies here as well:

$$i_m = \frac{1}{r_i + r_o} \frac{\partial^2 V_m}{\partial x^2} \qquad (3.42)$$

In an axon with radius a, the membrane current per unit length is

$$i_m = 2\pi a I_m \; [\mu\text{A/cm axon length}] \qquad (4.26)$$

The figure illustrates the model for a unit length of axon. In the model the quantities r_i and r_o represent the resistances per unit length inside and outside the axon, respectively. Between the inside and outside of the membrane,

Table 4.1   HODGKIN-HUXLEY EQUATIONS

TRANSMEMBRANE CURRENT

$$I_m = C_m \frac{dV_m}{dt} + (V_m - V_{Na})G_{Na} + (V_m - V_K)G_K + (V_m - V_L)G_L$$

IONIC CONDUCTANCES

$$G_{Na} = G_{Na\,max}m^3h \qquad \frac{dm}{dt} = \alpha_m(1 - m) - \beta_m m$$

$$\frac{dh}{dt} = \alpha_h(1 - h) - \beta_h h$$

$$G_K = G_{K\,max}n^4 \qquad \frac{dn}{dt} = \alpha_n(1 - n) - \beta_n n$$

$$G_L = \text{constant}$$

TRANSFER RATE COEFFICIENTS

$$\alpha_m = \frac{0.1 \cdot (25 - V')}{e^{(25-V')/10} - 1} \frac{1}{ms} \qquad \beta_m = \frac{4}{e^{(V'/18)}} \frac{1}{ms}$$

$$\alpha_h = \frac{0.07}{e^{V'/20}} \frac{1}{ms} \qquad \beta_h = \frac{1}{e^{(30-V')/10} + 1} \frac{1}{ms}$$

$$\alpha_n = \frac{0.01(10 - V')}{e^{(10-V')/10} - 1} \frac{1}{ms} \qquad \beta_n = \frac{0.125}{e^{V'/80}} \frac{1}{ms}$$

CONSTANTS

	$C_m = 1 \; \mu\text{F/cm}^2$
$V_r - V_{Na} = -115$ mV	$G_{Na\,max} = 120 \; \text{mS/cm}^2$
$V_r - V_K = +12$ mV	$G_{K\,max} = 36 \; \text{mS/cm}^2$
$V_r - V_L = -10.613$ mV	$G_L = 0.3 \; \text{mS/cm}^2$

where

I_m = membrane current per unit area [$\mu A/cm^2$].

The axoplasm resistance per unit length is:

$$r_i = \frac{\rho_i}{\pi a^2} \quad [k\Omega/cm] \quad (4.27)$$

where

ρ_i = axoplasm resistivity [$k\Omega cm$].

In practice, when the extracellular space is extensive, the resistance of the external medium per unit length, r_o, is so small that it may be omitted and thus from Equations 3.42, 4.26, and 4.27 we obtain:

$$I_m = \frac{i_m}{2\pi a} = \frac{1}{2\pi a(r_i + r_o)} \frac{\partial^2 V_m}{\partial x^2} \cong \frac{1}{2\pi a r_i} \frac{\partial^2 V_m}{\partial x^2}$$
$$= \frac{\pi a^2}{2\pi a \rho_i} \frac{\partial^2 V_m}{\partial x^2} = \frac{a}{2\rho_i} \frac{\partial^2 V_m}{\partial x^2} \quad (4.28)$$

Equation 4.10 evaluates the transmembrane current density based on the intrinsic properties of the membrane while Equation 4.28 evaluates the same current based on the behavior of the "load." Since these expressions must be equal, the Hodgkin-Huxley equation for the propagating nerve impulse may be written:

$$\frac{a}{2\rho_i} \frac{\partial^2 V_m}{\partial x^2} = C_m \frac{\partial V_m}{\partial t} + (V_m - V_{Na})G_{Na}$$
$$+ (V_m - V_K)G_K + (V_m - V_L)G_L \quad (4.29)$$

Under steady-state conditions the impulse propagates with a constant velocity and it maintains constant form; hence it obeys the wave equation:

$$\frac{\partial^2 V_m}{\partial x^2} = \frac{1}{\Theta^2} \frac{\partial^2 V_m}{\partial t^2} \quad (4.30)$$

where;

Θ = the velocity of conduction [m/s].

Substituting Equation 4.30 into 4.29 permits the equation for the propagating nerve impulse to be written in the form:

$$\frac{a}{2\rho_i\Theta^2} \frac{d^2 V_m}{dt^2} = C_m \frac{dV_m}{dt} + (V_m - V_{Na})G_{Na}$$
$$+ (V_m - V_K)G_K + (V_m - V_L)G_L \quad \textbf{(4.31)}$$

This is an ordinary differential equation which can be solved numerically if the value of Θ is guessed correctly. Hodgkin and Huxley ob-

tained numerical solutions that compared favorably with the measured values (18.8 m/s).

With modern computers it is now feasible to solve a parabolic partial differential equation, Equation 4.29, for V_m as a function of x and t (a more difficult solution than for Equation 4.31). This solution permits an examination of V_m during initiation of propagation and at its termination. One can observe changes in velocity and waveform under these conditions. The velocity in this case does not have to be guessed at initially, but can be deduced from the solution.

The propagation velocity of the nerve impulse may be written in the form:

$$\Theta = \sqrt{\frac{Ka}{2\rho_i}} \quad (4.32)$$

where

Θ = propagation velocity [m/s]
K = constant [1/s]
a = axon radius [cm]
ρ_i = axoplasm resistivity [Ωcm]

This can be deduced from Equation 4.31 by noting that the equation is unchanged if the coefficient of the first term is held constant (= $1/K$), it being assumed that the ionic conductances remain unaffected (Hodgkin, 1954). Equation 4.32 also shows that the propagation velocity of the nerve impulse is directly proportional to the square root of axon radius a in unmyelinated axons. This is supported by experiment; and, in fact, an empirical relation is:

$$\Theta = \sqrt{d} \quad (4.33)$$

where

Θ = propagation velocity [m/s]
d = axon diameter [μm]

This velocity contrasts with that observed in myelinated axons; there, the value is linearly proportional to the radius, as illustrated earlier in Figure 2.12. A discussion of the factors affecting the propagation velocity is given in Jack, Noble, and Tsien (1975).

Membrane Conductance Changes During a Propagating Nerve Impulse

K. S. Cole and H. J. Curtis (1939) showed that the impedance of the membrane decreased

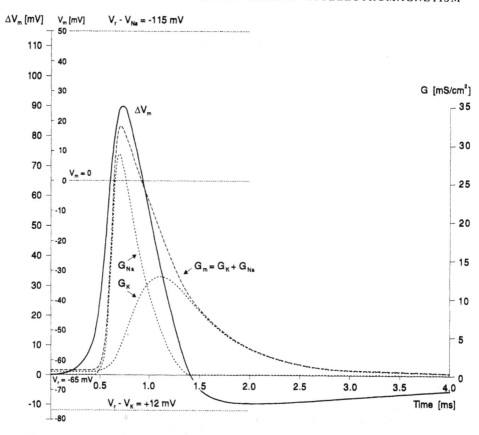

Fig. 4.19   Sodium and potassium conductances (G_{Na} and G_K), their sum (G_m), and the membrane voltage (V_m) during a propagating nerve impulse. This is a numerical solution of Equation 4.32. (After Hodgkin and Huxley, 1952d.)

greatly during activation and that this was due almost entirely to an increase in the membrane conductance. That is, the capacitance does not vary during activation. Figure 4.19 illustrates the components of the membrane conductance, namely G_{Na} and G_K, and their sum G_m during a propagating nerve impulse and the corresponding membrane voltage V_m. This is a numerical solution of Equation 4.31 (after Hodgkin and Huxley, 1952d).

The Components of the Membrane Current During the Propagating Nerve Impulse

Figure 4.20 illustrates the membrane voltage V_m during activation, the sodium and potassium conductances G_{Na} and G_K, the transmembrane

current I_m as well as its capacitive and ionic components I_{mC} and I_{mI}, which are illustrated for a propagating nerve impulse (Noble, 1966).

From the figure the following observations can be made:

1. The potential inside the membrane begins to increase before the sodium conductance starts to rise, owing to the local circuit current originating from the proximal area of activation. In this phase, the membrane current is mainly capacitive, because the sodium and potassium conductances are still low.

2. The local circuit current depolarizes the membrane to the extent that it reaches threshold and activation begins.

3. The activation starts with an increasing sodium conductance. As a result, sodium ions

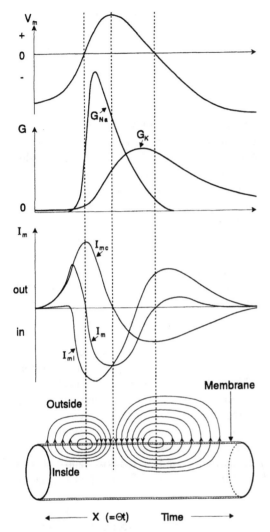

Fig. 4.20 Sodium and potassium conductances G_{Na} and G_K, the ionic and capacitive components I_{mI} and I_{mC} of the membrane current I_m, and the membrane voltage V_m during a propagating nerve impulse.

the capacitive current is zero ($dV/dt = 0$) and the membrane current is totally an ionic current.

6. The terminal phase of activation is governed by the potassium conductance which, through the outflowing potassium current, causes the membrane voltage to become more negative. Because the potassium conductance is elevated above its normal value, there will be a period during which the membrane voltage is more negative than the resting voltage—that is, the membrane is hyperpolarized.

7. Finally, when the conductances reach their resting value, the membrane voltage reaches its resting voltage.

4.4.7 Properties of the Hodgkin-Huxley Model

The Form of a Nonpropagating Nerve Impulse

Figure 4.21 shows both calculated (upper) and measured (lower) membrane voltages at 6°C temperature for an active membrane during a nonpropagating nerve impulse (space clamp) (Hodgkin and Huxley, 1952d). The calculated curves are numerical solutions of Equation 4.10. The values in the curves indicate the stimulus intensity and are expressed in [nC/cm^2].

We note from the figure that the calculated values differ very little from the measured values. There are, however, the following minor differences, namely that the calculated curves have:

1. Sharper peaks
2. A small downward deflection at the end of the recovery period

Effect of Temperature

Figure 4.22 shows both calculated (upper) membrane voltage at 18.5°C temperature and measured (lower) membrane voltage at 20.5°C temperature. Both curves have the same voltage axis, but the effect of temperature is corrected on the time axis. In this case, the same errors can be seen in the calculated membrane voltage as in the previous case. However, the correction of the rate constants with the factor 3.48 has maintained the equality of the curves.

flow inward, causing the membrane voltage to become less negative and finally positive.

4. The potassium conductance begins to increase later on; its time course is much slower than that for the sodium conductance.

5. When the decrease in the sodium conductance and the increase in the potassium conductance are sufficient, the membrane voltage reaches its maximum and begins to decrease. At this instant (the peak of V_m),

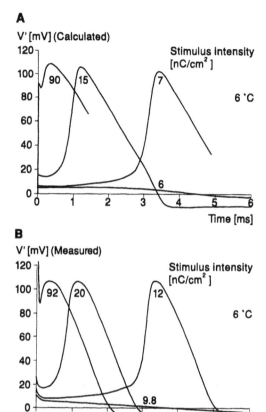

A

V' [mV] (Calculated)

Stimulus intensity [nC/cm²]

6 °C

Time [ms]

B

V' [mV] (Measured)

Stimulus intensity [nC/cm²]

6 °C

Time [ms]

Fig. 4.21 Membrane voltage during a nonpropagating nerve impulse of a squid axon: (A) calculated from Equation 4.10 with $I_m = 0$ and (B) measured (lower) at 6°C temperature. The numbers indicate the stimulus intensity in [nC/cm²]. Note the increasing latency as the stimulus is decreased until, finally, the stimulus falls below threshold.

The effect of the temperature is taken care in the model so that the right-hand sides of the Equations 4.12, 4.16, and 4.18 are multiplied by the factor

$$3^{(T-6.3)/10}$$

where T is the temperature in °C.

The Form of a Propagating Nerve Impulse

The propagating nerve impulse calculated from Equation 4.31 corresponds, accurately, to the measured one. The form of the simulated prop-

agating nerve impulse is illustrated in Figure 4.23A (Hodgkin and Huxley, 1952d). The corresponding membrane voltage measured at 18.5°C is given in Figure 4.23B.

Refractory Period

The Hodgkin-Huxley model also provides an explanation of the refractory period. Figures 4.17 and 4.18 show that the potassium conductance returns to the value corresponding to the resting state only after several milliseconds following initiation of activation. Since activation requires that the (inward) sodium current exceeds the (outward) potassium current, the sodium conductance must reach a relatively higher value during the recovery interval. This requires a stronger stimulus (i.e., the threshold must be elevated). The period being described is known as the *relative refractory period*. A second factor that explains the refractory behavior is the fact that following depolarization the sodium inactivation parameter, h, diminishes and recovers its resting value slowly. As a result, the likelihood of premature reexcitation of the membrane is further decreased.

Figure 4.24 illustrates the calculated and measured response for a stimulus during the refractory period (Hodgkin and Huxley, 1952d). The curves at Figure 4.24A show the response calculated from Equation 4.10 at 6°C temperature. The axon is first stimulated with a stimulus intensity of 15 nC/cm² which produces an action pulse (curve A in Figure 4.24A). Then after about 5 ms another stimulus pulse with an intensity of 90 nC/cm² is given. Because the axon is after the action pulse in refractory state, it does not produce an action pulse and only the stimulus artifact (curve B in Figure 4.24A is seen). If the 90 nC/cm² stimulus is given about 6 ms after the first 15 nc/cm² stimulus, the axon produces an activation (curve C) though with a lower amplitude than the first one. If the second stimulus is given 8 ms after the first one, the response (curve D) is close to the first one. Curve E represents the calculated response to a 90 nC/cm² stimulus when the axon is in the resting state (without the preceding 15 nC/cm² stimulus pulse). (In curves B–E of Fig. 4.24A the values of the response are calculated only for a time of about two milliseconds.) The

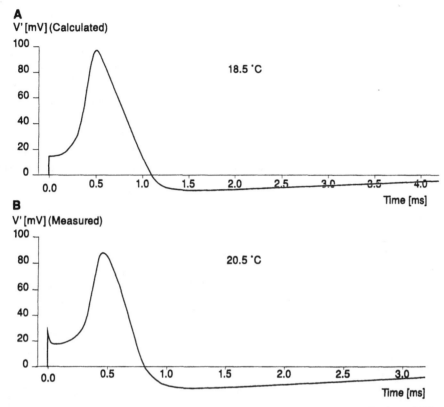

Fig. 4.22 The membrane voltage (A) calculated for the initial depolarization of 15 mV at a temperature of 18.5°C, and (B) measured at 20.5°C. Vertical scales are the same. The horizontal scales differ by a factor appropriate to the temperature difference.

curves in Figure 4.24B show the corresponding experiments performed with a real axon at 9°C temperature. The time scale is corrected to reflect the temperature difference.

Threshold

Figure 4.25 shows both the calculated and measured threshold at 6°C for short stimulus pulses. The calculated curves in Figure 4.25A are numerical solutions of Equation 4.10. The values shown indicate the stimulus intensity and are expressed in [nC/cm²]. The figure indicates that the stimulus intensities of 6 nC/cm² or less, or a negative value of −10 nC/cm², cannot produce an action pulse while the stimulus intensity of 7 nC/cm² produces it. In the measured data the threshold is 12 nC/cm². The behavior of the model corresponds to a real axon for stimuli both over and under the threshold (Hodgkin and Huxley, 1952d).

Anode Break

If the membrane voltage is hyperpolarized with a stimulus whose duration exceeds all ionic time constants and then the hyperpolarization is suddenly terminated, the membrane may elicit an action impulse. The Hodgkin-Huxley model illustrates this phenomenon which is called *anode break excitation* ("anode breakdown" in the original publication). This is described in Figure 4.26. Curve A, the numerical solution of Equation 4.10, illustrates the inside potential of the model when it is made 30 mV more negative than the resting potential at 6°C. In curve B the resting potential of an actual cell is made 26.5 mV more negative in 18.5°C (Hodgkin and Huxley, 1952d).

In the Hodgkin-Huxley model, the inactivation parameter *increases* from its normal value of around 0.6 to perhaps 1.0 during the long hyperpolarization. When the voltage is allowed

A

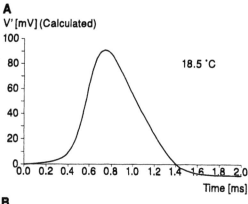

B

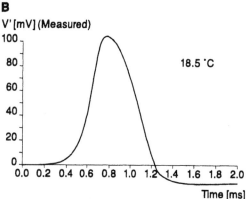

Fig. 4.23 The membrane voltage of a propagating nerve impulse. (A) Calculated from Equation 4.31. The temperature is 18.5°C and the constant K in Equation 4.32 has the value 10.47 [1/ms]. (B) Measured membrane voltage for an axon at the same temperature as (A).

to return to its resting value, its rise causes the sodium activation parameter m to be elevated. But h has a long time constant and tends to remain at its elevated level. The net result is an elevated sodium conductance and elevated sodium current, which can reach the excitatory regenerative behavior even at the normal resting transmembrane voltage. It is also relevant that the potassium conductance (steady-state value of n) is reduced during hyperpolarization, and recovers only with a time course comparable to that of sodium inactivation.

4.4.8   The Quality of the Hodgkin-Huxley Model

A. L. Hodgkin and A. F. Huxley showed that their membrane model describes the following

properties of the axon without any additional assumptions (all of these properties were not discussed here):

1. The form, amplitude, and threshold of the membrane voltage during activation as a function of temperature
2. The form, amplitude, and velocity of the propagating nerve impulse
3. The change, form, and amplitude of the membrane impedance during activation

A

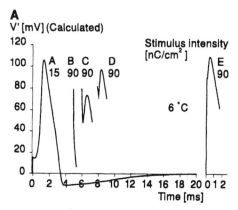

B

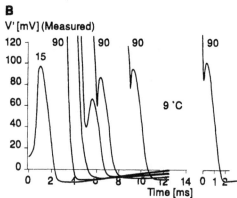

Fig. 4.24   (A) The response during the refractory period calculated from Equation 4.10 at 6°C temperature. The axon is first stimulated with a stimulus intensity of 15 nC/cm², curve A. Curves B, C, and D represent the calculated response to a 90 nC/cm² stimulus at various instants of time after the curve A. Curve E represents the calculated response to a 90 nC/cm² stimulus for an axon in the resting state. (B) The set of curves shows the corresponding experiments performed with a real axon at 9°C temperature. The time scale is corrected to reflect the temperature difference.

4. The total sodium inflow (influx) and potassium outflow (efflux) during activation
5. Threshold and response during the refractory period
6. The amplitude and form of the subthreshold response
7. Anode break response
8. Adaptation (accommodation)

On the basis of the facts given in this chapter, the Hodgkin-Huxley model is, without doubt, the most important theoretical model describing the excitable membrane.

A

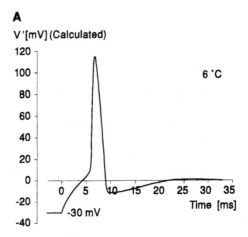

A

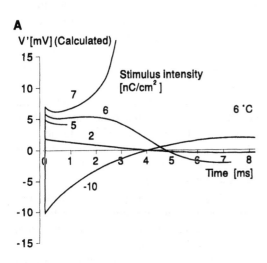

B

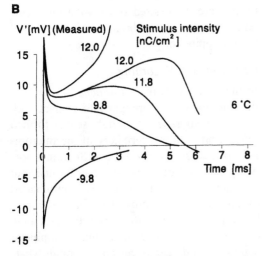

Fig. 4.25 (A) Calculated and (B) measured thresholds. The calculated curves are numerical solutions of Equation 4.10. The stimulus intensity is expressed in [nC/cm²].

B

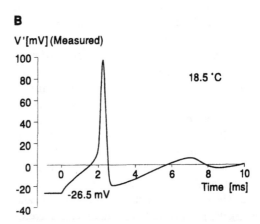

Fig. 4.26 Anode break phenomenon (A) calculated from Equation 4.10 and (B) measured from a squid axon at 6°C temperature. The numbers attached to the curves give the initial depolarization in [mV]. The hyperpolarization is released at $t = 0$.

4.5   PATCH CLAMP METHOD

4.5.1   Introduction

To elucidate how an ion channel operates, one needs to examine the factors that influence its opening and closing as well as measure the resulting current flow. For quite some time, the challenges involved in isolating a very small membrane area containing just a few (or a single) ion channels, and measuring the extraordinarily small ionic currents proved to be insurmountable.

Two cell physiologists, Edwin Neher and Bert Sakmann of the Max Planck Institute (in Göttingen, Germany), succeeded in developing a technique that allowed them to measure the membrane current of a single ion channel. They used a glass microelectrode, called a micropipette, having a diameter of the order of 1 μm. It is said that by accident they placed the electrode very close to the cell membrane so that it came in tight contact with it. The impedance of the measurement circuit then rose to about 50 GΩ (Neher and Sakmann, 1976). The current changes caused by single ion channels of the cell could then be measured by the voltage clamp method. This device came to be known as a *patch clamp* since it examined the behavior of a "patch" of membrane; it constitutes an excellent "space clamp" configuration.

The patch clamp method was further developed to measure the capacitance of the cell membrane (Neher and Marty, 1982). Since the membrane capacitance is proportional to the membrane surface, an examination of minute changes in membrane surface area became possible. This feature has proven useful in studying secretory processes. Nerve cells, as well as hormone-producing cells and cells engaged in the host defense (like mast cells), secrete different agents. They are stored in vesicles enclosed by a membrane. When the cell is stimulated, the vesicles move to the cell surface. The cell and vesicle membranes fuse, and the agent is liberated. The mast cell secretes histamine and other agents that give rise to local inflammatory reactions. The cells of the adrenal medulla liberate the stress hormone adrenaline, and the beta cells in the pancreas liberate insulin. Neher elucidated the secretory processes in these cell types through the development of the new technique which records the fusion of the vesicles with the cell membrane. Neher realized that the electric properties of a cell would change if its surface area increased, making it possible to record the actual secretory process. Through further developments of their sophisticated equipment, its high resolution finally permitted recording of individual vesicles fusing with the cell membrane. In 1991 Neher and Sakmann received the Nobel Prize for their work.

4.5.2 Patch Clamp Measurement Techniques

We discuss here the principles of the patch clamp measurement technique (Sakmann and Neher, 1984; Neher and Sakmann, 1992). We do not present the technical details, which can be found in the original literature (Hamill et al., 1981; Sakmann and Neher, 1984).

There are four main methods in which a patch clamp experiment may be performed. These are:

1. Cell-attached recording
2. Whole cell configuration
3. Outside-out configuration
4. Inside-out configuration

These four configurations are further illustrated in Figure 4.27 and discussed in more detail below.

If a heat-polished glass microelectrode, called a micropipette, having an opening of about 0.5–1 μm, is brought into close contact with an enzymatically cleaned cell membrane, it forms a seal on the order of 50 MΩ. Even though this impedance is quite high, within the dimensions of the micropipette the seal is too loose, and the current flowing through the micropipette includes leakage currents which enter around the seal (i.e., which do not flow across the membrane) and which therefore mask the desired (and very small) ion-channel transmembrane currents.

If a slight suction is applied to the micropipette, the seal can be improved by a factor of 100–1000. The resistance across the seal is then 10–100 GΩ ("G" denotes "giga" $\equiv 10^9$). This tight seal, called *gigaseal*, reduces the leakage currents to the point where it becomes possible to measure the desired signal—the ionic currents through the membrane within the area of the micropipette.

Cell-Attached Recording

In the basic form of *cell-attached recording*, the micropipette is brought into contact with the cell membrane, and a tight seal is formed by suction with the periphery of the micropipette orifice, as described above. Suction is normally released once the seal has formed, but all micropipette current has been eliminated except that flowing across the delineated membrane patch. As a consequence, the exchange of ions between the inside of the micropipette and the outside can occur only through whatever ion channels lie in the membrane fragment. In view of the small size, only a very few channels may lie in the patch of membrane under

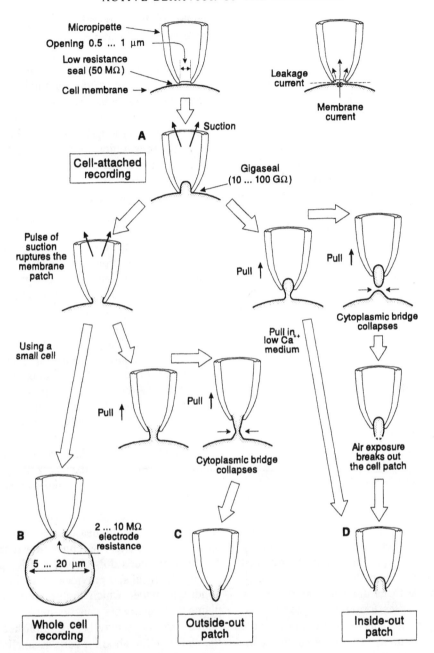

Fig. 4.27 Schematic illustration of the four different methods of patch clamp: (A) cell-attached recording, (B) whole cell configuration, (C) outside-out configuration, and (D) inside-out configuration. (Modified from Hamill et al., 1981.)

observation. When a single ion channel opens, ions move through the channel; these constitute an electric current, since ions are charged particles.

Whole Cell Recording

In the whole cell recording, the cell membrane within the micropipette in the cell-attached con-

figuration is ruptured with a brief pulse of suction. Now the micropipette becomes directly connected to the inside of the cell while the gigaseal is maintained; hence it excludes leakage currents. In contrast, the electric resistance is in the range of 2–10 MΩ. In this situation the microelectrode measures the current due to the ion channels of the whole cell. While the gigaseal is preserved, this situation is very similar to a conventional microelectrode penetration. The technique is particularly applicable to small cells in the size range of 5–20 μm in diameter, and yields good recordings in cells as small as red blood cells.

Outside-Out Configuration

The outside-out configuration is a microversion of the whole cell configuration. In this method, after the cell membrane is ruptured with a pulse of suction, the micropipette is pulled away from the cell. During withdrawal, a cytoplasmic bridge surrounded by membrane is first pulled from the cell. This bridge becomes more and more narrow as the separation between pipette and cell increases, until it collapses, leaving behind an intact cell and a small piece of membrane, which is isolated and attached to the end of the micropipette. The result is an attached membrane "patch" in which the former cell exterior is on the outside and the former cell interior faces the inside of the micropipette. With this method the outside of the cell membrane may be exposed to different bathing solutions; therefore, it may be used to investigate the behavior of single ion channels activated by extracellular receptors.

Inside-Out Configuration

In the inside-out configuration the micropipette is pulled from the cell-attached situation without rupturing the membrane with a suction pulse. As in the outside-out method, during withdrawal, a cytoplasmic bridge surrounded by the membrane is pulled out from the cell. This bridge becomes more and more narrow and finally collapses, forming a closed structure inside the pipette. This vesicle is not suitable for electric measurements. The part of the membrane outside the pipette may, however, be broken with a short exposure to air, and thus the cytoplasmic side of the membrane becomes open to the outside (just the reverse of the outside-out configuration). Inside-out patches can also be obtained directly without air exposure if the withdrawal is performed in Ca-free medium. With this configuration, by changing the ionic concentrations in the bathing solution, one can examine the effect of a quick change in concentration on the cytoplasmic side of the

membrane. It can therefore be used to investigate the cytoplasmic regulation of ion channels.

Formation of an outside-out or inside-out patch may involve major structural rearrangements of the membrane. The effects of isolation on channel properties have been determined in some cases. It is surprising how minor these artifacts of preparation are for most of the channel types of cell membranes.

4.5.3   Applications of the Patch Clamp Method

From the four patch clamp techniques, the *cell-attached configuration* disturbs least the structure and environment of the cell membrane. This method provides a current resolution several orders of magnitude larger than previous current measurement methods. The membrane voltage can be changed without intracellular microelectrodes, and both transmitter- and voltage-activated channels can be studied in their normal ionic environment. Figure 4.28 shows recording of the electric current of a single ion channel at the neuromuscular endplate of frog muscle fiber.

In the *whole cell configuration* a conductive pathway of very low resistance as (i.e., 2–10 MΩ) is formed between the micropipette and the interior of the cell. When the whole cell configuration is utilized with large cells, it allows the researcher to measure membrane voltage and current, just as conventional microelectrode methods do. But when it is applied to very small cells, it provides, in addition, the conditions under which high-quality voltage clamp measurements can be made. Voltage clamp recordings may be accomplished with the whole cell method for cells as small as red blood cells. Many other cell types could be studied for the first time under voltage clamp conditions in this way. Among them are bovine chromaffin cells, sinoatrial node cells isolated from rabbit heart, pancreatic islet cells, cultured neonatal heart cells, and ciliary ganglion cells.

A chromaffin cell of 10 μm in diameter can serve to illustrate the electric parameters that may be encountered. This cell has a resting-state input resistance of several gigaohms (GΩ) and active currents of about a few hundred pi-

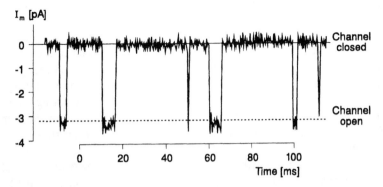

Fig. 4.28 Registration of the flow of current through a single ion channel at the neuromuscular endplate of frog muscle fiber with patch clamp method. (From Sakmann and Neher, 1984.)

coamperes (pA). If the electrode has a series resistance R_s of about 5 MΩ, that represents a negligible series resistance in the measurement configuration. The membrane capacitance C_m is about 5 pF and thus the time constant $\tau_m = R_s \cdot C_m$ is about 25 μs. Thus a voltage clamp measurement may be performed simply by applying a voltage to the micropipette and measuring the current in the conventional way.

The *outside-out configuration* is particularly well suited to those experiments where one wants to examine the ionic channels controlled by externally located receptors. The extracellular solution can be changed easily, allowing testing of effects of different transmitter substances or permeating ions. This configuration has been used to measure the dependence of conductance states of the AChR channel in embryonic cells on the permeating ion. The outside-out patches have also been used to isolate transmitter-gated Cl⁻ channels in the soma membrane of spinal cord neurones, in *Aplysia* neurones, and in the muscle membrane of *Ascaris*.

The *inside-out configuration* is suitable for experiments where the effects of the intracellular components of the ionic channels are under study. Such control over the composition of solutions on both sides of a membrane has been possible, in the past, only with quite involved techniques. Patch clamp methods with the inside-out configuration is a simple way to achieve this goal. Most of the studies to date have involved the role of intracellular Ca^{2+}. This configuration has also been used for per-

meability studies, and for exposing the inner surface of electrically excitable membranes to agents that remove Na^+ channel inactivation.

4.6 MODERN UNDERSTANDING OF THE IONIC CHANNELS

4.6.1 Introduction

Although the Hodgkin-Huxley formalism was published over 40 years ago, in many ways it continues to be satisfactory in its quantitative predictability and its conceptual structure. Still the Hodgkin-Huxley equations are empirically derived from a series of carefully devised experiments to measure total and component membrane ionic currents of the squid axon. To obtain the desired data on these currents, space and voltage clamping were introduced. The voltage clamp eliminated capacitive currents, whereas the space clamp eliminated otherwise confounding axial current flow. The measured quantity was the total current of a macroscopic membrane patch which, when divided by the membrane area, gave the ionic current density. Since the result is an integrated quantity, it leaves open the behavior of discrete membrane elements that contribute to the total.

Hodgkin and Huxley were aware that the membrane was primarily lipid with a dielectric constant in the neighborhood of 5 and an electric resistivity of 2×10^9 Ωcm, an obviously excellent insulator. Two leading hypotheses were advanced to explain ion currents through such a medium, namely carrier-mediated transport and flow through pores (or channels). Hodgkin and Huxley did not distinguish between these two possibilities, though in their final paper (Hodgkin and Huxley, 1952d, p. 502) they did note that the most straightforward form of the carrier hypothesis was inconsistent with their observations.

At this time, researchers have studied membrane proteins with sufficient care to know that they are much too large to catalyze ion fluxes known to exceed 10^6 ions per "channel" per second. Although these proteins have been investigated by a number of techniques their structure is still not definitively established; nevertheless, many features, including the presence of aqueous channels, are reasonably well understood. In the remainder of this section we describe some of the details of structure and function. Our treatment here is necessarily brief

and only introductory; the interested reader will find extensive material in Hille (1992).

Before proceeding it is useful to introduce a general description of a channel protein (illustrated in Fig. 4.29). Although based on recognized channel features, the figure is nevertheless only a "working hypothesis." It contains in cartoon form the important electrophysiological properties associated with "selectivity" and "gating," which will be discussed shortly. The overall size of the protein is about 8 nm in diameter and 12 nm in length (representing 1800–4000 amino acids arranged in one or several polypeptide chains); its length substantially exceeds the lipid bilayer thickness so that only a small part of the molecule lies within the membrane. Of particular importance to researchers is the capacity to distinguish protein structures that lie within the membrane (i.e., hydro*phobic* elements) from those lying outside (i.e., hydro*philic* extracellular and cytoplasmic elements). We have seen that mem-

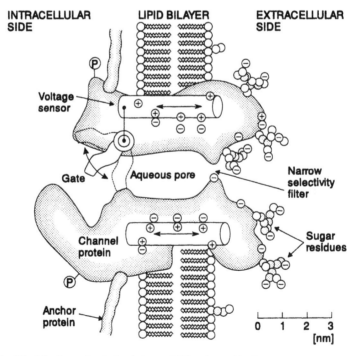

Fig. 4.29 Working hypothesis for a channel. The channel is drawn as a transmembrane macromolecule with a hole through the center. The functional regions—namely selectivity filter, gate, and sensor—are deducted from voltage clamp experiments and are only beginning to be charted by structural studies. (Redrawn from Hille, 1992.)

brane voltages are on the order of 0.1 V; these give rise to transmembrane electric fields on the order of 10^6 V/m. Fields of this intensity can exert large forces on charged residues within the membrane protein, as Figure 4.29 suggests, and also cause the conformational changes associated with transmembrane depolarization (the alteration in shape changes the conductance of the aqueous pore). In addition, ionic flow through aqueous channels, may be affected by fixed charges along the pore surface.

4.6.2   Single-Channel Behavior

As noted previously, it is currently believed that membrane proteins that support ion flux contain water-filled pores or *channels* through which ion flow is assumed to take place. The application of patch-clamp techniques has made it possible to observe the behavior of a single channel. In that regard, such studies have suggested that these channels have only two states: either fully open or fully closed. (Measurements such as those performed by Hodgkin-Huxley can thus be interpreted as arising from the *space-average behavior* of a very large number of individual channels).

In fact, most channels can actually exist in *three states* that may be described functionally as

Resting $\rightleftharpoons$ Open $\rightleftharpoons$ Inactivated

An example is the sodium channel, mentioned earlier in this chapter. At the single-channel level, a transthreshold change in transmembrane potential increases the probability that a resting (closed) channel will open. After a time following the opening of a channel, it can again close as a result of a new channel process—that of *inactivation*. Although inactivation of the squid axon potassium channel was not observed on the time scale investigated, new information on single channels is being obtained from the *shaker* potassium channel from *Drosophila melanogaster* which obeys the more general scheme described above (and to which we return below). In fact, this preparation has been used to investigate the mechanism of inactivation. Thus a relative good picture has emerged.

4.6.3   The Ionic Channel

There are many types of channels, but all have two important properties in common: *gating* and *selective permeability*. Gating refers to the opening and closing of the channel, depending on the presence of external "forces." Channels fall into two main classes: (1) *ligand-gated channels*, which respond to neurotransmitters (e.g., the acetylcholine-sensitive channel at the neuromuscular junction); and (2) *voltage-gated channels*, regulating flux of electrolytes (e.g., sodium, potassium, and calcium). The second feature, selective permeability, describes the ability of a channel to permit flow of only a single ion type (or perhaps a family of ions).

Neurotoxins that can block specific channel types are important tools in the study of membrane proteins. The first neurotoxin used in this way was tetrodotoxin (TTX) (see Section 4.3.3), a highly selective and powerful inhibitor of sodium channel conductance. Since TTX can eliminate (inactivate) sodium currents selectively from the total ionic current, it can be useful in studies attempting to identify the individual ionic membrane current components. The fact that TTX eliminates sodium flux exclusively also lends support to the idea that sodium ions pass only through specific sodium channels. By using a saturating amount of a radioactively labeled toxin; one can evaluate the target channel density. (For sodium, the channel density is quite sparse: 5–500 per μm^2 of membrane.) These labeled toxins are useful also in purifying channel preparations, making possible structural studies.

We now describe briefly three types of techniques useful for elucidating channel structure: (1) *biophysical*, (2) *molecular biological*, and (3) *electron microscopical* and *electron diffraction*. Although a fairly consistent picture emerges, much remains speculative, and an accurate picture of channel structure remains to emerge.

4.6.4   Channel Structure: Biophysical Studies

The Hodgkin-Huxley equations provide excellent simulations under a variety of conditions; these equations have been discussed in the ear-

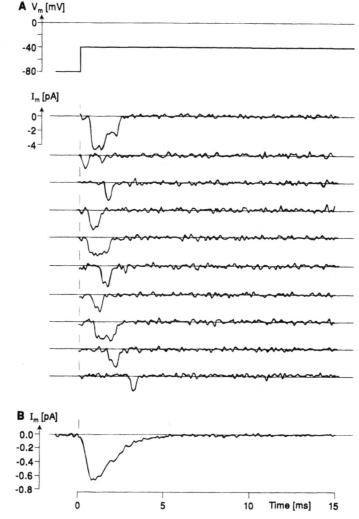

Fig. 4.30 Gating in single sodium channels: Patch clamp recording of unitary Na currents in a toe muscle of adult mouse during a voltage step from -80 to -40 mV. Cell-attached recording from a Cs-depolarized fiber. (A) Ten consecutive trials filtered at 3-kHz bandwidth. Two simultaneous channel openings have occurred in the first record; the patch may contain over 10 sodium channels. The dashed line indicates the current level when channels are all closed (background current). (B) The ensemble mean of 352 repetitions of the same protocol. $T = 15°C$. (From Hille, 1992, as provided by J. B. Patlak; see also Patlak and Ortiz, 1986.)

lier sections of this chapter and are summarized in Sections 4.4.3 and 4.4.4. Hodgkin and Huxley considered the physical implications of the results obtained with these equations. Thus the variables m, n, and h, rather than being considered abstract parameters, were thought to reflect actual physical quantities and were therefore interpreted to describe charged particles in the membrane that would be found at either the inner or outer surface and were required to open or close membrane "channels." This literal interpretation of the Hodgkin-Huxley equations is presented earlier in this chapter. Hodgkin and Huxley however, were aware of the limitations of such speculations (Hodgkin and Huxley, 1952d): ''Certain features of our equations are capable of physical interpretation, but the success of our equation is no evidence in favor of the mechanism of permeability change we tentatively had in mind when formulating them.'' More definitive studies, including true single channel recordings, are now available.

Figures 4.30 and 4.31 show single-channel recordings obtained in response to a voltage clamp; Figure 4.30 indicates the response of a sodium channel to a depolarization of 40 mV; whereas Figure 4.31 shows the response of a squid axon potassium channel to a change in voltage from −100 mV to 50 mV. If one dis-

regards the noise, then clearly the channel is either in a conducting or nonconducting condition. (In fact, although the transitions are obviously stochastic, careful study shows that the openings and closings themselves are sudden in all situations). The average of 40 sequential trials, given at the bottom of Figure 4.30, can be interpreted also as the total current from 40 simultaneous sodium channels (assuming statistically independent channel behavior). The latter approaches what would be measured in

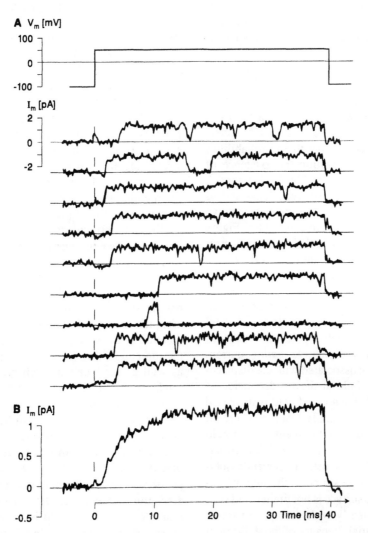

Fig. 4.31 Gating in single potassium channels: Patch clamp recording of unitary K currents in a squid giant axon during a voltage step from −100 to +50 mV. (A) Nine consecutive trials showing channels of 20 pS conductance filtered at 2 kHz bandwidth. (B) Ensemble mean of 40 trials. $T = 20°C$. (From Hille, 1992, based on data from Bezanilla and Augustine, 1986.)

an Hodgkin-Huxley procedure where a large number of channels would be simultaneously measured. The same observations apply to the potassium channels illustrated in Figure 4.31. The averages shown bear a striking resemblance to Hodgkin-Huxley voltage clamp data.

The single-channel behavior illustrated in Figure 4.31 demonstrates the stochastic nature of single-channel openings and closings. Consistent with the Hodgkin-Huxley model is the view that this potassium channel has the probability n^4 of being open. As a result, if $G_{K \, max}$ is the conductance when *all* of the channels are open, then the conductance under other conditions $G_K = G_{K \, max} \cdot n^4$. And, of course, this is precisely what the Hodgkin-Huxley equation (4.13) states.

One can interpret n as reflecting two probabilities: (1) that a subunit of the potassium channel is open, and (2) that there are four such subunits, each of which must be in the open condition for the channel itself to be open. Hodgkin and Huxley gave these probabilities specific form by suggesting the existence of gating *particles* as one possible physical model. Such particles have never been identified as such; however, the channel *proteins* are known to contain charged "elements" (see Figure 4.29), although in view of their overall electroneutrality, may be more appropriately characterized as *dipole* elements. The application of a depolarizing field on this dipole distribution causes movement (i.e., conformational changes) capable of opening or closing channel gates. In addition, such dipole movement, in fact, constitutes a capacitive *gating* current which adds to that associated with the displacement of charges held at the inside/outside of the membrane. If the applied field is increased gradually, a point is finally reached where all dipoles are brought into alignment with the field and the gating current reaches a maximum (saturation) value. In contrast, the current associated with the charge stored at the internal/external membrane surface is not limited and simply increases linearly with the applied transmembrane potential. Because of these different characteristics, measurements at two widely different voltage clamps can be used to separate the two components and reveal the gating currents themselves (Bezanilla and Augustine, 1986).

4.6.5 Channel Structure: Studies in Molecular Genetics

In recent years, gene cloning methods have been used in those investigations of channel structure designed to determine the primary amino acid sequence of channel proteins. One can even test the results by determining whether a cell that does not normally make the protein in question will do so when provided the cloned message or gene. Oocytes of the African toad *Xenopus laevis* are frequently used to examine the *expression* of putative channel mRNA. The resulting channels can be patch clamped and their voltage and ligand gating properties investigated to confirm whether the protein synthesized is indeed the desired channel protein.

Although the *primary* structures of many channels have now been determined, the rules for deducing secondary and tertiary structure are not known. Educated guesses on the folding patterns for a protein chain can be made, however. One approach involves searching for a stretch of 20 or so *hydrophobic* amino acids since this would most probably extend across the membrane and exhibit the appropriate intramembrane (intralipid) behavior. In this way, the linear amino acid sequence can be converted into a sequence of loops and folds based on the location of those portions of the molecule lying within the membrane, within the cytoplasm, and within the extracellular space. The hydrophobic stretches of the amino acid sequence assigned to the membrane might provide indication of the structure and the boundaries of the ion-conducting (i.e., pore-forming) region, as well as the location of charge groups that might be involved in voltage-sensing gating charge movement.

This approach was successfully used in the study of *shaker* potassium ion inactivation. Following activation of this channel, the ensuing inactivation was found to be voltage-independent. One can therefore deduce that the inactivation process must lie *outside* the membrane; otherwise it would be subjected to the effects of the membrane electric field. For this reason as well as other reasons, the amino-terminal cytoplasmic domain of the membrane protein was investigated by constructing *deletion mutants* whose channel gating behavior could then be examined. The results demonstrated that inactivation is controlled by 19 amino acids at the amino-terminal cytoplasmic side of the channel and that these constitute a *ball and chain* (Hoshi, Zagotta, and Aldrich, 1990). What appears to be happening is that associated with channel activation is the movement of negative charge into the cytoplasmic mouth of the channel, which then attracts the positively charged ball; movement of the ball (which exceeds the channel mouth in size) then results in closure of the channel.

Some hypotheses can be tested by *site-directed mutagenesis*, by which specific protein segments are deleted or inserted as just illustrated, or other such manipulations are performed (Krueger, 1989). By examining the altered properties of the channel expressed in *Xenopus* oocytes, one can make educated guesses on the function of certain segments of the protein. Of course, since the changes can have complex effects on the (unknown) tertiary structure, the conclusions must be considered as tentative.

4.6.6 Channel Structure:
Imaging Methods

Direct imaging of membrane proteins would, indeed, provide the structural information so greatly desired. X-ray crystallography is used to study macromolecules at atomic resolution, but it can be used only when the molecule is repeated in a regular lattice. It has generally not been possible to crystallize membrane proteins; however, two-dimensional arrays of concentrated purified proteins have been assembled into lipid bilayers with reasonably regular spacing. X-ray diffraction and electron microscopy (EM) have been used in such investigations, and images with modest resolution have been obtained. One example is the EM examination of the *Torpedo* neuromuscular junction acetylcholine receptor (nAChR) (Toyoshima and Unwin, 1988). The molecule was found to be 8 nm in diameter, with a central well of 2.5 nm. Viewed on face, the protein has a rosette-like appearance with five subunits. The subunits function like barrel staves in delineating the aqueous channel. Unfortunately, the resolution

of the image is too large to identify the central pore and its shape with any certainty.

It is thought that the central pore is actually nonuniform in diameter and, as described in Figure 4.29, has a narrow part which acts as a selectivity filter. Since the intramembrane subunits appear to be oriented as barrel staves with the pore resulting from a geometrically defined space, this space will be very sensitive to the tilt of the subunits. A small change in tilt arising from a change in transmembrane potential (i.e., a change in electrostatic force) could thereby quickly switch the channel from open to closed and vice versa. Such a hypothesis is developed by Zampighi and Simon (1985).

4.6.7 Ionic Conductance Based
on Single-Channel Conductance

The equivalent electric circuit of the single channel is a resistance in series with a battery and switch. (There is, of course, a parallel capacitance, representing the associated patch of lipid-bilayer dielectric.) The battery represents the Nernst potential of the ion for which the channel is selectively permeable while the switch reflects the possible states discussed above (namely open, closed, and inactivated). Referring to Figure 4.29 from which the aqueous pore dimension of 2.0 nm diameter and 12.0 nm length is suggested, then the ohmic conductance of such a cylinder, assuming a bulk resistivity of 250 Ωcm, is 105 pS, a value that lies in the range of those experimentally determined. (Since the channel is of atomic dimensions, the model used here is highly simplified and the numerical result must be viewed as fortuitous. A more detailed consideration of factors that may be involved is found in Hille (1992).) Based on this model one determines the channel current to be $i_K = \gamma_K (V_m - V_K)$, where γ_K is the channel conductivity and V_K the Nernst potential (illustrated here for potassium). Under normal conditions the channel conductance is considered to be a constant so that the macroscopic variation in ionic conductance arises from changes in the fraction of open channels (exactly the effect of the gating variables n, m, and h for the squid axon ionic conductances).

The statistical behavior of the single channel

can be obtained from an examination of the behavior of a large number of identical and independent channels and their subunits (the single subunit being a sample member of an ensemble). If N_c are the number of closed subunits in the ensemble and N_o the number that are open then assuming first-order rate processes with α the transfer rate coefficient for transitions from a closed to open state while β the rate from open to closed gives the equation

$$N_c \underset{\beta}{\overset{\alpha}{\rightleftharpoons}} N_o \qquad (4.34)$$

from which one obtains the differential equation

$$\frac{dN_c}{dt} = \beta N_o - \alpha N_c \qquad (4.35)$$

Since the total number of subunits, N, must satisfy $N = N_c(t) + N_o(t)$, where N is a fixed quantity, then the above equation becomes

$$\frac{dN_o}{dt} + (\alpha + \beta)N_o = \alpha N \qquad (4.36)$$

Dividing Equation 4.36 through by N and recognizing that $n = N_o/N$ as the statistical probability that any single subunit is open, we arrive at

$$\frac{dn}{dt} = \alpha - (\alpha + \beta)n \qquad (4.37)$$

which corresponds exactly to Equation 4.12. This serves to link the Hodgkin-Huxley description of a macroscopic membrane with the behavior of a single component channel. Specifically the transfer rate coefficients α and β describe the transition rates from closed to open (and open to closed) states. One can consider the movement of n-particles, introduced by Hodgkin and Huxley, as another way of describing in physical terms the aforementioned rates. (Note that n is a continuous variable and hence "threshold" is not seen in a single channel. Threshold is a feature of macroscopic membranes with, say, potassium, sodium, and leakage channels and describes the condition where the collective behavior of all channel types allows a regenerative process to be initiated which constitutes the upstroke of an action

pulse.) In the above the potassium channel probability of being open is, of course, n^4.

While the description above involved the simultaneous behavior of a large number of equivalent channels, it also describes the statistics associated with the sequential behavior of a single channel (i.e., assuming ergodicity). If a membrane voltage step is applied to the aforementioned ensemble of channels, then the solution to Equation 4.36 is:

$$N_o(t) = Ae^{-(\alpha+\beta)t} + \frac{\alpha}{\alpha + \beta} N \qquad (4.38)$$

It describes an exponential change in the number of open subunits and also describes the exponential rise in probability n for a single subunit. But if there is no change in applied voltage, one would observe only random opening and closings of a single channel. However, according to the *fluctuation-dissipation* theorem (Kubo, 1966), the same time constants affect these fluctuations as affect the macroscopic changes described in Equation 4.38. Much work has accordingly been directed to the study of membrane noise as a means of experimentally accessing single-channel statistics (DeFelice, 1981).

REFERENCES

Armstrong CW, Hille B (1972): The inner quaternary ammonium ion receptor in potassium channels of the node of Ranvier. *J. Gen. Physiol.* 59: 388–400.

Baker PF, Hodgkin AL, Shaw TI (1962): The effects of changes in internal ionic concentrations on the electrical properties of perfused giant axons. *J. Physiol. (Lond.)* 164: 355–74.

Bezanilla F, Augustine BH (1986): Voltage dependent gating. In *Ionic Channels in Cells and Model Systems*, ed. R Latorre, pp. 37–52, Plenum Press, New York.

Cole KS (1949): Dynamic electrical characteristics of squid axon membrane. *Arch. Sci. Physiol.* 3: 253–8.

Cole KS, Curtis HJ (1939): Electrical impedance of the squid giant axon during activity. *J. Gen. Physiol.* 22: 649–70.

Cole KS, Moore JW (1960): Potassium ion current in the squid giant axon: Dynamic characteristics. *Biophys. J.* 1: 1–14.

DeFelice LJ (1981): *Introduction to Membrane Noise*, 500 pp. Plenum Press, New York.

Hamill OP, Marty A, Neher E, Sakmann B, Sigworth FJ (1981): Improved patch clamp techniques for high resolution current recording from cells and cell-free membranes. *Pflüger Arch. ges. Physiol.* 391: 85–100.

Hille B (1970): Ionic channels in nerve membranes. *Prog. Biophys. Mol. Biol.* 21: 1–32.

Hille B (1992): *Ionic Channels of Excitable Membranes*, 2nd ed., 607 pp. Sinauer Assoc., Sunderland, Mass. (1st ed., 1984)

Hodgkin AL (1954): A note on conduction velocity. *J. Physiol. (Lond.)* 125: 221–4.

Hodgkin AL, Horowicz P (1959): The influence of potassium and chloride ions on the membrane potential of single muscle fibers. *J. Physiol. (Lond.)* 148: 127–60.

Hodgkin AL, Huxley AF (1952a): The components of membrane conductance in the giant axon of *Loligo. J. Physiol. (Lond.)* 116: 473–96.

Hodgkin AL, Huxley AF (1952b): Currents carried by sodium and potassium ions through the membrane of the giant axon of *Loligo. J. Physiol. (Lond.)* 116: 449–72.

Hodgkin AL, Huxley AF (1952c): The dual effect of membrane potential on sodium conductance in the giant axon of *Loligo. J. Physiol. (Lond.)* 116: 497–506.

Hodgkin AL, Huxley AF (1952d): A quantitative description of membrane current and its application to conduction and excitation in nerve. *J. Physiol. (Lond.)* 117: 500–44.

Hodgkin AL, Huxley AF, Katz B (1952): Measurement of current-voltage relations in the membrane of the giant axon of *Loligo. J. Physiol. (Lond.)* 116: 424–48.

Hoshi T, Zagotta WN, Aldrich RW (1990): Biophysical and molecular mechanisms of *shaker* potassium channel inactivation. *Science* 250: 533–68.

Huxley A (1993): Personal communication.

Jack JJB, Noble D, Tsien RW (1975): *Electric Current Flow in Excitable Cells*, 502 pp. Clarendon Press, Oxford.

Junge D (1992): *Nerve and Muscle Excitation*, 3rd ed., 263 pp. Sinauer Assoc., Sunderland, Mass.

Krueger BK (1989): Toward an understanding of structure and function of ion channels. *FASEB J.* 3: 1906–14.

Kubo R (1966): The fluctuation-dissipation theorem. *Rep. Prog. Phys. Lond.* 29: 255.

Marmont G (1949): Studies on the axon membrane. I. A new method. *J. Cell. Comp. Physiol.* 34: 351–82.

Moore JW, Blaustein MP, Anderson NC, Narahashi T (1967): Basis of tetrodotoxin's selectivity in blockage of squid axons. *J. Gen. Physiol.* 50: 1401–11.

Narahashi T, Moore JW, Scott WR (1964): Tetrodotoxin blockage of sodium conductance increase in lobster giant axons. *J. Gen. Physiol.* 47: 965–74.

Neher E, Marty A (1982): Discrete changes of cell membrane capacitance observed under conditions of enhanced secretion in bovine adrenal chromaffin cells. *Proc. Nat. Acad. Sci. USA* 79: 6712–6.

Neher E, Sakmann B (1976): Single-channel currents recorded from membrane of denervated frog muscle fibers. *Nature* 260: 799–802.

Neher E, Sakmann B (1992): The patch clamp technique. *Sci. Am.* 266:(3) 28–35.

Noble D (1966): Application of Hodgkin-Huxley equations to excitable tissues. *Physiol. Rev.* 46:(1) 1–50.

Patlak JB, Ortiz M (1986): Two modes of gating during late Na+ channel currents in frog sartorius muscle. *J. Gen. Physiol.* 87: 305–26.

Plonsey R (1969): *Bioelectric Phenomena*, 380 pp. McGraw-Hill, New York.

Sakmann B, Neher E (1983): *Single Channel Recording*, 496 pp. Plenum Press, New York.

Sakmann B, Neher E (1984): Patch clamp techniques for studying ionic channels in excitable membranes. *Annu. Rev. Physiol.* 46: 455–72.

Toyoshima C, Unwin N (1988): Ion channel of acetylcholine receptor reconstructed from images of postsynaptic membranes. *Nature* 336: 247–50.

Unwin PNT, Zampighi G (1980): Structure of the junctions between communicating cells. *Nature* 283: 545–9.

Young JZ (1936): The giant nerve fibers and epistellar body of cephalopods. *Q. J. Microsc. Sci.* 78: 367–86.

Zambighi GA, Simon SA (1985): The structure of gap junctions as revealed by electron microscopy. In *Gap Junctions*, ed. MVL Bennett, DC Spray, pp. 13–22, Cold Spring Harbor Laboratory, Cold Spring Harbor, N.Y.

5

Synapses, Receptor Cells, and Brain

5.1 INTRODUCTION

The focus of this book is primarily the electric activity of nerve and muscle and the extracellular electric and magnetic fields that they generate. It is possible to undertake such a study without considering the functional role of nerve and muscle in physiology. But without some life science background, the reader's evaluation of electrophysiological signals would necessarily be handicapped. For that reason, we have included an overview, with appropriate terminology, of relevant topics in physiology. This chapter is therefore devoted to a survey of the organization of the nervous system and its main components. It is hoped that the reader will find it helpful for understanding of the physiological function of the excitable tissues discussed in other chapters, and to know what to look for elsewhere. For further study, we suggest the following texts: Jewett and Rayner (1984); Kuffler, Nicholls, and Martin (1984); Nunez (1981); Patton et al. (1989); Schmidt (1981); Shepherd (1988); all of which appear in the list of references.

A discussion of the nervous system might logically begin with sensory cells located at the periphery of the body. These cells initiate and conduct signals to the brain and provide various sensory inputs such as vision, hearing, posture, and so on. Providing information on the environment to the body, these peripheral cells respond to stimuli with action pulses, which convey their information through encoded signals. These signals are conducted axonally through ascending pathways, across synapses, and finally to specific sites in the brain. Other neural cells in the brain process the coded signals, and direct the actions of muscles and other organs in response to the various sensory inputs. The entire *circuit* is recognized as a *reflex arc,* a basic unit in the nervous system. In some cases it is entirely automatic, and in others it is under voluntary control.

No neurons run directly from the periphery to the brain. Normally the initiated signal is relayed by several intermediate neural cells. The interconnection between neurons, called the *synapse,* behaves as a simple switch but also has a special role in information processing. The junction (synapse) between a neural cell and the muscle that it innervates, called the *neuromuscular junction,* has been particularly well studied and provides much of our quantitative understanding about synapses. Since it is impossible to discuss the structure of the nervous system without including synapses, we begin our discussion with an examination of that topic.

5.2 SYNAPSES

5.2.1 Structure and Function of the Synapse

The function of the synapse is to transfer electric activity (information) from one cell to another. The transfer can be from nerve to nerve (neuro-neuro), or nerve to muscle (neuro-myo). The region between the pre- and postsynaptic membrane is very narrow, only 30–50 nm. It is called the *synaptic cleft* (or *synaptic gap*). Direct electric communication between pre- and postjunctional cells does not take place; instead, a chemical mediator is utilized. The sequence of events is as follows:

1. An action pulse reaches the terminal endings of the presynaptic cell.
2. A neurotransmitter is released, which diffuses across the synaptic gap to bind to receptors in specialized membranes of the postsynaptic cell.

3. The transmitter acts to open channels of one or several ion species, resulting in a change in the transmembrane potential. If *depolarizing*, it is an *excitatory postsynaptic potential* (EPSP); if *hyperpolarizing*, an *inhibitory postsynaptic potential* (IPSP).

Figure 5.1 shows the synapse between a nerve and muscle cell, a neuromuscular junction.

In *cardiac muscle* the intercellular space between abutting cells is spanned by *gap junctions*, which provide a low-resistance path for the local circuit currents and may be regarded as an electric (myo-myo) synapse. (The gap, however, is *not* called a synaptic cleft.) This type of junction is discussed in a later chapter.

The presynaptic nerve fiber endings are generally enlarged to form *terminal buttons* or *synaptic knobs*. Inside these knobs are the vesicles that contain the chemical transmitters. The arrival of the action pulse opens voltage-gated Ca^{2+} channels that permit an influx of calcium ions. These in turn trigger the release into the

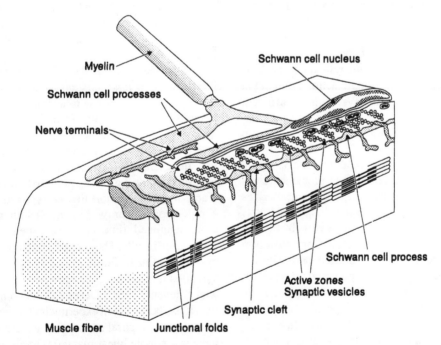

Fig. 5.1 The neuromuscular (synaptic) junction. Many features of this junction are also seen in the nerve-nerve synapse. The terminal ending of the prejunctional cell contains many vesicles, which are packages of the neurotransmitter acetylcholine (ACh). The gap between the pre- and postjunctional membrane is on the order of 15–30 nm. The transmitter is released by the arrival of an action impulse in the nerve; it diffuses and binds to receptors on the postjunctional muscle membrane, bringing about an EPSP and the initiation of a muscle action potential.

synaptic gap, by *exocytosis,* of a number of the "prepackaged" vesicles containing the neurotransmitter.

On average, each neuron divides into perhaps 1000 synaptic endings. On the other hand, a single spinal motor neuron may have an average of 10,000 synaptic inputs. Based on this data, it is not surprising that the ratio of synapse to neurons in the human forebrain is estimated to be around 4×10^4. In neuro-neuro synapses, the postjunctional site may be a dendrite or cell body, but the former predominates.

5.2.2 Excitatory and Inhibitory Synapses

In the neuromuscular junction, upon arrival of an action pulse at the motor neuron ending, *acetylcholine* (ACh) is released into the cleft. It diffuses across the gap to the muscle membrane where it binds to specialized receptors, resulting in a simultaneous increase in membrane permeability to both sodium and potassium ions. Because the relative effect on sodium exceeds that of potassium (described quantitatively later in this section), the membrane depolarizes and a postsynaptic action potential results. The process is *always* excitatory. Furthermore, arrival of a single action potential at the prejunctional site always results in sufficient release of transmitter to produce a *transthreshold* depolarization and initiate an action potential in the muscle.

Synaptic inhibition occurs at nerve-nerve (neuro-neuro) junctions when presynaptic activity releases a transmitter that hyperpolarizes the postsynaptic membrane (i.e., makes its membrane voltage more negative). In theory, hyperpolarization could result from elevation of either potassium or chloride permeability because the equilibrium potential of each is more negative than the normal resting potential (which is influenced in the positive direction by the presence of sodium). In actuality, however, inhibition is due to elevated chloride permeability.

In contrast with the neuromuscular (neuro-myo) junction, a single excitatory input to a neuro-neuro synapse is completely inadequate to depolarize the postjunctional membrane to threshold. In fact, with perhaps thousands of both excitatory and inhibitory inputs on the postjunctional cell, a *spatial* and *temporal summation* is continually taking place, and the membrane voltage will fluctuate. When, finally, a threshold of perhaps 10–15 mV is reached, an action potential results. In this way, an important integrative process takes place at the inputs to each nerve cell. The reader with computer science experience can appreciate the tremendous possibilities for information processing that can (and do!) take place, particularly when one considers that there are perhaps 10^{12} neurons and 10^{15} synapses in the human brain. This is indeed a *neural net.*

Presynaptic inhibition is another inhibition mechanism. In this case an inhibitory nerve ending (from another axon known as the presynaptic inhibitor) is synapsed to an *excitatory presynaptic* terminal. The inhibitory nerve releases a transmitter that partially depolarizes the presynaptic cell. As a consequence, activation arising in the presynaptic fiber is diminished, hence the release of transmitter is reduced. As a result, the degree of excitation produced in the *postsynaptic* cell is reduced (hence an inhibitory effect).

The *falling phase* of the EPSP is characterized by a single *time constant*—that is, the time required for the response to a single excitatory stimulus to diminish to $1/e$ of its maximum. This is an important value. If a sequence of afferent stimuli occurs in a very short time interval, then *temporal summation* of the EPSPs occurs, yielding a growing potential. Similarly, if activity occurs at more than one synaptic knob simultaneously (or within the length of the aforementioned time constant), then *spatial summation* results. The additive effect on a synapse is nonlinear. Furthermore, the individual synapses interact in an extremely complicated way (Stevens, 1968). Despite these complexities, it has been shown experimentally that both spatial and temporal summation generally behave in a simple linear manner (Granit, Haase, and Rutledge, 1960; Granit and Renkin, 1961).

Synaptic transmission has been compared to an electric information transfer circuit in the following way: In the nerve axon the information is transferred by means of nerve impulses in "digital" or, more accurately, "pulse-code modulated" form. In the synapse, information is conducted with the transmitter substance in analog form, to be converted again in the next neuron into "digital" form. Though this analogy is not correct in all aspects, it illustrates the character of the neural information chain.

5.2.3 Reflex Arc

The driver of a car receives visual signals via photoreceptors that initiate coded afferent impulses that ascend nerve fibers and terminate in the visual cortex. Once the brain has processed the information, it sends efferent signals to the muscles in the foot and hands. Thus the car is slowed down and can make a right turn. But if our hand is mistakenly brought to rest on a hot surface, a set of signals to the hand and arm muscles result that are *not* initiated in the higher centers; cognition comes into play only after the fact. We say that a *reflex path* is involved in both of these examples. The first is complex and involves higher centers in the central nervous system, whereas the second describes a simpler reflex at a lower level. In fact, a great deal of reflex activity is taking place *at all times* of which we are unaware. For example, input signals are derived from internal sensors, such as blood pressure, or oxygen saturation in the blood, and so on, leading to an adjustment of heart rate, breathing rate, etc.

The *reflex arc*, illustrated above, is considered to be the basic unit of integrated neural activity. It consists essentially of a sensory receptor, an afferent neuron, one or more synapses, an efferent neuron, and a muscle or other effector. The connection between afferent and efferent pathways is found, generally, in the spinal cord or the brain. The simplest reflex involves only a single synapse between afferent and efferent neurons (a *monosynaptic reflex*); an example is the familiar knee jerk reflex.

Homeostasis refers to the various regulatory processes in the body that maintain a normal state in the face of disturbances. The *autonomic nervous system* is organized to accomplish this automatically with regard to many organs of the body; its activity, like that of the somatic nervous system, is based on the reflex arc. In this case signals, which arise at visceral receptors, are conveyed via afferent neurons to the central nervous system, where integration takes place, resulting in efferent signals to visceral effectors (in particular, smooth muscle) to restore or maintain normal conditions. Integration of signals affecting blood pressure and respiration takes place in the *medulla oblongata;* those controlling pupillary response to light are integrated in the *midbrain,* whereas those responding to body temperature are integrated in the *hypothalamus*—to give only a few examples.

5.2.4 Electric Model of the Synapse

At the neuromuscular junction, Fatt and Katz (1951) showed that acetylcholine significantly increases the permeability of the cell membrane to small ions, whereas Takeuchi and Takeuchi (1960) demonstrated that chloride conductance was unaffected (in fact, $g_{Cl} \approx 0$). What happens if the membrane becomes equally permeable to sodium and potassium ions? Such a condition would alter the membrane potential from near the potassium Nernst potential to a value that approximates the average of the sodium and potassium equilibrium potentials. (This potential, in turn, is close to zero transmembrane voltage and is entirely adequate to initiate an activation.) If the postsynaptic region is voltage-clamped, the value that reduces the membrane current to zero during transmitter release is called the *reversal voltage* V_r. One can show that it equals the average Nernst potential of sodium and potassium, as mentioned above. In the neuromuscular junction in skeletal muscle, this reversal voltage is about -15 mV.

The electric behavior at a synapse can be estimated by examining an equivalent circuit of the postsynaptic membrane, such as that shown in Figure 5.2. Two regions are identified: One represents the membrane associated with receptors sensitive to the transmitter, and the other the normal excitable membrane of the cell. In Figure 5.2 these two regions are represented by discrete elements, but in reality these are distributed along the structure that constitutes the actual cell. This figure depicts a neu-

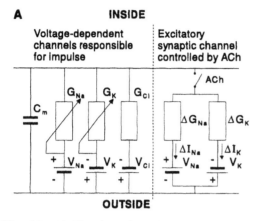

Fig. 5.2 (A) Electric model of the postsynaptic cell with excitatory synapse (a neuromuscular junction is specifically represented). Most of the cell is bounded by normal excitable membrane, as described on the left. In addition, a specialized postsynaptic region (end-plate) exists that is sensitive to the chemical transmitter ACh. When the ACh is released, it diffuses to receptor sites on the postjunctional membrane, resulting in the opening of potassium and sodium gates. This effect is mimicked in the model through closing of the switch, hence introducing the high transmembrane potassium and sodium conductance (ΔG_{Na} and ΔG_K). (B) The corresponding model with an inhibitory synapse.

romuscular junction, where the release of acetylcholine results in the elevation of sodium and potassium conductance in the target region, which is in turn depicted by the closing of the ACh switch. Upon closure of this switch,

$$\Delta I_{Na} = \Delta G_{Na} (V_m - V_{Na}) \quad (5.1)$$
$$\Delta I_K = \Delta G_K (V_m - V_K) \quad (5.2)$$

where

I_{Na}, I_K = sodium and potassium ion currents [μA/cm^2]
$\Delta G_{Na}, \Delta G_K$ = additional sodium and potassium conductances following activation by ACh (i.e., nearly equal large conductances) [mS/cm^2]
V_{Na}, V_K = the Nernst voltages corresponding to the sodium and potassium concentrations [mV]
V_m = membrane voltage [mV]

If we now introduce and maintain the reversal voltage across the postsynaptic membrane through a voltage clamp, Equations 5.1 and 5.2 are replaced by:

$$\Delta I_{Na} = \Delta G_{Na} (V_R - V_{Na}) \quad (5.3)$$
$$\Delta I_K = \Delta G_K (V_R - V_K) \quad (5.4)$$

since the transmembrane voltage V_m takes the value V_R, the reversal voltage.

For the conditions described by Equations 5.3 and 5.4, since the total current at the reversal voltage is zero, it follows that the sodium and potassium ion currents are equal and opposite in sign (i.e., $\Delta I_{Na} = -\Delta I_K$). Consequently, applying this condition to Equations 5.3 and 5.4 results in the following:

$$\Delta G_{Na} (V_R - V_{Na}) = -\Delta G_K (V_R - V_K) \quad (5.5)$$

Collecting terms in Equation 5.5 gives

$$(\Delta G_{Na} + \Delta G_K) V_R = \Delta G_{Na} V_{Na} + \Delta G_K V_K \quad (5.6)$$

and solving for the reversal voltage results in

$$V_R = \frac{\Delta G_{Na} V_{Na} + \Delta G_K V_K}{\Delta G_{Na} + \Delta G_K} \quad (5.7)$$
$$= \frac{\dfrac{\Delta G_{Na}}{\Delta G_K} V_{Na} + V_K}{\dfrac{\Delta G_{Na}}{\Delta G_K} + 1}$$

From Equation 5.7 it is easy to see that if the introduction of ACh causes an equal increase in the sodium and potassium conductances—that is, if

$$\frac{\Delta G_{Na}}{\Delta G_K} = 1 \quad (5.8)$$

then

$$V_R = \frac{V_{Na} + V_K}{2} \qquad (5.9)$$

as noted previously. For the frog's neuromuscular junction the reversal voltage comes to around -25 mV. In practice, the reversal voltage is a little closer to zero, which means that ACh increases the sodium conductance a little more than it does the potassium conductance. It is also clear that the increase of these sodium and potassium conductances must occur simultaneously. The differences in the mechanisms of the membrane activation and synaptic voltages are described in Table 5.1.

Returning to Figure 5.2, and applying Thevenin's theorem, we can simplify the receptor circuit to consist of a single battery whose *emf* is the average of V_{Na} and V_K (hence V_R), and with a conductivity $g_R = g_{Na} + g_K$. Its effect on the normal membrane of the postsynaptic cell can be calculated since the total current at any node is necessarily zero—that is, there are no applied currents. Consequently,

$$G_R (V_m - V_R) + G_K (V_m - V_K)$$
$$+ G_{Na} (V_m - V_{Na}) = 0 \qquad (5.10)$$

The chloride path in Figure 5.2 is not included in Equation 5.10, since $g_{Cl} \approx 0$, as noted above. Solving for the postsynaptic potential V_m results in

$$V_m = \frac{G_R V_R + G_K V_K + G_{Na} V_{Na}}{G_R + G_K + G_{Na}} \qquad (5.11)$$

This expression is only approximate since the distributed membrane is represented by a discrete (lumped) membrane. In addition, if the membrane is brought to or beyond threshold, then the linear circuit representation of Figure 5.2 becomes invalid. Nevertheless, Equation 5.11 should be a useful measure of whether the postsynaptic potential is likely to result in excitation of the postsynaptic cell.

5.3 RECEPTOR CELLS

5.3.1 Introduction

To begin the overview of the nervous system, we consider the sensory inputs to the body and how they are initiated. There are many specialized receptor cells, each characterized by a modality to which it is particularly sensitive and to which it responds by generating a train of action pulses. We are particularly interested in the structure and function of these receptor cells and focus on the *Pacinian corpuscle* as an example.

5.3.2 Various Types of Receptor Cells

One of the most important properties required to maintain the life of the living organism is the ability to react to external stimuli. Sense organs are specialized for this task. The es-

Table 5.1 Comparison of the mechanisms of membrane activation with synaptic voltage change for the postsynaptic neuromuscular junction

Feature	Membrane region	Synaptic region
Early effect	depolarization	arrival of acetylcholine
Changes in membrane conductance during		
rising phase	specific increase in G_{Na}	simultaneous increase in G_{Na} and G_K
falling phase	specific increase in G_K	passive decay
Equilibrium voltage of active membrane	$V_{Na} = +50$ mV	reversal voltage close to 0 mV
Other features	regenerative ascent followed by refractory period	no evidence for regenerative action or refractoriness
Pharmacology	blocked by TTX, not influenced by curare	blocked by curare, not influenced by TTX

Source: After Kuffler, Nicholls, and Martin, 1984.

sential element of these organs is the receptor cell, which responds to physical and chemical stimuli by sending information to the central nervous system. In general, a receptor cell may respond to several forms of energy, but each is specialized to respond primarily to one particular type. For instance, the *rods* and *cones* in the eye (photoreceptors) can respond to pressure, but they have a particularly low threshold to electromagnetic energy in the certain frequency band of electromagnetic radiation, namely visible light. In fact, they are the only receptor cells with such low thresholds to light stimulus.

There are at least a dozen conscious sense modalities with which we are familiar. In addition, there are other sensory receptors whose information processing goes on without our awareness. Together these may be classified as (1) *extroreceptors,* which sense stimuli arising external to the body; (2) *introreceptors,* which respond to physical or chemical qualities within the body; and (3) *proprioceptors,* which provide information on the body's position. Examples in each of these categories include the following:

1. Extroreceptors
   a. Photoreceptors in the retina for, vision
   b. Chemoreceptors for sensing of smell and taste
   c. Mechanoreceptors for sensing sound, in the cochlea, or in the skin, for touch sensation
   d. Thermoreceptors (i.e., Krause and Ruffini cells), for sensing cold and heat
2. Introreceptors
   a. Chemoreceptors in the carotid artery and aorta, responding to the partial pressure of oxygen, and in the breathing center, responding to the partial pressure of carbon dioxide
   b. Mechanoreceptors in the labyrinth
   c. Osmoreceptors in the hypothalamus, registering the osmotic pressure of the blood
3. Proprioceptors
   a. Muscle spindle, responding to changes in muscle length
   b. Golgi tendon organ, measuring muscle tension

The sensory receptor contains membrane regions that respond to one of the various forms of incident stimuli by a depolarization (or hyperpolarization). In some cases the receptor is actually part of the afferent neuron but, in others it consists of a separate specialized cell. All receptor cells have a common feature: They are *transducers*—that is, they change energy from one form to another. For instance, the sense of touch in the skin arises from the conversion of mechanical and/or thermal energy into the electric energy (ionic currents) of the nerve impulse. In general, the receptor cells do not generate an activation impulse themselves. Instead, they generate a gradually increasing potential, which triggers activation of the afferent nerve fiber to which they are connected.

The electric events in receptors may be separated into two distinct components:

1. Development of a *receptor voltage,* which is the graded response of the receptor to the stimulus. It is the initial electric event in the receptor.
2. Subsequent buildup of a *generator voltage,* which is the electric phenomenon that triggers impulse propagation in the axon. It is the final electric event before activation, which, in turn, follows the "all-or-nothing" law.

These voltage changes are, however, one and the same in a receptor such as the Pacinian corpuscle, in which there are no specialized receptor cells. But in cases like the retina where specialized receptor cells (i.e., the rods and cones) do exist, these voltages are separate. In the following, we consider the Pacinian corpuscle in more detail (Granit, 1955).

Because the neural output is carried in the form of all-or-nothing action pulses, we must look to another form of signal than one that is amplitude modulated. In fact, the generator or receptor potentials cause repetitive firing of action pulses on the afferent neuron, and the firing rate (and rate of change) is reflective of the sensory input. This coded signal can be characteristic of the modality being transduced.

In a process of *adaptation,* the frequency of action potential firing decreases in time with respect to a steady stimulus. One can separate the responses into fast and slow rates of adaptation, depending on how quickly the frequency reduction takes place (i.e., muscle spindle is slow whereas touch is fast).

5.3.3 The Pacinian Corpuscle

The Pacinian corpuscle is a touch receptor which, under the microscope, resembles an onion (see Fig. 5.3). It is 0.5–1 mm long and 0.3–0.7 mm thick and consists of several concentric layers. The center of the corpuscle includes the core, where the unmyelinated terminal part of the afferent neuron is located. The first node of Ranvier is also located inside the core. Several mitochondria exist in the corpuscle, indicative of high energy production.

Werner R. Loewenstein (1959) stimulated the corpuscle with a piezoelectric crystal and measured the generator voltage (from the unmyelinated terminal axon) and the action potential (from the nodes of Ranvier) with an external electrode. He peeled off the layers of the corpuscle, and even after the last layer was removed, the corpuscle generated signals similar to those observed with the capsule intact (see recordings shown in Fig. 5.4).

The *generator voltage* has properties similar to these of the excitatory postsynaptic voltage. (The generator voltage is a graded response

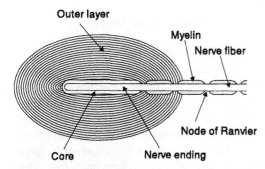

Fig. 5.3 The Pacinian corpuscle consists of a myelinated sensory neuron whose terminal portion is unmyelinated. The unmyelinated nerve ending and the first node lie within a connective tissue capsule, as shown.

whereby a weak stimulus generates a low generator voltage whereas a strong stimulus generates a large generator voltage.) Even partial destruction of the corpuscle did not prevent it from producing a generator voltage. But when Loewenstein destroyed the nerve ending itself, a generator voltage could no longer be elicited. This observation formed the basis for supposing that the transducer itself was located in the nerve ending. The generator voltage does not propagate on the nerve fiber (in fact, the nerve ending is electrically inexcitable) but, rather, triggers the activation process in the first node of Ranvier by electrotonic (passive) conduction. If the first node is blocked, no activation is initiated in the nerve fiber.

The ionic flow mechanism underlying the generator (receptor) voltage is the same as that for the excitatory postsynaptic voltage. Thus deformation of the Pacinian corpuscle increases both the sodium and potassium conductances such that their ratio (P_{Na}/P_K) increases and depolarization of the membrane potential results. As a result, the following behavior is observed:

1. Small *(electrotonic)* currents flow from the depolarized unmyelinated region of the axon to the nodes of Ranvier.
2. On the unmyelinated membrane, local graded generator voltages are produced independently at separate sites.
3. The aforementioned separate receptor voltages are summed in the first node of Ranvier.
4. The summed receptor voltages, which exceed threshold at the first node of Ranvier, generate an action impulse. This is evidence of *spatial summation,* and is similar to the same phenomenon observed in the excitatory postsynaptic potential.

5.4 ANATOMY AND PHYSIOLOGY OF THE BRAIN

5.4.1 Introduction

Action pulses generated at the distal end of sensory neurons propagate first to the cell body and then onward, conveyed by long axonal

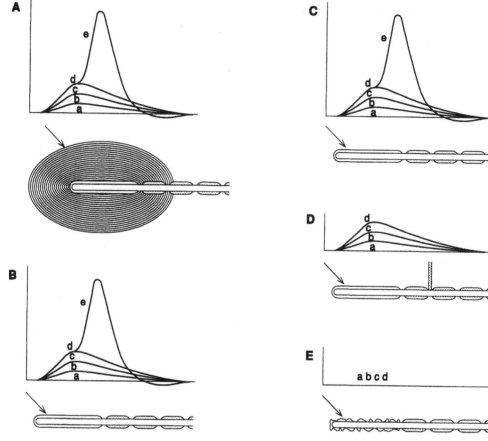

Fig. 5.4 Loewenstein's experiments with the Pacinian corpuscle. (A) The normal response of the generator voltage for increasing applied force (a)–(e). (B) The layers of the corpuscle have been removed, leaving the nerve terminal intact. The response to application of mechanical force is unchanged from A. (C) Partial destruction of the core sheath does not change the response from A or B. (D) Blocking the first node of Ranvier eliminates the initiation of the activation process but does not interfere with the formation of the generator voltage. (E) Degeneration of the nerve ending prevents the creation of the generator voltage.

pathways. These ascend the spinal cord (dorsal root) until they reach the lower part of the central nervous system. Here the signals are relayed to other neurons, which in turn relay them onward. Three or four such relays take place before the signals reach particular loci in the cerebral cortex. Signal processing takes place at all levels, resulting in the state of awareness and conscious recognition of the various signals that characterize human physiology. The important integrative activity of the brain has been the subject of intense study, but its complexity has slowed the rate of progress. In this section a brief description is given of both the anatomy and the physiology of the brain.

5.4.2   Brain Anatomy

The brain consists of 10^{10}–10^{11} neurons that are very closely interconnected via axons and dendrites. The neurons themselves are vastly outnumbered by glial cells. One neuron may receive stimuli through synapses from as many as 10^3 to 10^5 other neurons (Nunez, 1981). Embryologically the brain is formed when the front end of the central neural system has folded. The brain consists of five main parts, as described in Figure 5.5:

1. The cerebrum, including the two cerebral hemispheres

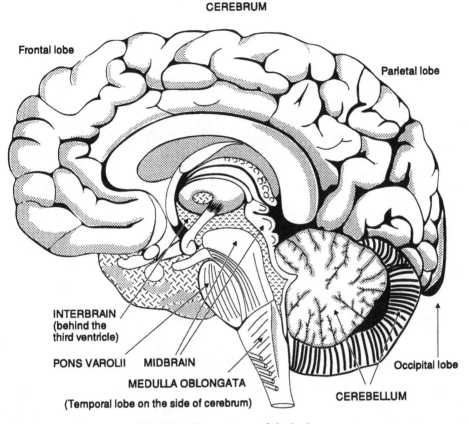

CEREBRUM

Frontal lobe

Parietal lobe

INTERBRAIN
(behind the
third ventricle)

PONS VAROLII   MIDBRAIN

MEDULLA OBLONGATA

(Temporal lobe on the side of cerebrum)

Occipital lobe

CEREBELLUM

Fig. 5.5   The anatomy of the brain.

2. The interbrain (diencephalon)
3. The midbrain
4. The pons Varolii and cerebellum
5. The medulla oblongata

The entire human brain weighs about 1500 g (Williams and Warwick, 1989). In the brain the *cerebrum* is the largest part. The surface of the cerebrum is strongly folded. These folds are divided into two hemispheres which are separated by a deep *fissure* and connected by the *corpus callosum*. Existing within the brain are three *ventricles* containing *cerebrospinal fluid*. The hemispheres are divided into the following lobes: *lobus frontalis, lobus parietalis, lobus occipitalis,* and *lobus temporalis.* The surface area of the cerebrum is about 1600 cm², and its thickness is 3 mm. Six layers, or *laminae,* each consisting of different neuronal types and populations, can be observed in this surface layer. The higher cerebral functions, accurate

sensations, and the voluntary motor control of muscles are located in this region.

The *interbrain* or *diencephalon* is surrounded by the cerebrum and is located around the third ventricle. It includes the *thalamus,* which is a bridge connecting the sensory paths. The *hypothalamus,* which is located in the lower part of the interbrain, is important for the regulation of autonomic (involuntary) functions. Together with the *hypophysis,* it regulates hormonal secretions. The *midbrain* is a small part of the brain. The *pons Varolii* is an interconnection of neural tracts; the *cerebellum* controls fine movement. The *medulla oblongata* resembles the spinal cord to which it is immediately connected. Many reflex centers, such as the vasomotor center and the breathing center, are located in the medulla oblongata.

In the cerebral cortex one may locate many different areas of specialized brain function (Penfield and Rasmussen, 1950; Kiloh, Mc-

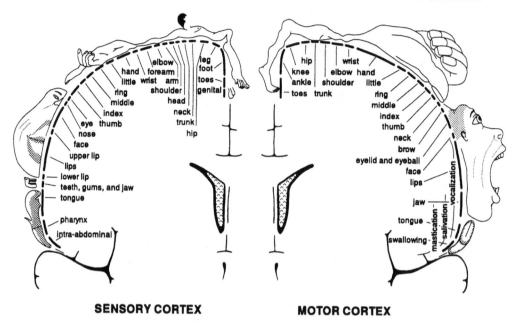

Fig. 5.6   The division of sensory (left) and motor (right) functions in the cerebral cortex. (From Penfield and Rasmussen, 1950.)

Comas, and Osselton, 1981). The higher brain functions occur in the frontal lobe, the visual center is located in the occipital lobe, and the sensory area and motor area are located on both sides of the central fissure. There are specific areas in the sensory and motor cortex whose elements correspond to certain parts of the body. The size of each such area is proportional to the required accuracy of sensory or motor control. These regions are described in Figure 5.6. Typically, the sensory areas represented by the lips and the hands are large, and the areas represented by the midbody and eyes are small. The visual center is located in a different part of the brain. The motor area, the area represented by the hands and the speaking organs, is large.

5.4.3   Brain Function

Most of the information from the sensory organs is communicated through the spinal cord to the brain. There are special tracts in both spinal cord and brain for various modalities. For example, touch receptors in the trunk synapse with interneurons in the dorsal horn of the spinal cord. These interneurons (sometimes referred to as second sensory neurons) then usually cross to the other side of the spinal cord and ascend the white matter of the cord to the brain in the lateral spinothalamic tract. In the brain they synapse again with a second group of interneurons (or third sensory neuron) in the thalamus. The third sensory neurons connect to higher centers in the cerebral cortex.

In the area of vision, afferent fibers from the photoreceptors carry signals to the brain stem through the optic nerve and optic tract to synapse in the lateral geniculate body (a part of the thalamus). From here axons pass to the occipital lobe of the cerebral cortex. In addition, branches of the axons of the optic tract synapse with neurons in the zone between thalamus and midbrain which is the pretectal nucleus and superior colliculus. These, in turn, synapse with preganglionic parasympathetic neurons whose axons follow the oculomotor nerve to the ciliary ganglion (located just behind the eyeball). The reflex loop is closed by postganglionic fibers which pass along ciliary nerves to the iris muscles (controlling pupil aperture) and to muscles controlling the lens curvature (adjusting its refractive or focusing qualities). Other reflexes concerned with head and/or eye movements may also be initiated.

Motor signals to muscles of the trunk and periphery from higher motor centers of the cerebral cortex first travel along upper motor neurons to the medulla oblongata. From here most of the axons of the upper motor neurons cross to the other side of the central nervous system and descend the spinal cord in the lateral corticospinal tract; the remainder travel down the cord in the anterior corticospinal tract. The upper motor neurons eventually synapse with lower motor neurons in the ventral horn of the spinal cord; the lower motor neurons complete the path to the target muscles. Most reflex motor movements involve complex neural integration and coordinate signals to the muscles involved in order to achieve a smooth performance.

Effective integration of sensory information requires that this information be collected at a single center. In the cerebral cortex, one can indeed locate specific areas identified with specific sensory inputs (Penfield and Rasmussen, 1950; Kiloh, McComas, and Osselton, 1981). While the afferent signals convey information regarding stimulus strength, recognition of the modality depends on pinpointing the anatomical classification of the afferent pathways. (This can be demonstrated by interchanging the afferent fibers from, say, auditory and tactile receptors, in which case sound inputs are perceived as of tactile origin and vice versa.)

The higher brain functions take place in the frontal lobe, the visual center is in the occipital lobe, the sensory area and motor area are located on both sides of the central fissure. As described above, there is an area in the sensory cortex whose elements correspond to each part of the body. In a similar way, a part of the brain contains centers for generating command (efferent) signals for control of the body's musculature. Here, too, one finds projections from specific cortical areas to specific parts of the body.

5.5 CRANIAL NERVES

In the central nervous system there are 12 *cranial nerves*. They leave directly from the cranium rather than the spinal cord. They are listed in Table 5.2 along with their functions. The following cranial nerves have special importance: the *olfactory* (I) and *optic* (II) nerves, which carry sensory information from the nose and eye; and the *auditory-vestibular* (VIII) nerve, which carries information from the ear and the balance organ. Sensory information from the skin of the face and head is carried by the *trigeminal* (V) nerve. Eye movements are controlled by three cranial nerves (III, IV, and VI). The *vagus* nerve (X) controls heart

Table 5.2 The cranial nerves

Number	Name	Sensory/ Motor	Functions	Origin or terminus in the brain
I	olfactory	s	smell	cerebral hemispheres (ventral part)
II	optic	s	vision	thalamus
III	oculomotor	m	eye movement	midbrain
IV	trochlear	m	eye movement	midbrain
V	trigeminal	m	masticatory movements	midbrain and pons
		s	sensitivity of face and tongue	medulla
VI	abducens	m	eye movement	medulla
VII	facial	m	facial movement	medulla
VIII	auditory	s	hearing	medulla
	vestibular	s	balance	
IX	glossopharyngeal	s,m	tongue and pharynx	medulla
X	vagus	s,m	heart, blood vessels, viscera	medulla
XI	spinal accessory	m	neck muscles and viscera	medulla
XII	hypoglossal	m		medulla

function and internal organs as well as blood vessels.

REFERENCES

Fatt P, Katz B (1951): An analysis of the end-plate potential recorded with an intracellular electrode. *J. Physiol. (Lond.)* 115: 320–70.

Granit R, Haase J, Rutledge LT (1960): Recurrent inhibition in relation to frequency of firing and limitation of discharge rate of extensor motoneurons. *J. Physiol. (Lond.)* 154: 308–28.

Granit R, Renkin B (1961): Net depolarization and discharge rate of motoneurons, as measured by recurrent inhibition. *J. Physiol. (Lond.)* 158: 461–75.

Hille B (1970): Ionic channels in nerve membranes. *Prog. Biophys. Mol. Biol.* 21: 1–32.

Loewenstein WR (1959): The generation of electric activity in a nerve ending. *Ann. N.Y. Acad. Sci.* 81: 367–87.

Schmidt RF (ed.) (1981): *Fundamentals of Sensory Physiology,* 2nd ed., 286 pp. Springer-Verlag, New York, Heidelberg, Berlin.

Stevens CF (1968): Synaptic physiology. *Proc. IEEE* 56:(6) 916–30. (Special issue on studies of neural elements and systems).

Takeuchi A, Takeuchi N (1960): On the permeability of end-plate membrane during the action of transmitter. *J. Physiol. (Lond.)* 154: 52–67.

REFERENCES, BOOKS

Granit R (1955): *Receptors and Sensory Perception,* 369 pp. Yale University Press, New Haven.

Hille B (1992): *Ionic Channels of Excitable Membranes,* 2nd ed., 607 pp. Sinauer Assoc., Sunderland, Mass. (1st ed., 1984)

Jewett DL, Rayner, MD (1984): *Basic Concepts of Neuronal Function,* 411 pp. Little Brown, Boston.

Kiloh LG, McComas AJ, Osselton JW (1981): *Clinical Electroencephalography,* 4th ed., 239 pp. Butterworth, London.

Kuffler SW, Nicholls JG, Martin AR (1984): *From Neuron to Brain,* 2nd ed., 651 pp. Sinauer Assoc., Sunderland, Mass.

Nunez PL (1981): *Electric Fields of the Brain: The Neurophysics of EEG,* 484 pp. Oxford University Press, New York.

Patton HD, Fuchs AF, Hille B, Scher AM, Steiner R (eds.) (1989): *Textbook of Physiology,* 21st ed., 1596 pp. W. B. Saunders, Philadelphia.

Penfield W, Rasmussen T (1950): *The Cerebral Cortex of Man: A Clinical Study of Localization of Function,* 248 pp. Macmillan, New York.

Schmidt RF (ed.) (1981): *Fundamentals of Sensory Physiology,* 2nd ed., 286 pp. Springer-Verlag, New York, Heidelberg, Berlin.

Shepherd GM (1988): *Neurobiology,* 689 pp. Oxford University Press, New York.

Williams PL, Warwick R (eds.) (1989): *Gray's Anatomy,* 37th ed., 1598 pp. Churchill Livingstone, Edinburgh.

6

The Heart

6.1 ANATOMY
AND PHYSIOLOGY
OF THE HEART

6.1.1 Location of the Heart

The heart is located in the chest between the lungs behind the sternum and above the diaphragm. It is surrounded by the pericardium. Its size is about that of a fist, and its weight is about 250–300 g. Its center is located about 1.5 cm to the left of the midsagittal plane. Located above the heart are the great vessels: the superior and inferior vena cava, the pulmonary artery and vein, as well as the aorta. The aortic arch lies behind the heart. The esophagus and the spine lie further behind the heart. An overall view is given in Figure 6.1 (Williams and Warwick, 1989).

6.1.2 Anatomy of the Heart

The walls of the heart are composed of cardiac muscle, called *myocardium*. It also has *striations* similar to skeletal muscle. It consists of four compartments: the *right* and *left atria* and *ventricles*. The heart is oriented so that the anterior aspect is the right ventricle while the posterior aspect shows the left atrium (see Fig. 6.2). The atria form one unit and the ventricles an-

other. This has special importance to the electric function of the heart, which will be discussed later. The left ventricular free wall and the *septum* are much thicker than the right ventricular wall. This is logical since the left ventricle pumps blood to the systemic circulation, where the pressure is considerably higher than for the pulmonary circulation, which arises from right ventricular outflow.

The cardiac muscle fibers are oriented spirally (see Fig. 6.3) and are divided into four groups: Two groups of fibers wind around the outside of both ventricles. Beneath these fibers a third group winds around both ventricles. Beneath these fibers a fourth group winds only around the left ventricle. The fact that cardiac muscle cells are oriented more tangentially than radially, and that the resistivity of the muscle is lower in the direction of the fiber has importance in electrocardiography and magnetocardiography.

The heart has four valves. Between the right atrium and ventricle lies the *tricuspid valve,* and between the left atrium and ventricle is the *mitral valve.* The *pulmonary valve* lies between the right ventricle and the pulmonary artery, while the *aortic valve* lies in the outflow tract of the left ventricle (controlling flow to the aorta).

The blood returns from the systemic circu-

119

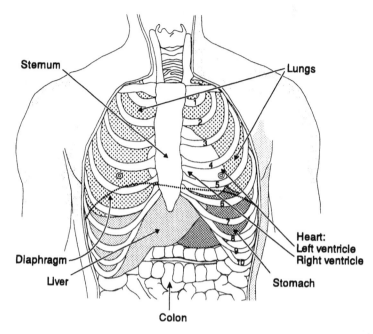

Fig. 6.1 Location of the heart in the thorax. It is bounded by the diaphragm, lungs, esophagus, descending aorta, and sternum.

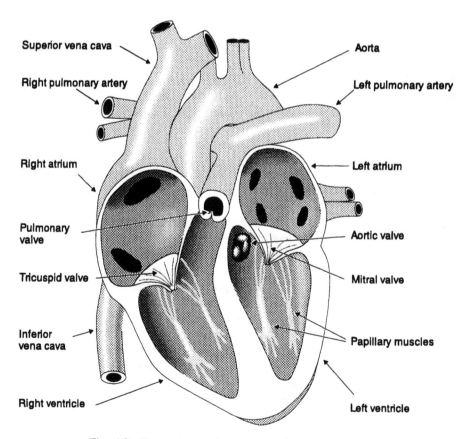

Fig. 6.2 The anatomy of the heart and associated vessels.

120

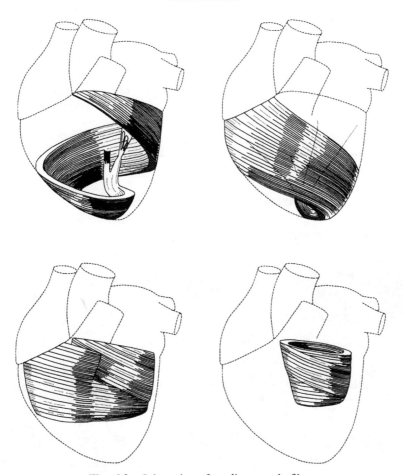

Fig. 6.3 Orientation of cardiac muscle fibers.

lation to the right atrium and from there goes through the tricuspid valve to the right ventricle. It is ejected from the right ventricle through the pulmonary valve to the lungs. Oxygenated blood returns from the lungs to the left atrium, and from there through the mitral valve to the left ventricle. Finally blood is pumped through the aortic valve to the aorta and the systemic circulation.

6.2 ELECTRIC ACTIVATION OF THE HEART

6.2.1 Cardiac Muscle Cell

In the heart muscle cell, or *myocyte,* electric activation takes place by means of the same mechanism as in the nerve cell—that is, from the inflow of sodium ions across the cell mem-

brane. The amplitude of the action potential is also similar, being about 100 mV for both nerve and muscle. The duration of the cardiac muscle impulse is, however, two orders of magnitude longer than that in either nerve cell or skeletal muscle. A *plateau phase* follows cardiac depolarization, and thereafter repolarization takes place. As in the nerve cell, repolarization is a consequence of the outflow of potassium ions. The duration of the action impulse is about 300 ms, as shown in Figure 6.4 (Netter, 1971).

Associated with the electric activation of cardiac muscle cell is its mechanical contraction, which occurs a little later. For the sake of comparison, Figure 6.5 illustrates the electric activity and mechanical contraction of frog sartorius muscle, frog cardiac muscle, and smooth muscle from the rat uterus (Ruch and Patton, 1982).

An important distinction between cardiac

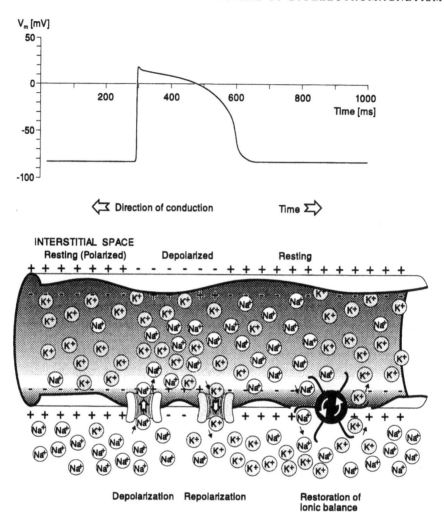

Fig. 6.4 Electrophysiology of the cardiac muscle cell.

muscle tissue and skeletal muscle is that in cardiac muscle, activation can propagate from one cell to another in any direction. As a result, the activation wavefronts are of rather complex shape. The only exception is the boundary between the atria and ventricles, which the activation wave normally cannot cross except along a special conduction system, since a nonconducting barrier of fibrous tissue is present.

6.2.2   The Conduction System of the Heart

Located in the right atrium at the superior vena cava is the *sinus node* (*sinoatrial* or *SA node*) which consists of specialized muscle cells. The

sinoatrial node in humans is in the shape of a crescent and is about 15 mm long and 5 mm wide (see Fig. 6.6). The SA nodal cells are self-excitatory, *pacemaker cells*. They generate an action potential at the rate of about 70 per minute. From the sinus node, activation propagates throughout the atria, but cannot propagate directly across the boundary between atria and ventricles, as noted above.

The *atrioventricular node* (AV node) is located at the boundary between the atria and ventricles; it has an intrinsic frequency of about 50 pulses/min. However, if the AV node is triggered with a higher pulse frequency, it follows this higher frequency. In a normal heart, the AV node provides the only conducting path

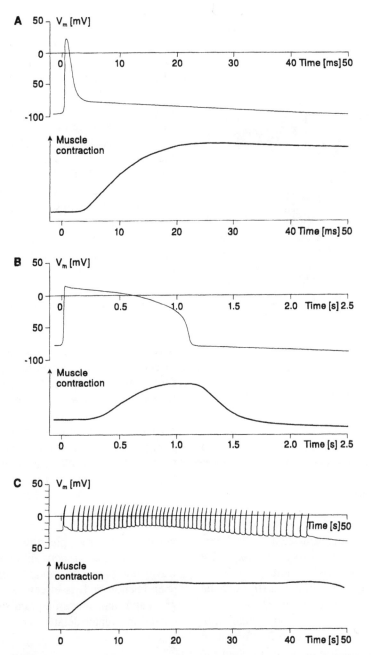

Fig. 6.5 Electric and mechanical activity in (A) frog sartorius muscle cell, (B) frog cardiac muscle cell, and (C) rat uterus wall smooth muscle cell. In each section the upper curve shows the transmembrane voltage behavior, whereas the lower one describes the mechanical contraction associated with it.

from the atria to the ventricles. Thus, under normal conditions, the latter can be excited only by pulses that propagate through it.

Propagation from the AV node to the ventricles is provided by a specialized conduction system. Proximally, this system is composed of a common bundle, called the *bundle of His* (named after German physician Wilhelm His, Jr., 1863–1934). More distally, it separates into two *bundle branches* propagating along each

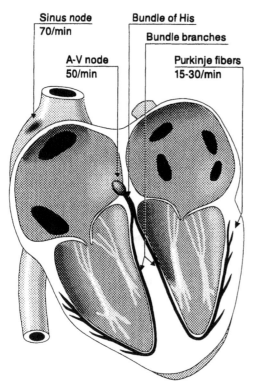

Fig. 6.6 The conduction system of the heart.

ity appears as if it were propagating from epicardium toward the endocardium.

Because the intrinsic rate of the sinus node is the greatest, it sets the activation frequency of the whole heart. If the connection from the atria to the AV node fails, the AV node adopts its intrinsic frequency. If the conduction system fails at the bundle of His, the ventricles will beat at the rate determined by their own region that has the highest intrinsic frequency. The electric events in the heart are summarized in Table 6.1. The waveforms of action impulse observed in different specialized cardiac tissue are shown in Figure 6.7.

A classical study of the propagation of excitation in human heart was made by Durrer and his co-workers (Durrer et al., 1970). They isolated the heart from a subject who had died of various cerebral conditions and who had no previous history of cardiac diseases. The heart was removed within 30 min post mortem and was perfused. As many as 870 electrodes were placed into the cardiac muscle; the electric activity was then recorded by a tape recorder and played back at a lower speed by the ECG writer; thus the effective paper speed was 960 mm/s, giving a time resolution better than 1 ms.

Figure 6.8 is redrawn from these experimental data. The ventricles are shown with the anterior wall of the left and partly that of the right ventricle opened. The isochronic surfaces show clearly that ventricular activation starts from the inner wall of the left ventricle and proceeds radially toward the epicardium. In the terminal part of ventricular activation, the excitation wavefront proceeds more tangentially. This phenomenon and its effects on electrocardiogram and magnetocardiogram signals are discussed in greater detail later.

side of the septum, constituting the *right* and *left bundle branches*. (The left bundle subsequently divides into an anterior and posterior branch.) Even more distally the bundles ramify into *Purkinje fibers* (named after Jan Evangelista Purkinje (Czech; 1787–1869)) that diverge to the inner sides of the ventricular walls. Propagation along the conduction system takes place at a relatively high speed once it is within the ventricular region, but prior to this (through the AV node) the velocity is extremely slow.

From the inner side of the ventricular wall, the many activation sites cause the formation of a wavefront which propagates through the ventricular mass toward the outer wall. This process results from cell-to-cell activation. After each ventricular muscle region has depolarized, repolarization occurs. Repolarization is not a propagating phenomenon, and because the duration of the action impulse is much shorter at the *epicardium* (the outer side of the cardiac muscle) than at the *endocardium* (the inner side of the cardiac muscle), the termination of activ-

6.3   THE GENESIS OF THE ELECTROCARDIOGRAM

6.3.1   Activation Currents in Cardiac Tissue

Section 6.2.1 discussed cardiac electric events on an intracellular level. Such electric signals

Table 6.1 Electric events in the heart

Location in the heart	Event	Time [ms]	ECG-terminology	Conduction velocity [m/s]	Intrinsic frequency [1/min]
SA node	impulse generated	0		0.05	70–80
atrium, Right	depolarization*	5	P	0.8–1.0	
Left	depolarization	85	P	0.8–1.0	
AV node	arrival of impulse	50	P-Q	0.02–0.05	
	departure of impulse	125	interval		
bundle of His	activated	130		1.0–1.5	
bundle branches	activated	145		1.0–1.5	
Purkinje fibers	activated	150		3.0–3.5	
endocardium					20–40
Septum	depolarization	175		0.3–(axial)	
Left ventricle	depolarization	190			
			QRS	0.8	
epicardium				(transverse)	
Left ventricle	depolarization	225			
Right ventricle	depolarization	250			
epicardium					
Left ventricle	repolarization	400			
Right ventricle	repolarization				
			T	0.5	
endocardium					
Left ventricle	repolarization	600			

*Atrial repolarization occurs during the ventricular depolarization; therefore, it is not normally seen in the electrocardiogram.

(as illustrated in Figs. 6.4, 6.5, and 6.7) may be recorded with a microelectrode, which is inserted inside a cardiac muscle cell. However, the electrocardiogram (ECG) is a recording of the electric potential, generated by the electric activity of the heart, on the surface of the thorax. The ECG thus represents the extracellular electric behavior of the cardiac muscle tissue. In this section we explain the genesis of the ECG signal via a highly idealized model.

Figure 6.9A and B show a segment of cardiac tissue through which propagating depolarization (A) and repolarization (B) wavefront planes are passing. In this illustration the wavefronts move from right to left, which means that the time axis points to the right. There are two important properties of cardiac tissue that we shall make use of to analyze the potential and current distribution associated with these propagating waves. First, cells are interconnected by low-resistance pathways (gap junctions), as a result of which currents flowing in the intracellular space of one cell pass freely

into the following cell. Second, the space between cells is very restrictive (accounting for less than 25% of the total volume). As a result, both intracellular and extracellular currents are confined to the direction parallel to the propagation of the plane wavefront.

The aforementioned conditions are exactly those for which the linear core conductor model, introduced in Section 3.4, fully applies; that is, both intracellular and extracellular currents flow in a linear path. In particular, when using the condition $I_i + I_o = 0$ and Equation 3.41.

$$\frac{\partial \Phi_i}{\partial x} = -I_i r_i, \qquad \frac{\partial \Phi_o}{\partial x} = -I_o r_o \qquad (3.41)$$

one obtains

$$\frac{\partial \Phi_i}{\partial x} = I_o r_i, \qquad \frac{\partial \Phi_o}{\partial x} = -I_o r_o \qquad (6.1)$$

Integrating from $x = -\infty$, to $x = x$ gives

$$\Phi_i = r_i \int I_o dx, \qquad \Phi_o = -r_o \int I_o dx \qquad (6.2)$$

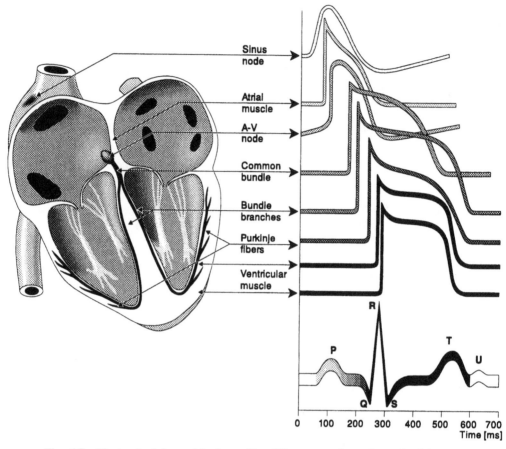

Fig. 6.7 Electrophysiology of the heart. The different waveforms for each of the specialized cells found in the heart are shown. The latency shown approximates that normally found in the healthy heart.

Subtracting the second of Equations 6.2 from the first and applying $V_m = \Phi_i - \Phi_o$, the definition of the transmembrane potential, we obtain:

$$V_m = (r_i + r_o) \int I_o dx \qquad (6.3)$$

From Equation 6.3 we obtain the following important relationships valid for linear core conductor conditions, namely that

$$\Phi_i = \frac{r_i}{r_i + r_o} V_m \qquad (6.4)$$

and

$$\Phi_o = -\frac{r_o}{r_i + r_o} V_m \qquad (6.5)$$

These equations describe "voltage divider" conditions and were first pointed out by Hodg-

kin and Rushton (1946). Note that they depend on the validity of Equation 3.36 which, in turn, requires that there be no external (polarizing) currents in the region under consideration.

6.3.2   Depolarization Wave

We may now apply Equation 6.5 to the propagating wave under investigation. The variation in the value of $V_m(x)$ is easy to infer from Figure 6.9C (dashed line) since in the *activated* region it is at the plateau voltage, generally around +40 mV, whereas in the *resting* region it is around −80 mV. The *transition* region is usually very narrow (about 1 mm, corresponding to a depolarization of about 1 ms and a velocity < 1 m/s), as the figure suggests. Application of Equation 6.4 results in the extracellular

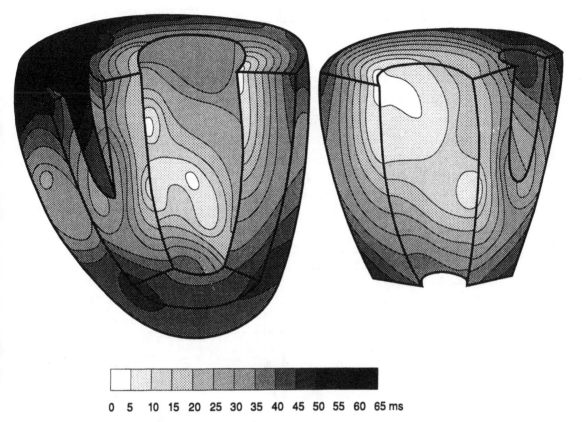

Fig. 6.8. Isochronic surfaces of the ventricular activation. (From Durrer et al., 1970.)

potential (Φ_o) behavior shown in Figure 6.9C (solid line). In Figure 6.9, the ratio $r_o/(r_o + r_i) = 0.5$ has been chosen on the basis of experimental evidence for propagation along the cardiac fiber axis (Kléber and Riegger, 1986).

The transmembrane current I_m can be evaluated from $V_m(x)$ in Figure 6.9C by applying the general cable equation (Equation 3.45):

$$\frac{\partial^2 V_m}{\partial x^2} = (r_i + r_o) \, i_m \qquad (3.45)$$

The equation for the transmembrane current i_m is thus

$$i_m = \frac{1}{r_i + r_o} \frac{\partial^2 V_m}{\partial x^2} \qquad (6.6)$$

This current is confined to the depolarization zone. As shown in Figure 6.9A, just to the right of the centerline it is inward (thick arrows), and just to the left it is outward (thin arrows). The inward portion reflects the sodium influx, trig-

gered by the very large and rapid rise in sodium permeability. The current outflow is the "local circuit" current which initially depolarizes the resting tissue, and which is advancing to the left (i.e., in the direction of propagation). The course of the transmembrane current is approximated in Figure 6.9E using Equation 6.6.

An examination of the extracellular potential Φ_o shows it to be uniform except for a rapid change across the wavefront. Such a change from plus to minus is what one would expect at a double-layer source where the dipole direction is from right to left (from minus to plus as explained in Section 11.2). So we conclude that for the depolarization (activation) of cardiac tissue a double layer appears at the wavefront with the dipole orientation in the direction of propagation. One can also approximate the source as proportional to the transmembrane current—estimated here by a lumped negative point source (on the right) and a lumped positive

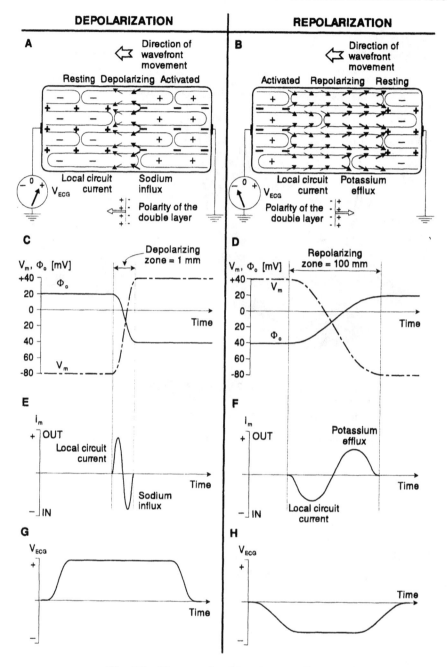

Fig. 6.9 The genesis of the electrocardiogram.

point source (on the left) which taken together constitute a dipole in the direction of propagation (to the left).

Finally, a double layer, whose positive side is pointing to the recording electrode (to the left), produces a positive (ECG) signal (Fig. 6.9G).

6.3.3 Repolarization Wave

The nature of the repolarization wave is in principle very different from that of the depolarization wave. Unlike depolarization, the repolarization is not a propagating phenomenon. If we examine the location of repolarizing cells at consecutive time instances, we can, however, approximate the repolarization with a proceeding wave phenomenon.

As stated previously, when a cell depolarizes, another cell close to it then depolarizes and produces an electric field which triggers the depolarization phenomenon. In this way, the depolarization proceeds as a propagating wave within cardiac tissue.

Repolarization in a cell occurs because the action pulse has only a certain duration; thus the cell repolarizes at a certain instant of time after its depolarization, not because of the repolarization of an adjoining cell. If the action pulses of all cells are of equal duration, the repolarization would of course accurately follow the same sequence as depolarization. In reality, however, this is not the case in ventricular muscle. The action pulses of the epicardial cells (on the outer surface) are of shorter duration than those of the endocardial cells (on the inner surface). Therefore, the "isochrones" of repolarizing cells proceed from the epicardium to the endocardium, giving the illusion that the repolarization proceeds as a wave from epicardium to endocardium.

If the cardiac action pulse were always of the same shape, then following propagation of depolarization from right to left, the recovery (repolarization) would also proceed from right to left. This case is depicted in the highly idealized Figure 6.9B, where the cells that were activated earliest must necessarily recover first. The recovery of cardiac cells is relatively slow, requiring approximately 100 ms (compare this with the time required to complete activation—roughly 1 ms). For this reason, in Figure 6.9B we have depicted the recovery interval as much wider than the activation interval.

The polarity of $V_m(x)$ decreases from its plateau value of +40 mV on the left to the resting value of −80 mV on the right (Fig. 6.9D (dashed line)). Again, Equation 6.5 may be applied, in this case showing that the extracellular potential Φ_o (solid line) increases from minus to plus. In this case the double layer source is directed from left to right. And, it is spread out over a wide region of the heart muscle. (In fact, if activation occupies 1 mm, then recovery occupies 100 mm, a relationship that could only

be suggested in Fig. 6.9B, since in fact, it encompasses the entire heart!)

The transmembrane current I_m can be again evaluated from $V_m(x)$ in Figure 6.9D by applying Equation 6.6. As shown in Figure 6.9B, to the right of the centerline it is outward (thick arrows) and just to the left it is inward (thin arrows). The outward portion reflects the potassium efflux due to the rapid rise of potassium permeability. The current inflow is again the "local circuit" current. The course of the transmembrane current during repolarization is approximated in Figure 6.9F.

Thus, during repolarization, a double layer is formed that is similar to that observed during depolarization. The double layer in repolarization, however, has a polarity opposite to that in depolarization, and thus its negative side points toward the recording electrode; as a result, a negative (ECG) signal is recorded (Figure 6.9H).

In real heart muscle, since the action potential duration at the epicardium is actually shorter than at the endocardium, the recovery phase appears to move from epicardium to endocardium, that is, just the opposite to activation (and opposite the direction in the example above). As a consequence, the recovery dipole is in the same direction as the activation dipole (i.e., reversed from that shown in Fig. 6.9B). Since the recovery and activation dipoles are thus in the same direction one can explain the common observation that the normal activation and recovery ECG signal has the same polarity.

REFERENCES

Durrer D, van Dam RT, Freud GE, Janse MJ, Meijler FL, Arzbaecher RC (1970): Total excitation of the isolated human heart. *Circulation* 41:(6) 899–912.

Fozzard HA, Haber E, Jennings RB, Katz AM, Morgan HI (eds.) (1991): *The Heart and Cardiovascular System*, 2193 pp. Raven Press, New York.

Hodgkin AL, Rushton WA (1946): The electrical constants of a crustacean nerve fiber. *Proc. R. Soc. (Biol.)* B133: 444–79.

Kléber AG, Riegger CB (1986): Electrical constants

of arterially perfused rabbit papillary muscle. *J. Physiol. (Lond.)* 385: 307–24.

Netter FH (1971): *Heart,* Vol. 5, 293 pp. The Ciba Collection of Medical Illustrations, Ciba Pharmaceutical Company, Summit, N.J.

Ruch TC, Patton HD (eds.) (1982): *Physiology and Biophysics,* 20th ed., 1242 pp. W. B. Saunders, Philadelphia.

Williams PL, Warwick R (eds.) (1989): *Gray's Anatomy,* 37th ed., 1598 pp. Churchill Livingstone, Edinburgh.

REFERENCES, BOOKS

Hurst JW, Schlant RC, Rackley CE, Sonnenblick EH, Wenger NK (eds.) (1990): *The Heart: Arteries and Veins,* 7th ed., 2274 pp. McGraw-Hill, New York.

Macfarlane PW, Lawrie TDV (eds.) (1989): *Comprehensive Electrocardiology: Theory and Practice in Health and Disease,* 1st ed., Vols. 1, 2, and 3, 1785 pp. Pergamon Press, New York.

II

Bioelectric Sources and Conductors
and their Modeling

A practical way to investigate the function of living organisms is to construct a simple model that follows their operation with reasonable accuracy. Thus, to investigate the function of bioelectric sources and conductors, we need to construct models that accurately describe the bioelectric behavior of the tissue they represent and that can be mathematically analyzed.

Chapter 7 of Part II first characterizes the nature of bioelectric sources and conductors. It points out that in contrast to electronic circuits, in which the electric properties of the components are concentrated, the biological organs are *distributed volume sources* and *volume conductors*. The standard equations describing the electric field of a volume source in a volume conductor are derived. The electric properties of the human body as a volume conductor are then characterized. This is followed by an introductory discussion of modeling of the biological volume sources and volume conductors. The fundamental concepts of *forward* and *inverse problems* are then defined and their solvability is discussed.

Chapter 8 provides a detailed theoretical discussion of various source-field models and their mathematical basis. Chapter 9 follows with a discussion of a model of the biological tissue as a volume conductor. This is called the *bidomain* model.

Chapter 10 further explores the modeling of biological sources in regard to electronic neuron models. The bioelectric behavior of neural cells and the electric concepts used in this discussion are further exemplified with electronic circuits. The discussion on electronic neuron models may also serve as a basic introduction to neurocomputers, which are a fascinating example of applying biological principles to technological systems. That topic is, however, far beyond the scope of this book.

7

Volume Source and Volume Conductor

7.1 CONCEPTS OF VOLUME SOURCE AND VOLUME CONDUCTOR

The field of science and engineering most relevant to electrophysiology and bioelectromagnetism is electrical engineering. However, the electrical engineering student will quickly note some important distinctions in emphasis between these disciplines. Much of electrical engineering deals with networks made up of batteries, resistances, capacitances, and inductors. Each of these elements, while actually comprising a physical object, is considered to be discrete. Electric circuits and electric networks have been extensively studied to elucidate the properties of their structures.

In electrophysiology and bioelectromagnetism there are no inductors, while resistances, capacitances, and batteries are not discrete but *distributed*. That is, the conducting medium extends continuously; it is *three-dimensional* and referred to as a *volume conductor*. Although the capacitance is localized to cellular membranes, since normally our interest is in multicellular preparations (e.g., brain tissue or cardiac muscle) which extend continuously throughout a three-dimensional region, the capacitance must also be deemed to be distributed. In fact, this is true as well for the "batteries,"

which are also continuously distributed throughout these same membranes.

Although the classical studies in electricity and magnetism are relevant, it is the area of electromagnetic fields that is the most pertinent. Such application to volume conductors is discussed later in detail in Chapter 11, where it is shown that they form an independent and logical discipline. Wherever possible, results from the simple sources discussed in the earlier chapters will be applied under more realistic conditions.

A major object of this chapter is to introduce the bioelectric sources and the electric fields arising from the sources. Another important task is to discuss the concept of modeling. It is exemplified by modeling the bioelectric volume sources, like those within the entire heart, and volume conductors, like the entire human body. This chapter provides also a preliminary discussion of the fundamental problems concerning the bioelectric or biomagnetic fields arising from the sources, called the solutions to the *forward problem*, and the general preconditions for the determination of the sources giving a description of the field, called the solutions to the *inverse problem*. The discussion on bioelectric sources and the fields that they produce is continued on a theoretical basis in Chapter 8.

133

7.2 BIOELECTRIC SOURCE AND ITS ELECTRIC FIELD

7.2.1 Definition of the Preconditions

The discussions in each section that follows are valid under a certain set of conditions—that is, for certain types of electric sources within certain types of volume conductors. Therefore, some limiting assumptions, or *preconditions*, are given first. One should note that when the preconditions are more stringent than the actual conditions the discussion will necessarily be valid. For instance, if the preconditions indicate the discussion is valid in an infinite homogeneous volume conductor, then it is not valid in a finite inhomogeneous volume conductor. On the other hand, if the preconditions indicate the discussion is valid in a finite inhomogeneous volume conductor, then it is also valid in a finite homogeneous volume conductor because the latter is a special case of the former.

It should be noted that all volume conductors are assumed to be linear (consistent with all experimental evidence). If the volume conductor is presumed to be homogeneous, it is assumed to be isotropic as well. The various types of sources and conductors are characterized later in this chapter.

7.2.2 Volume Source in a Homogeneous Volume Conductor

PRECONDITIONS

Source: *Volume source*

Conductor: *Infinite, homogeneous*

Let us introduce the concept of the *impressed current density* $\bar{J}^i$ *(x,y,z,t)*. This is a nonconservative current that arises from the bioelectric activity of nerve and muscle cells due to the conversion of energy from chemical to electric form. The individual elements of this bioelectric source behave as electric current dipoles. Hence the impressed current density equals the *volume dipole moment density* of the source. Note that $\bar{J}^i$ is zero everywhere outside the region of active cells (Plonsey, 1969). (Note also that bioelectric sources were formerly modeled by dipoles or double layers formed by the com-

ponent electric charges. Today we think of the *current source* as the basic element.)

If the volume conductor is infinite and homogeneous and the conductivity is σ, the primary sources $\bar{J}^i$ establish an electric field $\bar{E}$ and a conduction current $\sigma\bar{E}$. As a result, the total current density $\bar{J}$ (Geselowitz, 1967) is given by:

$$\bar{J} = \bar{J}^i + \sigma\bar{E} \qquad (7.1)$$

The quantity $\sigma\bar{E}$ is often referred to as the *return current*. This current is necessary to avoid buildup of charges due to the source current.

Because the electric field $\bar{E}$ is *quasistatic* (see Section 7.2.4), it can be expressed at each instant of time as the negative gradient of a scalar potential Φ, and Equation 7.1 may be rewritten

$$\bar{J} = \bar{J}^i - \sigma\nabla\Phi \qquad (7.2)$$

Since the tissue capacitance is negligible (quasistatic conditions), charges redistribute themselves in a negligibly short time in response to any source change. Since the divergence of $\bar{J}$ evaluates the rate of change of the charge density with respect to time, and since the charge density must be zero, the divergence of $\bar{J}$ is necessarily zero. (We refer to the total current $\bar{J}$ as being solenoidal, or forming closed lines of current flow.) Therefore, Equation 7.1 reduces to Poisson's equation:

$$\nabla \cdot \bar{J}^i = \nabla \cdot \sigma\nabla\Phi + \nabla \cdot \bar{J} = \sigma\nabla^2\Phi \quad (7.3)$$

Equation 7.3 is a partial differential equation satisfied by Φ in which $\nabla \cdot \bar{J}^i$ is the *source function* (or *forcing function*).

The solution of Equation 7.3 for the scalar function $\sigma\Phi$ for a region that is uniform and infinite in extent (Stratton, 1941) is:

$$4\pi\sigma\Phi = - \int_v \left(\frac{1}{r}\right) \nabla \cdot \bar{J}^i \, dv \qquad (7.4)$$

Since a source element $-\nabla \cdot \bar{J}^i \, dv$ in Equation 7.4 behaves like a *point source*, in that it sets up a field, that varies as $1/r$ (as will be explained in more detail later in Equation 8.35), the expression $-\nabla \cdot \bar{J}^i$ is defined as a *flow source density* (I_F). Because we seek the solution for field points outside the region occupied by the volume source, Equation 7.4 may be transformed (Stratton, 1941) to:

$$4\pi\sigma\Phi = \int_v \bar{J}^i \cdot \nabla \left(\frac{1}{r}\right) dv \qquad \mathbf{(7.5)}$$

This equation represents the distribution of potential Φ due to the bioelectric source $\bar{J}^i$ within an infinite, homogeneous volume conductor having conductivity σ. Here $\bar{J}^i \, dv$ behaves like a *dipole element* (with a field that varies as its dot product with $\nabla(1/r)$, and hence $\bar{J}^i$ can be interpreted as a *volume dipole density*).

In this section we started with a formal definition of $\bar{J}^i$ as an impressed current density (a nonconservative vector field) and developed its role as a source function of potential fields. These are expressed by Equations 7.4 and 7.5. But identical expressions will be obtained in Chapter 8 (namely Equations 8.34 and 8.32) based on an interpretation of $\bar{J}^i$ as a dipole moment per unit volume. This underscores the dual role played by the distribution $\bar{J}^i$, and provides alternative ways in which it can be evaluated from actual experiments. (One such approach will be illustrated in Chapter 8.) These alternate interpretations are, in fact, illustrated by Equations 7.4 and 7.5.

7.2.3 Volume Source in an Inhomogeneous Volume Conductor

PRECONDITIONS:

Source: *Volume source*

Conductor: *Inhomogeneous*

In Section 7.2.2 it was assumed that the medium is uniform (i.e., infinite and homogeneous). Such an assumption allowed the use of simple expressions that are valid only for uniform homogeneous media of infinite extent. However, even an in vitro preparation that is reasonably homogeneous is nevertheless bounded by air, and hence globally inhomogeneous. One can take such inhomogeneities into account by adding additional terms to the solution. In this section we consider inhomogeneities by approximating the volume conductor by a collection of regions, each one of which is homogeneous, resistive, and isotropic, where the current density $\bar{J}^i$ is linearly related to the electric field intensity $\bar{E}$ (Schwan and Kay, 1956). We show that such inhomogeneities can be taken into account while at the same time retaining the results obtained in Section 7.2.2 (which were based on the assumption of uniformity).

An inhomogeneous volume conductor can be divided into a finite number of homogeneous regions, each with a boundary S_j. On these boundaries both the electric potential Φ and the normal component of the current density must be continuous:

$$\Phi'(S_j) = \Phi''(S_j) \qquad (7.6)$$

$$\sigma_j' \nabla\Phi'(S_j) \cdot \bar{n}_j = \sigma_j'' \nabla\Phi''(S_j) \cdot \bar{n}_j \qquad (7.7)$$

where the primed and double-primed notations represent the opposite sides of the boundary and $\bar{n}_j$ is directed from the primed region to the double-primed one.

If dv is a volume element, and ψ and Φ are two scalar functions that are mathematically well behaved in each (homogeneous) region, it follows from Green's theorem (Smyth, 1968) that

$$\sum_j \int_{S_j} [\sigma_j' (\psi'\nabla\Phi' - \Phi'\nabla\psi')$$
$$- \sigma_j'' (\psi''\nabla\Phi'' - \Phi''\nabla\psi'')] \cdot d\bar{S}_j \qquad (7.8)$$
$$= \sum_j \int_{v_j} (\psi\nabla \cdot \sigma_j\nabla\Phi - \Phi\nabla \cdot \sigma_j\nabla\psi) \, dv_j$$

If we make the choice of $\psi = 1/r$, where r is the distance from an arbitrary field point to the element of volume or area in the integration, and Φ is the electric potential, and substitute Equations 7.3, 7.6, and 7.7 into Equation 7.8, then we obtain the following useful result (Geselowitz, 1967):

$$4\pi\sigma\Phi(r) = \int_v \bar{J}^i \cdot \nabla\left(\frac{1}{r}\right) dv$$
$$+ \sum_j \int_{S_j} (\sigma_j'' - \sigma_j') \Phi\nabla\left(\frac{1}{r}\right) \cdot d\bar{S}_j \qquad \textbf{(7.9)}$$

This equation evaluates the electric potential anywhere within an inhomogeneous volume conductor containing internal volume sources.

The first term on the right-hand side of Equation 7.9 involving $\bar{J}^i$ corresponds exactly to Equation 7.5 and thus represents the contribution of the volume source. The effect of inhomogeneities is reflected in the second integral, where $(\sigma_j'' - \sigma_j') \Phi\bar{n}_j$ is an equivalent double-layer source ($\bar{n}_j$ is in the direction of $d\bar{S}_j$). The double-layer direction, that of $\bar{n}_j$ or $d\bar{S}_j$, is the outward surface normal (from the prime to double-prime region). This can be emphasized by rewriting Equation 7.9 as

$$4\pi\sigma\Phi(r) = \int_v \bar{J}^i \cdot \nabla \left(\frac{1}{r}\right) dv$$
$$+ \sum_j \int_{S_j} (\sigma_j'' - \sigma_j') \Phi \bar{n}_j \cdot \nabla \left(\frac{1}{r}\right) dS_j \quad (7.10)$$

Note that the expression for the field from $\bar{J}^i$ (involving $\nabla(1/r)$) is in exactly the same form as $(\sigma_j'' - \sigma_j') \Phi \bar{n}_j$, except that the former is a *volume source density* (volume integral) and the latter a *surface source density* (surface integral). In Equations 7.9 and 7.10, and previous equations, the gradient operator is expressed with respect to the source coordinates whereupon $\nabla(1/r) = \bar{a}_r/r^2$ and $\bar{a}_r$ is from the source to field. The volume source $\bar{J}^i$ is the *primary source*, whereas the surface sources that are invoked by the field established by the primary source (therefore secondary to that source) are referred to as *secondary sources*.

We want to point out once again that the first term on the right-hand side of Equation 7.9 describes the *contribution of the volume source*, and the second term the contribution of boundaries separating regions of different conductivity—that is, the *contribution of the inhomogeneities* within the volume conductor. This may be exemplified as follows: If the conductivity is the same on both sides of each boundary S_j—that is, if the volume conductor is homogeneous—the difference $(\sigma_j'' - \sigma_j')$ on each boundary S_j in the second term is zero, and Equation 7.9 (applicable in an inhomogeneous volume conductor) reduces to Equation 7.5 (applicable in a homogeneous volume conductor).

The purpose of measuring bioelectric signals is to measure their *source,* not the properties of the volume conductor with the aid of the source inside it. Therefore, the clinical measurement systems of bioelectric events should be designed so that the contribution of the second term in Equation 7.9 is as small as possible. Later, Chapter 11 introduces various methods for minimizing the effect of this term.

Equation 7.9 includes a special case of interest in which the preparation of interest (e.g., the human body) lies in air, whereupon $\sigma_j'' = 0$ corresponding to the bounding nonconducting space.

7.2.4 Quasistatic Conditions

In the description of the volume conductor constituted by the human body, the capacitive component of tissue impedance is negligible in the frequency band of internal bioelectric events, according to the experimental evidence of Schwan and Kay (1957). They showed that the volume conductor currents were essentially conduction currents and required only specification of the tissue resistivity. The electromagnetic propagation effect can also be neglected (Geselowitz, 1963).

This condition implies that time-varying bioelectric currents and voltages in the human body can be examined in the conventional *quasistatic* limit (Plonsey and Heppner, 1967). That is, all currents and fields behave, at any instant, as if they were stationary. The description of the fields resulting from applied current sources is based on the understanding that the medium is resistive only, and that the phase of the *time variation can be ignored* (i.e., all fields vary synchronously).

7.3 THE CONCEPT OF MODELING

7.3.1 The Purpose of Modeling

A practical way to investigate the function of living organisms is to construct a model that follows the operation of the organism as accurately as possible. The model may be considered to represent a hypothesis regarding physiological observations. Often the hypothesis features complicated interactions between several variables, whose mutual dependence is difficult to determine experimentally. The behavior of the model should be controlled by the basic laws of science (e.g., Ohm's law, Kirchhoff's law, thermodynamic laws, etc.).

The purpose of the model is to facilitate deduction and to be a manipulative representation of the hypothesis. It is possible to perform experiments with the model that are not possible with living tissues; these may yield outputs based on assumed structural parameters and various inputs (including, possibly, noise). One can better understand the real phenomenon by comparing the model performance to experimental results. The model itself may also be improved in this way. A hypothesis cannot be accepted before it has been sufficiently analyzed and proven in detail.

Models have been criticized. For instance, it is claimed that models, which are not primary by construction, cannot add new information to the biological phenomenon they represent. In other words, models do not have scientific merit. We should note, however, that all of our concepts of our surroundings are based on models. Our perception is limited both methodically and conceptually. If we should abandon all "models of models," we would have to relinquish, for example, all the electric heart models in the following chapters of this textbook. They have been the basis for meritorious research in theoretical electrocardiology, which has been essential for developing clinical electrocardiology to its present status. Similarly, the electronic neuron models, which will be briefly reviewed in Chapter 10, serve as an essential bridge from neurophysiology to neurocomputers. Neurocomputers are a fascinating new field of computer science with a wide variety of important applications.

In addition to the *analysis* of the structure and function of organic nature, one should include *synthesis* as an important method—that is, the investigation of organic nature by model construction.

7.3.2 Basic Models of the Volume Source

Let us now consider some basic volume source models and their corresponding number of undetermined coefficients or degrees of freedom. (The reader should be aware that there are a large number of other models available, which are not discussed here.) These are:

Dipole

The (fixed-) dipole model is based on a single dipole with fixed location and variable orientation and magnitude. This model has three independent variables: the magnitudes of its three components x, y, and z in Cartesian coordinates (or the dipole magnitude and two direction angles, M, Θ, and ϕ, in the spherical coordinates).

Moving Dipole

The moving-dipole model is a single dipole that has varying magnitude and orientation, like the fixed dipole, and additionally variable location. Therefore, it has six independent variables.

Multiple Dipole

The multiple-dipole model includes several dipoles, each representing a certain anatomical region of the heart. These dipoles are fixed in location and have varying magnitude and varying orientation. If also the orientation is fixed, each dipole has only one independent variable, the magnitude. Then the number of independent variables is equal to the number of the dipoles.

Multipole

Just as the dipole is formed from two equal and opposite monopoles placed close together, a *quadrupole* is formed from two equal and opposite dipoles that are close together. One can form higher-order source configurations by continuing in this way (the next being the *octapole*, etc.). Each such source constitutes a *multipole*. What is important about multipoles is that it can be shown that any given source configuration can be expressed as an infinite sum of multipoles of increasing order (i.e., dipole, quadrupole, octapole, etc.). The size of each component multipole depends on the particular source distribution. Each multipole component, in turn, is defined by a number of coefficients. For example, we have already seen that the dipole is described by three coefficients (which can be identified as the strength of its x, y, and z components). It turns out that the quadrupole has five coefficients—the octapole seven, and so on. The multipole may be illustrated in different ways. One of them is the *spherical harmonic multipoles*, which is given in Figure 7.1.

A summary of these source models and the number of their independent variables are presented in Table 7.1, and the structure of the models is schematically illustrated in Figure 7.2.

MONOPOLE

DIPOLE

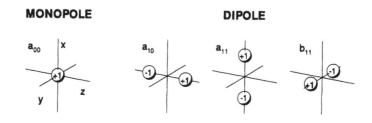

QUADRUPOLE

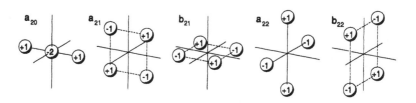

OCTAPOLE

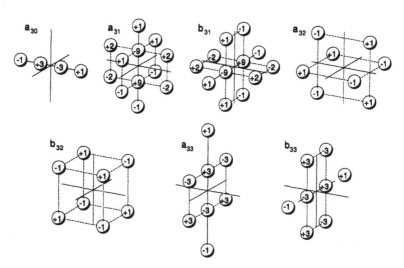

Fig. 7.1 Source-sink illustration of spherical harmonic multipole components (Wikswo and Swinney, 1984). The figure shows the physical source-sink configurations corresponding to the multipole components of the dipole (three components), quadrupole (five components), and octapole (seven components).

Table 7.1 Various source models and the number of their independent variables

Model	Number of variables
Dipole	3
Moving dipole	6
Multiple dipole	n, $(3n)$*
Multipole	
Dipole	3
Quadrupole	5
Octapole	7

*n for dipoles with fixed orientation and $3n$ for dipoles with variable orientation.

7.3.3 Basic Models of the Volume Conductor

The volume conductor can be modeled in one of the following ways, which are classified in order of increasing complexity:

Infinite, Homogeneous

The homogeneous model of the volume conductor with an infinite extent is a *trivial case,* which completely ignores the effects of the conductor boundary and internal inhomogeneities.

Finite, Homogeneous

Spherical. In its most simple form the finite homogeneous model is a spherical model (with the source at its center). It turns out that for a dipole source the field at the surface has the same form as in the infinite homogeneous volume conductor at the same radius except that its magnitude is three times greater. Therefore, this can also be considered a trivial case.

Realistic Shape, Homogeneous. The finite or bounded homogeneous volume conductor with real shape takes into consideration the actual outer boundary of the conductor (the thorax, the head, etc.) but ignores internal inhomogeneities.

Finite, Inhomogeneous

The finite inhomogeneous model takes into consideration the finite dimensions of the conductor and one or more of the following internal inhomogeneities.

Torso.

Cardiac muscle tissue

High-conductivity intracardiac blood mass

Low-conductivity lung tissue

Surface muscle layer

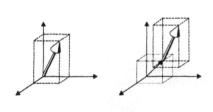

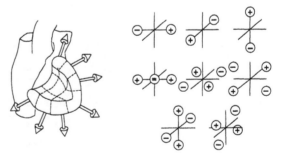

1) DIPOLE

Fixed location
Free direction
Free magnitude
3 variables

2) MOVING DIPOLE

Free location
Free direction
Free magnitude
3 + 3 = 6 variables

3) MULTIPLE DIPOLE

Number of dipoles = N
Fixed location
Free direction
Free magnitude
3N variables

If direction is fixed:
N variables

4) MULTIPOLE

Higher order
multipole expansion

Number of variables:
dipole   3
quadrupole   5
octapole   7

Fig. 7.2 Models used for representing the volume source.

Table 7.2 Various conductor models and their properties

Source model	Properties
Infinite homogeneous	the trivial case; does not consider the volume conductor's electric properties or its boundary with air
Finite homogeneous	
a. Spherical	another trivial case if the source is a dipole
b. Realistic shape	considers the shape of the outer boundary of the thorax but no internal inhomogeneities
Finite inhomogeneous	considers the outer boundary of the thorax and internal inhomogeneities

Nonconducting bones such as the spine and the sternum

Other organs such as the great vessels, the liver, etc.

Head. The specific conducting regions that are ordinarily identified for the head as a volume conductor are:

Brain

Cerebrospinal fluid

Skull

Muscles

Scalp

The volume conductor models are summarized in Table 7.2. The resistivities of various tissues are given in Table 7.3.

7.4   THE HUMAN BODY AS A VOLUME CONDUCTOR

7.4.1   Tissue Resistivities

The human body may be considered as a resistive, piecewise homogeneous and linear volume conductor. Most of the tissue is isotropic. The muscle is, however, strongly anisotropic, and the brain tissue is anisotropic as well. Figure 7.3 illustrates the cross section of the thorax, and Table 7.3 summarizes the tissue resistivity values of a number of components of the human body. More comprehensive lists of tissue resistivities are given in Geddes and Baker (1967), Barber and Brown (1984), and Stuchly and Stuchly (1984).

The resistivity of blood depends strongly on the hematocrit, *Hct* (which denotes the percent volume of the red blood cells in whole blood) (Geddes and Sadler, 1973). This dependence

Table 7.3 Resistivity values for various tissues

Tissue	$\rho[\Omega m]$	Remarks	Reference
Brain	2.2	gray matter	Rush and Driscoll, 1969
	6.8	white matter	Barber and Brown, 1984
	5.8	average	
Cerebrospinal fluid	0.7		Barber and Brown, 1984
Blood	1.6	*Hct* = 45	Geddes and Sadler, 1973
Plasma	0.7		Barber and Brown, 1984
Heart muscle	2.5	longitudinal	Rush, Abildskov, and McFee, 1963
	5.6	transverse	
Skeletal muscle	1.9	longitudinal	Epstein and Foster, 1982
	13.2	transverse	
Liver	7		Rush, Abildskov, and McFee, 1963
Lung	11.2		Schwan and Kay, 1956
	21.7		Rush, Abildskov, and McFee, 1963
Fat	25		Geddes and Baker, 1967
Bone	177		Rush and Driscoll, 1969
	15	longitudinal	Saha and Williams, 1992
	158	circumferential	
	215	radial (at 100 kHz)	

has an exponential nature and is given in Equation 7.11:

$$\rho = 0.537\ e^{0.025Hct} \qquad (7.11)$$

Hugo Fricke studied theoretically the electric conductivity of a suspension of spheroids (Fricke, 1924). When applying this method to the conductivity of blood, we obtain what is called the Maxwell-Fricke equation:

$$\rho = 0.586\ \frac{1 + 0.0125Hct}{1 - 0.01Hct} \qquad (7.12)$$

where

$$\rho = \text{resistivity of blood } [\Omega m]$$
$$Hct = \text{hematocrit } [\%]$$

Both of these equations give very accurate values. The correlation coefficient of Equation 7.11 to empirical measurements is $r = 0.989$. Because the best fitting curve to the measured resistivity values is slightly nonlinear in a semi-logarithmic plot, Equation 7.12 gives better values with very low or very high hematocrit values. The resistivity of blood is also a function

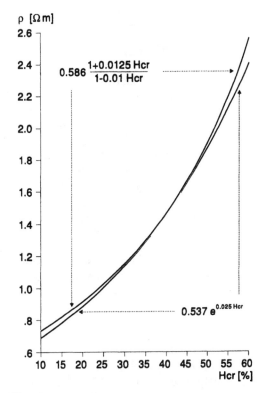

Fig. 7.4   Resistivity of blood as a function of hematocrit (*Hct*). Equations 7.11 and 7.12 are depicted in graphical form.

of the movement of the blood (Liebman, Pearl, and Bagnol, 1962; Tanaka et al., 1970). This effect is often neglected in practice. Equations 7.11 and 7.12 are presented in Figure 7.4.

7.4.2   Modeling the Head

The brain is composed of excitable neural tissue, the study of which is of great interest in view of the vital role played by this organ in human function. Its electric activity, readily measured at the scalp, is denoted the *electroencephalogram* (EEG). Brain tissue not only is the location of electric sources (generators), but also constitutes part of the volume conductor which includes also the skull and scalp.

Regarding volume conductor models, the head has been successfully considered to be a series of concentric spherical regions (the aforementioned brain, skull, and scalp), as illustrated in Figure 7.5 (Rush and Driscoll, 1969). In this model, the inner and outer radii of the skull are

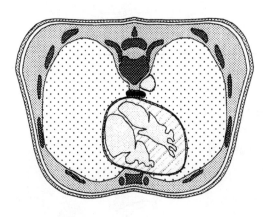

Tissue	Resistivity [Ω m]	
Blood	1.6	
Heart muscle	2.5	(parallel to fibers)
	5.6	(normal to fibers)
Skeletal muscle	1.9	(parallel to fibers)
	13.2	(normal to fibers)
Lungs	20	
Fat	25	
Bone	177	

Fig. 7.3   Cross section of the thorax. The resistivity values are given for six different types of tissues.

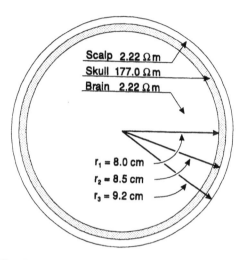

Fig. 7.5 Concentric spherical head model by Rush and Driscoll (1969). The model contains a region for the brain, scalp, and skull, each of which is considered to be homogeneous.

chosen to be 8 and 8.5 cm, respectively, while the radius of the head is 9.2 cm. For the brain and the scalp a resistivity of 2.22 Ωm is selected, whereas for the skull a resistivity of 80 $\times$ 2.22 Ωm = 177 Ωm is assigned. These numerical values are given solely to indicate typical (mean) physiological quantities. Because of the symmetry, and simplicity, this model is easy to construct as either an electrolytic tank model or a mathematical and computer model. It is also easy to perform calculations with a spherical geometry. Though this simple model does not consider the anisotrophy and inhomogeneity of the brain tissue and the cortical bone (Saha and Williams, 1992), it gives results that correspond reasonably well to measurements.

7.4.3   Modeling the Thorax

The applied electrophysiological preparation that has generated the greatest interest is that of electrocardiography. The electric sources (generators) lie entirely within the heart, whereas the volume conductor is composed of the heart plus remaining organs in the thorax. Rush, Abildskov, and McFee (1963) introduced two simple models of the thorax. In both, the outer boundary has the shape of a human thorax. In the simpler model, the resistivity of the lungs

is selected at 10 Ωm. The intracardiac blood is assigned a resistivity of 1 Ωm. In the more accurate model, the resistivity of the lungs is chosen to be 20 Ωm. In addition, the cardiac muscle and intercostal muscles are modeled with a resistivity of 4 Ωm, and the intracardiac blood is assigned a resistivity of 1.6 Ωm, as described in Figure 7.6. Because the experimentally found tissue resistivity shows a considerable variation, a similarly wide choice of values are used in thorax models.

In a first-order electrocardiographic (and particularly in a magnetocardiographic) model, the

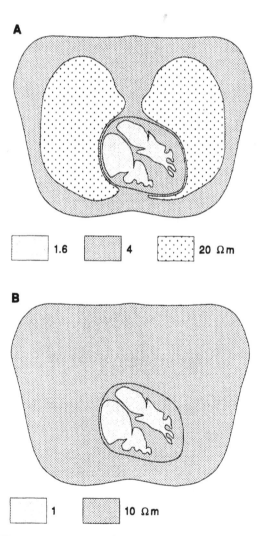

Fig. 7.6 Simplified thorax models by Rush (1971). (A) Heart, lung, and blood regions are identified. (B) The lung region is made uniform with the heart and surface muscle.

whole heart can be considered to be uniform and spherical. In a second-order model, the left ventricular chamber can be modeled with a sphere of a radius of 5.6 cm and hence a volume of 736 cm^3; the cavity is assumed to be filled with blood.

In more recent years, several models have been developed which take into account both shape as well as conductivity of the heart, intracavitary blood, pericardium, lungs, surface muscle and fat, and bounding body shape. These include models by Rudy and Plonsey (1979) and Horáček (1974). A physical inhomogeneous and anisotropic model of the human torso was constructed and described by Rush (1971). This has also been used as the basis for a computer model by Hyttinen et al. (1988).

7.5 FORWARD AND INVERSE PROBLEMS

7.5.1 Forward Problem

The problem in which the source and the conducting medium are known but the field is unknown and must be determined, is called the *forward problem*. The forward problem has a unique solution. It is always possible to calculate the field with an accuracy that is limited only by the accuracy with which we can describe the source and volume conductor. However, this problem does not arise in clinical (diagnostic) situations, since in this case only the field can be measured (noninvasively) at the body surface.

7.5.2 Inverse Problem

The problem in which the field and the conductor are known but the source is unknown, is called the *inverse problem* (see Fig. 7.7). In medical applications of bioelectric phenomena, it is the inverse problem that has clinical importance. For instance, in everyday clinical diagnosis the cardiologist and the neurologist seek to determine the source of the measured bioelectric or biomagnetic signals. The possible pathology affecting the source provides the basis for their diagnostic decisions—that is, the

To determine the FIELD from the known source and conductor is called the

FORWARD PROBLEM

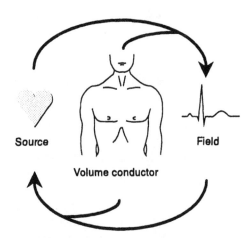

Source   Field

Volume conductor

To determine the SOURCE from the known field and conductor is called the

INVERSE PROBLEM

Fig. 7.7 Forward and inverse problems.

clinical status of the corresponding organ. What is the feasibility of finding solutions to the inverse problem? This will be discussed in the next section.

7.5.3 Solvability of the Inverse Problem

Let us discuss the solvability of the inverse problem with a simplified example of a source and a conductor (Fig. 7.8). In this model the source is represented by a single battery, and the conductor by a network of two resistors (McFee and Baule, 1972). Three cases are presented in which the voltage source is placed in different locations within the network and given different values. Note that although the magnitude of the battery voltage is different in each case, the output voltage in all three cases is the same, namely 2 V.

One may examine each network with Thevenin's theorem (or its dual Norton's theorem), which states that it is always possible to replace a combination of voltage sources and associated circuitry with a single equivalent source and a

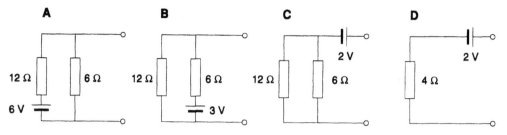

Fig. 7.8 Demonstration of the lack of uniqueness in the inverse problem.

series impedance. The equivalent emf is the open-circuit voltage, and the series resistance is the impedance looking into the output terminals with the actual sources short-circuited.

With this approach, we can evaluate the Thevenin equivalent for the three given circuits. In all cases the equivalent network is the same, namely an emf of 2 V in series with a resistance of 4 Ω. This demonstrates that based on external measurements one can evaluate only the Thevenin network. In this example, we have shown that this network is compatible with (at least) three *actual, but different,* networks. One cannot distinguish among these different inverse candidates without measurements within the source region itself. The example demonstrates the lack of uniqueness in constructing an inverse solution.

The solvability of the inverse problem was discussed through the use of a simple electronic circuit as an example. The first theoretical paper, which stated that the inverse problem does not have a unique solution, was written by Hermann von Helmholtz (1853).

7.5.4 Possible Approaches to the Solution of the Inverse Problem

Cardiac electric activity can be measured on the surface of the thorax as the *electrocardiogram.* Similarly, the electromyogram, electroencephalogram, and so on, are signals of muscular, neural, and other origins measured noninvasively at the body surface. The question facing the clinician is to determine the electric source (generator) of the measured signal and then to observe whether such source is normal or in what way it is abnormal.

To find the source, given the measured field, is the statement of the inverse problem. As noted above, a unique solution cannot be found based on external measurements alone. One may therefore ask how it is possible to reach a clinical diagnosis. Despite the discouraging demonstration in the previous section of the theorem regarding the lack of uniqueness of the inverse problem, there are several approaches that overcome this dilemma. Four of these approaches are discussed below:

1. An empirical approach based on the recognition of typical signal patterns that are known to be associated with certain source configurations.
2. Imposition of physiological constraints is based on the information available on the anatomy and physiology of the active tissue. This imposes strong limitations on the number of available solutions.
3. Examining the lead-field pattern, from which the sensitivity distribution of the lead and therefore the statistically most probable source configuration can be estimated.
4. Modeling the source and the volume conductor using simplified models. The source is characterized by only a few degrees of freedom (for instance a single dipole which can be completely determined by three independent measurements).

We discuss these approaches in more detail in the following:

The Empirical Approach

The empirical approach is based on the experience of the physician to recognize typical signal patterns associated with certain disorders. This means, that the diagnosis is based on the comparison of the recorded signal to a catalog of patterns associated with clinical disorders. If the signal is identified, the diagnosis can be made. This process has been formalized using a diagnostic tree. The diagnosis is reached through a sequence of logical steps that are derived statistically from the accumulated data base. This very same procedure may also be followed in creating a computer program to automate the diagnostic process (Macfarlane and Lawrie, 1974).

Imposition of Physiological Constraints

As noted, there is no unique solution to the inverse problem. By this we mean that more than one source configuration will generate fields that are consistent with the measurements (as demonstrated in Section 7.5.3). However, it may be possible to select from among these competing solutions one that at the same time meets physiological expectations. We say that this procedure involves the imposition of *physiological constraints*. Those that have been used successfully include a requirement that dipole sources point outward, that the activation sequence be continuous, that the signal and noise statistics lie in expected ranges, and so on (Pilkington and Plonsey, 1982).

Lead Field Theoretical Approach

It is possible to determine what is known as the *sensitivity distribution* of the lead. (To obtain it, we consider the relative voltage that would be measured at a lead as a function of the position and orientation of a unit dipole source; the lead sensitivity at a point is the relative lead voltage for a dipole whose direction is adjusted for maximum response.) One can then make decisions about the activity of the source based upon this information. This approach depends on the fact that each lead detects the component of the activation dipoles that are in the direction of the sensitivity of the lead.

For all leads and for a statistically homogeneously distributed source, the source of the detected signal is most probably located at that region of the source where the lead sensitivity is highest and oriented in the direction of the lead sensitivity. If the lead system is designed to detect a certain *equivalent* source like dipole, quadrupole, etc., the detected signal represents

SOLUTION OF THE INVERSE PROBLEM WITH THE MODELING METHOD

(1) A MODEL IS CONSTRUCTED FOR THE SOURCE

The model should have a limited number of independent variables

(2) A MODEL IS CONSTRUCTED FOR THE VOLUME CONDUCTOR

The accuracy of the conductor model must be as good as or better than that of the source model

(3) AT LEAST AS MANY INDEPENDENT MEASUREMENTS ARE MADE AS THE SOURCE MODEL HAS INDEPENDENT VARIABLES

Now we have as many equations as we have independent variables and the source model may be evaluated

BUT NOW WE HAVE A NEW QUESTION, NAMELY:

(4) HOW WELL DOES THE CONSTRUCTED MODEL REPRESENT ITS PHYSIOLOGICAL COUNTERPART?

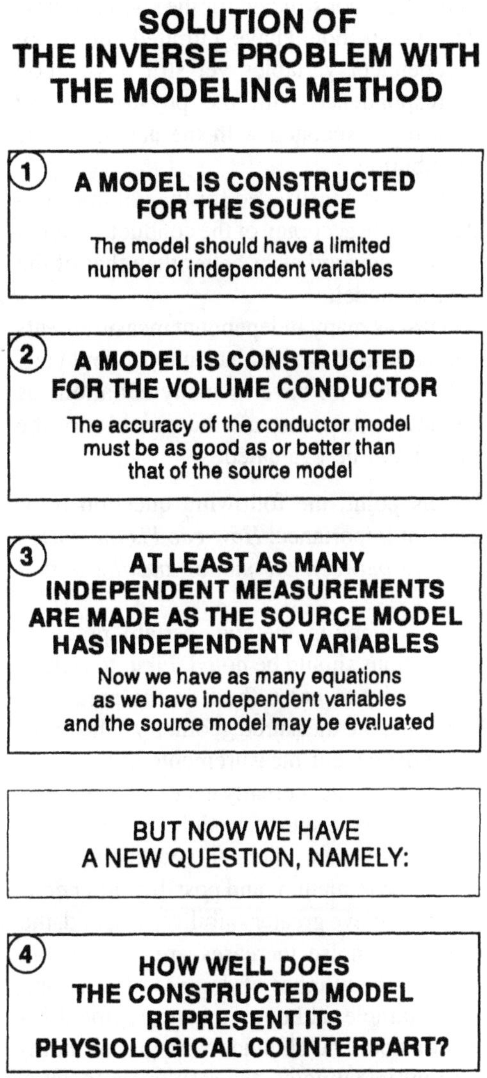

Fig. 7.9 Solution of the inverse problem based on the modeling method.

this equivalent source which is a simplified model of the real source. It must be pointed out that while this simplified model is not necessarily the source, it probably represents the main configuration of the source. This approach is discussed in detail later.

Simplified Source Model

The inverse problem may be solved by modeling the source of the bioelectric or biomagnetic signal and the volume conductor in the following way (Malmivuo, 1976; see Fig. 7.9):

1. A model is constructed for the signal source. The model should have a limited number of independent variables yet still have good correspondence with the physiology and anatomy associated with the actual source distribution.
2. A model is constructed for the volume conductor. The accuracy of the conductor model must be as good as or better than that of the source model.
3. At least as many independent measurements are made as the model has independent variables. Now we have as many equations as we have unknowns, and the variables of the model can be evaluated.

At this point, the following question is of paramount importance: *How good is the correspondence between the model and the actual physiology?*

In the modeling method, certain practical considerations should be noted. First, to reduce the sensitivity to noise (both in the measured voltages and the measured geometry), the number of independent measurements at the body surface usually must greatly exceed the number of variables in the source model. The overspecified equations are then solved using least squares approximation (and possibly other constraints to achieve greater stability). Second, the sensitivity to noise increases greatly with an increase in the number of degrees of freedom. So, for example, although greater regional information could be obtained with greater number of multiple dipoles, the results could actually become useless if too large a number were selected. At present, the number of dipoles that can be satisfactorily described in an inverse process, in electrocardiography, is under 10.

7.5.5 Summary

In Section 7.5 we have described the problem of clinical interest in electrocardiography, magnetocardiography, electroencephalography, magnetoencephalography, etc. as the solution of an inverse problem. This solution involves determination of the source configuration responsible for the production of the electric signals that are measured. Knowledge of this distribution permits clinical diagnoses to be made in a straightforward deterministic way.

As pointed out previously, from a theoretical standpoint the inverse problem has no unique solution. Added to this uncertainty is one based on the limitations arising from the limited data points and the inevitable contamination of noise. However, solutions are possible based on approximations of various kinds, including purely empirical recognition of signal patterns. Unfortunately, at this time, generalizations are not possible. As might be expected, this subject is currently under intense study.

REFERENCES

Barber DC, Brown BH (1984): Applied potential tomography. *J. Phys. E.: Sci. Instrum.* 17: 723–33.

Epstein BR, Foster KR (1983): Anisotropy as a dielectric property of skeletal muscle. *Med. & Biol. Eng. & Comput.* 21:(1) 51–5.

Fricke H (1924): A mathematical treatment of the electric conductivity and capacity of disperse systems. *Physiol. Rev.* 4: 575–87. (Series 2).

Geddes LA, Baker LE (1967): The specific resistance of biological material—A compendium of data for the biomedical engineering and physiologist. *Med. Biol. Eng.* 5: 271–93.

Geddes LA, Sadler C (1973): The specific resistance of blood at body temperature. *Med. Biol. Eng.* 11:(5) 336–9.

Geselowitz DB (1963): The concept of an equivalent cardiac generator. *Biomed. Sci. Instrum.* 1: 325–30.

Geselowitz DB (1967): On bioelectric potentials in an inhomogeneous volume conductor. *Biophys. J.* 7:(1) 1–11.

Helmholtz HLF (1853): Ueber einige Gesetze der Vertheilung elektrischer Ströme in körperlichen Leitern mit Anwendung auf die thierisch-elektrischen Versuche. *Ann. Physik und Chemie* 89: 211–33, 354–77.

Horáček BM (1974): Numerical model of an inhomogeneous human torso. In *Advances in Cardiology*, Vol. 10, ed. S Rush, E Lepeshkin, pp. 51–7, S. Karger, Basel.

Hyttinen JA, Eskola HJ, Sievänen H, Malmivuo JA (1988): Atlas of the sensitivity distribution of the common ECG-lead systems. *Tampere Univ. Techn., Inst. Biomed. Eng., Reports* 2:(2) 25+67.

Liebman FM, Pearl J, Bagnol S (1962): The electrical conductance properties of blood in motion. *Phys. Med. Biol.* 7: 177–94.

Macfarlane PW, Lawrie TDV (1974): *An Introduction to Automated Electrocardiogram Interpretation*, 115 pp. Butterworths, London.

Malmivuo JA (1976): On the detection of the magnetic heart vector—An application of the reciprocity theorem. *Helsinki Univ. Tech.*, Acta Polytechn. Scand., El. Eng. Series. Vol. 39, pp. 112. (Dr. tech. thesis)

McFee R, Baule GM (1972): Research in electrocardiography and magnetocardiography. *Proc. IEEE* 60:(3) 290–321.

Pilkington TC, Plonsey R (1982): *Engineering Contributions to Biophysical Electrocardiography*, 248 pp. IEEE Press, John Wiley, New York.

Plonsey R (1969): *Bioelectric Phenomena*, 380 pp. McGraw-Hill, New York.

Plonsey R, Heppner DB (1967): Considerations of quasistationarity in electrophysiological systems. *Bull. Math. Biophys.* 29:(4) 657–64.

Rudy Y, Plonsey R (1979): The eccentric spheres model as the basis of a study of the role of geometry and inhomogeneities in electrocardiography. *IEEE Trans. Biomed. Eng.* BME-26:(7) 392–9.

Rush S (1971): An inhomogeneous anisotropic model of the human torso for electrocardiographic studies. *Med. Biol. Eng.* 9:(5) 201–11.

Rush S, Abildskov JA, McFee R (1963): Resistivity of body tissues at low frequencies. *Circulation* 22:(1) 40–50.

Rush S, Driscoll DA (1969): EEG-electrode sensitivity—An application of reciprocity. *IEEE Trans. Biomed. Eng.* BME-16:(1) 15–22.

Saha S, Williams PA (1992): Electric and dielectric properties of wet human cortical bone as a function of frequency. *IEEE Trans. Biomed. Eng.* BME-39:(12) 1298–304.

Schwan HP, Kay CF (1956): Specific resistance of body tissues. *Circ. Res.* 4:(6) 664–70.

Schwan HP, Kay CF (1957): Capacitive properties of body tissues. *Circ. Res.* 5:(4) 439–43.

Smyth WR (1968): *Static and Dynamic Electricity*, 3rd ed., 623 pp. McGraw-Hill, New York.

Stratton JA (1941): *Electromagnetic Theory*, McGraw-Hill, New York.

Stuchly MA, Stuchly SS (1984): Electrical properties of biological substance. In *Biological Effects and Medical Applications of Electromagnetic Fields*, ed. OP Gandhi, Academic Press, New York.

Tanaka K, Kanai H, Nakayama K, Ono N (1970): The impedance of blood: The effects of red cell orientation and its application. *Jpn. J. Med. Eng.* 8: 436–43.

Wikswo JP, Swinney KR (1984): Comparison of scalar multipole expansions. *J. Appl. Phys.* 56:(11) 3039–49.

8

Source-Field Models

8.1 INTRODUCTION

In this chapter, we develop expressions for electric sources of bioelectric origin. These sources are generated by the passage of current across the membrane of active (excitable) cells, which may be either nerve or muscle. We consider excitable tissue with very simple models—mainly single cylindrical fibers. But the results are useful in later chapters when considering whole organs which can be thought of as composed of many such elements. We see that bioelectric sources can be described as surface/volume distributions of two types of source element, namely the *monopole* and/or *dipole*. Because of the fundamental importance of the monopole and dipole source, we first proceed to a description of the fields generated by each.

8.2 SOURCE MODELS

8.2.1 Monopole

PRECONDITIONS:

Source: *Monopole in a fixed location*
Conductor: *Infinite, homogeneous*

The simplest source configuration is the *point source* or *monopole*. If we consider a point current source of magnitude I_0 lying in a uniform conducting medium of infinite extent and conductivity σ, then current flow lines must be uniform and directed radially. As a consequence, for a concentric spherical surface of arbitrary radius r, the current density J crossing this surface must be uniform and will equal I_0 divided by the total surface area. That is

$$J = \frac{I_0}{4\pi r^2} \tag{8.1}$$

since the total current is conserved. Because the current is everywhere in the radial direction, the current density expressed as a vector is

$$\bar{J} = \frac{I_0}{4\pi r^2}\,\bar{a}_r \tag{8.2}$$

where

$\bar{a}_r$ = unit vector in the radial direction, where the origin is at the point source

Associated with the current flow field defined by Equation 8.2 is a scalar potential field Φ. Since the field is everywhere radial, there should be no variation of potential along a transverse direction, namely that on which r is a constant. Consequently, we expect isopotential surfaces to be a series of concentric spheres surrounding the point source with diminishing potentials for increasing values of r. In a formal sense, it is known from field theory that the

148

electric field $\overline{E}$ is related to a scalar potential Φ by

$$\overline{E} = -\nabla\Phi \qquad (8.3)$$

From Ohm's law it follows that

$$\overline{J} = \sigma\overline{E} \qquad (8.4)$$

Applying Equations 8.3 and 8.4 to 8.2 results in

$$\overline{J} = \frac{I_0}{4\pi r^2} \, \overline{a}_r = -\sigma\nabla\Phi \qquad (8.5)$$

To satisfy Equation 8.5, only the component of $\nabla\Phi$ in the direction of r can arise. This leads to

$$-\sigma \frac{d\Phi}{dr} = \frac{I_0}{4\pi r^2} \qquad (8.6)$$

and integration with respect to r leaves us with

$$\Phi = \frac{I_0}{4\pi\sigma r} \qquad \mathbf{(8.7)}$$

As suspected above, Φ is a constant on surfaces where r is constant (i.e., concentric spheres). Normally the potential for $r \to \infty$ is set to zero, which accounts for having chosen the constant of integration in Equation 8.7 equal to zero. We note from Equation 8.7 that equipotential surfaces are indeed concentric spheres and that the potential magnitude is inversely proportional to the radius (with the origin at the monopole source).

It is not always convenient to place the coordinate system origin at the point source (e.g., when considering several such sources). In this case it is desirable to distinguish the coordinates of the point source(s) from that of the field point, and we do this by using primes for the field point coordinates. Equation 8.7 then applies with, r given by

$$r = \sqrt{(x - x')^2 + (y - y')^2 + (z - z')^2} \qquad (8.8)$$

where each monopole is located at (x, y, z) while the field point is at (x', y', z').

The field described by Equation 8.7 for a point current source is identical to the electrostatic field from a point charge, provided that I_0 is replaced by Q_0 (the charge magnitude), σ is replaced by ϵ (the permittivity), and $\overline{J}$ replaced by $\overline{E}$. This result is not surprising since if the aforementioned exchanges are made, the governing equations for current flow convert exactly into those for electrostatics. This means that simply by interchanging symbols, solutions to problems in electrostatics can be converted into solutions to equivalent problems in current flow (and vice versa).

The aforementioned is an example of *duality*. It can be a useful tool when there is an extensive literature already in existence. Sometimes there may be a limitation in physically realizing a condition in one or the other dual systems. For example, one can have zero conductivity, but the permittivity can never be less than that of vacuum. Also, while one can have a point charge, one cannot actually have a physical point source.

The reader may wonder why there is an interest in a point current source when such is not physically obtainable. One reason is that in a limited region, the fields may behave as if they arise from such a source (we say that the source is *equivalent*). Second, one can actually have two point sources of opposite polarity, in which case the field of interest can be found by the superposition of point source fields. In fact, this very situation is examined in the next section.

8.2.2 Dipole

PRECONDITIONS:

Source: *Dipole in a fixed location*

Conductor: *Infinite, homogeneous*

In bioelectricity one can never have a single isolated monopole current source because of the need to conserve charge. But collections of positive and negative monopole sources are physically realizable if the total sum is zero. The simplest collection, and one that reflects a fundamental bioelectric source, is the *dipole*. The dipole consists of two monopoles of opposite sign but equal strength I_0 (often termed *source* and *sink*) separated by a very small distance, d. In fact, the strict definition requires $d \to 0$, $I_0 \to \infty$ with $p = I_0 d$ remaining finite in the limit. The quantity p is the *dipole moment* or dipole magnitude. The dipole is a vector whose direction is defined from the negative point source to the positive. In fact, if $\overline{d}$ is the *displacement* from negative to positive point source and $\bar{a}_d$ a unit vector in that direction, then

$$\bar{p} = I_0 \bar{d} = I_0 d\bar{a}_d \qquad (8.9)$$

where

$$\bar{p} = \text{the dipole vector}$$

A dipole of arbitrary orientation is illustrated in Figure 8.1, where the coordinate system origin is placed at the negative pole. If the positive pole were also at the origin, the sources would cancel each other and their field would be zero. Consequently, the field arising from the displacement of the positive pole from the origin to its actual position (shown in Fig. 8.1) is, in fact, the dipole field. But this can be found by examining the expression describing the potential of the positive monopole and evaluating the change in potential brought about by moving the monopole from the origin to its dipole position. And this, in turn, can be approximated from the first derivative of the monopole's potential field with respect to the source coordinates evaluated at the origin (as in a Taylor series representation). Specifically, to obtain the dipole field, a derivative of Φ (as given in Equation 8.7) is taken with respect to the direction $\bar{d}$ (a directional derivative) and then multiplied by the magnitude of d. Thus, de-

noting the dipole field Φ_d, and based on Equation 8.7, we have

$$\Phi_d = \frac{\partial\left(\dfrac{I_0}{4\pi\sigma r}\right)}{\partial d}d \qquad (8.10)$$

The directional derivative in Equation 8.10 equals the component of the gradient in the direction $\bar{d}$ so that

$$\Phi_d = \nabla\left(\frac{I_0}{4\pi\sigma r}\right) \cdot \bar{d} \qquad (8.11)$$

and, finally since $I_0 d = p$

$$\Phi_d = \frac{p}{4\pi\sigma} \nabla\left(\frac{1}{r}\right) \cdot \bar{a}_d \qquad (8.12)$$

The accuracy of Equation 8.10 improves as $d \to 0$, and in fact, p (as noted earlier) is normally defined in the limit that $d \to 0$, $I \to \infty$, such that the product $I_0 d$ is finite and is equal to p. Consequently, Equation 8.12 is a rigorous (exact) expression for a mathematically defined dipole.

If the coordinate axes are oriented so that the dipole is directed along z- (the polar) axis and the dipole is placed at the origin, then carrying out the gradient operation in Equation 8.12 and noting that

$$\nabla\left(\frac{1}{r}\right) = \frac{1}{r^2}\bar{a}_r \qquad (8.13)$$

where $\bar{a}_r$ is oriented from the source point to field point, we obtain for the field of a dipole

$$\Phi_d = \frac{p}{4\pi\sigma r^2} \bar{a}_r \cdot \bar{a}_z \qquad (8.14)$$

and

$$\Phi_d = \frac{p \cos\theta}{4\pi\sigma r^2} \qquad \textbf{(8.15)}$$

In Equation 8.15 the angle θ is the polar angle. The above expressions can be confirmed by noting that the gradient operator (in Equation 8.13) acts on the *source* (unprimed) coordinates in Equation 8.8.

A comparison of the dipole field to a monopole field, by contrasting Equation 8.15 with Equation 8.7, shows that the dipole field varies as $(1/r)^2$ whereas the monopole field varies as $(1/r)$. In addition, the dipole equipotential sur-

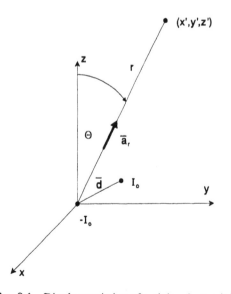

Fig. 8.1 Dipole consisting of a sink $-I_0$ at origin and a source I_0 at radius vector $\bar{d}$, where $d \to 0$. Also illustrated is a field point at radius vector $r\bar{a}_r$ and polar (colatitude) angle θ.

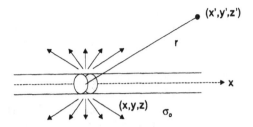

Fig. 8.2 A long thin fiber is shown embedded in a uniform conducting medium of conductivity σ_o and infinite in extent. The transmembrane current density is described by $i_m(x)$ so that $i_m(x)dx$, illustrated, behaves as a point source in the extracellular medium.

faces are not concentric spheres but, rather, are more complicated, because of the factor cos θ. The maximum dipole potential, for a given value of r, is on the polar axis (z axis).

8.2.3 Single Isolated Fiber: Transmembrane Current Source

PRECONDITIONS:

Source: *Active fiber of finite or infinite length with circular cross section*

Conductor: *Infinite, homogeneous*

Figure 8.2 illustrates a long, thin excitable fiber lying in a uniform conducting medium of conductivity σ_o and of unlimited extent. If we assume the existence of a propagating nerve impulse, then the activation currents are associated with a transmembrane current distribution $i_m(x)$. Since the fiber is very thin and there is axial symmetry, we can describe the transmembrane current as a function of the axial variable x only. Thus the source description is *one-dimensional*. The dimension of $i_m(x)$ is current per unit length. A small element of current $i_m(x)dx$ can, therefore, be considered to behave like a point current source (a monopole) within the extracellular medium. Consequently, from Equation 8.7, we have

$$d\Phi_o = \frac{i_m dx}{4\pi\sigma_o r} \qquad (8.16)$$

where r is given by Equation 8.8, Φ_o is the potential field and σ_o is the conductivity outside the fiber (i.e., extracellular conductivity). Integration over the fiber (i.e., with respect to x) gives the total field as

$$\Phi_o = \frac{1}{4\pi\sigma_o} \int \frac{i_m(x)dx}{\sqrt{(x - x')^2 + y'^2 + z'^2}} \qquad (8.17)$$

where the source is assumed to lie on the fiber axis, at $(x, 0, 0)$, and the (fixed) field point is at (x', y', z').

We may apply the equations derived in Chapter 3, Section 3.4.2, to the fiber in Figure 8.2. We may approximate that the resistance of the interstitial medium $r_o \approx 0$ and that similarly the potential in the interstitial medium $\Phi_o \approx 0$. Using these approximations and Equation 3.42 and noting that $\Phi_i - \Phi_o \approx V_m$ we obtain

$$i_m = \frac{1}{r_i} \frac{\partial^2 V_m}{\partial x^2} \qquad (8.18)$$

so that Equation 8.17 may be written

$$\Phi_o = \frac{1}{4\pi\sigma_o} \frac{1}{r_i} \int \frac{\partial^2 V_m/\partial x^2}{r} dx \qquad (8.19)$$

In Equation 8.19, r is given by

$$r = \sqrt{(x - x')^2 + y'^2 + z'^2} \qquad (8.20)$$

Using the cylindrical resistance formula for $r_i = 1/(\pi a^2 \sigma_i)$ based on a conductivity σ_i inside the cell, converts Equation 8.19 into

$$\Phi_o = \frac{a^2 \sigma_i}{4\sigma_o} \int \frac{\partial^2 V_m/\partial x^2}{r} dx \qquad \mathbf{(8.21)}$$

where a = the fiber radius.

The reader will note that initially Φ_o was set equal to zero and now we have found a solution for Φ_o which, of course, is not zero. The underlying explanation of this apparent paradox is that Φ_o was ignored in deriving Equation 8.18 in comparison with Φ_i. Since the latter is perhaps 100 times larger, dropping Φ_o at that point should have negligible consequences. The interested reader can pursue the matter by introducing the value Φ_o found in Equation 8.21 into the rigorous version of Equation 8.18, namely

$$i_m = \frac{1}{r_i} \frac{\partial^2(V_m + \Phi_o)}{\partial x^2} \qquad (8.18b)$$

and then recalculating Φ_o. This will produce an improved Φ_o. In fact, this iterative procedure can be repeated until a desired degree of convergence results. Such a procedure is followed in Henriquez and Plonsey (1988), and is seen to converge very rapidly, demonstrating that for typical physiological situations the first-order approximation (given by Equation 8.21) is entirely satisfactory.

Equation 8.21 may be integrated by parts. Since at the boundaries of the spatial activation, resting conditions are present, $\partial V_m/\partial x = 0$ and the integrated term drops out. Accordingly, we are left with

$$\Phi_o = \frac{a^2\sigma_i}{4\sigma_o} \int \frac{\partial V_m}{\partial x} \frac{\partial(1/r)}{\partial x} \qquad (8.22)$$

or

$$\Phi_o = \frac{a^2\sigma_i}{4\sigma_o} \int \frac{\partial V_m}{\partial x} \nabla \left(\frac{1}{r}\right) \cdot \bar{a}_x dx \qquad \textbf{(8.23)}$$

where

$\bar{a}_x$ = unit vector in the x-direction

Since both Equations 8.23 and 8.21 are mathematically the same, they necessarily evaluate the same field Φ_o. The physical interpretation of these expressions is that in Equation 8.21 the source is a (monopole) current density that lies on the axis, whereas in Equation 8.23 it is an axial dipole also lying along the axis. These are, of course, equivalent sources. Which source is prefeable to use depends on the shape of $V_m(x)$; this will be illustrated in the following sections.

8.2.4   Discussion of Transmembrane Current Source

The expression in Equation 8.17 describes the field in the extracellular volume arising from transmembrane current elements. It is therefore limited to the evaluation of potentials outside the cell and is not valid for describing intracellular fields.

There are two approximations that underlie Equation 8.17 and that should be kept in mind. First, the configuration of the current element is approximated as a point source, but the current actually emerges from the membrane surface rather than a point (see Fig. 8.2), and an axial segment could be characterized as a "ring source." For thin fibers this should be an acceptable simplification. Second, the field expression in Equation 8.17 is strictly for a point source in an *unbounded* space, whereas in reality the space is occluded by the fiber itself. This approximation is normally satisfactory. If,

however, the extracellular space is itself limited, then the fiber probably cannot be ignored and the actual boundary value problem must be solved (Rosenfalck, 1969).

The unbounded extracellular space is important to justify not only the use of the "free-space" point source field of Equation 8.7 but also the linear core-conductor expression of Equation 8.18, which is based on the assumption that $r_o \approx 0$ and $\Phi_i - \Phi_o \approx V_m$. For the isolated fiber of "small" radius, Equations 8.21 and 8.23 appear to be well justified (Trayanova, Henriquez, and Plonsey, 1990).

8.3   EQUIVALENT VOLUME SOURCE DENSITY

PRECONDITIONS:

Source: *Active fiber of finite or infinite length with circular cross section*

Conductor: *Infinite, homogeneous*

8.3.1   Equivalent Monopole Density

A physical interpretation can be given to Equation 8.21 based on the description of the field of a monopole source given by Equation 8.7. We note that $(\pi a^2 \sigma_i \partial^2 V_m/\partial x^2)dx$ behaves like a point current source. Accordingly, the term $(\pi a^2 \sigma_i \partial^2 V_m/\partial x^2)$ has the dimensions of current per unit length. This is a function of x, in general; the variation with x constitutes a description of the source density strength. Since, in fact, the source is considered as lying on the axis, one can interpret the term $(\pi a^2 \sigma_i \partial^2 V_m/\partial x^2)$ as a *line source density*. This is a conceptual as well as a quantitative view of the origins of the volume conductor field (arising from the action potential described by $V_m(x)$).

Alternatively, one can group the terms in Equation 8.21 as

$$\Phi_o = \frac{\sigma_i}{4\pi\sigma_o} \int \frac{(\partial^2 V_m/\partial x^2)\,(\pi a^2 dx)}{r} \qquad (8.24)$$

and $\sigma_i \partial^2 V_m/\partial x^2$ now has the dimensions of a *volume source density (flow source density)* since $\pi a^2 dx$ is a volume element. In fact, the interpretation of Equation 8.24 is that the source fills the intracellular fiber volume, where each source element is a disk of volume $\pi a^2 dx$. The source density is uniform over any disk cross section.

Of course, neither the volume nor line source is physically real. These sources are therefore designated as *equivalent sources*. That is, they are equivalent to the real sources in that the *extracellular fields* calculated from them are correct. For the calculation of *intracellular fields* the true sources (or some other equivalent source) would be required. We return to this topic in a subsequent section of this chapter.

8.3.2 Equivalent Dipole Density

A comparison of Equation 8.23 with Equation 8.12 identifies the equivalent source of the former expression as a *line dipole density* source. This association is highlighted by rewriting Equation 8.23 as

$$\Phi_o = \frac{1}{4\pi\sigma_o} \int \left(-\sigma_i \, \pi a^2 \, \frac{\partial V_m}{\partial x}\right) \nabla \left(\frac{1}{r}\right) \cdot \bar{a}_x \, dx$$

$$(8.25)$$

One can now identify a dipole element as $(-\sigma_i \pi a^2 \partial V_m/\partial x) dx \, \bar{a}_x$. The dipole is oriented in the positive *x*-direction, and the *line dipole density* is $(-\sigma_i \pi a^2 \partial V_m/\partial x)$.

Alternatively, the dipole source can be grouped as $(-\sigma_i \partial V_m/\partial x) \bar{a}_x (\pi a^2 dx)$, which identifies $(-\sigma_i \partial V_m/\partial x)$ as a *volume dipole density;* this fills the intracellular space of the fiber, is oriented in the *x*-direction, and is uniform in any cross section. Hence, a dipole element also can be thought of as a disk of volume $(\pi a^2 dx)$ with the vector magnitude of $(-\pi a^2 dx \sigma_i \partial V_m/\partial x) \bar{a}_x$.

8.3.3 Lumped Equivalent Sources: Tripole Model

Now consider a typical action potential, $V_m(x)$ (the membrane voltage during activation), and its second derivative with respect to *x*. As we have learned, the equivalent volume source density is proportional to $\partial^2 V_m/\partial x^2$, which is shown schematically in Figure 8.3. Note that positive sources lie in the region $x_1 < x < x_2$ and $x_3 < x < x_4$, where the function $\partial^2 V_m/\partial x^2 > 0$, whereas negative sources lie in the region $x_2 < x < x_3$, where $\partial^2 V_m/\partial x^2 < 0$. The sum of the positive sources equals the net negative source. That the field outside the cell, is

generated by this source, is observed to be triphasic (two regions of one polarity separated by a region of opposite polarity) is not surprising in view of the triphasic source distribution.

When the distance to the field point is large compared to the axial extent of each positive or negative source region, then each such source can be approximated by a single (lumped) monopole at the "center of gravity" of the respective source distribution. This is illustrated in Figure 8.3. The resultant model is referred to as a *tripole source* model (since it consists of three monopoles). Intuitively we expect it to be valid, provided a representative distance from each source distribution to the field point r_i satisfies

$$\frac{r_1}{(x_2 - x_1)} > 1, \quad \frac{r_2}{(x_3 - x_2)} > 1, \quad \frac{r_3}{(x_4 - x_3)} > 1$$

$$(8.26)$$

where r_1, r_2, and r_3 as well as x_1, x_2, and x_3 are as described in Figure 8.3. On the basis of Equation 8.24, we can express the tripole field as

$$\Phi_o = \frac{a^2\sigma_i}{4\sigma_o} \left[\frac{\left.\frac{\partial V_m}{\partial x}\right|_{x_2} - \left.\frac{\partial V_m}{\partial x}\right|_{x_1}}{r_1} \right.$$

$$- \frac{\left.\frac{\partial V_m}{\partial x}\right|_{x_3} - \left.\frac{\partial V_m}{\partial x}\right|_{x_2}}{r_2}$$

$$\left. + \frac{\left.\frac{\partial V_m}{\partial x}\right|_{x_4} - \left.\frac{\partial V_m}{\partial x}\right|_{x_3}}{r_3} \right] \quad (8.27)$$

8.3.4 Mathematical Basis for Double-Layer Source (Uniform Bundle)

PRECONDITIONS:

Source: *Active-fiber bundle of finite or infinite length with circular cross section*

Conductor: *Infinite, homogeneous*

The expression for volume dipole density in Section 8.3.2 was given as $(-\sigma_i \partial V_m/\partial x)$, but this was derived for an *isolated* fiber. For the fiber bundle this can be shown to be $(-\sigma_i C \partial V_m/\partial x)$ (Plonsey and Barr, 1987), where

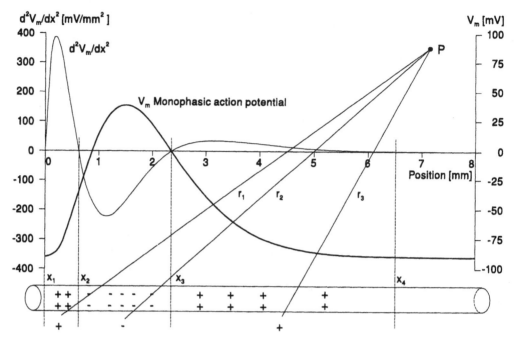

Fig. 8.3 The monophasic action potential (the spatial transmembrane voltage of a propagating activation wave) $V_m(x)$ and its second axial derivative $\partial^2 V_m/\partial x^2$ are shown. As explained in the text, the volume source density is proportional to $\partial^2 V_m/\partial x^2$. Consequently, positive sources lie in the region $x_1 < x < x_2$ and $x_3 < x < x_4$ while negative sources are present in the region $x_2 < x < x_3$. The sources within the fiber are illustrated below. When the extent of each source distribution is small compared to the distance to the field, each distribution can be summed into the lumped source as shown. The distances r_1, r_2, and r_3 are from each lumped source to the distant field point P.

C is a constant that depends on conductivities inside and outside the cell and the fiber bundle geometry. Its value is normally ≈ 0.4.

Figure 8.4 illustrates propagation of the rising phase of a cardiac action potential along a uniform bundle of fibers. In this figure the leading and trailing edges of the active region (where $\partial V_m/\partial x \neq 0$) are assumed to be planar. All fibers in the bundle are assumed to be parallel and carrying similar action potentials; consequently, each fiber will contain a similar equivalent source density. This is shown as a dipole density and hence proportional to $-\partial V_m/\partial x$. Note that in the aforementioned region the function $-\partial V_m(x)/\partial x$ is monophasic, and hence the dipole sources are all oriented in the same direction.

When the extent of the rising phase of the action potential ($x_2 - x_1$ in Fig. 8.4) is small compared to the distance to the field point P, then the axial dipole distribution in a small lateral cross section can be replaced by a lumped dipole. In this case, the source arising in the bundle as a whole can be approximated as a dipole sheet, or *double layer*. For cardiac muscle, because cells are highly interconnected, the fiber bundle of Figure 8.4 is a good approximation to the *behavior* of a propagating wave in any cardiac muscle region regardless of the actual physical fiber orientation.

Measurements on laboratory animals permit the determination at successive instants of time of the surface marking the furthest advance of propagation. Based upon the foregoing, these *isochronal* surfaces may also be viewed, at each instant, as the site of double-layer source. Since the thickness of the rising phase of the propagated cardiac action pulse is only around 0.5 mm (1 ms rise time multiplied by 50 cm/s propagation velocity), the condition that it be small as compared to the distance to the field point is nearly always satisfied when considering

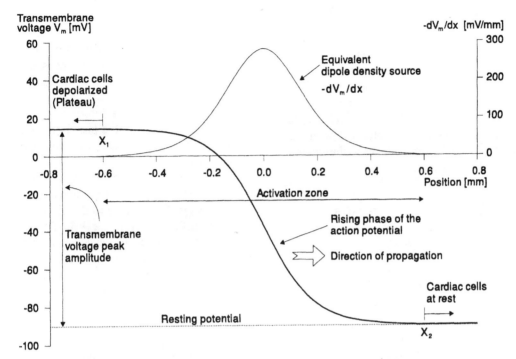

Fig. 8.4 The rising phase of an idealized propagated transmembrane action potential for a cardiac cell is designated V_m. The wave is propagating to the right. The tissue is at rest to the right of the activation zone and in a condition of uniform plateau to the left. The equivalent dipole density source is proportional to $-\partial V_m/\partial x$, which is shown. A physical representation of this dipole distribution is also shown. The dipoles lie in the range $x_1 < x < x_2$.

electrocardiographic voltages at the body surface. The double-layer source model is considered by many to be fundamental to electrocardiography.

8.4 RIGOROUS FORMULATION

8.4.1 Field of a Single Cell of Arbitrary Shape

PRECONDITIONS:

Source: *Single cell of arbitrary shape*
Conductor: *Infinite, homogeneous*

The source-field relationship for an isolated fiber is described by Equation 8.17, which identifies the source density as the transmembrane current. It was pointed out that when this expression was obtained, the source was approximated as a point (rather than a ring), and that

the effect of the fiber itself within the volume conductor was ignored. For the isolated fiber, where the spatial extent of the nerve impulse is large compared to the fiber radius, it can be shown that the line-source formula of Equation 8.17 is very satisfactory (Trayanova, Henriquez, and Plonsey, 1990).

When these conditions are not satisfied, it is desirable to have a rigorous (exact) source expression. One can show that for an arbitrarily shaped active cell of surface S, the field generated by it at point P, outside or inside the cell, is

$$\Phi_P = \frac{1}{4\pi\sigma_P} \int_S (\sigma_o\Phi_o - \sigma_i\Phi_i) \, \nabla\left(\frac{1}{r}\right) \cdot d\bar{S} \tag{8.28}$$

where

Φ_P = field at point P
Φ_i = potential just inside the membrane
Φ_o = potential just outside the membrane
σ_i = conductivity inside the membrane

σ_o = conductivity outside the membrane
σ_P = conductivity at the field point

The source identified by Equation 8.28 is a double layer lying on the membrane surface, whose strength is $(\sigma_o\Phi_o - \sigma_i\Phi_i)dS$ and whose orientation is along the outward surface normal (Plonsey, 1974). The field point P in Equation 8.28 can be intracellular as well as extracellular; however, the coefficient σ_P takes on the conductivity at the field point.

8.4.2 Field of an Isolated Cylindrical Fiber

PRECONDITIONS:

Source: *Isolated cylindrical fiber*
Conductor: *Infinite, homogeneous*

If one applies Equation 8.28 to an isolated cylindrical fiber, then assuming only $\Phi_o \approx 0$ (hence $\Phi_i - \Phi_o \approx V_m$) leads to

$$\Phi_o = \frac{1}{4\pi\sigma_o} \iint \frac{\partial^2 V_m/\partial x^2}{r} \, dA\,dx \quad \textbf{(8.29)}$$

where the integration proceeds over the cross-sectional area A, as well as axially. If the field point is at a large distance compared to the radius, then Equation 8.29 reduces to Equation 8.21 and Equation 8.17, thus confirming the earlier work when these approximations are satisfied.

8.5 MATHEMATICAL BASIS FOR MACROSCOPIC VOLUME SOURCE DENSITY (FLOW SOURCE DENSITY) AND IMPRESSED CURRENT DENSITY

PRECONDITIONS:

Source: *Layer of dipole source elements $\bar{J}^i$*
Conductor: *Infinite, homogeneous*

In this section we discuss the mathematical basis of the concepts of *volume source density (flow source density)*, I_F, and *impressed current density, $\bar{J}^i$*.

As a consequence of the activation process in cardiac tissue, the heart behaves as a source of currents and generates potentials in the surrounding volume conductor. These sources consist of layers of dipole source elements, which lie in the isochronal activation surfaces, as pointed out earlier. This description is only an approximation, since it is based on the assumption that cardiac tissue is homogeneous and isotropic.

In principle, Equation 8.28 can be applied to each active cell in the heart. Since a cardiac cell is very small compared to the distance of observation, the radius vector $\bar{r}$ in Equation 8.28 may be assumed to be constant in the integration over each cell. Thus each cell can be thought of as contributing a single lumped dipole source, which is simply the vector sum of its double-layer surface elements. That is, the dipole for the jth cell, $d\bar{p}_j$ is given by

$$d\bar{p}_j = \int (\sigma_o\Phi_o - \sigma_i\Phi_i)d\bar{S}_j \quad (8.30)$$

Since the heart contains around 5×10^{10} cells of which perhaps 5% are active at any moment during depolarization, the number of dipole source elements is extremely high. Under these conditions one can define a *volume dipole moment density function* (i.e., a dipole moment per unit volume) by averaging the dipole elements in each small volume. That is,

$$\bar{J}^i = \frac{\displaystyle\sum_{j=1}^{N} d\bar{p}_j}{\displaystyle\sum_{j=1}^{N} dv_j} \quad (8.31)$$

where the denominator is the total volume occupied by a group of N cells, and dS_j is the surface of each volume element dv_j. The idea is to make N small enough so that a good resolution is achieved (where the average is not smoothed unnecessarily), but large enough so that the function $\bar{J}^i$ is continuous from point to point (and does not reflect the underlying discrete cellular structure). Equation 8.31 is sometimes described as a *coarse-grained average*, since we do not let the volume, over which the average is taken, go to zero. The same considerations apply, for example, in electrostatics, where the *charge density* is normally consid-

Table 8.1 Summary of the equations for different sources and their fields (Equation number in text)

Source model	Source element description		Field Φ_o outside the source		Source density	
Monopole	I_0	(8.7)	$\dfrac{I_0}{4\pi\sigma r}$	(8.7)	[point source]	
Dipole	$\bar{p} = I_0\bar{d}$	(8.9)	$\dfrac{p\cos\theta}{4\pi\sigma r^2}$	(8.15)	[point (dipole) source]	
Single isolated fiber $r > a$ (where $a =$ fiber radius)	$i_m(x)dx$	(8.16)	$\dfrac{a^2\sigma_i}{4\sigma_o}\displaystyle\int\dfrac{\partial^2 V_m/\partial x^2}{r}\,dx$	(8.21)	$\dfrac{\sigma_i\pi a^2\partial^2 V_m}{\partial x^2}$	line source density
					$\dfrac{\sigma_i\partial^2 V_m}{\partial x^2}$	volume source density
			$-\dfrac{a^2\sigma_i}{4\sigma_o}\displaystyle\int\dfrac{\partial V_m}{\partial x}\nabla\left(\dfrac{1}{r}\right)\cdot\bar{a}_x\,dx$	(8.23)	$\dfrac{-\sigma_i\pi a^2\partial V_m}{\partial x}$	line dipole density
					$\dfrac{-\sigma_i\partial V_m}{\partial x}$	volume dipole density
Fiber bundle					$\dfrac{-\sigma_i C\partial V_m}{\partial x}$	volume dipole density, $C \approx 0.4$
Tripole	$\sigma_i\,\partial^2 V_m/\partial x^2$ $>0:x_1 < x < x_2$ $<0:x_2 < x < x_3$ $>0:x_3 < x < x_4$		$\dfrac{a^2\sigma_i}{4\sigma_o}\left[\dfrac{\dfrac{\partial V_m}{\partial x_1^2}}{r_1} - \dfrac{\dfrac{\partial V_m}{\partial x_2^3}}{r_2} + \dfrac{\dfrac{\partial V_m}{\partial x_3^4}}{r_3}\right]$ (8.27) V_m refers here to a triangular approximation of the actual transmembrane potential (exact form of the equation in the text).		Point sources on axis location: strength: x_1 $\left.\dfrac{\partial V_m}{\partial x}\right\|_1^2$ x_2 $\left.\dfrac{\partial V_m}{\partial x}\right\|_2^3$ x_3 $\left.\dfrac{\partial V_m}{\partial x}\right\|_3^4$	
Single cell (exact formulation)	$(\sigma_o\Phi_o - \sigma_i\Phi_i)\,dS$	(8.28)	$\dfrac{1}{4\pi\sigma_P}\displaystyle\int(\sigma_o\Phi_o - \sigma_i\Phi_i)\nabla\left(\dfrac{1}{r}\right)\cdot d\bar{S}$	(8.28)	Double layer with a strength of $(\sigma_o\Phi_o - \sigma_i\Phi_i)$ lying in the cell membrane, and oriented in the outward direction	
Isolated cylindrical fiber (exact formulation)	$(\sigma_o\Phi_o - \sigma_i\Phi_i)\,dS$	(8.28)	$\dfrac{1}{4\pi\sigma_o}\displaystyle\iint\dfrac{\partial^2 V_m/\partial x^2}{r}\,dA\,dx$	(8.29)	$\dfrac{\partial^2 V_m}{\partial x^2}$	volume source (flow source) density lying within the fiber
Multicellular tissue (brain or cardiac tissue)	$\bar{J}^i\,dV$		$\dfrac{1}{4\pi\sigma_o}\displaystyle\int\dfrac{-\nabla\cdot\bar{J}^i}{r}\,dv$	(8.34)	$\bar{J}^i$	volume dipole density
					$-\nabla\cdot\bar{J}^i$	volume source (flow source) density

157

ered to be a smooth, well-behaved function even though it reflects a discrete collection of finite point sources.

The source function $\bar{J}^i$ is a *(volume) dipole density function*. Consequently, the field it generates can be found by superposition, where $\bar{J}^i \, dv$ is a single dipole to which Equation 8.12 applies. Thus, summing the field from all such elements, one obtains

$$\Phi_o = \frac{1}{4\pi\sigma_o} \int \nabla \left(\frac{1}{r} \right) \cdot \bar{J}^i \, dv \qquad (8.32)$$

If one applies the vector identity $\nabla \cdot (\bar{J}^i/r) = \nabla (1/r) \cdot \bar{J}^i + (1/r) \nabla \cdot \bar{J}^i$ to Equation 8.32, then

$$\Phi_o = \frac{1}{4\pi\sigma_o} \int \nabla \cdot \left(\frac{\bar{J}^i}{r} \right) dv - \frac{1}{4\pi\sigma_o} \int \frac{\nabla \cdot \bar{J}^i}{r} \, dv$$

$$(8.33)$$

The divergence (or Gauss's) theorem can be applied to the first term on the right-hand side of Equation 8.33, and since $\bar{J}^i = 0$ at S (all source elements lie within the heart, and none are at the surface of integration), we get

$$\Phi_o = \frac{1}{4\pi\sigma_o} \int \frac{-\nabla \cdot \bar{J}^i}{r} \, dv \qquad \textbf{(8.34)}$$

Reference to Equation 8.7 identifies that

$$I_F = -\nabla \cdot \bar{J}^i \qquad \textbf{(8.35)}$$

is a *volume source (flow source) density*.

As was discussed in Section 7.2.2, one can interpret $\bar{J}^i$ as an impressed (i.e., an applied) current density. This current density is brought into being by the expenditure of chemical energy (i.e., the movement of ions due to concentration gradients); it is the primary cause for the establishment of an electric field. In contrast, we note that the current density, $\bar{J} = \sigma\bar{E}$, that is described by Ohm's law in Equation 8.4, is induced (i.e., it arises secondary to the presence of the aforementioned electric field $\bar{E}$). Impressed currents $\bar{J}^i$ are not established by the electric field $\bar{E}$, since they originate in a source of energy, which is nonelectric in nature.

8.6 SUMMARY OF THE SOURCE-FIELD MODELS

Table 8.1 gives the equations used in this chapter (with equation numbers) for the different sources and their fields in an infinite homogeneous volume conductor.

REFERENCES

Henriquez CS, Plonsey R (1988): The effect of the extracellular potential on propagation in excitable tissue. *Comments Theor. Biol.* 1: 47–64.

Plonsey R (1974): The formulation of bioelectric source-field relationships in terms of surface discontinuities. *J. Franklin Inst.* 297:(5) 317–24.

Plonsey R, Barr RC (1987): Interstitial potentials and their change with depth into cardiac tissue. *Biophys. J.* 51: 547–55.

Rosenfalck P (1969): Intra- and extracellular potential fields of active nerve and muscle fibers. *Acta Physiol. Scand.* 321:(Suppl) 1–168.

Trayanova N, Henriquez CS, Plonsey R (1990): Limitations of approximate solutions for computing the extracellular potential of single fibers and bundle equivalents. *IEEE Trans. Biomed. Eng.* BME-37: 22–35.

9

Bidomain Model of Multicellular Volume Conductors

9.1 INTRODUCTION

Many investigations in electrophysiology involve preparations that contain multiple cells. Examples include the nerve bundle, which consists of several thousand myelinated fibers; striated whole muscle, which may contain several thousand individual fibers; the heart, which has on the order of 10^{10} cells; and the brain, which also has about 10^{10} cells. In modeling the electric behavior of such preparations, the discrete cellular structure may be important (Spach, 1983). On the other hand, macroscopic (averaged) fields may adequately describe the phenomena of interest. In the latter case it is possible to replace the discrete structure with an averaged continuum that represents a considerable simplification. The goal of this chapter is to formulate a continuum representation of multicellular systems and then to explore its electric properties.

9.2 CARDIAC MUSCLE CONSIDERED AS A CONTINUUM

The individual cells of cardiac muscle are roughly circular cylinders with a diameter of around 10 μm and length of 100 μm. The cells are stacked together a lot like bricks and are held together by *tight junctions* (these behave like "spot welds" of abutting cellular membranes). In addition, there are *gap junctions,* which provide for intercellular communication. The latter introduce a direct intercellular link which permits the movement of small molecules and ions from the intracellular space of one cell to that of its neighbors.

The gap junction consists of hexagonal arrays of proteins called *connexons,* which completely penetrate the pre- and postjunctional abutting membranes. A central channel provides a resistive path for the movement of ions between the cells. Since such paths are limited in numbers and have very small cross-sectional areas, the effective junctional resistance is not negligible. In fact, the net junctional resistance between two adjoining cells is thought to be in the same order of magnitude as the end-to-end resistance of the myoplasm of either cell. On the other hand, this resistance is perhaps three orders of magnitude less than what it would be if current had to cross the two abutting membranes, highlighting the importance of the specialized gap-junctional pathway.

The length of the junctional channel is roughly that of the two plasma membranes (2 × 8.5 nm) through which it passes, plus the gap between membranes (3 nm)—or around 20 nm total. This length is very short in contrast with the length of a cell itself, since the ratio is roughly $20 \times 10^{-9}/100 \times 10^{-6} = 2 \times 10^{-4}$. Consequently, since the total junctional and myoplasmic resistances are approximately equal but are distributed over lengths that are in the ratio of 2×10^{-4}, one can think of the junctional resistance as if it were concentrated at a point (i.e., it is a discrete resistance), whereas the myoplasmic resistance is spread out (or distributed) in character. These two types of resistance structures affect a propagating wave differently, as we demonstrate below.

A simplified representation of the intracellular space is given in Figure 9.1. The current and potential distributions within a cell are continuous. However, the junction, in view of its relatively short length but sizable resistance, must be considered as relatively discrete (lumped), and it introduces jumps in the voltage patterns, which accounts for the representation given in Figure 9.1.

By confining our interest to potential and current field variations averaged over many cells, we can approximate the intracellular region described in Figure 9.1 by a continuous (averaged) volume conductor that fills the total space. The discrete and myoplasmic resistances are taken into account when the averaged values

are obtained. The result is an intracellular conducting medium that is continuous.

One can apply the same considerations to the interstitial space. Although there are no discrete elements in this case, the space is nevertheless broken up by the presence of the cells. The fields associated with this continuum may be considered averaged over a distance of several cells—just as for the intracellular space.

In summary, the complex cardiac tissue may be replaced by intracellular and interstitial continua, each filling the space occupied by the actual tissue. The parameters of the continua are derived by a suitable average of the actual structure. Both spaces are described by the same coordinate system. The membrane separates both domains at each point. This model has been described and has been designated as a *bidomain* (Miller and Geselowitz, 1978; Tung, 1978).

In a more accurate model one can introduce the potential and current field variations on a cellular scale which are superimposed on variations that take place over longer spatial distances. Usually the former are of little interest when one is studying the macroscopic behavior of the tissue, and an averaged, smoothed (continuum) associated with the averaged fields is an acceptable and even a desirable simplification.

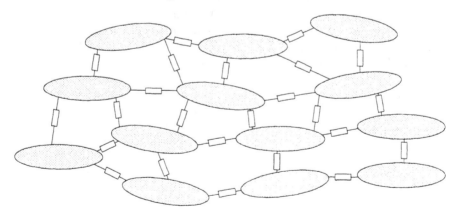

Fig. 9.1 Cells are represented as ellipsoidal-like regions within which the intracellular potential field is continuous. The intracellular spaces of adjoining cells are interconnected by junctional (discrete) resistances representing the effect of gap junctions. These introduce, on a cellular scale, discontinuities in the potential. If we confine our interest to variations on a macroscopic scale (compared to the size of a cell), then the medium can be considered to be continuous and fill all space. Such a medium is described by averaged properties, and the potentials that are evaluated must also be smoothed relative to a cellular dimension.

9.3 MATHEMATICAL DESCRIPTION OF THE BIDOMAIN AND ANISOTROPY

The verbal description of the bidomain, discussed above, leads to definitive mathematical expressions for currents and potentials which, in view of the continuous structure, are in analytical form.

We first introduce the concept of *bidomain conductivity* (σ^b). The intracellular and extracellular conductivities σ_i and σ_o, which we introduced earlier in this book, are *microscopic* conductivities. That is, they describe the conductivity at a point, and for an inhomogeneous medium they are functions of position. (Normally we consider σ_o a constant that tends to hide the fact that it is defined at each and every point.) The bidomain conductivities σ_i^b and σ_o^b are averaged values over several cells. That is why the bidomain conductivities depend on both the microscopic conductivity and the geometry.

We now generalize Equation 7.2 ($\bar{J} = -\sigma \nabla \Phi$) to an *anisotropic conducting medium* where the current density components in the x, y, and z directions are proportional to the gradient of the intracellular scalar potential function Φ_i in the corresponding directions. Thus, for the *intracellular* domain, application of Ohm's law gives

$$\bar{J}_i = - \left[\sigma_{ix}^b \frac{\partial \Phi_i}{\partial x} \bar{i} + \sigma_{iy}^b \frac{\partial \Phi_i}{\partial y} \bar{j} + \sigma_{iz}^b \frac{\partial \Phi_i}{\partial z} \bar{k} \right]$$

(9.1)

where

$\bar{J}_i$ = current density in the intracellular medium

Φ_i = electric potential in the intracellular medium

$\sigma_{ix}^b, \sigma_{iy}^b, \sigma_{iz}^b$ = intracellular bidomain conductivities in the x, y, and z directions

$\bar{i}, \bar{j}, \bar{k}$ = unit vectors in the x, y, and z directions

The proportionality constant (i.e., the bidomain conductivity) in each coordinate direction is considered to be different, reflecting the most general condition. Such anisotropicity is to be expected in view of the organized character of the tissue with preferential conducting directions. In fact, experimental observation has shown the conductivities to be highest along fiber directions relative to that in the cross-fiber direction.

Correspondingly, in the *interstitial* domain, assuming anisotropy here also, we have

$$\bar{J}_o = - \left[\sigma_{ox}^b \frac{\partial \Phi_o}{\partial x} \bar{i} + \sigma_{oy}^b \frac{\partial \Phi_o}{\partial y} \bar{j} + \sigma_{oz}^b \frac{\partial \Phi_o}{\partial z} \bar{k} \right]$$

(9.2)

where

$\bar{J}$ = current density in the interstitial medium

Φ_o = electric potential in the interstitial medium

$\sigma_{ox}^b, \sigma_{oy}^b, \sigma_{oz}^b$ = interstitial bidomain conductivities in the x, y, and z directions

In general, the conductivity coefficients in the intracellular and interstitial domains can be expected to be different since they are, essentially, unrelated. Macroscopic measurements performed by Clerc (1976) and by Roberts and Scher (1982), which evaluated the coefficients in Equations 9.1 and 9.2 for cardiac muscle, are given in Table 9.1. These represent the only available measurements of these important parameters; unfortunately they differ substantially (partly because different methods were used), leaving a degree of uncertainty regarding the correct values.

The fiber orientation (axis) in these determinations was defined as the x coordinate; because of uniformity in the transverse plane, the conductivities in the y and z directions are equal.

The intracellular current density $\bar{J}_i$ (Equation 9.1) and the interstitial current density $\bar{J}_o$ (Equation 9.2) are coupled by the need for current conservation. That is, current lost to one region

Table 9.1 Bidomain conductivities of cardiac tissue [mS/cm] measured by Clerc (1976) and Roberts and Scher (1982)

	Clerc (1976)	Roberts and Scher (1982)
σ_{ix}^b	1.74	3.44
$\sigma_{iy}^b, \sigma_{iz}^b$	0.193	0.596
σ_{ox}^b	6.25	1.17
$\sigma_{oy}^b, \sigma_{oz}^b$	2.36	0.802

must be gained by the other. The loss (or gain) is evaluated by the divergence; therefore,

$$-\nabla \cdot \bar{J}_\mathrm{i} = \nabla \cdot \bar{J}_\mathrm{o} = I_\mathrm{m} \qquad (9.3)$$

where

I_m = transmembrane current per unit volume [μA/cm^3].

In retrospect, the weakness in the bidomain model is that all fields are considered to be spatially averaged, with a consequent loss in resolution. On the other hand, the behavior of all fields is expressed by the differential Equations 9.1–9.3 which permits the use of mathematical approaches available in the literature on mathematical physics.

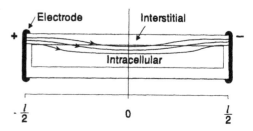

Fig. 9.2 A prototypical fiber of a fiber bundle lying in oil and its response to the application of a steady current. Since the fiber is sealed, current flow into the intracellular space is spread out along the cylinder membrane. The ratio of interstitial to intracellular cross-sectional area of the single fiber reflects that of the bundle as a whole. The Figure is not drawn to scale since usually the ratio of fiber length to fiber diameter is very large.

9.4 ONE-DIMENSIONAL CABLE: A ONE-DIMENSIONAL BIDOMAIN

PRECONDITIONS:

Source: *Bundle of parallel muscle fibers; a one-dimensional problem*

Conductor: *Finite, inhomogeneous, anisotropic bidomain*

Consider a large bundle of parallel striated muscle fibers lying in an insulating medium such as oil. If a large plate electrode is placed at each end and supplied a current step, and all fibers are assumed to be of essentially equal diameter, the response of each fiber will be the same. Consequently, to consider the behavior of the bundle, it is sufficient to model any single fiber, which then characterizes all fibers. Such a prototypical fiber and its associated interstitial space are described in Figure 9.2.

The cross-sectional area of the interstitial space shown in Figure 9.2 is $1/N$ times the total interstitial cross-sectional area of the fiber bundle, where N is the number of fibers. Usually, the interstitial cross-sectional area is less than the intracellular cross-sectional area, since fibers typically occupy 70–80% of the total area. Consequently, an electric representation of the preparation in Figure 9.2 is none other than the linear core-conductor model described in Figure 3.7 and Equations 3.41 and 3.42. In this case the model appropriately and correctly includes the interstitial axial resistance since current in that path is constrained to the axial direction (as it is for the intracellular space).

A circuit representation for steady-state subthreshold conditions is given in Figure 9.3. In this figure, r_i and r_o are the intracellular and interstitial axial resistances per unit length, respectively. Since steady-state subthreshold conditions are assumed, the membrane behavior can be described by a constant (leakage) resistance of r_m ohms times length (i.e., the capacitive membrane component can be ignored since $\partial V/\partial t = 0$ at steady state; hence the capacitive component of the membrane current $i_\mathrm{mC} = c_\mathrm{m}\partial V/\partial t = 0$.

The system, which is modeled by Figure 9.3, is in fact, a continuum. Accordingly it may be described by appropriate differential equations. In fact, these equations that follow, known as cable equations, have already been derived and commented on in Chapter 3. In particular, we found (Equation 3.46) that

$$\frac{\partial^2 V_\mathrm{m}}{\partial x^2} - \frac{V_\mathrm{m}}{\lambda^2} = 0 \qquad (9.4)$$

where the space constant, λ, is defined as

$$\lambda = \sqrt{\frac{r_\mathrm{m}}{r_\mathrm{i} + r_\mathrm{o}}} \qquad (9.5)$$

and has the dimension [cm]. This is the same as in Equation 3.48.

In Equation 9.4, and in the following equations of this chapter, V_m describes the membrane potential relative to the resting potential. Consequently V_m corresponds to the V' of

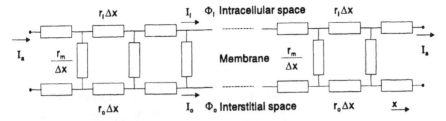

Fig. 9.3 Linear core-conductor model circuit that corresponds to the preparation shown in Figure 9.2. The applied steady-state current I_a enters the interstitial space on the left and leaves on the right (at these sites $I_i = 0$). The *steady-state* subthreshold response is considered; hence the membrane is modeled as a resistance. Only the first few elements at each end are shown explicitly.

Chapter 3. Since, under resting conditions, there are no currents or signals (though there is a transmembrane voltage), interest is usually confined entirely to the deviations from the resting condition, and all reference to the resting potential ignored. The literature will be found to refer to the potential difference from rest without explicitly stating this to be the case, because it has become so generally recognized. For this more advanced chapter we have adopted this common practice and have refrained from including the prime symbol with V_m.

For the preparation in Figure 9.2, we anticipate a current of I_a to enter the interstitial space at the left-hand edge ($x = -l/2$), and as it proceeds to the right, a portion crosses the membrane to flow into the intracellular space. The process is reversed in the right half of the fiber, as a consequence of symmetry. The boundary condition of $I_i = 0$ at $x = \pm l/2$ depends on the ends being sealed and the membrane area at the ends being a very small fraction of the total area. The argument is that although current may cross the end membranes, the relative area is so small that the relative current must likewise be very small (and negligible); this argument is supported by analytical studies (Weidmann, 1952). Since the transmembrane voltage is simply the transmembrane current per unit length times the membrane resistance times unit length (i.e., $V_m = i_m r_m$), the antisymmetric (i.e., equal but opposite) condition expected for i_m must also be satisfied by V_m. Since the solution to the differential equation of 9.4 is the sum of hyperbolic sine and cosine functions, only the former has the correct behavior, and the solution to Equation 9.4 is necessarily:

$$V_m = K_a \sinh(x/\lambda) \qquad (9.6)$$

where

K_a = a constant related to the strength of the supplied current, I_a

We found earlier for the axial currents inside and outside the axon, in Equation 3.41 that

$$I_i = \frac{1}{r_i}\frac{\partial \Phi_i}{\partial x} \qquad (9.7a)$$

$$I_o = \frac{1}{r_o}\frac{\partial \Phi_o}{\partial x} \qquad (9.7b)$$

If Equation 9.7 is applied at either end of the preparation ($x = \pm l/2$), where $\partial \Phi_i/\partial x = 0$ and where $I_o = I_a$, we get

$$I_o = \frac{1}{r_o}\frac{\partial V_m}{\partial x} = I_a \qquad (x = \pm l/2) \qquad (9.8)$$

Substituting Equation 9.6 into Equation 9.8 permits evaluation of K_a as

$$K_a = \frac{I_a r_o \lambda}{\cosh(l/2\lambda)} \qquad (9.9)$$

Consequently, substituting Equation 9.9 into Equation 9.6 results in

$$V_m = I_a r_o \lambda \frac{\sinh(x/\lambda)}{\cosh(l/2\lambda)} \qquad (9.10)$$

We are interested in examining the intracellular and interstitial current behavior over the length of the fiber. The intracellular and interstitial currents are found by substituting Equation 9.10 into Equations 9.7a,b, while noting that $V_m = \Phi_i - \Phi_o$ and that the intracellular and interstitial currents are constrained by the requirement that $I_i + I_o = I_a$ for all x due to conservation of current. The result is that

$$I_i = I_a \left[\frac{r_o}{r_i + r_o} - \frac{r_o}{r_i + r_o} \frac{\cosh(x/\lambda)}{\cosh(l/2\lambda)} \right] \quad (9.11)$$

$$I_o = I_a \left[\frac{r_i}{r_i + r_o} + \frac{r_o}{r_i + r_o} \frac{\cosh(x/\lambda)}{\cosh(l/2\lambda)} \right] \quad (9.12)$$

The intracellular and interstitial currents described by Equations 9.11 and 9.12 are plotted in Figure 9.4 for the case that $l = 20\lambda$ and where $r_i = r_o/2$. An important feature is that although the total current is applied to the interstitial space, a portion crosses the fiber membrane to flow in the intracellular space (a phenomenon described by *current redistribution*). We note that this redistribution of current from the interstitial to intracellular space takes place over an axial extent of several lambda. One can conclude that if the fiber length, expressed in lambdas, is say greater than 10, then in the central region, essentially complete redistribution has taken place. In this region, current-voltage relations appear as if the membrane were absent. Indeed, $V_m \approx 0$ and intracellular and interstitial currents are essentially axial and constant.

The total impedance presented to the electrodes by the fiber can be evaluated by dividing the applied voltage $V_a[\Phi_o(-l/2) - \Phi_o(l/2)]$ by the total current I_a. The value of V_a can be found by integrating I_oR_o from $x = -l/2$ to $x = l/2$ using Equation 9.12. The result is that this impedance Z is

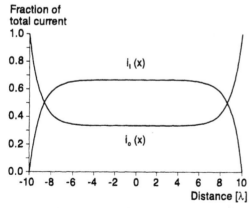

Fraction of
total current

Fig. 9.4 Distribution of intracellular axial current $i_i(x)$ and interstitial axial current $i_o(x)$ for the fiber described in Figure 9.2. The total length is 20λ and $r_i/r_o = 1/2$. Note that the steady-state conditions which apply for $-7\lambda < x < 7\lambda$, approximately suggest $\approx 3\lambda$ as an extent needed for current redistribution.

$$Z = \frac{r_o}{r_i + r_o} [r_i l + 2r_o \lambda \tanh(l/2\lambda)] \quad (9.13)$$

If $l > \lambda$ and if r_i and r_o are assumed to be of the same order of magnitude, then the second term in the brackets of Equation 9.13 can be neglected relative to the first and the load is essentially that expected if the membrane were absent (a single domain resistance found from the parallel contribution of r_o and r_i). And if $l < \lambda$, then $\tanh(l/2\lambda) \approx l/2\lambda$ and $Z = r_o l$, reflecting the absence of any significant current redistribution; only the interstitial space supplies a current flow path. When neither inequality holds, Z reflects some intermediate degree of current redistribution.

The example considered here is a simple illustration of the bidomain model and is included for two reasons. First, it is a one-dimensional problem and hence mathematically simple. Second, as we have noted, the preparation considered is, in fact, a continuum. Thus while cardiac muscle was approximated as a continuum and hence described by a bidomain, in this case a continuum is not just a simplifying assumption but, in fact, a valid description of the tissue.

Although we have introduced the additional simplification of subthreshold and steady-state conditions, the basic idea of current redistribution between intracellular and interstitial space should apply under less restrictive situations. It seems trivial to point out that whenever a multicellular region is studied, its separate intracellular and interstitial behavior needs to be considered in view of a possible discontinuity across the membrane (namely V_m). This is true whether the fibers are considered to be discrete or continuous.

9.5 SOLUTION FOR POINT-CURRENT SOURCE IN A THREE-DIMENSIONAL, ISOTROPIC BIDOMAIN

PRECONDITIONS:

Source: *Volume of muscle fibers; a three-dimensional problem*

Conductor: *Finite, inhomogeneous, anisotropic bidomain*

As a further illustration of the bidomain model, we consider a volume of cardiac muscle and assume that it can be modeled as a bidomain, which is uniform and isotropic. Consequently, in place of Equations 9.1 and 9.2 we may write:

$$\bar{J}_i = -\sigma_i^b \nabla \Phi_i \qquad (9.14)$$

$$\bar{J}_o = -\sigma_o^b \nabla \Phi_o \qquad (9.15)$$

Here σ_i^b and σ_o^b have the dimensions of conductivity, and we refer to them as the isotropic intracellular and interstitial bidomain conductivities. Their values can be found as follows. Since each domain is considered to fill the *total* tissue space, which is larger than the actual occupied space, σ_i^b and σ_o^b are evaluated from the *microscopic* conductivities σ_i and σ_o by multiplying by the ratio of the actual to total volume, thus

$$\sigma_i^b = \sigma_i v_c \qquad (9.16)$$

$$\sigma_o^b = \sigma_o (1 - v_c) \qquad (9.17)$$

where

v_c = the fraction of muscle occupied by the cells (= 0.70–0.85)

In these equations the conductivity on the left is a bidomain conductivity (and actually an averaged conductivity that could be measured only in an adequately large tissue sample), whereas the conductivity function on the right is the (microscopic) conductivity.

Now the divergence of $\bar{J}_o$ ordinarily evaluates the transmembrane current density, but we wish to include the possibility that an additional (applied) point current source has been introduced into the tissue. Assuming that an *interstitial* point source of strength I_a is placed at the coordinate origin requires

$$\nabla \cdot \bar{J}_o = I_m^b + I_a \delta_v \qquad (9.18)$$

where δ_v is a *three-dimensional Dirac delta function*, which is defined as

$$\int \delta_v dV = \int \delta_v 4\pi r^2 dr$$

= 1 if the volume includes the origin

= 0 if the volume excludes the origin

Equation 9.18 reduces to Equation 9.3 if $I_a = 0$.

Substituting Equation 9.15 into Equation 9.18 gives

$$-\sigma_o^b \nabla^2 \Phi_o = I_m^b + I_a \delta_v \qquad (9.19)$$

where

I_m^b = transmembrane current per unit volume [μA/cm^3]

We also require the conservation of current (Equation 9.3):

$$\nabla \cdot \bar{J}_i = -I_m^b \qquad (9.20)$$

and substituting Equation 9.14 into Equation 9.20 gives

$$\sigma_i^b \nabla^2 \Phi_i = I_m^b \qquad (9.21)$$

Now multiplying Equation 9.19 by $\rho_o^b (= 1/\sigma_o^b)$ and Equation 9.21 by $\rho_i^b (= 1/\sigma_i^b)$ and summing results, we get

$$\nabla^2 (\Phi_i - \Phi_o) = \nabla^2 V_m \qquad (9.22)$$
$$= (\rho_i^b + \rho_o^b) I_m^b + \rho_o I_a \delta_v$$

where

ρ_i^b = bidomain intracellular resistivity [k$\Omega \cdot$ cm]
ρ_o^b = bidomain interstitial resistivity [k$\Omega \cdot$ cm]
I_m^b = transmembrane current per unit volume [μA/cm^3]

Under subthreshold steady-state conditions, the capacitance can be ignored, and consequently, the membrane is purely resistive. If the surface-to-volume ratio of the cells is uniform and is designated χ, then the steady-state transmembrane current per unit volume (I_m^b) is

$$I_m^b = \frac{\chi V_m}{R_m} = \frac{V_m}{\rho_m^b} \qquad (9.23)$$

where

I_m^b = transmembrane current per unit volume [μA/cm^3]
χ = surface to volume ratio of the cell [1/cm]
V_m = membrane voltage [mV]
R_m = membrane resistance times unit area [k$\Omega \cdot$ cm^2]

and where

$$\rho_m^b = \frac{R_m}{\chi} \qquad (9.24)$$

is membrane resistance times unit volume [k$\Omega \cdot$ cm]. (The variable ρ_m^b has the dimension of resistivity, because it represents the contribution of the membranes to the leakage resistivity of a medium including intracellular and extracellular spaces and the membranes.)

Substituting Equation 9.23 into Equation 9.22 results in the desired differential equation for V_m, namely

$$\nabla^2 V_m = \frac{V_m}{\lambda^2} + \rho_o^b I_a \delta_v \qquad (9.25)$$

where

$$\lambda = \sqrt{\frac{\rho_m^b}{\rho_i^b + \rho_o^b}} \qquad (9.26)$$

The *three-dimensional isotropic space constant,* defined by Equation 9.26, is in the same form and has the same dimension [cm] as we evaluated for one-dimensional preparations described by Equation 9.5.

In view of the spherical symmetry, the Laplacian of V_m (in Equation 9.25) which in spherical coordinates has the form

$$\frac{1}{r^2}\frac{\partial}{\partial r}\left(r^2\frac{\partial}{\partial r}\right) + \frac{1}{r^2\sin\Theta}\frac{\partial}{\partial\Theta}\left(\sin\Theta\frac{\partial}{\partial\Theta}\right) + \frac{1}{r^2\sin^2\Theta}\frac{\partial}{\partial\Phi}$$

contains only an r dependence, so that we obtain

$$\frac{\partial^2 (rV_m)}{\partial r^2} = \frac{rV_m}{\lambda^2} + \rho_o^b r I_a \delta_v \qquad (9.27)$$

The solution when $r \neq 0$ is

$$V_m = K_B \frac{e^{-r/\lambda}}{r} \qquad (9.28)$$

One can take into account the delta function source δ_v by imposing a consistent boundary condition at the origin. With this point of view, K_B, in Equation 9.28, is chosen so that the behavior of V_m for $r \to 0$ is correct. This condition is introduced by integrating each term in Equation 9.25 through a spherical volume of radius $r \to 0$ centered at the origin. The volume integral of the term on the left-hand side of Equation 9.25 is performed by converting it to a surface integral using the divergence theorem of vector analysis. One finds that

$$\int_0^r (\nabla^2 V_m)\, 4\pi r^2 dr = 4\pi \int_0^r \nabla \cdot \nabla V_m r^2 dr$$

$$= \oint \nabla V \cdot d\bar{S} \qquad (9.29)$$

$$= \lim_{r \to 0}\left(4\pi r^2 \frac{\partial V_m}{\partial r}\right)$$

$$= -4\pi K_B$$

(The last step is achieved by substituting from Equation 9.28 for V_m.)

Substituting Equation 9.28 for V_m in the second term of Equation 9.25 gives

$$\int_0^r \frac{V_m}{\lambda^2}\, 4\pi r^2 dr = 4\pi K_B \int_0^r re^{-r/\lambda}\, dr = 0 \qquad (9.30)$$

whereas the third term

$$\int_0^r \rho_o^b I_a\, 4\pi r^2 \delta_v dr = \rho_o^b I_a \qquad (9.31)$$

Equation 9.31 follows from the definition of the Dirac delta function δ_v given for Equation 9.18. Substituting Equations 9.29–9.31 into Equation 9.25 demonstrates that V_m will have the correct behavior in the r neighborhood of the origin if K_B satisfies

$$K_B = -\frac{\rho_o^b I_a}{4\pi} \qquad (9.32)$$

Substituting Equation 9.32 into Equation 9.28 finally results in

$$V_m = -\frac{\rho_o^b I_a}{4\pi}\frac{e^{-r/\lambda_o^b}}{r} \qquad (9.33)$$

If the scalar function ψ is defined as

$$\psi = \frac{\rho_o^b \Phi_i}{\rho_o^b + \rho_i^b} + \frac{\rho_i^b \Phi_o}{\rho_o^b + \rho_i^b} \qquad (9.34)$$

then, from Equations 9.19 and 9.21, we have

$$\nabla^2 \psi = \frac{\rho_o^b \rho_i^b}{\rho_o^b + \rho_i^b} I_m - \frac{\rho_o^b \rho_i^b}{\rho_o^b + \rho_i^b} I_m - \frac{\rho_o^b \rho_i^b}{\rho_o^b + \rho_i^b} I_a \delta_v \qquad (9.35)$$

Consequently,

$$\nabla^2 \psi = -\rho_t^b I_a \delta_v \qquad (9.36)$$

where

$$\rho_t^b = \frac{\rho_o^b \rho_i^b}{\rho_o^b + \rho_i^b}$$

and ρ_t^b is the total tissue impedance in the absence of a membrane (referred to as a *bulk* impedance). We note, in Equation 9.36, that ψ satisfies a *(monodomain)* Poisson equation. In fact, ψ is the field of a point source at the origin and is given by

$$\psi = \frac{\rho_t^b I_a}{4\pi r} \qquad (9.37)$$

Since $V_m = \Phi_i - \Phi_o$, one can express either Φ_i or Φ_o in terms of V_m and ψ by using Equation 9.34. The result is

$$\Phi_i = \frac{\rho_i^b}{\rho_i^b + \rho_o^b} V_m + \psi = -\frac{\rho_t^b I_a}{4\pi} \frac{e^{-r/\lambda}}{r} + \frac{\rho_t^b I_a}{4\pi r}$$
$$(9.38)$$

$$\Phi_o = -\frac{\rho_o^b}{\rho_i^b + \rho_o^b} V_m + \psi = \frac{\rho_t^b \rho_o^b}{\rho_i^b} \frac{I_a}{4\pi} \frac{e^{-r/\lambda}}{r} + \frac{\rho_t^b I_a}{4\pi r}$$
$$(9.39)$$

where Equations 9.33 and 9.37 were substituted into Equation 9.38 and 9.39 to obtain the expressions following the second equal signs. This pair of equations describes the behavior of the component fields. Note that the boundary condition $\partial \Phi_i / \partial r = 0$ at $r \to 0$ is satisfied by Equation 9.38. This condition was implied in formulating Equation 9.19, where the total source current is described as interstitial.

9.6 FOUR-ELECTRODE IMPEDANCE METHOD APPLIED TO AN ISOTROPIC BIDOMAIN

For a homogeneous isotropic tissue, the experimental evaluation of its resistivity is often performed using the *four-electrode method* (Figure 9.5). In this method, four equally spaced electrodes are inserted deep into the tissue. We assume that the overall extent of the electrode system is small compared to its distance to a boundary, so that the volume conductor can be approximated as unlimited in extent (unbounded). The outer electrodes carry an applied current (i.e., I_a and $-I_a$) whereas the inner electrodes measure the resulting voltage. The resistivity ρ (Heiland, 1940) is given by

$$\rho = \frac{4\pi d V_Z}{I_a} \qquad (9.40)$$

where

$$V_Z = \text{measured voltage and}$$
$$d = \text{interelectrode spacing}$$

The advantage in the use of the four-electrode method arises from the separation of the current-driving and voltage-measuring circuits. In this arrangement the unknown impedance at the electrode-tissue interface is important only in the voltage-measuring circuit, where it adds a negligible error that depends on the ratio of electrode impedance to input impedance of the amplifier (ordinarily many times greater).

For an isotropic bidomain the four-electrode method also may be used to determine the intracellular and interstitial conductivities ρ_i^b and ρ_o^b. In this case, at least two independent observations must be made since there are two unknowns. If we assume that a current source of strength I_a is placed on the z axis at a distance of $3d/2$ (i.e., at $(0, 0, 1.5d)$) and source of strength $-I_a$ at $(0, 0, -1.5d)$ (as described in Fig. 9.5, where d is the spacing between adjacent electrodes), then the resulting interstitial electric fields can be calculated from Equation 9.39 using superposition. In particular, we are interested in the voltage (V_Z) that would be measured by the voltage electrodes, where

$$V_Z = V_1 - V_2 \qquad (9.41)$$
$$\equiv \Phi_o (0, 0, 0.5d) - \Phi_o(0, 0, -0.5d)$$

Application of Equation 9.39 to the point source I_a (imagine for this calculation that the origin of coordinates is at this point) shows that it contributes to V_Z an amount V_Z^s, namely

$$V_Z^s = \frac{\rho_t^b \rho_o^b}{\rho_i^b} \frac{I_a e^{-d/\lambda}}{4\pi d} + \frac{\rho_t^b I_a}{4\pi d}$$
$$- \frac{\rho_t^b \rho_o^b}{\rho_i^b} \frac{I_a e^{-2d/\lambda}}{4\pi(2d)} - \frac{\rho_t^b I_a}{4\pi(2d)} \qquad (9.42)$$

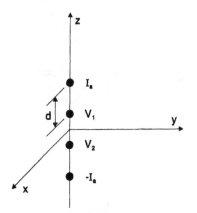

Fig. 9.5 Four-electrode method for the determination of tissue impedance. The electrode is embedded in the tissue. The outer elements carry the applied current $\pm I_a$ while the inner elements measure the resulting voltage $(V_Z = V_1 - V_2)$. The electrodes are spaced a distance (a) from each other (equispaced). For a uniform isotropic monodomain, the resistivity $\rho = 2\pi d V_Z / I_a$.

This result is, of course, independent of the actual coordinate origin since it is a unique physical entity. Correspondingly, the point *sink* (i.e., the negative source of $-I_a$) contributes an amount V_z^k given by

$$V_z^k = - \frac{\rho_t^b \rho_o^b}{\rho_i^b} \frac{I_a e^{-2d/\lambda}}{4\pi(2d)} - \frac{\rho_t^b I_a}{4\pi(2d)}$$
$$+ \frac{\rho_t^b \rho_o^b}{\rho_i^b} \frac{I_a e^{-d/\lambda}}{4\pi d} + \frac{\rho_t^b I_a}{4\pi d} \quad (9.43)$$

Summing Equations 9.42 and 9.43 yields the voltage that would be measured at the voltage electrodes, namely

$$V_z = \frac{\rho_t^b I_a}{4\pi d} - \frac{\rho_t^b \rho_o^b}{\rho_i^b} \frac{I_a}{4\pi d} e^{-2d/\lambda} + \frac{\rho_t^b \rho_o^b}{\rho_i^b} \frac{I_a}{2\pi d} e^{-d/\lambda}$$
$$(9.44)$$

or

$$V_z = \frac{\rho_t^b I_a}{4\pi d} \left[1 + \frac{\rho_o^b}{\rho_i^b} (2e^{-d/\lambda} - e^{-2d/\lambda}) \right] \quad (9.45)$$

If measurement of V_z and I_a is made with $d \gg \lambda$ then, according to Equation 9.45, this condition results in a relationship

$$\rho_t^b = \frac{4\pi d V_z}{I_a} \quad (d \gg \lambda) \quad (9.46)$$

and the bulk resistivity $\rho_t^b = \rho_o^b \rho_i^b / (\rho_o^b + \rho_i^b))$ is obtained. If a second measurement is made with $d \ll \lambda$, then according to Equation 9.45 we have

$$\rho_o^b = \frac{4\pi d V_z}{I_a} \quad (d \ll \lambda) \quad (9.47)$$

and only the interstitial resistivity is evaluated (as expected since over the relatively short distance no current is redistributed to the intracellular space, and hence only the interstitial resistivity influences the voltage-current behavior).

The two experiments permit determination of both ρ_o^b and ρ_i^b.

One important conclusion to be drawn from the work presented in this chapter is illustrated by the contrast of Equations 9.45 and 9.40. The interpretation of a four-electrode measurement depends on whether the tissue is a monodomain or bidomain. If it is a bidomain, then the monodomain interpretation can lead to considerable error, particularly if $d \ll \lambda$ or if $d \approx \lambda$. For such situations Equation 9.45 must be used. When the tissue is an anisotropic bidomain, it is even more important to use a valid (i.e., Equation 9.45) model in the analysis of four-electrode measurements (Plonsey and Barr, 1986).

REFERENCES

Clerc L (1976): Directional differences of impulse spread in trabecular muscle from mammalian heart. *J. Physiol. (Lond.)* 225:(2) 335–46.

Heiland CA (1940): *Geophysical Exploration,* 1013 pp. Prentice-Hall, Englewood Cliffs, N.J.

Miller WT, Geselowitz DB (1978): Simulation studies of the electrocardiogram, I. The normal heart. *Circ. Res.* 43:(2) 301–15.

Plonsey R, Barr RC (1986): A critique of impedance measurements in cardiac tissue. *Ann. Biomed. Eng.* 14: 307–22.

Roberts DE, Scher AM (1982): Effects of tissue anisotropy on extracellular potential fields in canine myocardium in situ. *Circ. Res.* 50: 342–51.

Spach MS (1983): The discontinuous nature of electrical propagation in cardiac muscle. *Ann. Biomed. Eng.* 11: 209–61.

Tung L (1978): A bidomain model for describing ischemic myocardial D-C potentials. *M.I.T. Cambridge, Mass.,* (Ph.D. thesis)

Weidmann S (1952): The electrical constants of Purkinje fibers. *J. Physiol. (Lond.)* 118: 348–60.

10

Electronic Neuron Models

10.1 INTRODUCTION

10.1.1 Electronic Modeling of Excitable Tissue

In Chapters 3 and 4, we discussed the electric behavior of excitable tissues—the nerve and the muscle cell. In that discussion we have used equations that describe the equivalent electric circuit of the membrane as well as electronic circuits that represent the passive electric properties of the tissue. From these equations and electric circuits we utilize the following:

1. *The Nernst equation* (Equation 3.21), which expresses the required membrane voltage to equilibrate the ion flux through the membrane for an existing concentration ratio of a particular ion species. Because the Nernst equation evaluates the ion moving force due to a concentration gradient as a voltage [V], this may be represented in equivalent electric circuits as a battery.

2. *The cable model of an axon,* which is composed of external and internal resistances as well as the electric properties of the membrane. This equivalent circuit may be used to calculate the general cable equation of the axon (Equation 3.45) describing the sub-threshold transmembrane voltage response to a constant current stimulation. The time-varying equations describing the behavior of the transmembrane voltage due to a step-impulse stimulation are also of interest (though more complicated). Their solutions were illustrated in Figure 3.11. The equivalent circuit for (approximate) derivation of the strength-duration equation, Equation 3.58, was shown in Figure 3.12.

3. *The equivalent electric circuits describing the behavior of the axon under conditions of nerve propagation,* or under space clamp and voltage clamp conditions, are shown in Figures 4.1, 4.2, and 4.3; the corresponding equations are 4.1, 4.2, and 4.3, respectively.

4. *The electric circuit for the parallel-conductance model of the membrane,* which contains pathways for sodium, potassium, and chloride ion currents, is illustrated in Figure 4.10, and its behavior described by Equation 4.10. This equation includes the following passive electric parameters (electronic components): membrane capacitance, Nernst voltages for sodium, potassium, and chloride ions, as well as the leakage conductance. Further, the circuit includes the behavior of the active parameters, the sodium and potassium conductances, as described by

the Hodgkin-Huxley equations (Equations 4.12–4.24).

Thus our understanding of the electric behavior of excitable tissue, and our methods to illustrate it are strongly tied to the concepts of electronic circuits and to the equations describing their behavior. From this standpoint it is possible to proceed to realize physically the electronic equivalent circuits for the excitable tissues. The physical realization of the electronic equivalent circuits of excitable tissues has two main purposes:

1. It provides us with an opportunity to verify that the models we have constructed really behave the same as the excitable tissue that they should model—that is, that the model is correct. If the behavior of the model is not completely correct, we may be able to adjust the properties of the model and thereby improve our understanding of the behavior of the tissue. This *analysis* of the behavior of the excitable tissue is one general purpose of modeling work.
2. There exists also the possibility of constructing, or *synthesizing* electronic circuits, whose behavior is similar to neural tissue, and which perform information processing in a way that also is similar to nature. In its most advanced form, it is called *neural computing*.

In Section 7.3 we discussed the concept of modeling in general. Various models in the neurosciences are discussed in Miller (1992). In this chapter, we discuss especially electronic neural modeling including representative examples of electronic neuron models developed to realize the electric behavior of neurons. A more comprehensive review of the electronic neuron models constructed with discrete electronic components may be found in Malmivuo (1973) and Reiss et al. (1964).

We should note that simulation of electric circuits with digital computers is another way to investigate the behavior of the electronic models. Despite this fact, electronic neural modeling is important because it is the bridge to construction of electronic circuits, which are the elements of neurocomputers.

10.1.2 Neurocomputers

The most important application of electronic neural modeling is the neurocomputer. Although this subject is beyond the scope of this book, and the theory of neural networks and neurocomputers is not discussed in this volume, we include here a brief description and include some references to this subject. A good introduction and short review is in Hecht-Nielsen (1988).

The first computers were called "electric brains." At that time there was a popular conception that computers could think, or that such computers would soon be available. In reality, however, even computers of today must be programmed exactly to do the desired task.

Artificial intelligence has been a popular buzzword for decades. It has produced some useful expert systems, chess-playing programs, and some limited speech and character recognition systems. These remain in the domain of carefully crafted algorithmic programs that perform a specific task. A self-programming computer does not exist. The *Turing test* of machine intelligence is that a machine is intelligent if in conversing with it, one is unable to tell whether one is talking to a human or a machine. By this criterion artificial intelligence does not seem any closer to realization than it was 30 years ago.

If we make an attempt to build an electronic brain, it makes sense to study how a biological brain works and then to try to imitate nature. This idea has not been ignored by scientists. Real brains, even those of primitive animals, are, however, enormously complex structures. The human brain contains about 10^{11} neurons, each capable of storing more than a single bit of data.

Computers are approaching the point at which they could have a comparable memory capacity. Whereas computer instruction times are measured in nanoseconds, mammalian information processing is done in milliseconds. However, this speed advantage for the computer is superseded by the massively parallel structure of the nervous system; each neuron processes information and has a large number of interconnections to other neurons. Multiprocessor computers are now being built, but making effective use of thousands of processors is a task that is still a challenge for computer theory (Tonk and Hopfield, 1987).

10.2 CLASSIFICATION OF NEURON MODELS

In general, neuron models may be divided into categories according to many different criteria. In the following, four different criteria are presented, to exemplify these classifications (Malmivuo, 1973):

1. The *structure* of the model may be expressed in terms of
   a. Mathematical equations (Hodgkin-Huxley equations, Section 4.4)
   b. An imaginary construction following the laws of physics (Eccles model, Section 3.5.4, Fig. 3.2)
   c. Constructions, which are physically different from but analogous to the original phenomenon, and which illustrate the function of their origin (electronic neuron model)
2. Models may describe a phenomenon in different *conceptual dimensions*. These model aspects include:
   a. Structure (usually illustrated with a mechanical model)
   b. Function (usually illustrated with an electronic or mathematical or computer model)
   c. Evolution
   d. Position in the hierarchy
3. Classification according to the *physiological level* of the phenomenon:
   a. Intraneuronal level
      (1) The membrane in the resting state
      (2) The mechanism generating the nerve impulse
      (3) The propagation of the nerve impulse in an axon
   b. Stimulus and response functions of single neurons
   c. Synaptic transmission
   d. Interactions between neurons and neuron groups, neuronal nets
   e. Psychophysiological level

4. The classification according to the *model parameters*. The variables included in a nervous system model have different time constants. On this basis the following classification may be obtained:
   a. Resting parameters
   b. Stimulus parameters
   c. Recovery parameters
   d. Adaptation parameters

This chapter considers representative examples of electronic neuron models (or neuromimes) that describe the generation of the action impulse, the neuron as an independent unit, and the propagation of the nerve impulse in the axon.

10.3 MODELS DESCRIBING THE FUNCTION OF THE MEMBRANE

Most of the models describing the excitation mechanism of the membrane are electronic realizations of the theoretical membrane model of Hodgkin and Huxley (Hodgkin and Huxley, 1952). In the following sections, two of these realizations are discussed.

10.3.1 The Lewis Membrane Model

Edwin R. Lewis published several electronic membrane models that are based on the Hodgkin-Huxley equations. The sodium and potassium conductances, synaptic connections, and other functions of the model are realized with discrete transistors and associated components. All these are parallel circuits connected between nodes representing the inside and outside of the membrane.

We discuss here the model published by Lewis in 1964. Lewis realized the sodium and potassium conductances using electronic hardware in the form of active filters, as shown in the block diagram of Figure 10.1. Since the output of the model is the transmembrane voltage V_m, the potassium current can be evaluated by multiplying the voltage corresponding to G_K by $(V_m - V_K)$. Figure 10.1 is consequently an

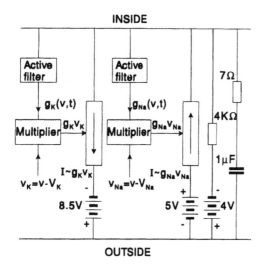

Fig. 10.1 The block diagram of the Lewis membrane model.

accurate physical analog to the Hodgkin-Huxley expressions, and the behavior of the output voltage V_m corresponds to that predicted by the Hodgkin-Huxley equations.

The electronic circuits in the Lewis neuromime had provision for inserting (and varying) not only such constants as $G_{K\,max}$, $G_{Na\,max}$, V_K, V_{Na}, V_{Cl}, which enter the Hodgkin-Huxley formulation, but also τ_h, τ_m, τ_n, which allow modifications from the Hodgkin-Huxley equations. The goal of Lewis's research was to simulate the behavior of a neuronal network, including coupled neurons, each of which is simulated by a neuromime; this is documented later in this chapter.

In the electronic realization the voltages of the biological membrane are multiplied by 100 to fit the electronic circuit. In other quantities, the original values of the biological membrane have been used. In the following, the components of the model are discussed separately.

Potassium Conductance

The circuit simulating the potassium conductance is shown in Figure 10.2. The potassium conductance function $G_K(V_m,t)$ is generated from the simulated membrane voltage through a nonlinear active filter according to the Hodgkin-Huxley model (in the figure separated with a dashed line). The three variable resistors in the filter provide a control over the delay time,

rise time, and fall time. The value of the potassium conductance is adjusted with a potentiometer, which is the amplitude regulator of a multiplier. The multiplier circuit generates the function $G_K(V_m,t) \cdot v_K$, where v_K is the difference between the potassium potential (V_K) and membrane potential (V_m). The multiplier is based on the quadratic function of two diodes.

Sodium Conductance

In the circuit simulating the sodium conductance, Lewis omitted the multiplier on the basis that the equilibrium voltage of sodium ions is about 120 mV more positive than the resting voltage. Because we are more interested in small membrane voltage changes, the gradient of sodium ions may be considered constant. The circuit simulating the sodium conductance is shown in Figure 10.3. The time constant of the inactivation is defined according to a varistor. The inactivation decreases monotonically with the depolarization, approximately following the Hodgkin-Huxley model.

Simulated Action Pulse

By connecting the components of the membrane model as in Figure 10.4 and stimulating

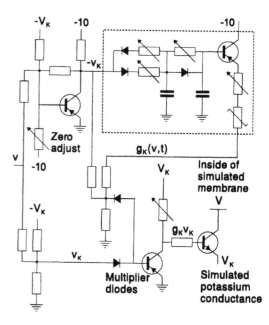

Fig. 10.2 The circuit simulating the potassium conductance of the Lewis membrane model.

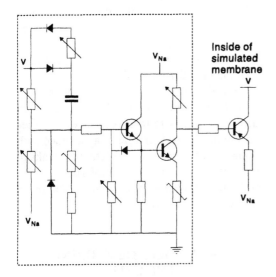

Fig. 10.3 Circuit simulating the sodium conductance of the Lewis membrane model.

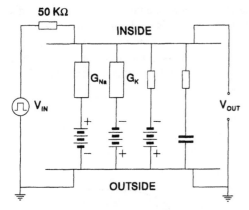

Fig. 10.4 The complete Lewis membrane model.

the model analogously to the real axon, the model generates a membrane action pulse. This simulated action pulse follows the natural action pulse very accurately. Figure 10.5A illustrates a single action pulse generated by the Lewis membrane model, and Figure 10.5B shows a series of action pulses.

10.3.2 The Roy Membrane Model

Guy Roy published an electronic membrane model in 1972 (Roy, 1972) and gave it the name "Neurofet." His model, analogous to Lewis's, is also based on the Hodgkin-Huxley model. Roy used FET transistors to simulate the sodium and potassium conductances. FETs are well known as adjustable conductors. So the multiplying circuit of Lewis may be incorporated into a single FET component (Fig. 10.6).

In the Roy model the conductance is controlled by a circuit including an operational amplifier, capacitors, and resistors. This circuit is designed to make the conductance behave according to the Hodgkin-Huxley model. Roy's main goal was to achieve a very simple model rather than to simulate accurately the Hodgkin-Huxley model. Nevertheless, the measurements resulting from his model, shown in Figures 10.7 and 10.8, are reasonably close to the results obtained by Hodgkin and Huxley.

Figure 10.7 illustrates the steady-state values for the potassium and sodium conductances as a function of applied voltage. Note that for potassium conductance the value given is the steady-state value, which it reaches in steady state. For sodium the illustrated value is $G'_{Na} = G_{Namax}m^3_\infty h_0$; it is the value that the

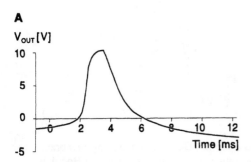

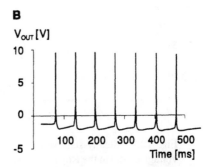

Fig. 10.5 (A) Single action pulse, and (B) a series of action pulses generated by the Lewis membrane model.

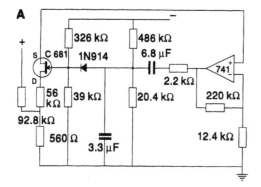

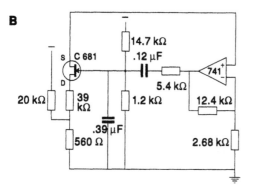

Fig. 10.6 The circuits simulating (A) sodium and (B) potassium conductances in the Roy membrane model.

sodium conductance would attain if h remained at its resting level (h_0). (The potassium and sodium conductance values of Hodgkin and Huxley are from tables 1 and 2, respectively, in Hodgkin and Huxley, 1952.)

The full membrane model was obtained by connecting the potassium and sodium conductances in series with their respective batteries and simulating the membrane capacitance with a capacitor of 4.7 nF and simulating the leakage conductance with a resistance of 200 kΩ. The results from the simulation of the action pulse are illustrated in Figure 10.8.

10.4 MODELS DESCRIBING THE CELL AS AN INDEPENDENT UNIT

10.4.1 The Lewis Neuron Model

In this section the neuron model described by Lewis in 1968 (Lewis, 1968) is briefly discussed. The Lewis model is based on the Hodgkin-Huxley membrane model and the theories of Eccles on synaptic transmission (Eccles, 1964). The model circuit is illustrated in Figure 10.9.

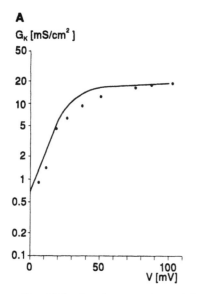

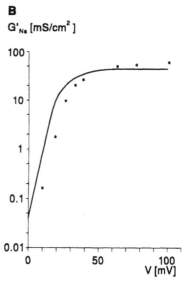

Fig. 10.7 Steady-state values of the (A) G_K and (B) G'_{Na} as a function of membrane voltage clamp in the Roy model (solid lines), compared to the measurements of Hodgkin and Huxley (dots). V_m, the transmembrane voltage, is related to the resting value of the applied voltage clamp. (See the text for details.)

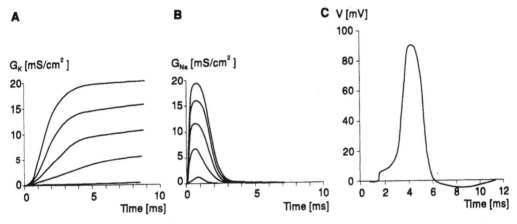

Fig. 10.8 Voltage-clamp measurements made for (A) potassium and (B) sodium conductances in the Roy model. The voltage steps are 20, 40, 60, 80, and 100 mV. (C) The action pulse simulated with the Roy model.

This neuron model is divided into two sections: the synaptic section and the section generating the action pulse. Both sections consist of parallel circuits connected to the nodes representing the intracellular and extracellular sites of the membrane.

The section representing the synaptic junction is divided into two components. One of these represents the inhibitory junction and the other the excitatory junction. The sensitivity of the section generating the action pulse to a stimulus introduced at the excitatory synaptic junction is reduced by the voltage introduced at the inhibitory junction. The section generating the

action pulse is based on the Hodgkin-Huxley model. As described earlier, it consists of the normal circuits simulating the sodium and potassium conductances, the leakage conductance, and the membrane capacitance. The circuit also includes an amplifier for the output signal.

This neuron model which is relatively complicated, is to be used in research on neural networks. However, it is actually a simplified version of Lewis's 46-transistor network having the same form. The purpose of this simplified Lewis model is to simulate the form of the action pulse, not with the highest possible

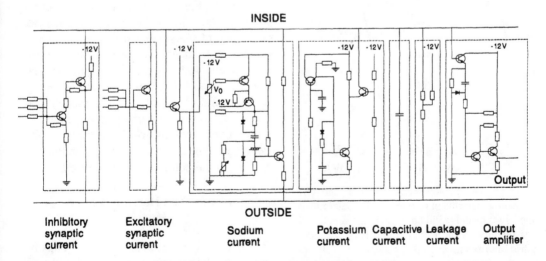

Fig. 10.9 The Lewis neuron model from 1968.

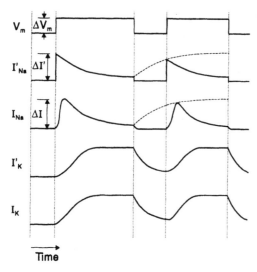

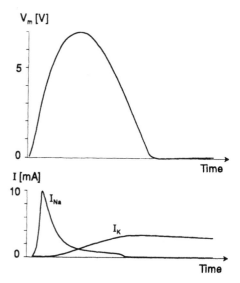

Fig. 10.10 The responses of the sodium and potassium current from the Lewis model (primed) and the biological neuron (as evaluated by the Hodgkin-Huxley model) to a voltage step. The applied transmembrane voltage is shown as V_m.

Fig. 10.12 The action pulse generated by the Lewis model. The corresponding sodium and potassium currents are also illustrated.

accuracy but, rather, with a sufficient accuracy provided by a simple model. Figures 10.10, 10.11, and 10.12 show the behavior of the model compared to the simulation based directly on the Hodgkin and Huxley model.

From Figure 10.10 we find that when the stimulation current begins, the sodium ion current determined by Lewis (I'_{Na}) rises to its peak

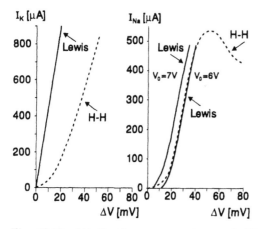

Fig. 10.11 (A) Steady-state potassium and (B) peak sodium currents in response to V_m determined in the Lewis model (solid line) and in the simulation based directly on the Hodgkin and Huxley model (dashed line) as a function of the membrane voltage. (V_o is the voltage applied by the potentiometer in the sodium current circuit.)

value almost immediately, whereas the sodium ion current of the Hodgkin-Huxley biological nerve (I_{Na}) rises much more slowly. The exponential decay of the current occurs at about the same speed in both. The behavior of the potassium ion current is very similar in both the model and the biological membrane as simulated by Hodgkin and Huxley.

Figure 10.11A and 10.11B compare the potassium and sodium ion currents of the Lewis model to those in the Hodgkin-Huxley model, respectively. Figure 10.12 illustrates the action pulse generated by the Lewis model. The peak magnitude of the simulated sodium current is 10 mA. This magnitude is equivalent to approximately 450 μA/cm^2 in the membrane, which is about half of the value calculated by Hodgkin and Huxley from their model. The maximum potassium current in the circuit is 3 mA, corresponding to 135 μA/cm^2 in the membrane. The author gave no calibration for the membrane potential or for the time axis.

10.4.2 The Harmon Neuron Model

The electronic realizations of the Hodgkin-Huxley model are very accurate in simulating the function of a single neuron. However, when

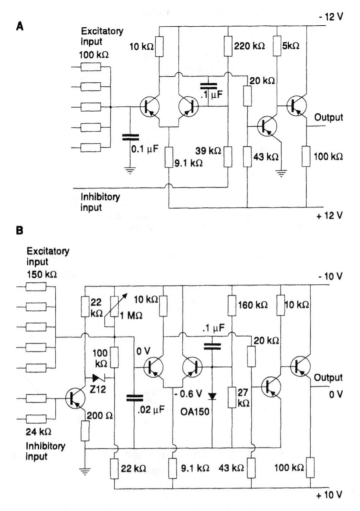

Fig. 10.13 Construction of the Harmon neuron model. (A) The preliminary and (B) the more advanced version of the circuit.

one is trying to simulate the function of neural networks, they become very complicated. Many scientists feel that when simulating large neural networks, the internal construction of its element may not be too important. It may be satisfactory simply to ensure that the elements produce an action pulse in response to the stimuli in a manner similar to an actual neuron. On this basis, Leon D. Harmon constructed a neuron model having a very simple circuit. With this model he performed experiments in which he simulated many functions characteristic of the neuron (Harmon, 1961).

The circuit of the Harmon neuron model is given in Figure 10.13. Figures 10.13A and 10.13B show the preliminary and more advanced versions of the circuit, respectively. The

model is equipped with five excitatory inputs which can be adjusted. These include diode circuits representing various synaptic functions. The signal introduced at excitatory inputs charges the 0.02 μF capacitor which, after reaching a voltage of about 1.5 V, allows the monostable multivibrator, formed by transistors T1 and T2, to generate the action pulse. This impulse is amplified by transistors T3 and T4. The output of one neuron model may drive the inputs of perhaps 100 neighboring neuron models. The basic model also includes an inhibitory input. A pulse introduced at this input has the effect of decreasing the sensitivity to the excitatory inputs.

Without external circuits, Harmon investigated successfully seven properties of his neu-

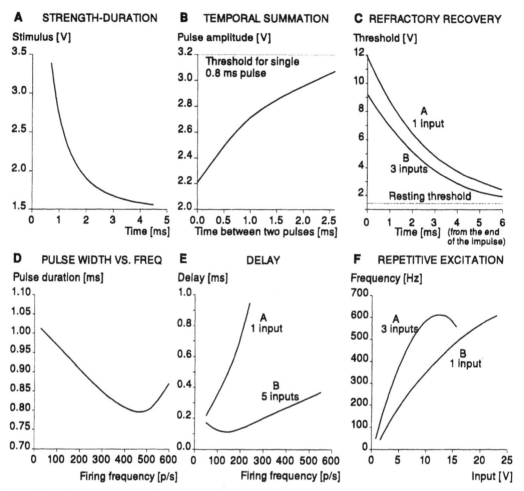

Fig. 10.14 Properties of the Harmon model. (A) strength-duration curve; (B) temporal summation of the stimulus; (C) refractory recovery; (D) the output pulse width as a function of the pulse frequency; (E) the delay between initiation of excitation and initiation of the action pulse as a function of firing frequency; and (F) the behavior of the model in repetitive excitation. The input frequency is 700 p/s.

ron model. These are illustrated in Figure 10.14 and are described briefly in the following.

Strength-Duration Curve

The Harmon model follows a strength-duration curve similar to that exhibited by the natural neuron. The time scale is approximately correct, but owing to the electric properties of circuit components, the voltage scale is much higher. The threshold voltage in the Harmon model is about $V_{th} = 1.5$ V, as described in Figure 10.14A.

Latency

Because the model contains no internal circuit that specifically generates a latency, this phe-nomenon is totally described by the strength-duration curve which is interpreted as a stimu-lus-latency curve. The action pulse is generated only when the stimulus has lasted long enough to generate the action pulse.

Temporal Summation

The model illustrates the stimulus threshold in the case of two consecutive stimulus pulses where the first pulse leaves the membrane hy-perexcitable to the second. Figure 10.14B shows the required amplitude of two 0.8 ms pulses as a function of their interval, and one notes that the threshold diminishes with a re-duced pulse interval, owing to temporal sum-mation. In all cases the pulse amplitude is reduced from the value required for activation from a single pulse.

Refractory Period (Recovery of Excitability)

The typical recovery of excitability of the model after an action pulse is shown in Figure 10.14C (curve A). This curve is similar to that for a biological neuron. The neuron model is absolutely refractory for about 1 ms—that is, the time of the output pulse. The relative refractory period starts after this ($t = 0$), and its time constant is about 1.7 ms. Curve A is obtained when the stimulus is applied at one input. Curve B represents the situation when the stimulus is simultaneously applied to three inputs (see Fig. 10.13).

Output Pulse, Action Impulse

The output pulse obeys the all-or-none law, and its amplitude is quite stable. Its width is, however, to some degree a function of the pulse frequency. This dependence is given in Figure 10.14D.

Delay

The delay refers, in this case, to the time between the onsets of the stimulus pulse and the output pulse. It is not the delay in the usual meaning of the term. In the model, the delay is a function of the integration in the input as well as the refractory condition. Curve A in Figure 10.14E represents the delay when a stimulus is applied to one input, and curve B when the stimulus is applied to all five excitatory inputs.

Repetitive Excitation

Repetitive excitation refers to the generation of output pulses with a constant input voltage and frequency. Figure 10.14F, curve A, shows the frequency of the output pulse when the input voltage is connected to three inputs, and curve B when the input voltage is connected to one input. The output frequency follows the input only for high voltage inputs. As the input is reduced, pulses drop out, and the resulting output frequency is reduced compared to the input.

By connecting capacitors between the input and output ports of the neuron model, it is possible to realize much more complex functions. Harmon performed experiments also with combinations of many neuron models. Furthermore, Harmon investigated propagation of the action pulse by chaining models together. These neuron models can be applied to simulate quite complex neural networks, and even to model brain waves.

10.5 A MODEL DESCRIBING THE PROPAGATION OF ACTION PULSE IN AXON

Using an iteration of the membrane section of his neuron model described in Section 10.3.1, Lewis simulated the propagation of an action pulse in a uniform axon and obtained interesting results (Lewis, 1968). The model structure, illustrated in Figure 10.15, can be seen to include a network of membrane elements as well as axial resistors representing the intracellular resistance. A total of six membrane elements are depicted in the figure. The model is an electronic realization of the linear core-conductor model with active membrane elements.

Figure 10.16A and 10.16B illustrate the simulation of propagation of an action pulse in a model consisting of a chain of axon units, as described in Figure 10.15. Curve A represents the case with a chain of six units, and curve B a continuous ring of 10 units. In the latter, the signals are recorded from every second unit. A six-unit model represents a section of a squid

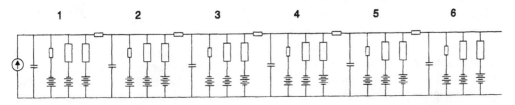

Fig. 10.15 The Lewis model that simulates the propagation of the action pulse.

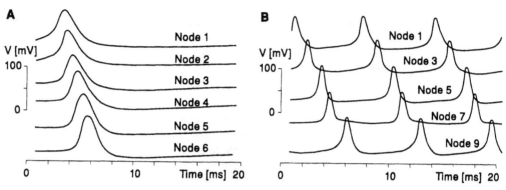

Fig. 10.16 Propagation of the action pulse in the Lewis model in (A) a six-unit chain and (B) a ten-unit ring.

axon 4 cm long and 1 mm in diameter. Figure 10.15A shows that the conduction time of the action pulse from unit three (where it has reached the final form) to unit six (i.e., three increments of distance) is 1.4 ms. Because the full six-unit model forms five increments of distance, the modeled conduction velocity was 17 m/s. This is comparable to spike conduction velocities (14 - 23 m/s) measured in squid giant axons.

10.6   INTEGRATED CIRCUIT REALIZATIONS

The development of the integrated circuit technology has made it possible to produce electronic neuron models in large quantities (Mahowald et al., 1992). This makes it possible to use electronic neuron models or neuron-like circuits as processing elements for electronic computers, called neurocomputers. In the following paragraphs, we give two examples of these.

Stefan Prange (1988, 1990) has developed an electronic neuron model that is realized with integrated circuit technology. The circuit includes one neuron with eight synapses. The chip area of the integrated circuit is 4.5 × 5 mm². The array contains about 200 NPN and 100 PNP transistors, and about 200 of them are used. The circuit is fabricated with one metal layer with a line width of 12 μm. Because the model is realized with integrated circuit technology, it is easy to produce in large quantities, which is

necessary for simulating neural networks. These experiments, however, have not yet been made with this model.

In 1991, Misha Mahowald and Rodney Douglas published an integrated circuit realization of electronic neuron model (Mahowald and Douglas, 1991). It was realized with complementary metal oxide semiconductor (CMOS) circuits using very large-scale integrated (VLSI) technology. Their model simulates very accurately the spikes of a neocortical neuron. The power dissipation of the circuit is 60 μW, and it occupies less than 0.1 mm². The authors estimate that 100–200 such neurons could be fabricated on a 1 cm × 1 cm die.

REFERENCES

Eccles JC (1964): *The Physiology of Synapses,* 316 pp. Springer-Verlag, Berlin.

Harmon LD (1961): Studies with artificial neurons, I: Properties and functions of an artificial neuron. *Kybernetik* Heft 3(Dez.): 89–101.

Hecht-Nielsen R (1988): Neurocomputing: Picking the human brain. *IEEE Spectrum* 25:(3(March)) 36–41.

Hodgkin AL, Huxley AF (1952): A quantitative description of membrane current and its application to conduction and excitation in nerve. *J. Physiol. (Lond.)* 117: 500–44.

Lewis ER (1964): An electronic model of the neuron based on the dynamics of potassium and sodium ion fluxes. In *Neural Theory and Modelling. Proceedings of the 1962 Ojai Symposium,* ed. RF Reiss, HJ Hamilton, LD Harmon, G Hoyle, D Kennedy, O Schmitt, CAG Wiersma, p. 427, Stanford University Press, Stanford.

Lewis ER (1968): Using electronic circuits to model simple neuroelectric interactions. *Proc. IEEE* 56:(6) 931–49. (Special issue on studies of neural elements and systems).

Mahowald MA, Douglas RJ (1991): A silicon neuron. *Nature* 354:(December) 515–8.

Mahowald MA, Douglas RJ, LeMoncheck JE, Mead CA (1992): An introduction to silicon neural analogs. *Semin. Neurosci.* 4: 83–92.

Malmivuo JA (1973): *Bioelectric Function of a Neuron and Its Description With Electronic Models,* 195 pp. Helsinki Univ. Techn., Dept. El. Eng. (In Finnish)

Prange S (1988): Aufbau eines Neuronenmodells mit hilfe einer analogen, kundenspezifischen Schaltung. *Institute of Microelectronics, Techn. Univ. Berlin, Berlin,* pp. 87. (Diploma thesis)

Prange S (1990): Emulation of biology-oriented neural networks. In *Proc. Int. Conf. On Parallel Processing in Neural Systems and Computers (ICNC),* ed. M Eckmiller, Düsseldorf.

Roy G (1972): A simple electronic analog of the squid axon membrane: The neurofet. *IEEE Trans. Biomed. Eng.* BME-19:(1) 60–3.

Tonk DW, Hopfield JJ (1987): Collective computation in neuronlike circuits. *Sci. Am.* 257:(6) 62–70.

REFERENCES, BOOKS

Aleksander I (ed.) (1989): *Neural Computing Architectures, The Design of Brain-Like Machines,* 401 pp. The MIT Press, Cambridge, Mass.

Andersson JA, Rosenfeld E (eds.) (1988): *Neurocomputing: Foundations of Research,* 729 pp. MIT Press, Cambridge, Mass.

Grossberg S (ed.) (1988): *Neural Networks and Natural Intelligence,* 637 pp. MIT Press, Cambridge, Mass.

Hecht-Nielsen R (1990): *Neurocomputing,* 432 pp. Addison-Wesley Publishing, Reading, Mass.

MacGregor RJ (1987): Neural and Brain Modelling, 643 pp. Academic Press, San Diego.

MacGregor RJ, Lewis ER (1977): *Neural Modelling: Electric Signal Processing in the Nervous System,* 414 pp. Plenum Press, New York.

Miller KD (1992): The Use of Models in the Neurosciences. *Semin. Neurosci.* 4:(1) 92. (Special issue).

Reiss RF, Hamilton HJ, Harmon LD, Hoyle G, Kennedy D, Schmitt O, Wiersma CAG (eds.) (1964): *Neural Theory and Modelling. Proceedings of the 1962 Ojai Symposium,* 427 pp. Stanford University Press, Stanford.

Sejnowski T (ed.) (1989): *Neural Computation,* MIT Press, Cambridge, Mass.

III

Theoretical Methods
in Bioelectromagnetism

Chapters 11 and 12 examine theoretical methods that have been developed for analyzing the source-field relationships of bioelectric and biomagnetic phenomena. As discussed in Chapter 7, because bioelectric sources and conductors are *volume sources* and *volume conductors*, the theoretical methods that are used in analyzing electronic circuits are not applicable in bioelectromagnetism. Therefore, the contents of Part III are central to theoretical bioelectromagnetism.

In Part III, it is shown that the *reciprocity theorem* applies to the volume conductor. It serves as the basis for the *lead field theory*, which provides a powerful way of evaluating and interpreting measured signals in terms of their sources. The lead field theory ties together sensitivity distribution of the measurement of bioelectric sources, distribution of stimulation energy, and sensitivity distribution of impedance measurements. These points pertain in both electric and magnetic applications.

The two chapters of Part III are linked together by the fact that *the same electrophysiological sources generate both bioelectric and biomagnetic fields.* Since the fields behave differently, separate treatments are necessary. Furthermore, it is important to point out that from a theoretical point of view, the only difference between bioelectric and biomagnetic measurements is their different sensitivity distribution in regard to the bioelectric sources. The lead field theory clearly explains the similarities and differences between the electric and the corresponding magnetic methods. Because different instrumentation is employed, there are, of course, certain technical differences between these methods.

Although the ECG and MCG are the vehicles for explaining most of the theoretical methods discussed in Part III, application of these methods is, of course, not limited to electro- and magnetocardiography; this generalization is emphasized where appropriate.

11

Theoretical Methods for Analyzing Volume Sources and Volume Conductors

11.1 INTRODUCTION

The first two theoretical methods of this chapter (solid angle theorem and Miller-Geselowitz model) are used to evaluate the electric field in a volume conductor produced by the source—that is, to solve the *forward problem.* After this discussion is a presentation of methods used to evaluate the source of the electric field from measurements made outside the source, inside or on the surface of the volume conductor—that is, to solve the *inverse problem.* These methods are important in designing electrode configurations that optimize the capacity to obtain the desired information.

In fact, application of each of the following methods usually results in a particular ECG-lead system. These lead systems are not discussed here in detail because the purpose of this chapter is to show that these methods of analysis form an independent theory of bioelectricity that is not limited to particular ECG applications.

The biomagnetic fields resulting from the electric activity of volume sources are discussed in detail in Chapter 12.

11.2 SOLID ANGLE THEOREM

11.2.1 Inhomogeneous Double Layer

PRECONDITIONS:

Source: *Inhomogeneous double layer*

Conductor: *Infinite, homogeneous (finite, inhomogeneous)*

The solid angle theorem was developed by the German physicist Hermann von Helmholtz in the middle of the nineteenth century. In this theory, a double layer is used as the source. Although this topic was introduced in Chapter 8, we now examine the structure of a double layer in somewhat greater detail.

Suppose that a point current source and a current sink (i.e., a negative source) of the same magnitude are located close to each other. If their strength is i and the distance between them is d, they form a dipole moment id as discussed in Section 8.2.2. Consider now a smooth surface of arbitrary shape lying within a volume conductor. We can uniformly distribute many such dipoles over its surface, with each dipole placed normal to the surface. In addition, we choose the dipole density to be a well-behaved function of position—that is, we assume that the number of dipoles in a small area is great enough so that the density of dipoles can be well approximated with a continuous function. Such a source is called a *double layer* (Figure 11.1). If it is denoted by $p(S)\bar{n}$, then $p(S)$ denotes a dipole moment density (dipole moment per unit area) as a function of position, while its direction is denoted by $\bar{n}$, the surface normal. With this notation, $p(S)d\bar{S}$ is a dipole whose magnitude is $p(S)dS$, and its direction is normal to the surface at dS.

An alternative point of view is to recognize that on one side of the double layer, the sources form a current density J [A/m²] whereas on the other side the sinks form a current density $-J$ [A/m²], and that the conducting sheet between the surfaces of the double layer has a resistivity ρ. The resistance across this sheet (of thickness d) for a unit cross-sectional area is

$$R = \rho d \qquad (11.1)$$

where

R = double layer resistance times unit area [Ωm²]
ρ = resistivity of the medium [Ωm]
d = thickness of the double layer [m]

Of course, the double layer arises only in the limit that $d \to 0$ while $J \to \infty$ such that $Jd \to p$ remains finite.

From Ohm's law we note that the double layer has a potential difference of

$$V_d = \Phi_1 - \Phi_2 = J\rho d \qquad (11.2)$$

where

V_d = voltage difference over the double layer [V]
Φ_1, Φ_2 = potentials on both sides of the double layer [V]
J = double layer current density [A/m²]
ρ = resistivity of the medium [Ωm]
d = double layer thickness [m]

By definition, the double layer forms a dipole moment per unit surface area of

$$p = Jd \qquad (11.3)$$

where

p = dipole moment per unit area [A/m]
J = double layer current density [A/m²]
d = double layer thickness [m]

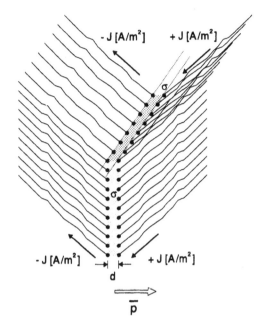

Fig. 11.1 Structure of a double layer. The double layer is formed when the dipole density increases to the point that it may be considered a continuum. In addition, we require that $J \to \infty$, $d \to 0$, and $Jd \to p$.

As noted, in the general case (nonuniform double layer), p and J are functions of position. Strictly we require $d \to 0$ while $J \to \infty$ such that $Jd = p$ remains finite. (In the case where d is not uniform, then for Equation 11.2 to be a good approximation it is required that $\Delta\Phi$ not vary significantly over lateral distances several times d.)

Since $\bar{p} \equiv p\bar{n}$ is the dipole moment per unit area (with the direction from negative to positive source), $\bar{p}dS$ is an elementary dipole. Its field, given by Equation 8.12 is:

$$d\Phi = \frac{p}{4\pi\sigma} \nabla \left(\frac{1}{r}\right) \cdot d\bar{S} \qquad (11.4)$$

since the direction of $\bar{p}$ and $d\bar{S}$ are the same. Now the *solid angle* $d\Omega$, as defined by Stratton (1941), is:

$$-d\Omega = \nabla \left(\frac{1}{r}\right) \cdot d\bar{S} \qquad (11.5)$$

Thus

$$\Phi = \frac{1}{4\pi\sigma} \int_S p(-d\Omega) \qquad (11.6)$$

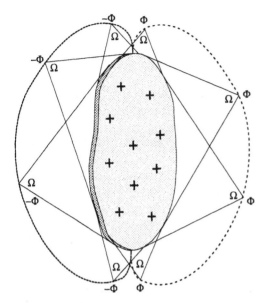

Fig. 11.2 A sketch of some isopotential points on an isopotential line of the electric field generated by a uniform double layer. That these points are equipotential is shown by the identity of the solid angle magnitudes. According to the convention chosen in Equation 11.5, the sign of the solid angle is negative.

The double layer generates a potential field given by Equation 11.6, where $d\Omega$ is the element of solid angle, as seen from the field point as the point of observation (Fig. 11.2). This figure provides an interpretation of the solid angle as a measure of the opening between rays from the field point to the periphery of the double layer, a form of three-dimensional angle. Equation 11.6 has a particularly simple form, which readily permits an estimation of the field configuration arising from a given double-layer source function.

This result was first obtained by Helmholtz, who showed that it holds for an infinite, homogeneous, isotropic, and linear volume conductor. Later the solid angle theorem was also applied to inhomogeneous volume conductors by utilizing the concept of secondary sources. As discussed in Section 7.2.3, the inhomogeneous volume conductor may be represented as a homogeneous volume conductor including secondary sources at the sites of the boundaries. Now the potential field of a double layer source in an inhomogeneous volume conductor may

be calculated with the solid angle theorem by applying it to the primary and secondary sources in a homogeneous volume conductor.

The Polarity of the Potential Field

We discuss shortly the polarity of the potential field generated by a double layer. This will clarify the minus sign in Equations 11.5 and 11.6.

If the double layer is uniform, then the field point's potential is proportional to the total solid angle subtended at the field point. It is therefore of interest to be able to determine this solid angle. One useful approach is the following: From the field point, draw lines (rays) to the periphery of the double layer surface. Now construct a unit sphere centered at the field point. The area of the sphere surface intercepted by the rays is the solid angle. If the negative sources associated with the double layer face the field point, then the solid angle will be positive, according to Equation 11.5. This polarity arises from the purely arbitrary way in which the sign in Equation 11.5 was chosen. Unfortunately, the literature contains both sign choices in the definition of the solid angle (in this book we adopted the one defined by Stratton, 1941).

For example, suppose a uniform double layer is a circular disk centered at the origin, whose dipoles are oriented in the x direction. For a field point along the positive x-axis, because the field point faces positive sources, the solid angle will be negative. However, because of the minus sign in Equation 11.5, the expression 11.6 also contains a minus sign. As a consequence, the potential, evaluated from Equation 11.6, will be positive, which is the expected polarity.

11.2.2   Uniform Double Layer

PRECONDITIONS:

Source: *Uniform double layer*

Conductor: *Infinite, homogeneous*

A uniform double layer exhibits some interesting properties that are discussed here in this section.

To begin with, we note that Equation 11.6 describes the potential field in an infinite volume conductor due to an inhomogeneous double layer; this reduces to the following simplified form when the double layer is uniform:

$$\Phi = \frac{1}{4\pi\sigma} p(-\Omega) \qquad (11.7)$$

Consider a closed uniform double layer. When such a double layer is seen from any point of observation, it can always be divided into two parts. One is seen from the positive side and the other is seen from the negative side, though each has exactly the same magnitude solid angle Ω, as described in Figure 11.3. (Double-layer sources having more complex form can, of course, be divided into more than two parts.) These both produce a potential of the same magnitude, but because they have opposite signs, they cancel each other. As a result, a closed uniform double layer produces a zero field, when considered in its entirety.

Wilson et al. (1931) applied this principle to electrocardiography, since he understood the cardiac double layer source formulation. Suppose that the double layer formed by the depolarization in the ventricles includes a single wavefront, which is represented by a uniform double layer, and has the shape of a cup. If this cup is closed with a ''cover'' formed by a double layer of similar strength, then a closed surface is formed, that does not generate any potential field. From this we can conclude that the double layer having the shape of a cup can be replaced with a double layer having the shape of the cup's cover, but with its double layer oriented in the same direction as the cup, as described in Figure 11.4. From this example one can assert that two uniform double layers with the same periphery generate identical potential fields.

The field generated by a double layer disk at distances that are much greater than the disk radius appears to originate from a single dipole. In fact, at large enough distances from any dipole distribution, the field will appear to originate from a single dipole whose strength and orientation are the vector sum of the source components, as if they were all located at the same point. This is the reason why the electric field of the heart during the activation has a dipolar form and the concept of a single *electric heart vector* (EHV), as a description of the cardiac source, has a wide application. This is par-

ticularly true when the activation involves only a single ventricle. The true situation, where the right and left ventricle are simultaneously active, is more accurately represented by two separate dipoles.

This same argument may be used in explaining the effect of an infarct on the electric field of the heart. The *infarct* is a region of dead tissue; it can be represented by the absence of a double layer (i.e., an opening in a double layer). As a consequence, closing the double layer surface in this case introduces an additional cover, as shown in Figure 11.4. The latter source is a direct reflection of the effect of the infarct. (The paradox in this deduction is that the region of *dead tissue* is represented by an *active dipole* directed inward.)

Finally, we summarize the two important properties of uniform double layers defined by the solid angle theorem:

1. A closed uniform double layer generates a zero external potential field.
2. The potential field of an open uniform double layer is completely defined by the rim of the opening (Wikswo et al., 1979).

11.3 MILLER-GESELOWITZ MODEL

PRECONDITIONS:

Source: *Distributed dipole, cellular basis*
Conductor: *Finite, homogeneous*

W. T. Miller and D. B. Geselowitz (1978) developed a source model that is based directly on the generators associated with the activation of each cell. Their basic expression is patterned after Equation 8.23, which assigns a dipole source density to the spatial derivative of transmembrane voltage. For three dimensions, instead of a derivative with respect to a single variable, a gradient (including all three variables) is required. Consequently,

$$\bar{J}^i = -\sigma\nabla V_m \qquad (11.8)$$

where

$\bar{J}^i$ = dipole source density [μA/cm^2]
σ = conductivity [mS/cm]
∇V_m = spatial derivative of transmembrane voltage [mV/cm]

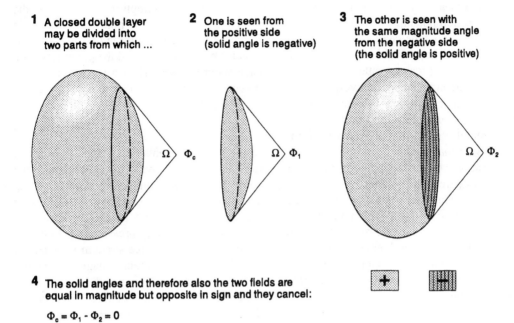

1 A closed double layer may be divided into two parts from which ...

2 One is seen from the positive side (solid angle is negative)

3 The other is seen with the same magnitude angle from the negative side (the solid angle is positive)

4 The solid angles and therefore also the two fields are equal in magnitude but opposite in sign and they cancel:

$$\Phi_c = \Phi_1 - \Phi_2 = 0$$

Fig. 11.3 A closed uniform double layer produces a zero potential field.

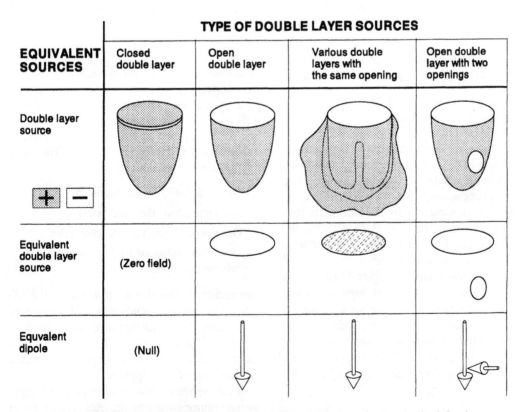

TYPE OF DOUBLE LAYER SOURCES

EQUIVALENT SOURCES	Closed double layer	Open double layer	Various double layers with the same opening	Open double layer with two openings
Double layer source				
Equivalent double layer source	(Zero field)			
Equivalent dipole	(Null)			

Fig. 11.4 The potential field of an open uniform double layer is completely defined by the rim of its opening.

Miller and Geselowitz used published data to evaluate action potential waveforms at various sites throughout the heart as well as times of activation. They could thus estimate $V_m(x,y,z,t)$ and as a result, could evaluate the "actual" dipole moment per unit volume at all points. For simplicity the heart was divided into a finite number of regions, and the net dipole source strength in each region found by summing $\bar{J}^i\, dV$ in that region.

In determining the surface potential fields the authors considered the number of dipole elements to be a small set (of 21) and evaluated the contribution from each. This part of their work constituted a relatively straightforward solution of the forward problem (dipole source in a bounded volume conductor). The reconstructed electrocardiograms showed very reasonable qualities.

11.4   LEAD VECTOR

11.4.1   Definition
of the Lead Vector

PRECONDITIONS:

Source: *Dipole in a fixed location*

Conductor: *Finite (infinite), inhomogeneous*

We examine the potential field at a point P, within or at the surface of a volume conductor, caused by a unit dipole $\bar{i}$ (a unit vector in the x direction) in a fixed location Q, as illustrated in Figure 11.5. (Though the theory, which we will develop, applies to both infinite and finite volume conductors, we discuss here is only finite volume conductors, for the sake of clarity.)

Suppose that at the point P the potential Φ_P due to the unit dipole $\bar{i}$ is c_x. (The potential at P must be evaluated relative to another local point or a remote reference point. Both choices are followed in electrophysiology, as is explained subsequently. For the present, we assume the existence of some unspecified remote reference point.) Because of our linearity assumption, the potential Φ_P corresponding to a dipole $p_x\bar{i}$ of arbitrary magnitude p_x is

$$\Phi_P = c_x p_x \qquad (11.9)$$

A similar expression holds for dipoles in the y and z directions.

The linearity assumption ensures that the principle of superposition holds, and any dipole $\bar{p}$ can be resolved into three orthogonal components $p_x\bar{i}$, $p_y\bar{j}$, $p_z\bar{k}$, and the potentials from each superimposed. Thus we can express the potential Φ_P at point P, due to any dipole $\bar{p}$ at the point Q

$$\Phi_P = c_x p_x + c_y p_y + c_z p_z \qquad (11.10)$$

where the coefficients c_x, c_y, and c_z are found (as described above) by energizing the corresponding unit dipoles at point Q along x-, y-, and z-axes, respectively, and measuring the corresponding field potentials. Equations 11.9 and 11.10 are expressions of linearity, namely that if the source strength is increased by a factor c, the resultant voltage is increased by the same factor c. Since no other assumptions were required, Equation 11.10 is valid for any linear volume conductor, even for an inhomogeneous conductor of finite extent.

Equation 11.10 can be simplified if the coefficients c_x, c_y, and c_z are interpreted as the components of a vector $\bar{c}$. This vector is called the *lead vector*. Consequently, Equation 11.10 can be written

$$\Phi_P = \bar{c} \cdot \bar{p} \qquad (11.11)$$

The lead vector is a three-dimensional transfer coefficient which describes how a dipole source at a fixed point Q inside a volume conductor influences the potential at a point within or on the surface of the volume conductor relative to the potential at a reference location. The value of the lead vector depends on:

The location Q of the dipole $\bar{p}$

The location of the field point P

The shape of the volume conductor

The (distribution of the) resistivity of the volume conductor

We tacitly assume that the potential at the reference is zero and hence does not have to be considered. Note that the value of the lead vector is a property of the lead and volume conductor and does not depend on the magnitude or direction of the dipole $\bar{p}$.

It can be shown that in an infinite, homogeneous volume conductor the lead vector is given by the sum of components along lines connecting the source point with each of the two

A LINEARITY

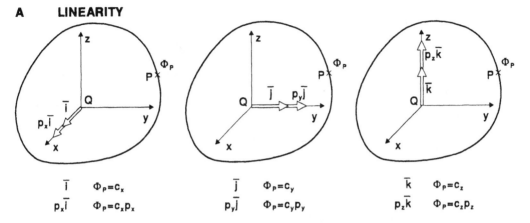

$\bar{i}$	$\Phi_P = c_x$	$\bar{j}$	$\Phi_P = c_y$	$\bar{k}$	$\Phi_P = c_z$
$p_x\bar{i}$	$\Phi_P = c_x p_x$	$p_y\bar{j}$	$\Phi_P = c_y p_y$	$p_z\bar{k}$	$\Phi_P = c_z p_z$

Because of linearity, in each case Φ_P is linearly proportional to the dipole magnitude

B SUPERPOSITION

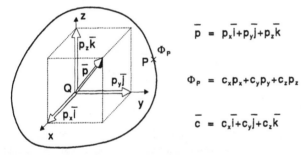

$$\bar{p} = p_x\bar{i} + p_y\bar{j} + p_z\bar{k}$$

$$\Phi_P = c_x p_x + c_y p_y + c_z p_z$$

$$\bar{c} = c_x\bar{i} + c_y\bar{j} + c_z\bar{k}$$

Because of superpositon, Φ_P is proportional to
the sum of the potentials of each dipole component.
The proportionality coefficient is three-dimensional.
It is the lead vector $\bar{c}$.

C VECTOR ALGEBRA

Mathematically, the potential Φ_P is
the scalar product of dipole $\bar{p}$
and the lead vector $\bar{c}$

$$\boxed{\Phi_P = \bar{c} \cdot \bar{p}}$$

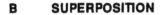

$$\Phi_P = \bar{c} \cdot \bar{p} = |\bar{c}|\,|\bar{p}|\cos\alpha$$

Fig. 11.5 Development of the lead vector concept.
(A) Because of linearity, the potential at a point P
in the volume conductor is linearly proportional to
dipoles in each coordinate direction. (B) By superposition the potential at the point P is proportional to
the sum of component dipoles in each coordinate
direction. This proportionality is three-dimensional
and can therefore be considered as a vector $\bar{c}$, called
lead vector. (C) The potential at the point P is the
scalar product of the source dipole $\bar{p}$ and the lead
vector $\bar{c}$.

electrode points (each scaled inversely to its
uphysical length). The same also holds for a
spherical, homogeneous volume conductor,
provided that the source is at the center.

11.4.2 Extending the Concept
of Lead Vector

In the previous section we considered the lead
voltage to be measured relative to a remote reference—as it is in practice in a so-called *unipolar lead*. In this section, we consider a *bipolar
lead* formed by a lead pair (where neither elec-

trode is remote), and examine the corresponding lead vector, as illustrated in Figure 11.6.

For each location $P_0 \ldots P_n$ of P, that lies
within or at the surface of the volume conductor,
we can determine a lead vector $\bar{c}_0 \ldots \bar{c}_n$ for
the dipole $\bar{p}$ at a fixed location, so that, according to Equation 11.11, we have

$$\Phi_i = \bar{c}_i \cdot \bar{p} \qquad (11.12)$$

Then the potential difference between any two
points P_i and P_j is

$$V_{ij} = \Phi_i - \Phi_j \qquad (11.13)$$

A

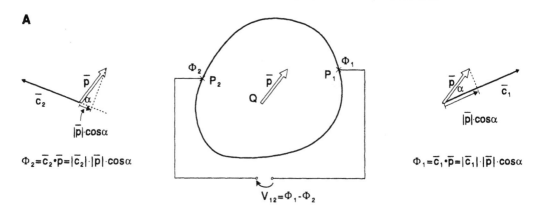

B

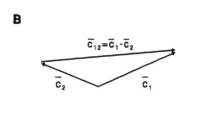

$$V_{12} = \Phi_1 - \Phi_2 = \bar{c}_1 \cdot \bar{p} - \bar{c}_2 \cdot \bar{p} = (\bar{c}_1 - \bar{c}_2) \cdot \bar{p} = \bar{c}_{12} \cdot \bar{p}$$

C

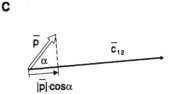

$$V_{12} = \bar{c}_{12} \cdot \bar{p} = |\bar{c}_{12}| \cdot |\bar{p}| \cdot \cos\alpha$$

Fig. 11.6 Determination of the voltage between two points at or within the surface of a volume conductor. (A) The potentials Φ_i and Φ_j at P_i and P_j due to the dipole $\bar{p}$ may be established with scalar products with the lead vectors $\bar{c}_i$ and $\bar{c}_j$, respectively.

(B) For determining the voltage V_{ij} between P_i and P_j, the lead vector $\bar{c}_{ij} = \bar{c}_i - \bar{c}_j$ is first determined. (C) The voltage V_{ij} is the scalar product of the lead vector $\bar{c}_{ij}$ and the dipole $\bar{p}$.

This describes the voltage that would be measured by the lead whose electrodes are at P_i and P_j. To what lead vector does this lead voltage correspond? Consider first the vector $\bar{c}_{ij}$ formed by

$$\bar{c}_{ij} = \bar{c}_i - \bar{c}_j \qquad (11.14)$$

Now the voltage between the points P_i and P_j given by Equation 11.13 can also be written, by substitution from Equation 11.12, as follows:

$$V_{ij} = \Phi_i - \Phi_j = \bar{c}_i \cdot \bar{p} - \bar{c}_j \cdot \bar{p} = \bar{c}_{ij} \cdot \bar{p} \qquad (11.15)$$

hence identifying $\bar{c}_{ij}$ as the lead vector for leads $P_i - P_j$. From this result we can express any bipolar lead voltage V as

$$V = \bar{c} \cdot \bar{p} \qquad \textbf{(11.16)}$$

where $\bar{c}$ is a lead vector. We note that Equation 11.16 for bipolar leads is in the same form as Equation 11.11 for monopolar leads. But Equations 11.14–11.16 can be interpreted as that we may first determine the lead vectors $\bar{c}_i$ and $\bar{c}_j$ corresponding to unipolar leads at P_i and P_j, respectively, and then form their vector difference, namely $\bar{c}_{ij}$. Then the voltage between the points P_i and P_j, as evaluated by a bipolar lead, is the scalar product of the vector $\bar{c}_{ij}$ and the dipole $\bar{p}$, as shown in Figure 11.6 and described by Equation 11.16.

11.4.3 Example of Lead Vector Application: Einthoven, Frank, and Burger Triangles

As an example of lead vector application, we introduce the concept of the Einthoven triangle.

It represents the lead vectors of the three limb leads introduced by Einthoven (1908). Einthoven did not consider the effect of the volume conductor on the lead vectors. The effect of the body surface on the limb leads was published by Ernest Frank (1954), and the effect of the internal inhomogeneities was published by Burger and van Milaan (1946). The corresponding lead vector triangles are called Frank triangle and Burger triangle. In this section we discuss these lead vector triangles in detail.

Einthoven Triangle

PRECONDITIONS:

Source: *Two-dimensional dipole (in the frontal plane) in a fixed location*

Conductor: *Infinite, homogeneous volume conductor or homogeneous sphere with the dipole in its center (the trivial solution)*

In Einthoven's electrocardiographic model the cardiac source is a two-dimensional dipole in a fixed location within a volume conductor that is either infinite and homogeneous, or a homogenous sphere with the dipole source at its center.

Einthoven first recognized that because the limbs are generally long and thin, no significant electrocardiographic currents from the torso would be expected to enter them. Accordingly, Einthoven realized that the potential at the wrist was the same as at the upper arm, while that at the ankle was the same as at the upper thigh. Einthoven consequently assumed that the functional position of the measurement sites of the right and left arm and the left leg corresponded to points on the torso which, in turn, bore a geometric relationship approximating the apices of an equilateral triangle. He further assumed that the heart generator could be approximated as a single dipole whose position is fixed, but whose magnitude and orientation could vary. The location of the heart dipole relative to the leads was chosen, for simplicity, to be at the center of the equilateral triangle. (In matter of fact, the Einthoven assumptions and model were not truly original, but were based on the earlier suggestions of Augustus Waller (1889).)

Because of the central location of the heart

dipole in the Einthoven model, the relationship between potentials at the apices of the triangle are the same whether the medium is considered uniform and infinite in extent, or the volume conductor is assumed to be spherical and bounded. For the unbounded case, we can apply Equation 8.12, which may be written $\Phi_P = \bar{p} \cdot \bar{a}_r/(4\pi\sigma r^2)$ from which we learn that the lead vector for a surface point P is $\bar{a}_r/(4\pi\sigma r^2)$—that is, along the radius vector to P. Point P is, according to Einthoven, at the apices of the equilateral triangle. Consequently, if the right and left arms and left foot are designated R, L, and F, respectively, then the three corresponding lead vectors $\bar{c}_R$, $\bar{c}_L$, and $\bar{c}_F$ are the radius vectors between the origin and the corresponding points on the equilateral triangle, as illustrated in Figure 11.7. From the aforementioned, the potentials at these points are:

$$\Phi_R = \bar{c}_R \cdot \bar{p}$$
$$\Phi_L = \bar{c}_L \cdot \bar{p} \qquad (11.17)$$
$$\Phi_F = \bar{c}_F \cdot \bar{p}$$

Einthoven defined the potential differences between the three pairs of these three points to

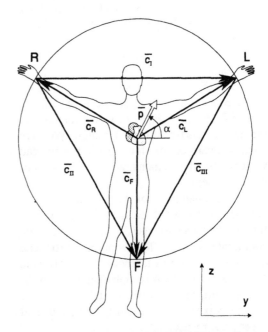

Fig. 11.7   Einthoven triangle. Note the coordinate system that has been applied (the frontal plane coordinates are shown). It is described in detail in Appendix A.

constitute the fundamental lead voltages in electrocardiography. These are designated V_I, V_{II}, and V_{III} and are given by

$$V_I = \Phi_L - \Phi_R = \bar{c}_L \cdot \bar{p} - \bar{c}_R \cdot \bar{p}$$
$$= (\bar{c}_L - \bar{c}_R) \cdot \bar{p} = \bar{c}_I \cdot \bar{p}$$
$$V_{II} = \Phi_F - \Phi_R = \bar{c}_F \cdot \bar{p} - \bar{c}_R \cdot \bar{p} \qquad (11.18)$$
$$= (\bar{c}_F - \bar{c}_R) \cdot \bar{p} = \bar{c}_{II} \cdot \bar{p}$$
$$V_{III} = \Phi_F - \Phi_L = \bar{c}_F \cdot \bar{p} - \bar{c}_L \cdot \bar{p}$$
$$= (\bar{c}_F - \bar{c}_L) \cdot \bar{p} = \bar{c}_{III} \cdot \bar{p}$$

Since $\bar{c}_R$, $\bar{c}_L$, and $\bar{c}_F$ are equal in magnitude and each is in the direction from the origin to an apex of the equilateral triangle, then $\bar{c}_I$, $\bar{c}_{II}$, and $\bar{c}_{III}$ must lie along a leg of the triangle (since $\bar{c}_I = \bar{c}_L - \bar{c}_R$, etc.) For example $\bar{c}_I$ is seen to lie oriented horizontally from the right arm to the left arm.

In summary, V_I, V_{II}, and V_{III} are the three standard limb leads (or scalar leads) in electro- cardiography. From Equation 11.18 one can confirm that the three lead vectors $\bar{c}_I$, $\bar{c}_{II}$, and $\bar{c}_{III}$ also form an equilateral triangle, the so- called *Einthoven triangle*, and these are shown in Figure 11.7.

The limb lead voltages are not independent, since $V_I + V_{III} - V_{II} = 0$, as can be verified by substituting for the left side of this equation the component potentials from Equation 11.18, namely $(\Phi_L - \Phi_R) + (\Phi_F - \Phi_L) - (\Phi_F - \Phi_R)$, and noting that they do, in fact, sum to zero. The above relationship among the stan- dard leads is also expressed by $\bar{c}_I \cdot \bar{p} + \bar{c}_{III} \cdot \bar{p} - \bar{c}_{II} \cdot \bar{p} = 0$, according to Equation 11.18. Since $\bar{p}$ is arbitrary, this can be satisfied only if $\bar{c}_I + \bar{c}_{III} - \bar{c}_{II} = 0$, which means that the lead vectors form a closed triangle. We were already aware of this for the Einthoven lead vectors, but the demonstration here is com- pletely general.

From the geometry of the equilateral (Eint- hoven) triangle, we obtain the following values for the three lead voltages. Please note that the coordinate system differs from that introduced by Einthoven. In this textbook, the coordinate system of Appendix A is applied. In this coordi- nate system, the positive directions of the x-, y-, and z-axes point anteriorly, leftward, and superiorly, respectively.

$$V_I = p \cos\alpha = p_y$$
$$V_{II} = \frac{p}{2} \cos\alpha - \frac{\sqrt{3}}{2} p \sin\alpha = \frac{1}{2} p_y - \frac{\sqrt{3}}{2} p_z$$
$$= 0.5\, p_y - 0.98\, p_z$$

$$V_{III} = -\frac{p}{2} \cos\alpha \frac{\sqrt{3}}{2} p \sin\alpha = -\frac{1}{2} p_y - \frac{\sqrt{3}}{2} p_z$$
$$= -0.5 p_y - 0.87 p_z$$

$$(11.19)$$

For the lead vectors we obtain:

$$\bar{c}_I = \bar{j}$$
$$\bar{c}_{II} = 0.5\bar{j} - 0.87\bar{k} \qquad (11.20)$$
$$\bar{c}_{III} = -0.5\bar{j} - 0.87\bar{k}$$

Frank Triangle

PRECONDITIONS:

Source: *(Three-dimensional) dipole in a fixed location*

Conductor: *Finite, homogeneous*

Ernest Frank measured the lead vectors of the scalar leads by constructing an electrolytic tank model of the human torso (Frank, 1954). The following values were obtained for the three lead vectors of the standard leads. Note that only the relative values of these lead vectors have any meaning because the measurement procedure was not calibrated.

$$\bar{c}_I = -14\bar{i} + 76\bar{j} + 27\bar{k}$$
$$\bar{c}_{II} = 16\bar{i} + 30\bar{j} - 146\bar{k} \qquad (11.21)$$
$$\bar{c}_{III} = 30\bar{i} - 46\bar{j} - 173\bar{k}$$

We noted earlier that since $V_I + V_{III} = V_{II}$, a condition dictated by Kirchhoff's law, the cor- responding lead vectors must form a closed tri- angle. One can confirm from Equation 11.21 that, indeed, $\bar{c}_I + \bar{c}_{II} - \bar{c}_{III} = 0$ and hence form a closed triangle. This triangle is called the *Frank triangle* and is illustrated in Figure 11.8.

Burger Triangle

PRECONDITIONS:

Source: *Dipole in a fixed location*

Conductor: *Finite, inhomogeneous*

Lead vector concept was first introduced by H. C. Burger and J. B. van Milaan (1946, 1947, 1948) (Burger, 1967), who also used an inho- mogeneous electrolyte tank model of the human torso to measure the lead vectors of standard leads.

The lead vectors, which they measured, are given below. Since these vectors must necessar- ily form a closed triangle (just as Einthoven and Frank triangles), this triangle has been

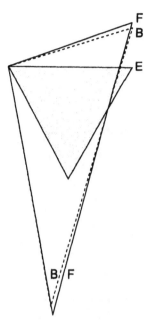

Fig. 11.8 Einthoven (E), Frank (F), and Burger (B) triangles. Note that the Einthoven triangle lies in the frontal plane, whereas the Frank and Burger triangles are tilted out of the frontal plane. Only their frontal projections are illustrated here.

Table 11.1 Comparison of the lead vectors for Einthoven (E), Frank (F), and Burger (B) Triangles

Lead	Triangle	c_x	c_y	c_z
c_I	Einthoven		100	
	Frank	−18	100	36
	Burger	−26	100	32
c_{II}	Einthoven		50	−87
	Frank	21	40	−192
	Burger	23	38	−185
c_{III}	Einthoven		−50	−87
	Frank	39	−61	−228
	Burger	49	−62	−217

called *Burger triangle;* it is shown in Figure 11.8. The absolute values of the lead vectors have no special meaning since no calibration procedure was carried out. The lead vectors obtained were

$$\bar{c}_I = -17\bar{i} + 65\bar{j} + 21\bar{k}$$
$$\bar{c}_{II} = 15\bar{i} + 25\bar{j} - 120\bar{k} \quad (11.22)$$
$$\bar{c}_{III} = 32\bar{i} - 40\bar{j} - 141\bar{k}$$

We may compare the three triangles described so far (i.e., the Einthoven, Frank, and Burger) by normalizing the y-component of each $\bar{c}_I$ vector to 100. This means that the values of the Einthoven triangle components must be multiplied by 100, those of the Frank triangle by $100/76 = 1.32$, and those of the Burger triangle by $100/65 = 1.54$. (The reader can confirm that in each case $c_I = 100$ results.) The resulting lead vector components are summarized in Table 11.1.

One may notice from the table that in the measurements of Frank and Burger, the introduction of the boundary of the volume conductor has a great influence on the lead vectors. As pointed out earlier, the lead vector also depends on the dipole location; thus these comparisons may also reflect differences in the particular choice that was made. Figure 11.8 illustrates the Einthoven, Frank, and Burger triangles standardized according to Table 11.1.

The shape of the Frank and Burger triangles was recently investigated by Hyttinen et al. (1988). Instead of evaluating the lead vectors for a single dipole location, they examined the effect of different dipole positions within the heart. According to these studies the shape of the Frank and Burger triangles varies strongly as a function of the location of the assumed heart dipole $\bar{p}$. They showed that the difference between the original Frank and Burger triangles is not necessarily so small if the dipole is placed at other locations. Figures 11.9 and 11.10 illustrate the variation of the Frank and Burger triangles as functions of the source location. Tables 11.2A and 11.2B compare the lead vectors for the Einthoven, Frank, and Burger triangles from two source locations.

11.5   IMAGE SURFACE

11.5.1   The Definition of the Image Surface

PRECONDITIONS:

Source: *Dipole in a fixed location*

Conductor: *Finite (infinite), inhomogeneous*

For a fixed-source dipole lying within a given volume conductor, the lead vector depends solely on the location of the field point. A lead vector can be found associated with each point on the volume conductor surface. The tips of

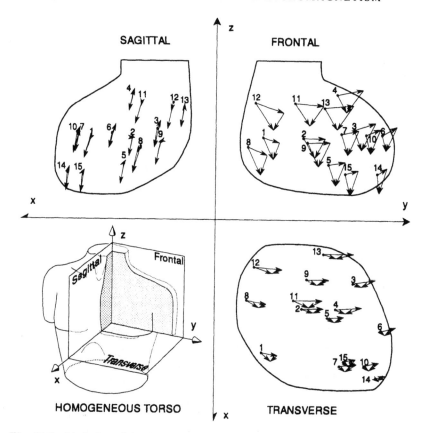

Fig. 11.9 Variation of the Frank triangle as a function of dipole location. The black circle in the miniature lead vector triangles arising from the Frank torso are superimposed on the site of the dipole origin. (From Hyttinen et al., 1988.)

these lead vectors sweep out a surface of its own. This latter surface is known as the *image surface.*

One could, in principle, consider a physical surface lying *within* a volume conductor of finite or infinite extent and evaluate an image surface for it in the same way as described above. However, most interest is concentrated on the properties of fields at the bounding surface of volume conductors, since this is where potentials are available for noninvasive measurement. Consequently, the preconditions adopted in this section are for a dipole source (multiple sources can be considered by superposition) lying in a bounded conducting region.

We accept, without proof, that any physical volume conductor surface has an associated image surface for each dipole source location. This seems, intuitively, to require only that no two points on the physical surface have the

same lead vector—a likely condition for convex surfaces. The image surface is a useful tool in characterizing the properties of the volume conductor, such as the effect of the boundary shape or of internal inhomogeneities, independent of the effect of the leads. That is, one could compare image surfaces arising with different inhomogeneities without having to consider any particular lead system.

A simple example of an image surface is given by a uniform spherical volume conductor with dipole source at its center. We have seen that for this situation the unipolar lead vector is proportional to the radius vector from the center of the sphere to the surface field point. Therefore, the image surface for a centric source in a uniform sphere is also a sphere.

We now describe how to construct the image surface for any linear volume conductor of arbitrary shape. It is done by placing a unit dipole

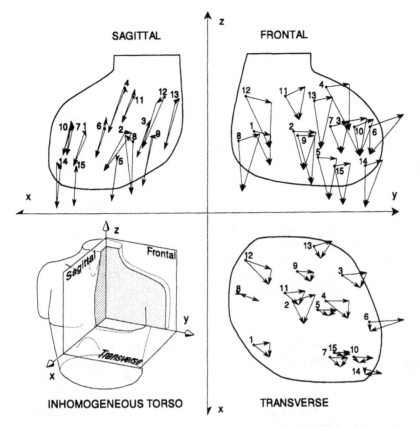

Fig. 11.10 Variation of the Burger triangle as a function of source location. (From Hyttinen et al., 1988.)

source at a chosen point within the conductor in the direction of each coordinate axis and then measuring the corresponding potential at every point on the surface. For the unit vector along the x-axis, the potentials correspond precisely to the lead vector component in the x direction,

as is clear from Equation 11.10. Similarly for the y and z directions, and therefore, the lead vectors can be determined in space from these measurements, and they form the image surface

Table 11.2A Dipole in the center of the heart (septum): coefficient for Frank = 1.546; Burger = 1.471

Lead	Triangle	c_x	c_y	c_z
c_I	Einthoven		100	
	Frank	−2.8	100	−1.8
	Burger	−31.2	100	−6.4
c_{II}	Einthoven		50	−87
	Frank	16	53	−88
	Burger	97	46	−162
c_{III}	Einthoven		−50	−87
	Frank	19	−47	−86
	Burger	135	−57	−163

Table 11.2B Dipole in the center of the transverse projection of the heart (0.5 cm anterior, 2 cm left and inferior from the dipole in Table 11.2A): coefficient for Frank = 1.976; Burger = 1.784

Lead	Triangle	c_x	c_y	c_z
c_I	Einthoven		100	
	Frank	−6.6	100	12
	Burger	−3.0	100	−8.2
c_{II}	Einthoven		50	−87
	Frank	23	44	−117
	Burger	33	62	−217
c_{III}	Einthoven		−50	−87
	Frank	30	−60	−130
	Burger	30	−39	−209

A   **B**   **C**

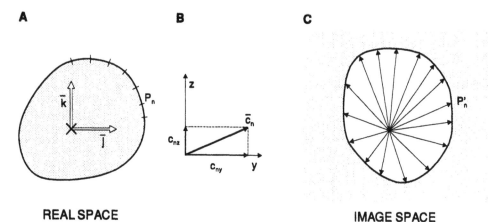

REAL SPACE   IMAGE SPACE

Fig. 11.11 Construction of the image surface for a source point at a volume conductor of arbitrary shape, illustrated in two dimensions. A one-to-one relation is established between points on the surface of the volume conductor and the image surface. (A)

Unit vectors are placed at the source location. (B) By measuring the corresponding potentials at each surface point, the lead vector can be determined. (C) The locus described by the family of lead vectors form the image surface.

for the chosen source location. This procedure and the resulting image surface are illustrated in Figure 11.11.

11.5.2 Points Located Inside the Volume Conductor

As noted above, it is not necessary to restrict the physical surface to points on the boundary of the volume conductor. If we examine the potential inside the volume conductor, we find that it is greater than on the surface; that is, the closer to the dipole the measurements are made, the larger the voltage, and therefore, the longer the corresponding lead vector. This means that points inside the volume conductor transform to points in the image space that lie outside the image surface. The dipole source location itself transforms to infinity in the image space.

Note that the shadings in Figures 11.11, 11.12, and 11.13 are not arbitrary; rather, they illustrate that for the region inside the volume conductor, the corresponding region in the image space is farther from the origin.

11.5.3 Points Located Inside the Image Surface

We now examine the real-space behavior of points that lie in the image space within the

image surface. Suppose that an image point is designated P' and that an arbitrary line has been drawn through it. The line intersects the image surface in points P_1' and P_2'. Further, the point P' divides this line inside the image surface as follows:

$$\frac{P_1'P'}{P'P_2'} = \frac{a}{b} \qquad (11.23)$$

From Figure 11.12 it is easy to see the following relationship between the lead vectors $\bar{c}_1$, $\bar{c}_2$, and $\bar{c}_s$:

$$\bar{c}_s = \bar{c}_1 + \frac{a}{a+b}(\bar{c}_2 - \bar{c}_1) = \bar{c}_2 - \frac{b}{a+b}(\bar{c}_2 - \bar{c}_1) \qquad (11.24)$$

Therefore, the voltage, measured in the real space from the point P must fulfill the requirement:

$$\Phi_s = \Phi_1 + \frac{a}{a+b}(\Phi_2 - \Phi_1)$$
$$= \Phi_2 - \frac{b}{a+b}(\Phi_2 - \Phi_1) \qquad (11.25)$$

The point that fulfills this requirement in the real space can be found in the following way: We connect between the points P_1 and P_2 two resistors in series having the resistance ratio of a/b. The point P is at the interconnection of these resistors. (We must choose R_a and R_b

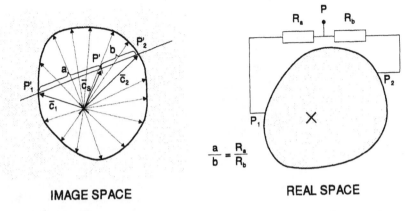

Fig. 11.12 Determination of the point P in the real space corresponding to an image space point P′ located inside the image surface.

large enough so that the current through this pathway has a negligible effect on Φ_1 and Φ_2.)

11.5.4 Application of the Image Surface to the Synthesis of Leads

In this section, we examine how the image surface concept can be applied to the identification

of an unknown dipole inside the volume conductor from measurements on the surface. Our initial task is to synthesize an *orthonormal* lead system for the measurement of the dipole. The concept "orthonormal" denotes that a lead system is both (1) orthogonal *and* (2) normalized; that is, the three measured components of the dipole are orthogonal and their magnitudes are

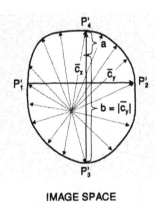

IMAGE SPACE

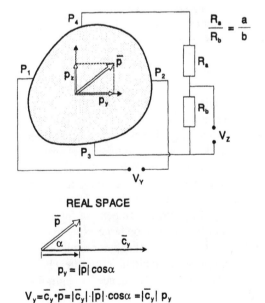

REAL SPACE

Fig. 11.13 Construction of an orthonormal lead system utilizing the image surface. The lead $\bar{c}_{34}$ for surface points $P_3 - P_4$ is solely in the z direction, whereas lead $\bar{c}_{12}$ established for surface points $P_1 - P_2$ is solely in the y direction. Since $|\bar{c}_{34}|/|\bar{c}_{12}| =$

$(a + b)/b$, the resistor network R_a and R_b is inscribed to reduce the voltage from $(P_3 - P_4)$ by $b/(a + b)$, hence making the effective z-lead equal to the y-lead in magnitude.

measured with equal sensitivity. That means, the lead voltage corresponding to equal-value components of the dipole source is the same.

To begin, we construct the image surface of the volume conductor in relation to the known location of the dipole. Now we want to find two points on the surface of the volume conductor such that the voltage between them is proportional only to the y-component of the dipole. Mathematically, this can be formulated as:

$$V_{21} = \bar{c}_{21} \cdot \bar{p} = c_{21x}p_x + c_{21y}\,p_y + c_{21z}p_z$$
$$(11.26)$$

and we seek a lead vector $\bar{c}_{21}$, which both lies in the image space and is oriented solely in the direction of the y-axis. This corresponds to identifying any pair of points on the image surface that are located at the intersections of a line directed parallel to the y-axis. The voltage measured between those points in real space is consequently proportional only to the y-component of the dipole. To obtain the largest possible signal (in order to minimize the noise), we select from all image space points that fulfill the requirement discussed above, the one with the longest segment (maximum lead vector), as illustrated in Figure 11.13.

If we want to measure all three orthogonal components of the dipole source, we repeat this procedure for the z and x directions. Because the resulting (maximum) lead vectors are usually not of equal length, we equalize the measured signals with a resistor network to obtain both an orthogonal and a normalized lead system. Such a normalizing procedure is described in Figure 11.13 for a two-dimensional system. In this case two resistors, R_A and R_B, form a simple voltage-divider, and the output voltage is reduced from the input by $R_B/(R_A + R_B)$. We choose this ratio to compensate for a lead vector amplitude that is too large. Note that the assumed voltage-divider behavior requires that the voltage-measuring circuit (amplifier) has a sufficiently high input impedance for negligible loading.

11.5.5   Image Surface
of Homogeneous Human Torso

We consider here the image surface of the homogeneous human torso, as determined by Er-

nest Frank (1954). Frank constructed a tank model having the form of the thorax. It was oriented upside down because it was easier to insert and manipulate the source dipole from the larger opening of the model at the level of the abdomen. The model was filled with a salt solution and therefore formed a finite, homogeneous model.

Frank adopted the following coordinate system for the model: The model was divided into 12 levels with horizontal planes at increments of 5 cm (2 inches). The center of the heart was located on level 6 about 4 cm to the front of the plane located at the midline of the right and left arms, and about 2.5 cm to the left of the sagittal plane located at the midline of the model. On each horizontal plane, 16 points were established by drawing 8 lines through the midline of the model (within increments of 22.5°). The intersections of these lines on the surface of the model were labeled with letters A through P in a clockwise direction starting from the left side, as shown in Figure 11.14. Note that the coordinate axis nomenclature used here is not the same as that adopted by Frank, since the consistent coordinate system of Appendix A has been used.

Figures 11.15, 11.16, and 11.17 illustrate the image surface measured by Frank in the three projections—the frontal, sagittal, and transverse planes. The figures also show the points corresponding to the Einthoven limb leads, which in this case form the Frank triangle.

11.5.6   Recent Image
Surface Studies

In recent years the image surface for the human torso has been investigated using computer models. In these models one can introduce not only the effect of body shape but also inhomogeneities such as the lungs, intracavitary blood masses, surface muscle layers, and so on. One such study is that of Horáček (1971), who included the effect of body shape, lungs, and intracavitary blood. Horáček observed that the lungs and the intracavitary blood masses can substantially distort the image surface and consequently cause variations in the body surface potential distribution. However, because of the complexity of the effect, no simple universal

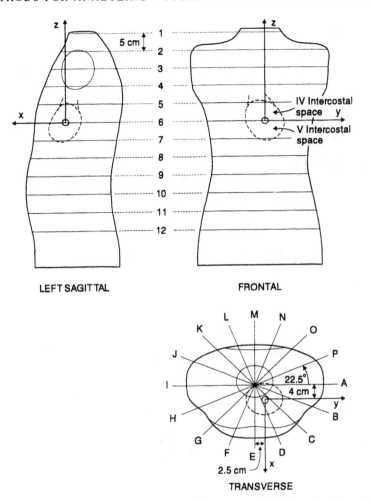

Fig. 11.14 The Frank torso model and coordinate system. (The latter has been related to correspond with the system adopted in this text and discussed in Appendix A.)

statement can be made to describe the influence of the inhomogeneities.

A modified Horáček model that includes the skeletal muscle was developed and studied by Gulrajani and Mailloux (1983). The latter authors chose to examine the effects of modifications introduced by inhomogeneities in terms of effects on body surface potentials rather than on the image surface per se.

11.6   LEAD FIELD

11.6.1   Concepts Used in Connection with Lead Fields

It is useful to start a discussion of the lead field by first introducing the concept of *sensitivity*

distribution. As noted in Section 11.4.3, the lead vector has different values for different source locations. In other words, for a given field point, the length and direction of the lead vector vary as a function of the source location. For a fixed field point location, one can assign to each possible source point the value of the lead vector. In this way we establish a lead vector field, which is distributed throughout the volume conductor. Because the lead vector indicates the sensitivity of the lead to the dipole source through $V = \bar{c} \cdot \bar{p}$ (Equation 11.16), the distribution of the magnitude and the direction of the lead vector is at the same time the *distribution of the sensitivity of the lead* to the dipole source as a function of its location and orientation. This is further illustrated in Figure 11.18. (It should be emphasized that the concept

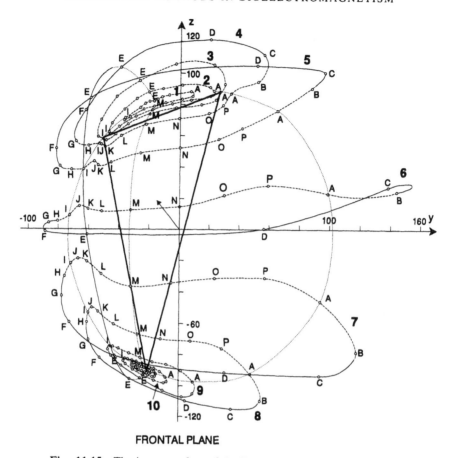

FRONTAL PLANE

Fig. 11.15 The image surface of the Frank torso model in frontal view.

of sensitivity distribution is not limited to the detection of bioelectric sources. The same concept is applicable also to the measurement of tissue impedance.)

For later use we will define the concepts of *isosensitivity surface* or *isosensitivity line* and *half-sensitivity volume*. An isosensitivity surface is a surface in the volume conductor where the absolute value of the sensitivity is constant. When sensitivity distributions are illustrated with two-dimensional figures, the isosensitivity surface is illustrated with isosensitivity line(s). The concept of isosensitivity surface is used to enhance our view of the distribution of the magnitude of the sensitivity. The isosensitivity surface where the absolute value of the sensitivity is one half of its maximum value within the volume conductor separates a volume called half-sensitivity volume. This concept can be

used to indicate how concentrated the detector's sensitivity distribution is.

11.6.2   Definition of the Lead Field

PRECONDITIONS:

Source: *Volume source*

Conductor: *Finite (infinite), inhomogeneous*

The concept of *lead field* is a straightforward extension of the concept of lead vector. In the evaluation of a lead field, one follows a procedure that is just the reverse of that followed in obtaining the image surface. These may be contrasted as follows (see Fig. 11.19).

In our definition of the *image surface* (Section 11.5.1):

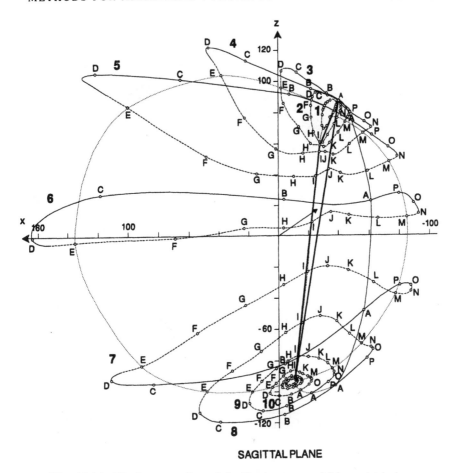

Fig. 11.16   The image surface of the Frank torso model in sagittal view.

1. The source was a dipole $\bar{p}$ located at a fixed point.
2. The measurement point was varied over the surface of the volume conductor (Fig. 11.11A).

The image surface was generated by the tips of the lead vectors $\bar{c}$ associated with all surface sites (Fig. 11.11C).

In evaluating the *lead field* we proceed the other way around:

1. We assume a fixed electrode pair defining a lead (fixed measurement sites).
2. We observe the behavior of the lead vector $\bar{c}$ as a function of the location of the dipole source $\bar{c}$ varying throughout the volume conductor (Fig. 11.19A)

3. We assign $\bar{c}$ to the location of $\bar{p}$ (which for a volume source is a field of dipole elements $\bar{p}_k$).

With this latter procedure, it is possible to evaluate the variation of the lead vector $\bar{c}$ within the volume conductor. This *field of lead vectors* is called the *lead field* $\bar{J}_L$, as noted earlier and illustrated in Figure 11.19A. Therefore, the lead field theory applies to distributed volume sources. The procedure may be carried out with a finite or an infinite volume conductor. In any physically realizable system, the volume conductor is necessarily finite, of course. Thus the preconditions for the discussion on the lead field are those defined above.

From the behavior of the lead vector $\bar{c}$ as a function of the location k of the dipole source

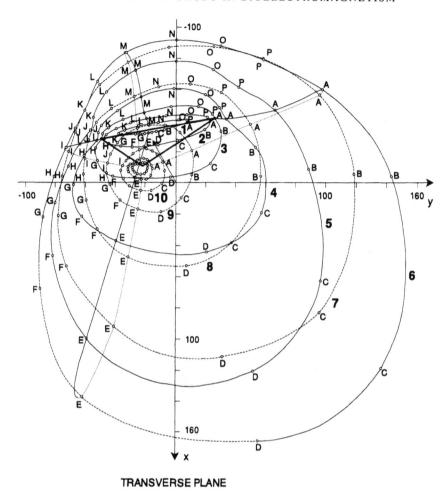

TRANSVERSE PLANE

Fig. 11.17 The image surface of the Frank torso model in transverse view.

$\bar{p}$, we can easily determine the lead voltage V_L generated by a distributed volume source (see Fig. 11.19B). The contribution V_k of each elementary dipole $\bar{p}_k$ to the lead voltage is obtained, as was explained in Section 11.4.1, with Equation 11.16 by forming the scalar product of the dipole element $\bar{p}_k$ and the lead vector $\bar{c}_k$ at that location, namely $V_k = \bar{c}_k \cdot \bar{p}_k$. The total contribution of all dipole elements—that is, the total lead voltage—is, according to the principle of superposition, the sum of the contributions of each dipole element $\bar{p}_k$, namely $V_L = \Sigma \bar{c}_k \cdot \bar{p}_k$. Mathematically this will be described later by Equations 11.30 and 11.31, where the dipole element $\bar{p}_k$ is replaced by the impressed current source element $\bar{J}^i dV$ (where $\bar{J}^i$ has the dimensions of dipole moment per unit volume).

The lead field has a very important property, which arises from the *reciprocity theorem of Helmholtz*. It is that for any lead, the lead field $\bar{J}_{LE}$ is *exactly the same* as the current flow field resulting from the application of a unit current $\bar{I}_r$, called the *reciprocal current*, to the lead (Fig. 11.19C). In this procedure the lead is said to be *reciprocally energized*. It is this correspondence that makes the lead field concept so very powerful in the following way:

1. With the concept of lead field it is possible both to visualize and to evaluate quantitatively the sensitivity distribution of a lead within a volume conductor, since it is the same as the field of a reciprocal current.

2. The actual measurement of sensitivity distribution (using either a torso-shaped tank

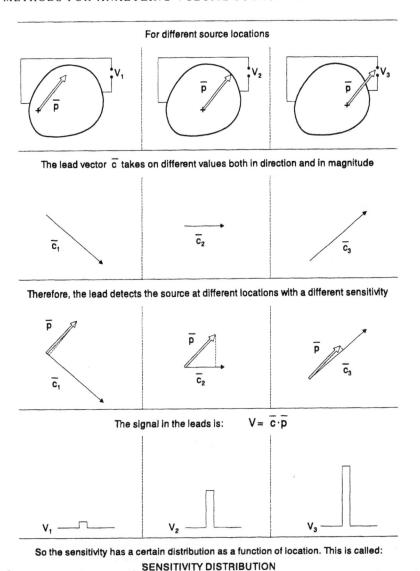

For different source locations

The lead vector $\bar{c}$ takes on different values both in direction and in magnitude

Therefore, the lead detects the source at different locations with a different sensitivity

The signal in the leads is: $V = \bar{c} \cdot \bar{p}$

So the sensitivity has a certain distribution as a function of location. This is called:
SENSITIVITY DISTRIBUTION

Fig. 11.18   The concept of sensitivity distribution.

model or a computer model) can be accomplished more easily using reciprocity.

3. Because the reciprocal current corresponds to the stimulating current introduced by a lead in electric stimulation, they have exactly the same distribution.

4. The sensitivity distribution in the measurement of electric impedance of the tissue may be similarly determined with the concept of lead field.

5. Because the principle of reciprocity and the concept of lead field are valid also in magnetic fields, all of these points are true for

the corresponding magnetic methods as well.

6. Furthermore, the concept of lead field easily explains the similarities and differences in the sensitivity distributions between the corresponding electric and magnetic methods.

The lead field may be visualized either as a field of lead vectors, as in Figure 11.19C, or with lead field current flow lines, as in Figure 11.19D. The relationship between these two methods is, obviously, that the lead vectors are tangents to the lead field current flow lines and

A

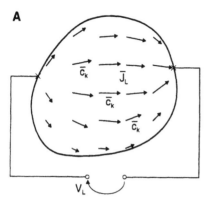

The field of the lead vectors $\bar{c}_k$ is the lead field $\bar{J}_L$

B

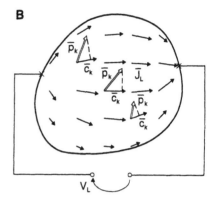

Each dipole element p_k contributes to the lead voltage by $V_k = \bar{c}_k \bullet \bar{p}_k$
The total lead voltage is the sum of the lead voltage elements $V_L = \sum_k \bar{c}_k \bullet \bar{p}_k$

C   RECIPROCITY

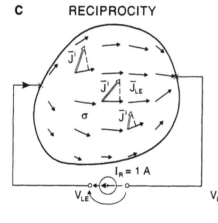

$$V_{LE} = \int \frac{1}{\sigma} \bar{J}_{LE} \bullet \bar{J}^i dv$$

Because of reciprocity, the field of lead vectors $\bar{J}_L$ is the same as the current field $\bar{J}_{LE}$ raised by feeding a reciprocal current of 1 A to the lead.

D

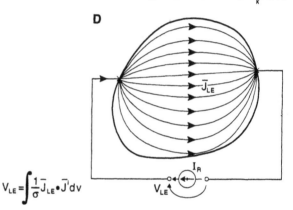

The lead field may also be illustrated with lead field current flow lines.

Fig. 11.19 The definition of the lead field and different ways to illustrate it. (A) When defining the lead field, we assume a fixed electrode pair constituting a lead, and we observe the behavior of the lead vector $\bar{c}$ as a function of the location k of the dipole source within the volume conductor. This field of lead vectors is the lead field $\bar{J}_L$. (B) When we know the lead vector $\bar{c}$ at each location k, we obtain the contribution of each dipole element $\bar{p}_k$ to the lead voltage: $V_k = \bar{c}_k \cdot \bar{p}_k$. Due to superposition, the total lead voltage V_L is the sum of the lead voltage elements. (C) Based on the reciprocity theorem, the lead field $\bar{J}_{LE}$ is the same as the electric current field if a (reciprocal) current I_r of 1A is introduced to the lead. The lead voltage due to a volume source of distribution $\bar{J}^i$ is obtained through integrating the dot product of the lead field current density and the source density throughout the volume source. (D) The lead field may also be illustrated with the lead field current flow lines.

that their length is proportional to the density of the flow lines. The reciprocity theorem is further discussed in the next section in greater detail.

11.6.3 Reciprocity Theorem: the Historical Approach

The lead field theory that is discussed in this section is based on a general *theory of reciproc-*

ity, introduced by Hermann von Helmholtz in 1853 (Helmholtz, 1853). Its application to the formulation of lead field theory was carried out 100 years later by Richard McFee and Franklin D. Johnston (1953, 1954a,b) as well as by Robert Plonsey (1963) and by Jaakko Malmivuo (1976). Before describing the lead field theory in more detail, we consider first the reciprocity theorem of Helmholtz.

Though Helmholtz introduced the principle

of reciprocity in connection with bioelectricity, it is a general property of linear systems, not limited only to bioelectricity. Helmholtz described the principle of reciprocity, in its original form, with the following example, which, it should be noted, also includes (for the first time) the *principle of superposition*.

A galvanometer is connected to the surface of the body. Now every single element of a biological electromotive surface produces such a current in the galvanometer circuit as would flow through that element itself if its electromotive force were impressed on the galvanometer wire. If one adds the effects of all the electromotive surface elements, the effect of each of which are found in the manner described, he will have the value of the total current through the galvanometer.

In other words, it is possible to swap the location of the (dipole) source and the detector without any change in the detected signal amplitudes. (Note that Helmholtz used a *voltage double layer source* and measured the *current* produced by it, whereas in our case the source is considered to be a *current dipole or a collection of dipoles such as implied in a double layer source*, whereas the measured signal is a *voltage*.)

Helmholtz illustrated the leading principle of the reciprocity theorem with the following example, described in Figure 11.20. This example includes two cases: case 1 and case 2.

We first consider case 1: A galvanometer (i.e., an electric current detector) G is connected at the surface of the volume conductor. Inside the conductor there is a differential element of double layer source, whose voltage is V_d and which causes a current I_L in the galvanometer circuit.

We now consider case 2: The double layer source element is first removed from the volume conductor. Then the galvanometer is replaced by an electromotive force of the same magnitude V_d as the voltage of the double layer source. This produces a reciprocal current i_r through the same differential area at the (removed) double layer source element in the volume conductor.

Now the reciprocity theorem of Helmholtz asserts that *the current I_L flowing in case 1 through the galvanometer is equal to the current i_r flowing in case 2 through the differential area located at the (removed) double layer source element*. This result is expressed in equation form as:

$$\frac{I_L}{V_d} = \frac{i_r}{V_d} \qquad (11.27)$$

where the left-hand side of the equation denotes case 1 and the right-hand side case 2.

Demonstration of the Consistency of the Reciprocity Theorem

It is easy to demonstrate that Equation 11.27 does not depend on the area of the double layer source. This is illustrated by the following examples.

If we make the area of the double layer K

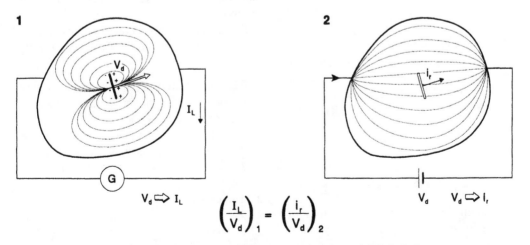

Fig. 11.20   Illustration of the reciprocity theorem of Helmholtz.

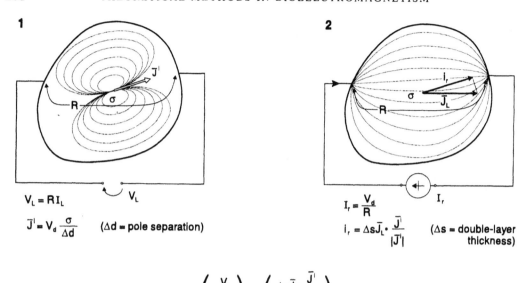

1

$V_L = R I_L$ $\overset{\frown}{} V_L$

$\bar{J}^i = V_d \dfrac{\sigma}{\Delta d}$ (Δd = pole separation)

2

$I_r = \dfrac{V_d}{R}$ I_r

$i_r = \Delta s \bar{J}_L \cdot \dfrac{\bar{J}^i}{|\bar{J}^i|}$ (Δs = double-layer thickness)

$$\left(\begin{matrix} \dfrac{V_L}{R} \\[2mm] \dfrac{J^i \Delta d}{\sigma} \end{matrix} \right)_1 = \left(\begin{matrix} \Delta s \bar{J}_L \cdot \dfrac{\bar{J}^i}{|\bar{J}^i|} \\[2mm] I_r R \end{matrix} \right)_2$$

Fig. 11.21 Derivation of the equation for lead field theory.

times larger, the current I_L through the galvanometer in case 1 is now (by the application of superposition) K times larger—that is, KI_L. In case 2, the electromotive force V_d in the galvanometer wire remains the same, because it represents the (unchanged) voltage over the double layer source in case 1. Therefore, it still produces the same current density in the source area. But because the source area is now K times larger, the total current through it is also K times larger—that is, Ki_r. Consequently, Equation 11.27 becomes

$$\frac{KI_L}{V_d} = \frac{Ki_r}{V_d} \qquad (11.27A)$$

and dividing both sides by K returns it to the expression arising from the original area. (In the above one should keep in mind that the original area A and KA are assumed to be very small so that i_r and V_d can be considered uniform.)

11.6.4 Lead Field Theory: the Historical Approach

In this section we derive the basic equation of the lead field from the original formulation of

Helmholtz (expressed by Equation 11.27) based on a description of current double layer source and lead voltage. As stated before, Helmholtz described the source as a voltage double layer element V_d, whose effect is evaluated by a measured lead current I_L. Alternatively, as is done presently, the source may be described as a current dipole layer element $\bar{J}^i$, whereas the signal is the lead voltage V_L produced by it. We can directly obtain these expressions from those of Helmholtz by application of the *principle of duality*. The result, illustrated in Figure 11.21, is discussed below.

Since Helmholtz's theorem applies to a discrete source, we make the following assumptions:

1. The lateral extent of the voltage double-layer element V_d is differential—that is, Δs.
2. The separation of the poles of the corresponding dipole element $\bar{J}^i \Delta s$ is Δd, where $\bar{J}^i$ is an applied current density so that $\bar{J}^i \Delta d$ has the dimensions of a double layer source.
3. The conductivity at the source point is σ.
4. The resistance of the galvanometer circuit between the measurement points equals R.

In case 1 and case 2 we may further evaluate the following expressions. For case 1:

1. Instead of the current I_L measured by the galvanometer, we can examine the related lead voltage $V_L = RI_L$, or $I_L = V_L/R$. (To prevent the galvanometer from affecting the volume conductor currents and voltages in a real situation, $R \rightarrow \infty$ should be chosen, but this choice does not affect the validity of this expression.)
2. Instead of reference to a voltage source V_d, we now emphasize the concomitant current source $J^i = V_d\sigma/\Delta d$ (Equation 11.2), where by rearranging we have $V_d = J^i\Delta d/\sigma$.

For case 2:

1. Instead of examining the reciprocal current density i_r at the (removed) source point we can evaluate the related lead field current density $\bar{J}_L = i_r/\Delta s$. These are connected by $i_r = \overline{\Delta s} \cdot \bar{J}_L$. The dot product is required here because the current i_r is the component of the reciprocal current flowing through the source area in the direction of the source $\bar{J}^i$. This can also be written $i_r = \Delta s\bar{J}_L \cdot \bar{J}^i/|\bar{J}^i|$.
2. The required voltage source V_d in the circuit connected to the conductor can be achieved if we use a reciprocal current source $I_r = V_d/R$, since then we have $V_d = I_rR$.

Substituting these equivalencies into the equation of Helmholtz, namely Equation 11.27, we obtain:

$$\frac{\dfrac{V_L}{R}}{\dfrac{J^i \, \Delta d}{\sigma}} = \frac{\Delta s\bar{J}_L \cdot \dfrac{\bar{J}^i}{|\bar{J}^i|}}{I_rR} \qquad (11.28)$$

where the left-hand side of the Equation 11.28 denotes case 1 and the right-hand side case 2 in the Helmholtz procedure, respectively. Solving for the lead voltage V_L in Equation 11.28, we obtain

$$V_L = \frac{1}{I_r}\frac{1}{\sigma}\bar{J}_L \cdot \bar{J}^i \, \Delta s \, \Delta d \qquad (11.29)$$

where $\Delta s \, \Delta d = \Delta v$, which is the volume element of the source. (In the limit, $\Delta v \rightarrow dv$.) By extending Equation 11.29 throughout all

source elements, and choosing the reciprocal current to be a *unit current* $I_r = 1$ A, we may write:

$$V_{LE} = \int \frac{1}{\sigma}\bar{J}_{LE} \cdot \bar{J}^i dv \qquad (11.30)$$

where $\bar{J}_{LE}$ denotes an electric lead field due to unit reciprocal current. Note that although $\bar{J}^i$ was originally defined as a current density, it may also be interpreted as a volume dipole density, as is clear in Equation 11.30 and by their similar dimensions. Equation 11.30 is the most important equation in the lead field theory, as it describes the lead voltage (the electric signal in a lead) produced by an arbitrary volume source described by $\bar{J}^i$ (x,y,z). It may be stated in words as follows:

To determine the lead voltage produced by a volume source, we first generate the lead field in the volume conductor by feeding a unit (reciprocal) current to the lead. Every element of the volume source contributes to the lead voltage a component equal to the scalar product of the lead field current density and the volume source element divided by the conductivity.

If the volume conductor is homogeneous throughout the source region, we may move the coefficient $1/\sigma$ outside the integral and write:

$$V_{LE} = \frac{1}{\sigma} \int \bar{J}_{LE} \cdot \bar{J}^i \, dv \qquad (11.31)$$

According to Equation 11.31, the lead field has an important property: it equals the lead sensitivity distribution. This means that at each point of the volume conductor, the absolute value of the lead field current density equals to the magnitude of the lead sensitivity, and the direction of the lead field current equals the direction of the lead sensitivity. It should be noted that the lead field fully takes into account the effect of the volume conductor boundary and internal inhomogeneities; hence these have an effect on the form of the lead field. (The concept of secondary sources is contained within lead field theory through the effect of the inhomogeneities on the form of the lead field.)

Lead field theory is a very powerful tool in bioelectromagnetism. It ties together the sensitivity distribution of the measurement of bioelectric sources, distribution of stimulation energy, and sensitivity distribution of impedance measurements, as is explained later. In general, if the lead and the volume conductor are known, the distribution of the lead sensitivity may be determined, based upon lead field theory. On the other hand, if the source and the volume conductor are known, the distribution of the actual field may be determined directly without using the lead field concept. All this holds for corresponding biomagnetic phenomena as well.

11.6.5 Field Theoretic Proof of the Reciprocity Theorem

A brief explanation of Helmholtz's reciprocity theorem was given in Section 11.6.3, without offering a mathematical proof. That explanation was based on the ideas of the original publication of Helmholtz (1853). The field-theoretic proof of the reciprocity theorem as described by Plonsey (1963) is presented below.

Proof of the Reciprocity Theorem
Consider an arbitrary volume v bounded by the surface S and having a conductivity σ (which may be a function of position). If Φ_1 and Φ_2 are any two scalar fields in v, the following vector identities must be satisfied:

$$\nabla \cdot \Phi_1 (\sigma \nabla \Phi_2) = \Phi_1 \nabla \cdot (\sigma \nabla \Phi_2) + \sigma \nabla \Phi_1 \cdot \nabla \Phi_2$$
$$\nabla \cdot \Phi_2 (\sigma \nabla \Phi_1) = \Phi_2 \nabla \cdot (\sigma \nabla \Phi_1) + \sigma \nabla \Phi_2 \cdot \nabla \Phi_1$$
$$(11.32)$$

If we subtract the second equation from the first one, integrate term by term over the volume v, and use the divergence theorem, we obtain

$$\int_S \Phi_1 (\sigma \nabla \Phi_2) \cdot d\bar{S} - \int_S \Phi_2 (\sigma \nabla \Phi_1) \cdot d\bar{S}$$
$$= \int_v \Phi_1 \nabla \cdot (\sigma \nabla \Phi_2) \, dv - \int_v \Phi_2 \nabla \cdot (\sigma \nabla \Phi_1) \, dv$$
$$(11.33)$$

Since $\nabla \Phi_1 \cdot \nabla \Phi_2 = \nabla \Phi_2 \cdot \nabla \Phi_1$, these terms cancel out in deriving Equation 11.33 from 11.32. The derivation of Equation 11.33 is well known in the physical sciences; it is one of a number of forms of *Green's theorem*.

Now we assume that Φ_1 is the scalar potential

in volume v due to sources within it specified by the equation

$$I_F = -\nabla \cdot \bar{J}^i \qquad (11.34)$$

(Thus I_F is a *flow source*, as defined earlier in Equation 8.35.) We assume further that Φ_2 is the scalar potential produced solely by current caused to cross the surface S with a current density J [A/m^2]. Usually we assume that J flows from conducting electrodes of high conductivity compared with σ, so that the direction of J is normal to the bounding surface. In this case J can be specified as a scalar corresponding to the flow into v. (The scalar potential Φ_2 is later identified as the *reciprocal electric scalar potential* due to the reciprocal current I_r fed to the lead.) Since the current J is solenoidal, it satisfies

$$\oint J \, dS = 0 \qquad (11.35)$$

The scalar fields Φ_1 and Φ_2 satisfy the following equations:

$$\nabla \cdot (\sigma \nabla \Phi_1) = -I_F \qquad (11.36)$$

since I_F is a source of Φ_1 and

$$\sigma \nabla \Phi_2 \cdot d\bar{S} = J \, dS \qquad (11.37)$$

since the field Φ_2 is established by the applied current J.

Since $-\sigma \nabla \Phi_2$ carries the direction of the current $(= \bar{J}_L)$ and $d\bar{S}$ is the outward surface normal, Equation 11.37 shows that for our chosen signs J is positive for an inflow of current. No current due to the source I_F crosses the boundary surface (since in this case it is totally insulating), and hence

$$\nabla \Phi_1 \cdot d\bar{S} = 0 \qquad (11.38)$$

For the source J at the surface, the current must be solenoidal everywhere in v; hence:

$$\nabla \cdot (\sigma \nabla \Phi_2) = 0 \qquad (11.39)$$

We may rewrite Equation 11.33 by substituting Equations 11.38 and 11.37 into its left-hand side, and Equations 11.38 and 11.36 into its right-hand side, obtaining

$$\int_S \Phi_1 J \, dS = \int_v \Phi_2 I_F \, dv \qquad (11.40)$$

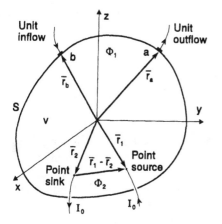

Fig. 11.22 Geometry for deriving the reciprocity theorem.

which is the desired form of the reciprocity theorem.

The Reciprocity Theorem of Helmholtz

The reciprocity theorem of Helmholtz can be derived from Equation 11.40 in the following way. Consider that Φ_2 (the *reciprocal electric scalar potential*) arises from a particular distribution J, where an inflow of a unit (reciprocal) current is concentrated at point $\bar{r}_b$ on the surface and an outflow of a unit (reciprocal) current at point $\bar{r}_a$ on the surface, where $\bar{r}_a$ and $\bar{r}_b$ are position vectors shown in Figure 11.22. Note that this is opposite to the current flow direction given in Plonsey (1963). (With this sign notation, current dipoles in the direction of the lead field current produce a positive signal in the lead, as will be seen later in Equation 11.50 (Malmivuo, 1976).)

The above can be expressed mathematically:

$$J = \delta_s (\bar{r}_b - \bar{r}) - \delta_s (\bar{r}_a - \bar{r}) \quad (11.41)$$

where δ_s is a two-dimensional unit Dirac delta function on the bounding surface, and hence the magnitude of both inflow and outflow is unity.

Consider I_F to consist of a point source of current I_0 at $\bar{r}_1$ and a point sink of equal magnitude at $\bar{r}_2$, where $\bar{r}_1$ and $\bar{r}_2$ are the position vectors shown in Figure 11.22. Now I_F can be written:

$$I_F = I_0 [\delta_v (\bar{r}_1 - \bar{r}) - \delta_v (\bar{r}_2 - \bar{r})] \quad (11.42)$$

where δ_v is a three-dimensional Dirac delta function.

Substituting Equations 11.41 and 11.42 into Equation 11.40, we obtain

$$\Phi_1 (r_a) - \Phi_1 (r_b) = I_0 [\Phi_2 (r_2) - \Phi_2 (r_1)] \quad (11.43)$$

If we choose I_0 to be unity, then this equation shows that *the voltage between two arbitrary surface points* a *and* b *due to a unit current supplied internally between points 1 and 2 equals the voltage between these same points 2 and 1 due to a unit current applied externally (reciprocally) between points* a *and* b. This is essentially the reciprocity theorem of Helmholtz.

Deriving the Equations for Lead Field

The value of $\Phi_2(r_1)$ can be specified in terms of the field at $\bar{r}_2$ by means of a Taylor series expansion:

$$\Phi_2 (\bar{r}_1) = \Phi_2 (\bar{r}_2) + \nabla\Phi_2 \cdot (\bar{r}_1 - \bar{r}_2) + \cdots \quad (11.44)$$

Note that since the field Φ_2 is established by currents introduced at the surface into a source-free region, it is well behaved internally and a Taylor series can always be generated. If we let $(\bar{r}_1 - \bar{r}_2)$ approach zero and the current I_0 approach infinity, such that their product remains constant, then a dipole moment of $I_0 (\bar{r}_1 - \bar{r}_2) = \bar{p}_0$ is created. Under these conditions the higher-order terms in Equation 11.44 can be neglected, and we obtain

$$I_0 [\Phi_2 (\bar{r}_2) - \Phi_2 (\bar{r}_1)] = \\ - I_0 \nabla\Phi_2 \cdot (\bar{r}_1 - \bar{r}_2) = -\nabla\Phi_2 \cdot \bar{p}_0 \quad (11.45)$$

Denoting the voltage between the points a and b as

$$V_{LE} = \Phi_1 (\bar{r}_a) - \Phi_1 (\bar{r}_b) \quad (11.46)$$

and substituting Equations 11.45 and 11.46 into Equation 11.43, we obtain

$$V_{LE} = -\nabla\Phi_2 \cdot \bar{p}_0 \quad (11.47)$$

Note that $-\nabla\Phi_2$ corresponds precisely to a description of the sensitivity distribution associated with this particular lead, and is in fact the lead vector (field). Since no assumption has been made concerning the volume conductor, we have found a powerful method for quantitatively evaluating lead vector fields of arbitrary leads on arbitrary shaped inhomogeneous volume conductors.

The actual bioelectric sources may be characterized as a volume distribution $\bar{J}^i$ with dimensions of current dipole moment per unit volume. Equation 11.47 may be generalized to the case of such a volume distribution of current dipoles with a dipole moment density of $\bar{J}^i$ to obtain

$$V_{LE} = - \int_v \nabla\Phi_2 \cdot \bar{J}^i \, dv \qquad (11.48)$$

The quantity Φ_2 was earlier defined as the reciprocal electric potential field in the volume conductor due to unit reciprocal current flow in the pickup leads a and b and is designated in the following as Φ_{LE}. Plonsey (1963) has termed this potential field as the lead field in his field-theoretic proof of the reciprocity theorem. In this text, however, the term ''lead field'' denotes the *current density field* due to reciprocal application of current in the lead. They are related, of course, by $\bar{J}_{LE} = -\sigma\nabla\Phi_{LE}$).

Using the vector identity $\nabla \cdot (\Phi_{LE}\bar{J}^i) = \nabla\Phi_{LE} \cdot \bar{J}^i + \Phi_{LE}\nabla \cdot \bar{J}^i$ and the divergence theorem, we obtain from Equation 11.48

$$V_{LE} = - \int_S \Phi_L \bar{J}^i \cdot d\bar{S} + \int_v \Phi_{LE}\nabla \cdot \bar{J}^i \, dv \qquad (11.49)$$

Because the impressed current sources are totally contained within S, the integrand is zero everywhere on S, and the first term on the right-hand side of Equation 11.49 is zero; thus we obtain

$$V_{LE} = \int_v \Phi_{LE} \nabla \cdot \bar{J}^i \, dv \qquad (11.50)$$

The quantity $-\nabla \cdot \bar{J}^i$ is the strength of the impressed current source and is called the *flow* (or *flux*) *source* I_F as defined in Equation 8.35. Thus Equation 11.50 can be expressed as

$$V_{LE} = - \int_v \Phi_{LE}I_F dv \qquad (11.51)$$

McFee and Johnston (1953) designated the vector field $\bar{J}_{LE} = -\sigma\nabla\Phi = \sigma\bar{E}_{LE}$ the lead field.

Here the symbol E_{LE} denotes the reciprocal electric field due to unit reciprocal current, and σ the conductivity of the volume conductor. Using this formulation, we may rewrite Equation 11.48 as:

$$V_{LE} = \int_v \frac{1}{\sigma} \bar{J}_{LE} \cdot \bar{J}^i \, dv \qquad (11.52)$$

where $\bar{J}_{LE}$ is the lead field arising from unit reciprocal current (the reader should review the definition of J in Equation 11.41). But Equation 11.52 corresponds precisely to Equation 11.30 (assuming $I_r = 1$ [A]). Consequently, Equation 11.52 confirms Equation 11.30, which is the equation characterizing lead field theory, introduced earlier.

11.6.6 Summary of the Lead Field Theory Equations

In this section we summarize the equations of the lead field theory for electric leads. (Equations for magnetic leads are given in the next chapter.) We consider the situation in Figure 11.23, where two disklike electrodes in a volume conductor form the bipolar electric lead.

To determine the lead field, a *unit* reciprocal current I_r is fed to the lead. It generates a reciprocal electric potential field Φ_{LE} in the volume conductor (this potential field was defined as Φ_2 in Section 11.6.5 in the proof of the reciprocity theorem). If the electrodes are parallel and their lateral dimensions are large compared to their separation, Φ_{LE} is uniform in the central region. The negative gradient of this electric potential field Φ_{LE} is the *reciprocal electric field*, $\bar{E}_{LE}$:

$$\bar{E}_{LE} = -\nabla\Phi_{LE} \qquad (11.53)$$

The reciprocal electric field is related to the *reciprocal current field* by the conductivity of the medium:

$$\bar{J}_{LE} = \sigma\bar{E}_{LE} \qquad (11.54)$$

This reciprocal current field $\bar{J}_{LE}$ is defined as the *lead field*.

Now, when we know the lead field $\bar{J}_{LE}$, we can remove the reciprocal current generator (of unit current) from the lead. The electric signal V_{LE} in the lead due to current sources $\bar{J}^i$ in the volume conductor is obtained from the equation

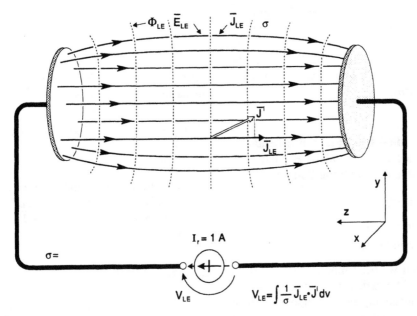

Fig. 11.23 Basic form of a bipolar electric lead, where: I_r = unit reciprocal current; Φ_{LE} = reciprocal electric scalar potential field; $\bar{E}_{LE}$ = reciprocal electric field; $\bar{J}_{LE}$ = lead field; V_{LE} = voltage in the lead due to the volume source $\bar{J}^i$ in the volume conductor; and σ = conductivity of the medium.

$$V_{LE} = \int \frac{1}{\sigma} \bar{J}_{LE} \cdot \bar{J}^i \, dv \qquad (11.30)$$

If the volume conductor is homogeneous, the conductivity σ may be taken in front of the integral operation, and we obtain

$$V_{LE} = \frac{1}{\sigma} \int \bar{J}_{LE} \cdot \bar{J}^i \, dv \qquad (11.31)$$

Section 11.6.1 introduced the concept of *isosensitivity surface* and its special case *half-sensitivity surface* which bounds a *half-sensitivity volume*. The isosensitivity surfaces, including the half-sensitivity surface, are surfaces where the lead field current density $\bar{J}_{LE}$ is constant. In a homogeneous region of a volume conductor, where σ is constant, the isosensitivity surfaces are, of course, surfaces where the reciprocal electric field $\bar{E}_{LE}$ is constant. In certain cases the isosensitivity surfaces coincide with the isopotential surfaces. These cases include those where all isopotential surfaces are parallel planes, concentric cylinders, or concentric spheres. Then the surfaces where the electric field is constant (i.e., where two adjoining isopotential surfaces are separated by a constant distance) have the same form as well. But in

a general case, where the isopotential surfaces are irregular so that two adjacent surfaces are not a constant distance apart, the surfaces of constant electric field do not have the same form.

As summarized in Figure 11.23, as a consequence of the reciprocal energization of an electric lead, the following three fields are created in the volume conductor: electric potential field Φ_{LE} (illustrated with isopotential surfaces); electric field $\bar{E}_{LE}$ (illustrated with field lines); and current field $\bar{J}_{LE}$ (illustrated with current flow lines and called the lead field). In addition to these three fields we defined a fourth field of surfaces (or lines): the field of isosensitivity surfaces. When the conductivity is isotropic, the electric field lines coincide with the current flow lines. In a symmetric case where all isopotential surfaces are parallel planes, concentric cylinders, or concentric spheres, the isopotential surfaces and the isosensitivity surfaces coincide.

In an ideal lead field for detecting the equivalent dipole moment of a volume source (see the following section) the isopotential surfaces are parallel planes. To achieve this situation, the volume conductor must also be homogeneous. Thus, in such a case from the aforementioned four fields, the electric field lines coincide with the lead field flow lines and the isopotential surfaces coincide with the isosensitivity surfaces.

11.6.7 Ideal Lead Field of a Lead Detecting the Equivalent Electric Dipole of a Volume Source

PRECONDITIONS:

Source: *Volume source*

Conductor: *Infinite, homogeneous*

In this section we determine the desired form of the lead field of a detector that measures the equivalent (resultant) electric dipole moment of a distributed volume source located in an infinite, homogeneous volume conductor.

As discussed in Section 7.3.2, a dipole in a fixed location has three independent variables, the magnitudes of the x-, y-, and z-components. These can be measured with either unipolar or bipolar electrodes located at the coordinate axes. The vectorial sum of these measurements is the dipole moment of the dipole.

Because a volume source is formed from a distribution of dipole elements, it follows from the principle of superposition that the dipole moment of a volume source equals the sum of the dipole moments of its dipole elements. This can be determined by measuring the x-, y-, and z-components of all the elementary dipoles and their sums are the x-, y-, and z-components of the equivalent dipole moment of the volume source, respectively. In introducing these important equations, we also show this fact mathematically.

The equivalent electric dipole moment of a volume source may be evaluated from its flow source description. It was shown in Equation 8.35 (Section 8.5) that the flow source density I_F is defined by the impressed current density (Plonsey, 1971) as

$$I_F = -\nabla \cdot \bar{J}^i \qquad (8.35)$$

The resultant (electric) dipole moment of such a source can be shown to be

$$\bar{p} = \int_v \bar{r} I_F dv \qquad (11.55)$$

This dipole moment has three components. Because $\bar{r} = x\bar{i} + y\bar{j} + z\bar{k}$, these three components may be written as:

$$\bar{p} = \int_v x\bar{i} I_F dv + \int_v y\bar{j} I_F dv + \int_v z\bar{k} I_F dv \qquad (11.56)$$

We consider the x-component of the dipole moment. Noting Equation 8.35 and using the vector identity $\nabla \cdot (x\bar{J}^i) = x\nabla \cdot \bar{J}^i + \bar{J}^i \cdot \nabla x$, we obtain

$$p_x = \int_v x I_F dv = -\int_v x\nabla \cdot \bar{J}^i dv$$
$$= -\int_v \nabla \cdot (x\bar{J}^i)dv + \int_v \bar{J}^i \cdot \nabla x \, dv \qquad (11.57)$$

Using the divergence theorem, we may rewrite the first term on the right-hand side of Equation 11.57 as

$$-\int_V \nabla \cdot (x\bar{J}^i)dv = -\int_S x\bar{J}^i \cdot d\bar{S} = 0 \qquad (11.58)$$

Since there can be no impressed current density on the surface, this term vanishes. Therefore, and because $\nabla x = \bar{i}(\partial x/\partial x) + \bar{j}(\partial x/\partial y) + \bar{k}(\partial x/\partial z) = \bar{J}^i$, we obtain for the x-component of the dipole moment

$$p_x = \int_v \bar{J}^i \cdot \nabla x \, dv = \int_v \bar{J}^i \cdot \bar{i} dv = \int_v J_x^i dv \qquad (11.59)$$

In fact, recalling the dual identity of $\bar{J}^i$ as a dipole moment per unit volume, we can write Equation 11.59 directly.

Equation 11.59 can be described as follows: *one component of the equivalent electric dipole (moment) of a volume source may be evaluated from the sum of corresponding components of the distributed dipole elements of the volume source independent of their location.* A comparison of Equation 11.59 with Equation 11.49 identifies Φ_L with $-x$. Consequently, we see

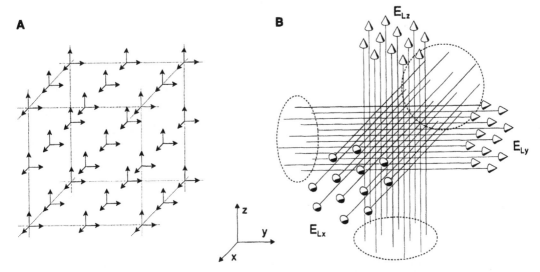

Fig. 11.24 Ideal lead field (sensitivity distribution) for detecting the electric dipole moment of a volume source. Each component is uniform in one direction throughout the source region, and the components are mutually orthogonal. (A) Lead field current density vector presentation. (B) Lead field current flow line presentation. This is the *physiological meaning* of the measurement of the electric dipole. (See the text for details.)

that this summation is, in fact, accomplished with a lead system with the following properties (see Fig. 11.24):

1. The lead field current density is given by $\bar{J}_L = \nabla x = \bar{i}$ (so that it is everywhere in the x direction only).
2. The lead field current density is uniform throughout the source area.
3. Three such identical, mutually perpendicular lead fields form the three orthogonal components of a complete lead system.

Physiological Meaning of Electric Dipole

The sensitivity distribution (i.e., the lead field), illustrated in Figure 11.24, is the *physiological meaning* of the measurement of the (equivalent) electric dipole of a volume source.

The concept "physiological meaning" can be explained as follows: When considering the forward problem, the lead field illustrates what is the contribution (effect) of each active cell on the signals of the lead system. When one is considering the inverse problem, the lead field illustrates similarly the most probable distribution and orientation of active cells when a signal is detected in a lead.

11.6.8 Application of Lead Field Theory to the Einthoven Limb Leads

PRECONDITIONS:

Source: *Volume source*

Conductor: *Infinite, homogeneous*

To build a bridge between lead field and lead vector and to clarify the result of Equation 11.59 illustrated in Figure 11.24, we apply lead field theory to the Einthoven limb leads.

Previously, in Section 11.4.3, the Einthoven triangle was discussed as an application of the lead vector concept. The volume source of the heart was modeled with a (two-dimensional) dipole in the frontal plane. It was shown that the signal in each limb lead V_I, V_{II}, and V_{III} is proportional to the projections of the equivalent dipole on the corresponding lead vectors.

Instead of modeling the volume source of the heart with the resultant of its dipole elements, we could have determined the contribution of each dipole element to the limb leads and

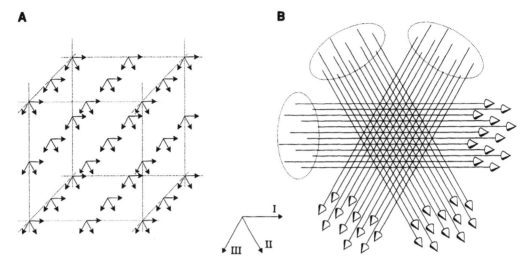

Fig. 11.25   The ideal lead field (sensitivity distribution) of Einthoven limb leads V_I, V_{II}, and V_{III}. This is the physiological meaning of the measurement of the limb leads.

summed up these contributions. In this procedure one can use the lead field theory to illustrate the lead fields—that is, the sensitivities of the limb leads. The idealized lead fields of the limb leads are uniform in the directions of the edges of the Einthoven triangle. Figure 11.25 illustrates the sensitivity distribution of the (ideal) Einthoven limb leads within the area of the heart.

This is the *physiological meaning* of the measurement of the Einthoven limb leads (see the previous section).

11.6.9   Synthesization of the Ideal Lead Field for the Detection of the Electric Dipole Moment of a Volume Source

Synthesization of the Ideal Lead Fields in Infinite, Homogeneous Volume Conductors

PRECONDITIONS:

Source: *Volume source*

Conductor: *Infinite, homogeneous*

We begin the discussion on the synthesis of ideal lead fields for detecting the equivalent dipole moment of a volume source by discussing the properties of unipolar and bipolar leads in *infinite, homogeneous* volume conductors.

If the dimensions of a distributed volume source are small in relation to the distance to the point of observation, we can consider it to be a lumped (discrete) dipole. The detection of such an electric dipole can be accomplished through unipolar measurements on each coordinate axis, as illustrated on the left-hand side of Figure 11.26A. If the dimensions of the distributed volume source are large in relation to the measurement distance, the lead field of a unipolar measurement is not directed in the desired direction in different areas of the volume source and the magnitude of the sensitivity is larger in the areas closer to the electrode than farther away. This is illustrated on the right-hand side of Figure 11.26A.

The quality of the lead field both in its direction and its magnitude is considerably improved when using a bipolar lead, where the electrodes are located symmetrically on both sides of the volume source, as illustrated in Figure 11.26B. (Note also that in the bipolar measurement the difference in potential between the electrodes is twice the unipolar potential relative to the center.)

The quality of the lead field of a bipolar lead in measuring volume sources with large dimensions is further increased by using large electrodes, whose dimensions are comparable to the source dimensions. This is illustrated in Figure 11.26C.

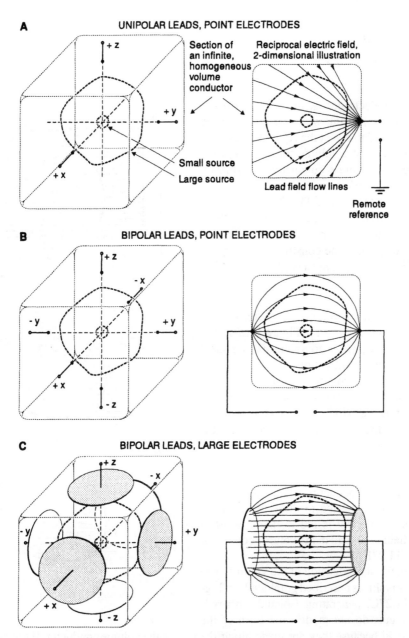

Fig. 11.26 Properties of unipolar and bipolar leads in detecting the equivalent electric dipole moment of a volume source. (A) If the dimensions of the volume source are small compared to the measurement distance the simplest method is to use point electrodes and unipolar leads on the coordinate axes. (B) For volume sources with large dimensions the quality of the lead field is considerably improved with the application of bipolar leads. (C) Increasing the size of the electrodes further improves the quality of the leads.

Synthesization of Ideal Lead Fields in Finite, Homogeneous Volume Conductors

PRECONDITIONS:

Source: *Volume source*

Conductor: *Finite, homogeneous*

Using large electrodes is, in practice, impossible. In the following we describe a method to design a lead to detect the equivalent electric dipole moment of a volume source in a *finite, homogeneous* volume conductor of arbitrary shape (Brody, 1957).

According to Section 11.6.7, such a lead, when energized reciprocally, produces three orthogonal, uniform, and homogeneous lead fields. We consider the construction of one of them. This may be done according to the following steps:

1. Suppose that the volume conductor has the arbitrary shape shown in Figure 11.27A and that our purpose is to synthesize an ideal lead field in the *y* direction within this region.
2. We extend the volume conductor in the direction of the *y*-axis in both directions so that it forms a cylinder limited by two planes in the *zx* direction and having the cross section of the original volume conductor (Fig. 11.27B).
3. Then we plate the end planes of the cylinder with a well-conducting material. If electrodes are connected to these plates and a reciprocal current is fed to them, an ideal lead field is created in the volume conductor (Fig. 11.27B).
4. Thereafter the extension of the volume conductor is slit, as described graphically in Figure 11.27C, generating isolated "fibers." These cuts do not modify the form of the lead field because they are made along the flow lines which are nowhere intersected, as is clear in Figure 11.27C.
5. Each of the volume conductor "fibers" may now be replaced with discrete resistances of equal resistive value, as illustrated in Figure 11.27D.

The above procedure is repeated in the direction of the *z*- and *x*-axes. Corresponding to each discrete resistor, an electrode must be placed

A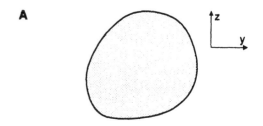

B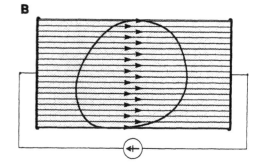

C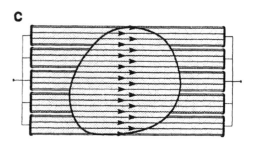

D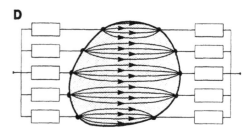

Fig. 11.27   Synthesizing an ideal lead field within a finite, homogeneous volume conductor.

on the volume conductor. If the number of electrodes is sufficiently large, the ideal lead field (requiring an infinite number of electrodes) will be well approximated. Since one wishes to keep the number of electrodes to a minimum, one must explore the acceptability of reduced numbers of electrodes, make the spacing of electrodes unequal to strengthen accuracy only in the heart region, and use the same electrode for more than a single component lead.

Note once again, that this method may be

applied to a *finite homogeneous volume conductor having an arbitrary shape*. In general, the effect of internal inhomogeneities cannot be corrected with electrodes located on the surface of the conductor with the method described above.

11.6.10 Special Properties of Electric Lead Fields

Two special properties of the lead fields are summarized as follows:

1. If the volume conductor is cut or an inhomogeneity boundary is inserted along a lead field current flow line, the form of the lead field does not change. Only the intensity of the field changes in relation to the conductivity.
2. The reciprocity theorem may be applied to the reciprocal situation. This means that it is possible in electrolytic tank models to feed a ''reciprocally reciprocal'' current to the dipole in the conductor and to measure the signal from the lead and interpret the result as having been obtained by feeding the reciprocal current to the lead and measuring the signal from the dipole.

The latter is easily proved by imagining that the lead field is a result of the mapping of the behavior of the lead vector as a function of the source location, as discussed in Section 11.6.2. This mapping is done by feeding unit currents in each coordinate direction at each point of the source area and by measuring the corresponding voltages at the lead, as explained in Section 11.4.1.

The benefit of this ''reciprocally reciprocal'' arrangement is that for technical reasons, the signal-to-noise ratio of the measurement may be improved while still having the advantage of the interpretations associated with the lead field current distribution.

The special properties of electric lead fields are discussed in more detail in connection with magnetic lead fields.

11.6.11 Relationship Between the Image Surface and the Lead Field

In this section, the relationship between the image surface and the lead field is described with the aid of Table 11.3 and Figure 11.28.

The *source* in the concept of the image sur-

Table 11.3 Relationship between the image surface and the lead field

	Image surface	Lead field
Preconditions		
Source	Dipole $\bar{p}$ in a fixed location	Volume source (dipole elements $\bar{J}^i$ distributed in a volume)
Conductor	Infinite or finite	Infinite or finite
Theory		
Basic principle	Measurement points P vary source point Q fixed, see Figure 11.28A	Measurement points P fixed source point Q varies, see Figure 11.28B
Procedure	Lead vectors are mapped as a function of the *measurement* point; their end points form the image surface	Lead vectors are mapped as a function of the *source* point; these lead vectors form the lead field
Geometric presentation	See Figure 11.28C	See Figure 11.28D and Figure 11.28E
Application of the theory	A lead, with a desired sensitivity in a certain direction, may be found from a lead vector in image space in that direction $$V_L = \bar{c} \cdot \bar{p}$$	The contribution of the source to the lead is evaluated from the equation $$V_{LE} = \int \frac{1}{\sigma} \bar{J}_{LE} \cdot \bar{J}^i dv$$

Note: (1) There is similarity between the variables: $\bar{c} \leftrightarrow \bar{J}_{LE}$ and $\bar{p} \leftrightarrow \bar{J}^i$.

(2) It follows from the reciprocity theorem that $\bar{J}_{LE}$ is the same as the current density field in the volume conductor due to feeding the reciprocal current I_r of 1 A to the lead.

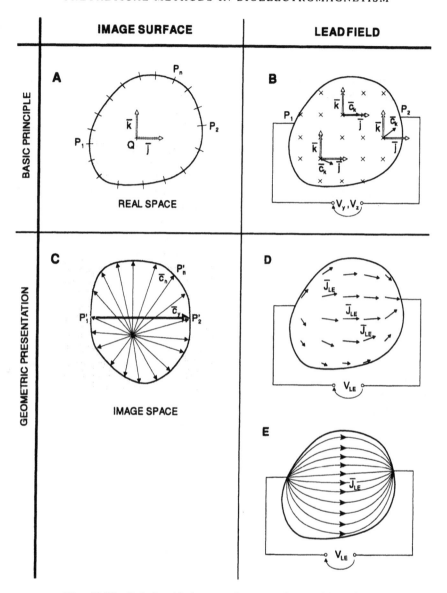

Fig. 11.28   Relationship between image surface and lead field.

face is a dipole. This can be a discrete dipole (at a point), or it can be a dipole element of a distributed volume source. In the lead field concept, the source may be a distributed volume source or a discrete dipole. The *conductor* in both cases was previously considered to be finite (and inhomogeneous). However, the theory holds for infinite volume conductors as well.

Source location in the image surface was fixed and the measurement points were variable and forming a continuum. In characterizing the

lead field, we note that the situation is the opposite: The measurement points are fixed while the source point varies (continuously). This means that in the image surface the lead vectors are mapped as a function of the measurement point, but in the lead field the mapping is a function of the source point. The image surface takes into account field points lying on a surface, whereas in the lead field the source point may lie within a three-dimensional volume.

Geometrically, in the image surface concept,

the ends of the lead vectors form the image surface. In the lead field concept, the field of lead vectors establish the lead field.

The equations for the application of the lead vector and image surface (Equation 11.16) and the lead field (Equations 11.30 and 11.31) are, in principle, of the same form. The main difference is that the equation for the lead field is in integral form. This comes from the fact that it is applied to a volume source.

An important consequence of the reciprocity theorem of Helmholtz is that the lead field is identical to the current field resulting from feeding the (unit) reciprocal current to the lead.

11.7 GABOR-NELSON THEOREM

PRECONDITIONS:

Source: *Moving (equivalent) dipole moment of a volume source (position, direction, and magnitude)*

Conductor: *Finite, homogeneous*

11.7.1 Determination of the Dipole Moment

In 1954, Dennis Gabor and Clifford V. Nelson presented a mathematical method that can be used in solving for the equivalent dipole of a volume source in a homogeneous volume conductor (Gabor and Nelson, 1954). The method, which also gives the location of the dipole, is based on potential measurements at the surface of the volume conductor and on the knowledge of the volume conductor's geometry. The details are provided in this section.

As described in Section 8.5 (Equation 8.35), the flow (flux) source density I_F of a distribution of impressed current density $\bar{J}^i$ is

$$I_F = -\nabla \cdot \bar{J}^i \tag{8.35}$$

and the resulting (electric) dipole moment of such a system is evaluated from the definition (Equation 11.55)

$$\bar{p} = \int_v \bar{r} I_F \, dv \tag{11.60}$$

where

$\bar{r}$ = the radius vector
dv = the volume element

The dipole moment has three components, as was illustrated by Equation 11.56. We now examine the x-component of this dipole moment. We develop it in the following way: The explanation for each step is given on the right-hand side of the column.

$$p_x = \int x I_F \, dv$$

from Equation 11.57

$$= -\int x\nabla \cdot \bar{J}^i \, dv$$

because $-I_F = \nabla \cdot \bar{J}^i$ (Equation 8.35)

$$= -\sigma \int x\nabla \cdot \nabla\Phi \, dv$$

from Equation 7.3 we have $\nabla \cdot \bar{J}^i = \nabla \cdot \sigma\nabla\Phi$; for a uniform conducting medium this reduces to $\nabla \cdot \bar{J}^i = \sigma\nabla \cdot \nabla\Phi$

$$= \sigma \int \nabla x \cdot \nabla\Phi \, dv$$

$\nabla \cdot (x\nabla\Phi) = x\nabla \cdot \nabla\Phi + \nabla x \cdot \nabla\Phi$ is a vector identity. Integrating each term through the entire volume, and applying Gauss's theorem to the first integral, we get

$$\oint x\nabla\Phi \cdot d\bar{S} =$$
$$\int x\nabla \cdot \nabla\Phi \, dv +$$
$$\int \nabla x \cdot \nabla\Phi \, dv$$

Since the boundary is insulated, $\nabla\Phi \cdot d\bar{S} = 0$. Thus

$$-\int x\nabla \cdot \nabla\Phi \, dv = \int \nabla x \cdot \nabla\Phi dv$$

$$= \sigma \int \frac{\partial\Phi}{\partial x} \, dv$$

$\nabla x \cdot \nabla\Phi = \bar{i} \cdot \left(\bar{i}\frac{\partial\Phi}{\partial x} + \bar{j}\frac{\partial\Phi}{\partial y} + \bar{k}\frac{\partial\Phi}{\partial z}\right) = \frac{\partial\Phi}{\partial x}$

$$= \sigma \int \Phi \, dy \, dz$$

because the volume integral may be transformed to a surface integral by integrating with respect to x

$$= \sigma \int \Phi \, dS_x \quad (11.61)$$

because the surface integral may be written in a more convenient form by using a vectorial surface element $d\overline{S}_x$ whose absolute value is $dS = dy \, dz$, and which is directed outward and normal to the surface defined by $dy \, dz$.

Summing Equation 11.61 and similar expressions for p_y and p_z and replacing the poten-

tial Φ with voltage V, we finally obtain the vector equation

$$\overline{p} = \sigma \int_S V \, d\overline{S} \quad (11.62)$$

which expresses the resultant dipole moment of a volume source in an arbitrary volume conductor.

We now explain in detail the meaning of Equation 11.62, as illustrated in Figure 11.29.

Figure 11.29A illustrates the homogeneous volume conductor including the volume source. In the illustration the Gabor-Nelson theorem is discussed in two dimensions. The equivalent dipole moment of the volume source is $\overline{p}$. The vectorial surface element $d\overline{S}$ is a vector attached to the surface element. It is directed outward and normal to the surface element, and its absolute value equals the area of the surface element. For clarity the volume conductor is

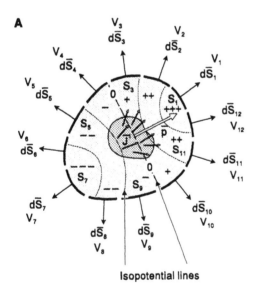
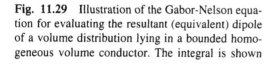
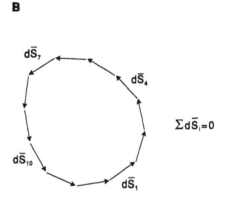
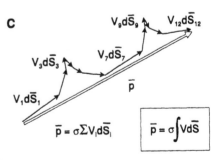

Fig. 11.29 Illustration of the Gabor-Nelson equation for evaluating the resultant (equivalent) dipole of a volume distribution lying in a bounded homogeneous volume conductor. The integral is shown approximated by discretizing the surface into 12 elements. The calculation of the integral is explained in detail in the text.

divided into 12 surface elements, S_1 through S_{12}. (When applying Equation 11.62, of course, one assumes that the number of surface elements is infinite.) A vector $d\bar{S}_1$ through $d\bar{S}_{12}$ is attached to each surface element. The volume source produces a potential, Φ_1 through Φ_{12}, at each surface element.

It is obvious that because the surface is closed, the sum of the vectorial surface elements is equal to zero; that is, $\Sigma d\bar{S}_i = 0$ (Fig. 11.29B).

If we multiply each vectorial surface element $d\bar{S}_i$ by the corresponding potential Φ_i (or actually with the voltage V_i measured at each surface element in relation to an indifferent reference), the sum of these products, $\Sigma V_i\, d\bar{S}_i$, is no longer zero. It is clear that when one is considering the surface potential due to the dipole $\bar{p}$ along the surface elements of increasing index, one finds that it is at its maximum at the surface elements S_1 and S_2. Then it decreases and reaches the value zero somewhere between the surface elements S_4 and S_5. Thereafter the surface potential turns to negative polarity and reaches its maximum at the surface element S_7. Thereafter the (negative) surface potential decreases to zero and increases again to the positive maximum in the area of S_1. Therefore, the sum $\Sigma V_i d\bar{S}_i$ is not zero; and according to Equation 11.62, if the number of the surface elements is infinite, one obtains $\bar{p}$. For clarity, the length of $\bar{p}$ is shown longer in Figure 11.29C than in Figure 11.29A.

11.7.2 The Location of the Equivalent Dipole

Next we describe the procedure for finding the position of the resultant dipole. If we actually had an equal point source and sink, $+I$ and $-I$, located at points

$$X + \frac{1}{2}\Delta x; \quad X - \frac{1}{2}\Delta x$$

the second moment of the source distribution is in the x direction and given by

$$-\int x^2 \nabla \cdot \bar{J}^i \, dv = I\left[(X + \frac{1}{2}\Delta x)^2 \right.$$
$$\left. - (X - \frac{1}{2}\Delta x)^2\right] = 2X(I\Delta x) \quad (11.63)$$

where upper-case X denotes the x-coordinate of the dipole location and lower-case x is the variable in this coordinate.

In the limit $\Delta x \to 0$ and $I\Delta x \to p_x$ we obtain

$$Xp_x = -\frac{1}{2}\int x^2 \nabla \cdot \bar{J}^i \, dv \quad (11.64)$$

We now transform this second moment integral, following the same steps as with the first moment, namely

$$\begin{aligned} Xp_x &= -\frac{1}{2}\int x^2 \nabla \cdot \bar{J}^i \, dv \\ &= -\frac{\sigma}{2}\int x^2 \nabla \cdot \nabla\Phi \, dv \\ &= \frac{\sigma}{2}\int \nabla(x^2) \cdot \nabla\Phi \, dv \\ &= \sigma \int x \frac{\partial\Phi}{\partial x} \, dv \end{aligned} \quad (11.65)$$

Integrating by parts with respect to x and again replacing the potential Φ with the measured voltage V gives

$$Xp_x = \sigma \int xV \, dS_x - \sigma \int V \, dv \quad (11.66)$$

In a similar way, we obtain equations for Yp_y and Zp_z. It is obvious that we cannot determine any of these by surface measurements alone because the second term in each expression requires a volume integral of the potential V. However, in the same way as one obtains Equation 11.66, one can show that

$$Xp_y + Yp_x = \int xyI_F dv = -\int xy\nabla \cdot \bar{J}^i \, dv \quad (11.67)$$

Two similar equations arise by cyclic permutation of the coordinates. We can also derive three new equations of the type

$$Xp_y + Yp_x = \sigma \int V(x \, dS_y + y \, dS_x) \quad (11.68)$$

in the same manner as Equations 11.61 and 11.66 were derived. We can now eliminate the unknown volume integral of V from the equations of the type 11.66, and, together with the three equations of the type 11.68, we are left with the five equations for the three quantities X, Y, and Z. Any three of these five equations can be used for finding the location of the dipole, and the other two for checking how well the assumption of one dipole accounts for the observation. One can also use the method of least squares to obtain the best fit.

11.8 SUMMARY OF THE THEORETICAL METHODS FOR ANALYZING VOLUME SOURCES AND VOLUME CONDUCTORS

We have discussed six different theoretical methods for analyzing volume sources and volume conductors. Two of them are used for solving the forward problem, and the other four for solving the inverse problem. These methods are:

1. For the forward problem:

   Solid angle theorem

   Miller-Geselowitz model

2. For the inverse problem:

   Lead vector

   Image surface

   Lead field

   Gabor-Nelson theorem

In various cases we had the following sources:

Double layer

Distributed dipole

Dipole (in a fixed location)

Moving dipole

Dipole moment of a volume source

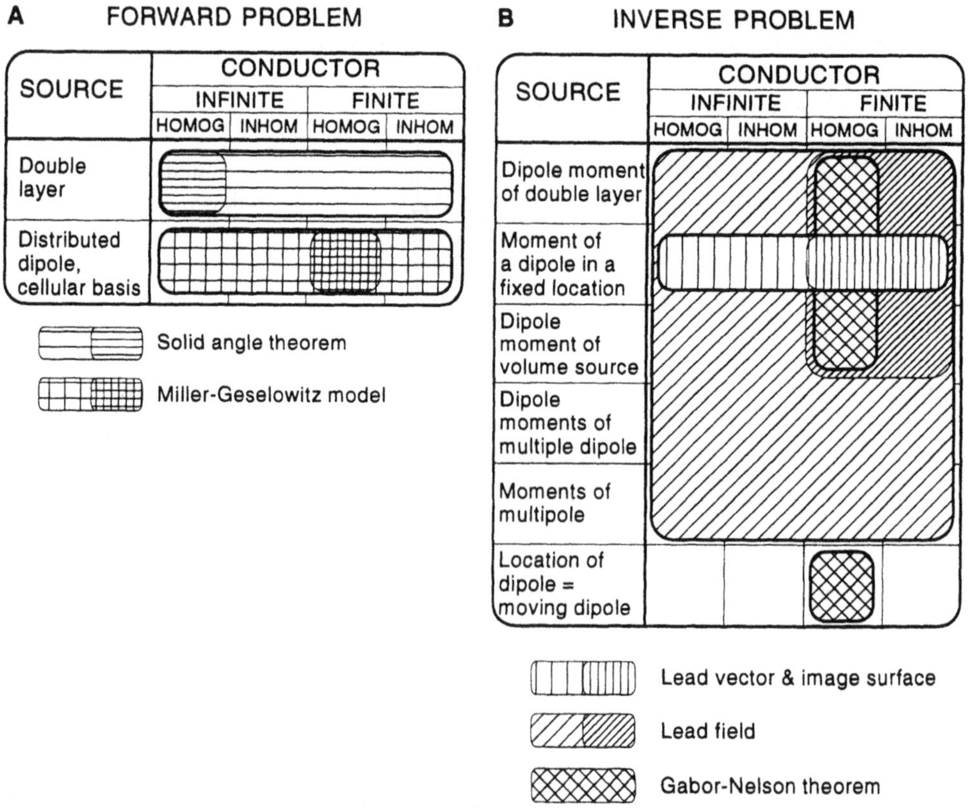

A   FORWARD PROBLEM

SOURCE	CONDUCTOR			
	INFINITE		FINITE	
	HOMOG	INHOM	HOMOG	INHOM
Double layer				
Distributed dipole, cellular basis				

Solid angle theorem

Miller-Geselowitz model

B   INVERSE PROBLEM

SOURCE	CONDUCTOR			
	INFINITE		FINITE	
	HOMOG	INHOM	HOMOG	INHOM
Dipole moment of double layer				
Moment of a dipole in a fixed location				
Dipole moment of volume source				
Dipole moments of multiple dipole				
Moments of multipole				
Location of dipole = moving dipole				

Lead vector & image surface

Lead field

Gabor-Nelson theorem

Fig. 11.30 (A) The source-conductor combinations where the solid angle theorem and Miller-Geselowitz model may be applied in solving the forward problem. (B) The source-conductor combinations where the lead vector, image surface, and lead field methods as well as Gabor-Nelson theorem may be applied in solving the inverse problem.

Multiple dipole

Multipole

These sources have been located in volume conductors that were:

Infinite, homogeneous

(Infinite, inhomogeneous, not discussed)

Finite, homogeneous

Finite, inhomogeneous

The application of each method is limited to certain source-conductor combinations, as expressed in the sets of preconditions in connection with the discussion of each method. We summarize these preconditions in Figure 11.30. The former one of these shows the application areas for the two methods used in solving the forward problem, and the latter one for those used in solving the inverse problem.

Figure 11.30A is quite obvious. The preconditions of the two methods are shown by locating the methods in the corresponding location in the source-conductor plane. The application area of the solid angle theorem is shown to be both the infinite homogeneous volume conductor, as derived first by Helmholtz, and the finite homogeneous and inhomogeneous conductors, where it can be extended with the concept of secondary sources.

Figure 11.30B needs some clarification, and certainly some details of this figure could perhaps be presented also in some other way.

The source for the lead vector and image surface methods is dipole. In Sections 11.4 and 11.5, these methods were discussed, for simplicity, in connection with finite conductors. There is, however, no theoretical reason, that would restrict their application only to finite conductors, but they are applicable to infinite conductors as well. Therefore, their application area is shown for both finite and infinite conductors, but more light shaded in infinite conductors.

The same holds also for the lead field theory. Section 11.6.4 did not discuss the application of the lead field theory for a multiple dipole or multipole source. The lead field theory may, however, be applied also in connection with

these sources. Therefore, they are included into the application area but with lighter shading.

The application area of the Gabor-Nelson theorem is clear. It can be applied for solving the dipole moment of a single dipole or a volume source in a finite homogeneous volume conductor. It also gives the location of this dipole moment.

REFERENCES

Brody DA (1957): A method for applying approximately ideal lead connections to homogeneous volume conductors of irregular shape. *Am. Heart J.* 53:(2) 174–82.

Burger HC (1967): *Heart and Vector,* (Series ed, HW Julius Jr.: Philips Technical Library.) 143 pp. Gordon & Breach Science Publishers, New York.

Burger HC, van Milaan JB (1946): Heart vector and leads—I. *Br. Heart J.* 8:(3) 157–61.

Burger HC, van Milaan JB (1947): Heart vector and leads—II. *Br. Heart J.* 9: 154–60.

Burger HC, van Milaan JB (1948): Heart vector and leads—III. *Br. Heart J.* 10: 233.

Einthoven W (1908): Weiteres über das Elektrokardiogram. *Pflüger Arch. ges. Physiol.* 122: 517–48.

Frank E (1954): The image surface of a homogeneous torso. *Am. Heart J.* 47: 757–68.

Gabor D, Nelson CV (1954): Determination of the resultant dipole of the heart from measurements on the body surface. *J. Appl. Phys.* 25:(4) 413–6.

Gulrajani RM, Mailloux GE (1983): A simulation study of the effects of torso inhomogeneities on electrocardiographic potentials using realistic heart and torso models. *Circ. Res.* 52: 45–56.

Helmholtz HLF (1853): Ueber einige Gesetze der Vertheilung elektrischer Ströme in körperlichen Leitern mit Anwendung auf die thierisch-elektrischen Versuche. *Ann. Physik und Chemie* 89: 211–33, 354–77.

Horáček BM (1971): The effect on electrocardiographic lead vectors of conductivity inhomogeneities in the human torso. *Dalhousie University, Halifax, Nova Scotia,* pp. 182. (Ph.D. thesis)

Hyttinen JA, Eskola HJ, Sievänen H, Malmivuo JA (1988): Atlas of the sensitivity distribution of the common ECG-lead systems. *Tampere Univ. Techn., Inst. Biomed. Eng., Reports* 2:(2) 25+67.

Malmivuo JA (1976): On the detection of the magnetic heart vector—An application of the reciprocity theorem. *Helsinki Univ. Tech.,* Acta Polytechn. Scand., El. Eng. Series. Vol. 39., pp. 112. (Dr. tech. thesis)

McFee R, Johnston FD (1953): Electrocardiographic leads I. Introduction. *Circulation* 8:(10) 554–68.

McFee R, Johnston FD (1954a): Electrocardiographic leads II. Analysis. *Circulation* 9:(2) 255–66.

McFee R, Johnston FD (1954b): Electrocardiographic leads III. Synthesis. *Circulation* 9:(6) 868–80.

Miller WT, Geselowitz DB (1978): Simulation studies of the electrocardiogram, I. The normal heart. *Circ. Res.* 43:(2) 301–15.

Plonsey R (1963): Reciprocity applied to volume conductors and the EEG. *IEEE Trans. Biomed. Electron.* BME-10:(1) 9–12.

Plonsey R (1971): The biophysical basis for electrocardiology. *CRC Crit. Rev. Bioeng.* 1: 1–48.

Stratton JA (1941): *Electromagnetic Theory,* McGraw-Hill, New York.

Waller AD (1889): On the electromotive changes connected with the beat of the mammalian heart, and on the human heart in particular. *Phil. Trans. R. Soc. (Lond.)* 180: 169–94.

Wikswo JP, Malmivuo JA, Barry WM, Leifer M, Fairbank WM (1979): The theory and application of magnetocardiography. In *Advances in Cardiovascular Physics,* Vol. 2, ed. DN Ghista, pp. 1–67, S. Karger, Basel.

Wilson FN, Macleod AG, Barker PS (1931): Potential variations produced by the heart beat at the apices of Einthoven's triangle. *Am. Heart J.* 7: 207–11.

12

Theory of Biomagnetic Measurements

12.1 BIOMAGNETIC FIELD

PRECONDITIONS:

Source: *Distribution of impressed current source elements $\bar{J}^i$ (volume source)*

Conductor: *Finite, inhomogeneous*

The current density $\bar{J}$ throughout a volume conductor gives rise to a magnetic field given by the following relationship (Stratton, 1941; Jackson, 1975):

$$4\pi\bar{H} = \int_{v} \bar{J} \times \nabla\left(\frac{1}{r}\right) dv \qquad (12.1)$$

where r is the distance from an external field point at which $\bar{H}$ is evaluated to an element of volume dv inside the body, $\bar{J}dv$ is a source element, and ∇ is an operator with respect to the source coordinates. Substituting Equation 7.2, which is repeated here,

$$\bar{J} = -\sigma \nabla\Phi + \bar{J}^i \qquad (7.2)$$

into Equation 12.1 and dividing the inhomogeneous volume conductor into homogeneous regions v_j, with conductivity σ_j, we obtain

$$4\pi\bar{H} = \int_{v} \bar{J}^i \times \nabla\left(\frac{1}{r}\right) dv$$
$$- \sum_{j} \int_{v_j} \sigma_j \nabla\Phi \times \nabla\left(\frac{1}{r}\right) dv \qquad (12.2)$$

If the vector identity $\nabla \times \Phi\bar{A} = \Phi\,\nabla \times \bar{A} + \nabla\Phi \times \bar{A}$ is used, then the integrand of the last term in Equation 12.2 can be written $\sigma_j\nabla \times [\Phi\,\nabla(1/r)] - \Phi\,\nabla \times \nabla(1/r)$. Since $\nabla \times \nabla\Phi = 0$ for any Φ, we may replace the last term including its sign by

$$- \sum_{j} \int_{v_j} \sigma_j\,\nabla \times \Phi\,\nabla\left(\frac{1}{r}\right) dv \qquad (12.3)$$

We now make use of the following vector identity (Stratton, 1941, p. 604):

$$\int_{v} \nabla \times \bar{C}\,dv = -\int_{s} \bar{C} \times d\bar{S} \qquad (12.4)$$

where the surface integral is taken over the surface S bounding the volume v of the volume integral. By applying 12.4 to Equation 12.3, the last term in Equation 12.2, including its sign, can now be replaced by

$$\sum_{j} \int_{S_j} \sigma_j\Phi\,\nabla\left(\frac{1}{r}\right) \times d\bar{S}_j \qquad (12.5)$$

Finally, applying this result to Equation 12.2 and denoting again the primed and double primed regions of conductivity to be inside and outside a boundary, respectively, and orienting $d\bar{S}_j$ from the primed to double-primed region, we obtain (note that each interface arises twice, once as the surface of v_j and secondly from surfaces of each neighboring region of v_j)

227

$$4\pi\overline{H}(r) = \int_v \overline{J}^i \times \nabla\left(\frac{1}{r}\right) dv$$
$$+ \sum_j \int_{S_j} (\sigma_j'' - \sigma_j')\Phi \nabla\left(\frac{1}{r}\right) \times d\overline{S}_j \quad (12.6)$$

This equation describes the magnetic field outside a finite volume conductor containing internal (electric) volume sources $\overline{J}^i$ and inhomogeneities $(\sigma_j'' - \sigma_j')$. It was first derived by David Geselowitz (Geselowitz, 1970).

It is important to notice that the first term on the right-hand side of Equation 12.6, involving $\overline{J}^i$, represents the contribution of the volume source, and the second term the effect of the boundaries and inhomogeneities. The impressed source $\overline{J}^i$ arises from cellular activity and hence has diagnostic value whereas the second term can be considered a distortion due to the inhomogeneities of the volume conductor. These very same sources were identified earlier when the electric field generated by them was being evaluated (see Equation 7.10). (Just, as in the electric case, these terms are also referred to as primary source and secondary source.)

Similarly, as discussed in connection with Equation 7.10, it is easy to recognize that if the volume conductor is homogeneous, the differences $(\sigma_j'' - \sigma_j')$ in the second expression are zero, and it drops out. Then the equation reduces to the equation of the magnetic field due to the distribution of a volume source in a *homogeneous* volume conductor. This is introduced later as Equation 12.20. In the design of high-quality biomagnetic instrumentation, the goal is to cancel the effect of the secondary sources to the extent possible.

From an examination of Equation 12.6 one can conclude that the discontinuity in conductivity is equivalent to a secondary surface source $\overline{K}_j$ given by $\overline{K}_j = (\sigma_j'' - \sigma_j')\Phi\overline{n}$ where Φ is the surface potential on S_j. Note that $\overline{K}_j$ is the same secondary current source for electric fields (note Equation 7.10) as for magnetic fields.

12.2 NATURE OF THE BIOMAGNETIC SOURCES

Equation 12.6 shows that the physiological phenomenon that is the source of the biomagnetic signal is the *electric* activity of the tissue $\overline{J}^i$

(described earlier). Thus, for instance, the source for the magnetocardiogram (MCG) or magnetoencephalogram (MEG) is the *electric* activity of the cardiac muscle or nerve cells, respectively, as it is the source of the electrocardiogram (ECG) and electroencephalogram (EEG). The theoretical difference between biomagnetic and bioelectric signals is the difference in the *sensitivity distribution* of these measurements. The sensitivity distribution (the form of the lead field) of electric measurements was discussed in detail in the previous chapter. The sensitivity distribution of magnetic measurements is discussed in detail in this chapter. (The technical distinctions in the electric and magnetic detectors introduce additional differences. These are briefly discussed later in connection with magnetocardiography in Chapter 20.)

The difference between biomagnetic and bioelectric signals may be also seen from the form of their mathematical equations. When comparing the Equations 12.6 and 7.10, one can note that the magnetic field arises from the curl and the electric field from the divergence of the source. This distinction holds both for the first component on the right-hand side of these equations arising from the distribution of impressed current, and for the second component arising from the boundaries of the inhomogeneities of the volume source.

It is pointed out that in the design of magnetic leads one must keep in mind the electric origin of the magnetic signal and the characteristic form of the sensitivity distribution of the magnetic measurement. If the lead of a magnetic measurement is not carefully designed, it is possible that the sensitivity distribution of a magnetic lead will be similar to that of another electric lead. In such a case the magnetic measurement does not provide any new information about the source.

Please note that the biomagnetic signal discussed above is assumed not to arise from magnetic material because such material does not exist in these tissues. There are special circumstances, however, where biomagnetic fields are produced by magnetic materials—for example, in the case of the signal due to the magnetic material contaminating the lungs of welders or the iron accumulating in the liver in certain dis-

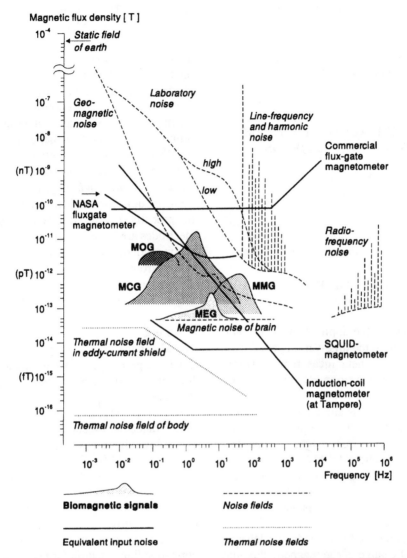

Fig. 12.1 Magnetic signals produced by various sources. *Biomagnetic signals:* MCG = magnetocardiogram, MMG = magnetomyogram, MEG = magnetoencephalogram, MOG = magneto-oculogram. *Noise fields:* static field of the Earth, geomagnetic fluctuations, laboratory noise, line frequency noise, radio frequency noise. *Equivalent input noise:* commercial flux-gate magnetometer, ring-core flux-gate (NASA), induction coil magnetometer, SQUID-magnometer. *Thermal noise fields:* eddy current shield, the human body.

eases. Such fields are not discussed in this textbook.

Biomagnetic fields have very low amplitude compared to the ambient noise fields and to the sensitivity of the detectors. A summary of these fields is presented in Figure 12.1 (Malmivuo et al., 1987). The figure indicates that it is possible to detect the MCG with induction coil magnetometers, albeit with a reasonably poor signal-to-noise ratio. However, even the most sensitive induction coil magnetometer built for biomagnetic purposes (Estola and Malmivuo, 1982) is not sensitive enough to detect the MEG for clinical use. Therefore, the Superconducting QUantum Interference Device (SQUID) is the only instrument that is sensitive enough for high-quality biomagnetic measurements. The instrumentation for measuring biomagnetic fields is not discussed further in this textbook. A good overview of the instrumentation is published by Williamson et al. (1983).

12.3   RECIPROCITY THEOREM FOR MAGNETIC FIELDS

PRECONDITIONS:

Source: *Distribution of impressed current source elements $\bar{J}^i$ (volume source)*

Conductor: *Infinite, homogeneous; or finite, inhomogeneous with cylindrical symmetry*

12.3.1   The Form of the Magnetic Lead Field

Plonsey extended the application of the reciprocity theorem to the time-varying conditions that arise in biomagnetic measurements (Plonsey, 1972). That development follows along lines similar to the proof of the reciprocity theorem for electric fields and therefore need not be repeated here. Only the equations for the reciprocity theorem for magnetic measurements are derived here. In this discussion subscript L denotes "lead," as in the previous chapter, but we add a subscript M to denote "magnetic leads" due to reciprocal current of unit time derivative.

The current induced in a conductor depends on the rate of change of the magnetic flux that links the current loop. In analogy to the electric field case (see Equations 11.30 and 11.52), the reciprocally energizing (time-varying) current I_r is normalized so that its *time derivative is unity* for all values of ω. The necessary equations for the lead field theory for biomagnetic measurements can then be readily obtained from the corresponding equations in electric measurements.

An elementary bipolar lead in magnetic measurements is a solenoid (coil) with a core and disklike terminals of infinite permeability, as illustrated in Figure 12.2. If the coil is energized with a current, a magnetic field is set up, which can be considered to result from magnetic charges (equal and opposite) at the terminals

of the core. These terminals are called *magnodes* (Baule and McFee, 1963). (The word *"electrode"* was introduced by Michael Faraday (1834).) This elementary bipolar magnetic lead is equivalent to the elementary bipolar electric lead illustrated in Figure 11.23.

When a reciprocal current I_r is fed to the elementary magnetic lead, it produces in an infinite space of uniform permeability a reciprocal magnetic scalar potential field Φ_{LM} of the *same spatial behavior as the reciprocal scalar electric potential field* Φ_{LE} in an infinite medium of uniform conductivity arising from a reciprocally energized electric lead, whose electrodes are located at sites corresponding to the magnodes. As noted in Section 11.6.6, if the electrodes or magnodes are parallel and their dimensions are large compared to their separation, both Φ_{LE} and Φ_{LM} are uniform in the central region.

An unbounded homogeneous medium is required for the conductivity to be dual to the magnetic permeability, where the latter is uniform in the body and in space. As in electric measurements, it is possible to create compound magnetic leads by connecting any number of detectors together.

We investigate now the nature of the magnetic lead field $\bar{J}_{LM}$ produced by reciprocal energization of the coil of the magnetic detector with a current I_r at an angular frequency ω. Using the same sign convention between the energizing current and the measured voltage as in the electric case, Figure 11.23, we obtain the corresponding situation for magnetic measurements, as illustrated in Figure 12.2.

The reciprocal magnetic field $\bar{H}_{LM}$ arising from the magnetic scalar potential Φ_{LM} has the form:

$$\bar{H}_{LM} = -\nabla\Phi_{LM} \qquad (12.7)$$

The reciprocal magnetic induction $\bar{B}_{LM}$ is

$$\bar{B}_{LM} = \mu\bar{H}_{LM} \qquad (12.8)$$

where μ is the magnetic permeability of the medium. We assume μ to be uniform (a constant), reflecting the assumed absence of discrete magnetic materials.

The reciprocal electric field $\bar{E}_{LM}$ arising from the reciprocal magnetic induction $\bar{B}_{LM}$ (resulting from the energized coil) depends on the

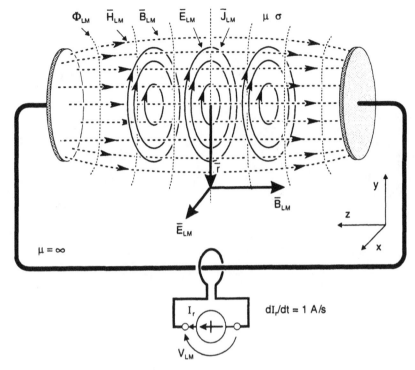

Fig. 12.2 Basic form of a bipolar magnetic lead, where: I_r = reciprocal current; Φ_{LM} = reciprocal magnetic scalar potential field; $\bar{H}_{LM}$ = reciprocal magnetic field; $\bar{B}_{LM}$ = reciprocal magnetic induction field; $\bar{E}_{LM}$ = reciprocal electric field; $\bar{J}_{LM}$ = lead field; V_{LM} = voltage in the lead due to the volume source $\bar{J}^i$ in the volume conductor; μ = magnetic permeability of the medium; σ = conductivity of the medium; and $\bar{r}$ = radius vector.

field and volume conductor configuration. For a magnetic field that is axially symmetric and uniform within some bounded region (cylindrically symmetric situation), $2\pi r E_\phi = \pi r^2 B_z$ within that region (ϕ and z being in cylindrical coordinates), or in vector notation:

$$\bar{E}_{LM} = \frac{1}{2}\bar{r} \times \bar{B}_{LM} = \frac{\mu}{2}\bar{r} \times \bar{H}_{LM}$$

$$= -\frac{\mu}{2}\bar{r} \times \nabla\Phi_{LM} \quad (12.9)$$

In this equation $\bar{r}$ is a radius vector in cylindrical coordinates measured from the symmetry axis (z) as the origin. As before, harmonic conditions are assumed so that all field quantities are complex phasors. In addition, as noted before, $I_r(\omega)$ is adjusted so that the magnitude of B_{LM} is independent of ω. The 90-degree phase lag of the electric field relative to the magnetic field, is assumed to be contained in the electric field phasor. The field config-

uration assumed above should be a reasonable approximation for practical reciprocal fields established by magnetic field detector.

The result in Equation 12.9 corresponds to the reciprocal electric field $\bar{E}_{LE} = -\nabla\Phi$ produced by the reciprocal energization of an electric lead (described in Equation 11.53 in the previous chapter).

The magnetic lead field current density may be calculated from Equation 12.9. Since

$$\bar{J}_{LM} = \sigma\bar{E}_{LM} \quad (12.10)$$

we obtain for the magnetic lead field $\bar{J}_{LM}$

$$\bar{J}_{LM} = \frac{\sigma}{2}\bar{r} \times \bar{B}_{LM} \quad \textbf{(12.11)}$$

As before, the quantity $\bar{B}_{LM}$ is the magnetic induction due to the reciprocal energization at a frequency ω of the pickup lead.

This magnetic lead field $\bar{J}_{LM}$ has the following properties:

1. The lead field current density $\bar{J}_{LM}$ is everywhere circular and concentric with the symmetry axis.
2. The magnitude of the lead field current density J_{LM} is proportional to the distance from

the symmetry axis r (so long as the field point remains within the uniform $\bar{B}_{LM}$ field).

3. As a consequence of (2), the sensitivity is zero on the symmetry axis. Therefore, the

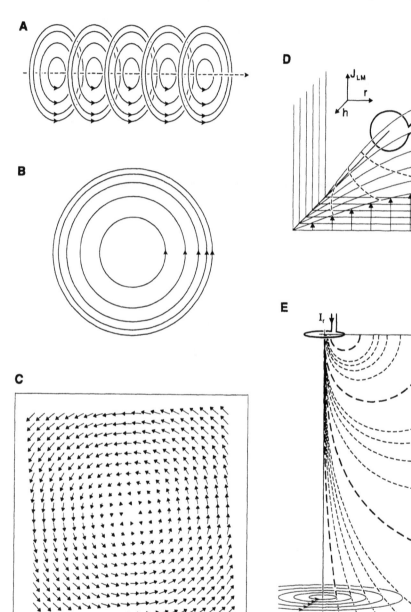

Fig. 12.3   Lead field current density of a magnetic lead. (A) The lead field current density—that is, the sensitivity—is directed tangentially, and its magnitude is proportional to the distance from the symmetry axis. Note that in this figure the dashed line represents the symmetry axis where the lead field

current density is zero. (B) Lead field current density shown on one plane with flow lines, and (C) with current density vectors. (D) Lead field current density as a function of distance from the symmetry axis. (E) Isosensitivity lines of the lead.

symmetry axis is called the *zero sensitivity line*.

Based upon Equation 11.30 and noting that also in the magnetic case the reciprocal current I_r is normalized so that it is unity for all values of ω, we evaluate the voltage V_{LM} in the magnetic lead produced by a current dipole moment density $\bar{J}^i$ as (Plonsey, 1972)

$$V_{LM} = \int_v \frac{1}{\sigma} \bar{J}_{LM} \cdot \bar{J}^i dv \qquad (12.12)$$

This equation is similar to Equation 11.30, which describes the sensitivity distribution of electric leads. The sensitivity distribution of a magnetic measurement is, however, different from that of the electric measurement because the magnetic lead field $\bar{J}_{LM}$ has a different form from that of the electric lead field $\bar{J}_{LE}$.

In the material above, we assumed that the conducting medium is uniform and infinite in extent. This discussion holds also for a uniform cylindrical conducting medium of finite radius if the reciprocally energized magnetic field is uniform and in the direction of the symmetry axis. This comes about because the concentric circular direction of $\bar{J}_{LM}$ in the unbounded case is not interfered with when the finite cylinder boundary is introduced. As in the infinite medium case, the lead field current magnitude is proportional to the distance r from the symmetry axis. On the axis of symmetry, the lead field current density is zero, and therefore, it is called the *zero sensitivity line* (Eskola, 1983; Eskola and Malmivuo, 1983).

The form of the magnetic lead field is illustrated in detail in Figure 12.3. For comparison, the magnetic lead field is illustrated in this figure with four different methods. Figure 12.3A shows the magnetic lead field current density in a perspective three-dimensional form with the lead field flow lines oriented tangentially around the symmetry axis. As noted before, because the lead field current density is proportional to the radial distance r from the symmetry axis, the symmetry axis is at the same time a zero sensitivity line. Figure 12.3B shows the projection of the lead field on a plane transverse to the axis. The flow lines are usually drawn so that a fixed amount of current is assumed to flow between two flow lines. Thus the flow line density is proportional to the current density. (In this case, the lead field current has a component normal to the plane of illustration, the flow lines are discontinuous, and some inaccuracy is introduced into the illustration, as may be seen later in Section 13.4.) Figure 12.3C illustrates the lead field with current density vectors, which are located at corners of a regular grid. Finally, Figure 12.3D shows the magnitude of the lead field current density J_{LM} as a function of the radial distance r from the symmetry axis with the distance from the magnetometer h as a parameter. This illustration does not show the direction of the lead field current density, but it is known that it is tangentially oriented. In Figure 12.3E the dashed lines join the points where the lead field current density has the same value, thus they are called the isosensitivity lines.

The relative directions of the magnetic field and the induced currents and detected signal are sketched in Figure 12.2. If the reciprocal magnetic field $\bar{B}_{LM}$ of Equation 12.11 is uniform and in the negative coordinate direction, as in Figure 12.2, the form of the resulting lead field current density $\bar{J}_{LM}$ is tangential and oriented in the positive direction of rotation. It should be remembered that harmonic conditions have been assumed so that since we are plotting the peak *magnitude* of $\bar{B}_{LM}$ versus J_{LM}, the sign chosen for each vector class is arbitrary. The instantaneous relationship can be found from Equation 12.11, if the explicit phasor notation is restored, including the 90-degree phase lag of $\bar{J}_{LM}$.

12.3.2 The Source of the Magnetic Field

This section provides an alternative description of the source of the magnetic field sensed by magnetic pickup coils (which is valid for the case of axial symmetry). By substituting Equation 12.9 into Equation 12.10, and then this equation into Equation 12.12, we obtain (note that $\bar{r}$ is in cylindrical coordinates)

$$V_{LM} = -\frac{\mu}{2} \int_v (\bar{r} \times \nabla \Phi_{LM}) \cdot \bar{J}^i dv \qquad (12.13)$$

$$= \frac{\mu}{2} \int_v \nabla \Phi_{LM} \cdot (\bar{r} \times \bar{J}^i) dv$$

Using the vector identity $\nabla \cdot (\Phi_{LM}\bar{r} \times \bar{J}^i) = \Phi_{LM}\nabla \cdot (\bar{r} \times \bar{J}^i) + \nabla\Phi_{LM} \cdot (\bar{r} \times \bar{J}^i)$, we obtain from Equation 12.13

$$V_{LM} = \frac{\mu}{2}\int_v \nabla \cdot (\Phi_{LM}\bar{r} \times \bar{J}^i)dv$$

$$- \frac{\mu}{2}\int_v \Phi_{LM}\nabla \cdot (\bar{r} \times \bar{J}^i)dv \quad (12.14)$$

Applying the divergence theorem to the first term on the right-hand side and using a vector expansion (i.e., $\nabla \cdot (\bar{r} \times \bar{J}^i) = \bar{J}^i \cdot \nabla \times \bar{r} - \bar{r} \cdot \nabla \times \bar{J}^i$) on the second term of Equation 12.14, and noting that $\nabla \times \bar{r} = 0$, we obtain

$$V_{LM} = \frac{\mu}{2}\int_s \Phi_{LM}(\bar{r} \times \bar{J}^i) \cdot d\bar{S}$$

$$+ \frac{\mu}{2}\int_v \Phi_{LM}\bar{r} \cdot \nabla \times \bar{J}^i dv \quad (12.15)$$

Since $\bar{J}^i = 0$ at the boundary of the medium, the surface integral equals zero, and we may write

$$V_{LM} = \frac{\mu}{2}\int_v \Phi_{LM}\bar{r} \cdot \nabla \times \bar{J}^i dv \quad \mathbf{(12.16)}$$

This equation corresponds to Equation 11.50 in electric measurements. The quantity Φ_{LM} is the magnetic scalar potential in the volume conductor due to the reciprocal energization of the pickup lead. The expression $\nabla \times \bar{J}^i$ is defined as the *vortex source*, $\bar{I}_V$:

$$\bar{I}_V = \nabla \times \bar{J}^i \quad (12.17)$$

In Equation 12.16 this is the strength of the magnetic field source.

The designation of *vortex* to this source arises out of the definition of *curl*. The latter is the circulation per unit area, that is:

$$\nabla \times \bar{A} = \frac{1}{\Delta S}\oint_{\Delta S} \bar{A} \cdot d\bar{l} \quad (12.18)$$

and the line integral is taken around ΔS at any point in the region of interest such that it is oriented in the field to maximize the integral (which designates the direction of the curl).

If one considers the velocity field associated with a volume of water in a container, then its flow source must be zero if water is neither added nor withdrawn. But the field is not necessarily zero in the absence of flow source because the water can be stirred up, thereby creating a nonzero field. But the vortex thus created leads to a nonzero curl since there obviously exists a circulation. This explains the use of the term "vortex" as well as its important role as the source of a field independent of the flow source.

12.3.3 Summary of the Lead Field Theoretical Equations for Electric and Magnetic Measurements

As summarized in Figure 12.2, as a consequence of the reciprocal energization of a magnetic lead, the following five reciprocal fields are created in the volume conductor: magnetic scalar potential field Φ_{LM} (illustrated with isopotential surfaces); magnetic field $\bar{H}_{LM}$ (illustrated with field lines); magnetic induction $\bar{B}_{LM}$ (illustrated with flux lines); electric field $\bar{E}_{LM}$ (illustrated with field lines); and current field $\bar{J}_{LM}$ (illustrated with current flow lines and called the lead field).

In addition to these five fields, we may define a sixth field for a magnetic lead: the field of *isosensitivity surfaces*. This is a similar concept as was defined for an electric lead in Section 11.6.6. When the magnetic permeability is isotropic (as it usually is in biological tissues), the magnetic field lines coincide with the magnetic induction flux lines. When the conductivity is isotropic, the electric field lines coincide with the current flow lines. Thus, in summary, in a lead system detecting the magnetic dipole moment of a volume source (see Section 12.6) from the aforementioned six fields, the magnetic field lines coincide with the magnetic flux lines and the electric field lines coincide with the lead field flow lines. Similarly, as in the electric case (see Section 11.6.6), the magnetic scalar isopotential surfaces coincide with the magnetic isofield and isoflux surfaces.

Table 12.1 summarizes the lead field theoretical equations for electric and magnetic measurements.

The spatial dependence of the electric and magnetic scalar potentials Φ_{LE} and Φ_{LM}, are found from Laplace's equation. These fields will have the same form (as will $\bar{E}_{LE}$ vs. $\bar{H}_{LM}$), if the shape and location of the electrodes and magnodes are similar and if there

Table 12.1 The equations for electric and magnetic leads

Quantity	Electric lead		Magnetic lead	
Field as a negative gradient of the scalar potential of the reciprocal energization	$\bar{E}_{LE} = -\nabla\Phi_{LE}$	(11.53)	$\bar{H}_{LM} = -\nabla\Phi_{LM}$	(12.7)
Magnetic induction due to reciprocal energization			$\bar{B}_{LM} = \mu\bar{H}_{LM}$	(12.8)
Reciprocal electric field*	$\bar{E}_{LE} (= -\nabla\Phi_{LE})$	(11.53)	$\bar{E}_{LM} = \frac{1}{2}\bar{r} \times \bar{B}_{LM}$	(12.9)
Lead field (current field)	$\bar{J}_{LE} = \sigma\bar{E}_{LE}$	(11.54)	$\bar{J}_{LM} = \sigma\bar{E}_{LM}$	(12.10)
Detected signal when: $I_{RE} = 1$ A $\dfrac{dI_{RM}}{dt} = 1$ A/s	$V_{LE} = \displaystyle\int \frac{1}{\sigma}\bar{J}_{LE} \cdot \bar{J}^i\, dv$	(11.30)	$V_{LM} = \displaystyle\int \frac{1}{\sigma}\bar{J}_{LM} \cdot \bar{J}^i\, dv$	(12.12)

*Note: The essential difference between the electric and magnetic lead fields is explained as follows: The reciprocal electric field of the electric lead has the form of the negative gradient of the electric scalar potential (as explained on the first line of this table). The reciprocal electric field of the magnetic lead has the form of the *curl* of the negative gradient of the magnetic scalar potential. (In both cases, the lead field, which is defined as the current field, is obtained from the reciprocal electric field by multiplying by the conductivity.) Numbers in parentheses refer to equation numbers in text.

is no effect of the volume conductor inhomogeneities or boundary with air. Similarly, the equations for the electric and magnetic signals V_{LE} and V_{LM}, as integrals of the scalar product (dot product) of the lead field and the impressed current density field, have the same form.

The difference in the sensitivity distributions of the electric and magnetic detection of the impressed current density $\bar{J}^i$ is a result of the difference in the form of the electric and magnetic lead fields $\bar{J}_{LE}$ and $\bar{J}_{LM}$. The first has the form of the reciprocal electric field, whereas the latter has the form of the *curl* of the reciprocal magnetic field.

We emphasize again that this discussion of the magnetic field is restricted to the case of axially symmetric and uniform conditions (which are expected to be applicable as a good approximation in many applications).

12.4 THE MAGNETIC DIPOLE MOMENT OF A VOLUME SOURCE

PRECONDITIONS:

Source: *Distribution of $\bar{J}^i$ forming a volume source*

Conductor: *Finite, inhomogeneous*

The magnetic dipole moment of a volume current distribution $\bar{J}$ with respect to an arbitrary origin is *defined* as (Stratton, 1941):

$$\bar{m} = \frac{1}{2}\int_v \bar{r} \times \bar{J}\, dv \qquad (12.19)$$

where $\bar{r}$ is a radius vector from the origin. The magnetic dipole moment of the total current density $\bar{J}$, which includes a distributed volume current source $\bar{J}^i$ and its conduction current,

$$\bar{J} = \bar{J}^i - \sigma\nabla\Phi \qquad (7.2)$$

is consequently

$$\bar{m} = \frac{1}{2}\int_v \bar{r} \times \bar{J}^i\, dv - \frac{1}{2}\int_v \bar{r} \times \sigma\,\nabla\Phi\, dv \qquad (12.20)$$

Assuming σ to be piecewise constant, we may use the vector identity $\nabla \times \bar{r}\Phi = \Phi\,\nabla \times \bar{r} + \nabla\Phi \times \bar{r} = -\bar{r} \times \nabla\Phi$ (because $\nabla \times \bar{r} = 0$), and convert the second term on the right-hand side of Equation 12.20 to the form:

$$\frac{1}{2}\int_v \nabla \times \bar{r}\sigma\,\Phi\, dv \qquad (12.21)$$

We now apply Equation 12.4 to 12.21 and note that the volume and hence surface integrals must be calculated in a piecewise manner for each region where σ takes on a different value. Summing these integrals and designating the value of conductivity σ with primed and double-primed symbols for the inside and outside of each boundary, we finally obtain from Equation 12.20:

$$\bar{m} = \tfrac{1}{2} \int_v \bar{r} \times \bar{J}^i \, dv$$

$$+ \tfrac{1}{2} \sum_j \int_{S_j} (\sigma_j'' - \sigma_j') \Phi \bar{r} \times d\bar{S}_j \quad \textbf{(12.22)}$$

This equation gives the magnetic dipole moment of a volume source $\bar{J}^i$ located in a finite inhomogeneous volume conductor. As in Equation 12.6, the first term on the right-hand side of Equation 12.22 represents the contribution of the volume source, and the second term the contribution of the boundaries between regions of different conductivity. This equation was first derived by David Geselowitz (Geselowitz, 1970).

12.5   IDEAL LEAD FIELD OF A LEAD DETECTING THE EQUIVALENT MAGNETIC DIPOLE OF A VOLUME SOURCE

PRECONDITIONS:

Source: *Distribution of $\bar{J}^i$ forming volume source (at the origin)*

Conductor: *Infinite (or spherical) homogeneous*

This section develops the form of the lead field for a detector that detects the equivalent magnetic dipole moment of a distributed volume source located in an infinite (or spherical) homogeneous volume conductor. We first have to choose the origin; we select this at the center of the source. (The selection of the origin is necessary, because of the factor r in the equation of the magnetic dipole moment, Equation 12.22.)

The total magnetic dipole moment of a volume source is evaluated in Equation 12.20 as a volume integral. We notice from this equation that a magnetic dipole moment density function is given by the integrand, namely

$$\bar{m} = \tfrac{1}{2}\bar{r} \times \bar{J}^i \quad (12.23)$$

Equation 12.14 provides a relationship between the (magnetic) lead voltage and the current source distribution $\bar{J}^i$, namely

$$V_{LM} = \tfrac{1}{2}\int \bar{r} \times \bar{B}_{LM} \cdot \bar{J}^i \, dv \quad (12.24)$$

$$= -\tfrac{1}{2}\int \bar{B}_{LM} \cdot \bar{r} \times \bar{J}^i dv$$

Substituting Equation 12.23 into Equation 12.24 gives the desired relationship between the lead voltage and magnetic dipole moment density, namely

$$V_{LM} = -\int \bar{B}_{LM} \cdot \bar{m} \, dv \quad \textbf{(12.25)}$$

This equation may be expressed in words as follows:

1. One component of the magnetic dipole moment of a volume source is obtained with a detector which, when energized, produces a homogeneous reciprocal magnetic field $\bar{B}_{LM}$ in the negative direction of the coordinate axis in the region of the volume source.

2. This reciprocal magnetic field produces a reciprocal electric field $\bar{E}_{LM} = \tfrac{1}{2}\bar{r} \times \bar{B}_{LM}$ and a magnetic lead field $\bar{J}_{LM} = \sigma\bar{E}_{LM}$ in the direction tangential to the symmetry axis.

3. Three such identical, mutually perpendicular lead fields form the three orthogonal components of a complete lead system detecting the magnetic dipole moment of a volume source.

Figure 12.4 presents the principle of a lead system detecting the magnetic dipole moment of a volume source. It consists of a bipolar coil system (Fig. 12.4A) which produces in its center the three components of the reciprocal magnetic field $\bar{B}_{LM}$ (Fig. 12.4B). Note that the region where the coils of Figure 12.4A produce linear reciprocal magnetic fields is rather small, as will be explained later, and therefore Figures 12.4A and 12.4B are not in scale. The three reciprocal magnetic fields $\bar{B}_{LM}$ produce the three components of the reciprocal electric field $\bar{E}_{LE}$ and the lead field $\bar{J}_{LE}$ that are illustrated in Figure 12.5. It is important to note that the reciprocal magnetic field $\bar{B}_{LM}$ has the same geometric form as the reciprocal electric field $\bar{E}_{LE}$ of a detector which detects the electric dipole moment of a volume source (Fig. 11.24).

A

B

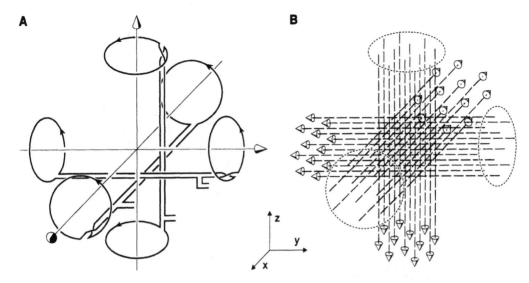

Fig. 12.4 The principle of a lead system detecting the magnetic dipole moment of a volume source. (A) The three orthogonal bipolar coils. (B) The three components of the reciprocal magnetic field $\overline{B}_{LM}$ in the center of the bipolar coil system. The region where the coils produce linear reciprocal magnetic fields is rather small and therefore Figures 12.4A and 12.4B are not to scale.

Similarly as in the equation of the electric field of a volume source, Equation 7.9, the second term on the right-hand side of Equation 12.22 represents the contribution of the boundaries and inhomogeneities to the magnetic dipole moment. This is equivalent to the effect of the boundaries and inhomogeneities on the form of the lead field. In general, a detector that produces an ideal lead field in the source region despite the boundaries and inhomogeneities of the volume conductor, detects the dipole moment of the source undistorted.

Physiological Meaning of Magnetic Dipole

The sensitivity distribution (i.e., the lead field), illustrated in Figure 12.5, is the *physiological meaning* of the measurement of the (equivalent) magnetic dipole of a volume source.

Similarly, as in the detection of the electric dipole moment of a volume source, the concept of ''physiological meaning'' can be explained in the detection of the magnetic dipole moment of a volume source as follows: When considering the forward problem, the lead field illustrates what is the contribution (effect) of each active cell to the signals of the lead system.

When one is considering the inverse problem, the lead field illustrates similarly the most probable distribution and orientation of active cells when a signal is detected in a lead.

12.6 SYNTHESIZATION OF THE IDEAL LEAD FIELD FOR THE DETECTION OF THE MAGNETIC DIPOLE MOMENT OF A VOLUME SOURCE

PRECONDITIONS:

Source: *Volume source (at the origin)*

Conductor: *Finite, homogeneous with spherical symmetry*

As in the case of the detection of the electric dipole moment of a volume source, Section 11.6.9, both unipolar and bipolar leads may be used in synthesizing the ideal lead field for detecting the magnetic dipole moment of a volume source. In the case of an infinite conducting medium and a uniform reciprocal magnetic field, the lead field current flows concentrically about the symmetry axis, as shown in Figure

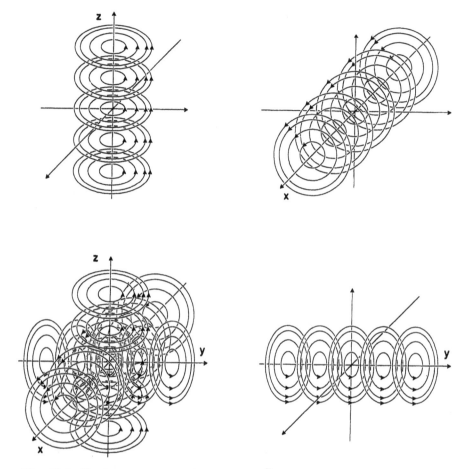

Fig. 12.5   The three components of the lead field $\bar{J}_{LM}$ of an ideal lead system detecting the magnetic dipole moment of a volume source.

12.3. No alteration then results if the conducting medium is terminated by a spherical boundary (since the lead current flow lines lie tangential to the surface). The spherical surface ensures lead current flow lines, as occurs in an infinite homogeneous medium, when a uniform reciprocal magnetic field is established along any x-, y-, and z-coordinate direction.

If the dimensions of the volume source are small in relation to the distance to the point of observation, we can consider the magnetic dipole moment to be a contribution from a point source. Thus we consider the magnetic dipole moment to be a discrete vector. The evaluation of such a magnetic dipole may be accomplished through unipolar measurements on each coordinate axis, as illustrated on the left-hand side of Figure 12.6A. If the dimensions of the vol-

ume source are large, the quality of the aforementioned lead system is not high. Because the reciprocal magnetic field decreases as a function of distance, the sensitivity of a single magnetometer is higher for source elements located closer to it than for source elements located far from it. This is illustrated on the right-hand side of Figure 12.6A. In Figure 12.6 the dashed lines represent the reciprocal magnetic field flux tubes. The thin solid circular lines represent the lead field flow lines. The behavior of the reciprocal magnetic field of a single magnetometer coil is illustrated more accurately in Figures 20.14, 20.15, and 22.3.

The result is very much improved if we use symmetric pairs of magnetometers forming bipolar leads, as in Figure 12.6B. This arrangement will produce a reciprocal magnetic field

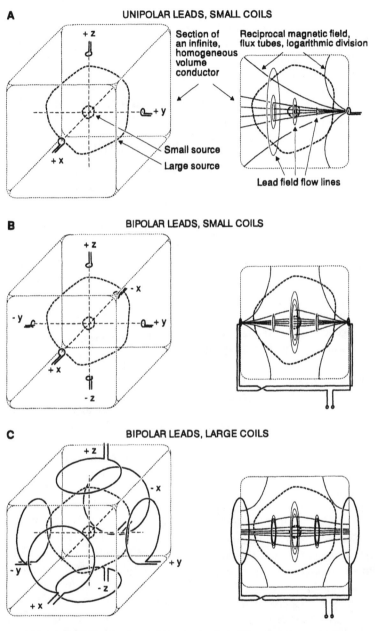

Fig. 12.6 Properties of unipolar and bipolar leads in detecting the equivalent magnetic dipole moment of a volume source. The dashed lines illustrate the reciprocal magnetic field flux tubes. The thin solid circular lines represent the lead field flow lines. (A) If the dimensions of the volume source are small compared to the measurement distance the most simple method is to make the measurement with unipolar leads on the coordinate axes. (B) For volume sources with large dimensions the quality of the lead field is considerably improved by using symmetric pairs of magnetometers forming bipolar leads. (C) Increasing the size of the magnetometers further improves the quality of the leads.

that is more uniform over the source region than is attained with the single coils of the unipolar lead system (Malmivuo, 1976).

Just as with the electric case, the quality of the bipolar magnetic lead fields in measuring volume sources with large dimensions is further improved by using large coils whose dimensions are comparable to the source dimensions. This is illustrated in Figure 12.6C.

The behavior of the reciprocal magnetic field and the sensitivity distribution of a bipolar lead as a function of coil separation are described in Figure 12.7 for two coil pairs with different separation. (Please note that the isosensitivity lines are not the same as the reciprocal magnetic field lines.) Figure 12.7A illustrates the reciprocal magnetic field as rotational flux tubes for the Helmholtz coils which are a coaxial pair of identical circular coils separated by the coil radius. With this coil separation, the radial component of the compound magnetic field at the center plane is at its minimum and the magnetic field is very homogeneous. Helmholtz coils cannot easily be used in detecting biomagnetic fields, but they can be used in magnetization or in impedance measurement. They are much used in balancing the gradiometers and for compensating the Earth's static magnetic field in the measurement environment. Figure 12.7B illustrates the reciprocal magnetic field flux tubes for a coil pair with a separation of $5r$. Figures 12.7C and 12.7D illustrate the isosensitivity lines for the same coils.

Later in Chapter 20, Figure 20.16 illustrates the isosensitivity lines for a coil pair with a separation of $32r$. Comparing these two bipolar leads to the Helmholtz coils one may note that in them the region of homogeneous sensitivity is much smaller than in the Helmholtz coils. Owing to symmetry, the homogeneity of bipolar leads is, however, much better than that of corresponding unipolar leads.

The arrangement of a bipolar lead must not be confused with the differential magnetometer or gradiometer system, which consists of two coaxial coils on the same side of the source wound in opposite directions. The purpose of such an arrangement is to null out the background noise, not to improve the quality of the lead field. The realization of the bipolar lead system with gradiometers is illustrated in Figure 12.8. Later, Figure 12.20 illustrates the effect of the second coil on the gradiometer sensitivity distribution for several baselines.

12.7 COMPARISON OF THE LEAD FIELDS OF IDEAL BIPOLAR LEADS FOR DETECTING THE ELECTRIC AND MAGNETIC DIPOLE MOMENTS OF A VOLUME SOURCE

PRECONDITIONS:

Source: *Electric and magnetic dipole moments of a volume source*

Conductor: *Infinite, homogeneous*

In summary, we note the following details from the lead fields of ideal bipolar lead systems for detecting the electric and magnetic dipole moments of a volume source:

12.7.1 The Bipolar Lead System for Detecting the Electric Dipole Moment

1. The lead system consists of three components.
2. For a spherically symmetric volume conductor, each is formed by a pair of electrodes (or electrode matrices), whose axis is in the direction of the coordinate axes. Each electrode is on opposite sides of the source, as shown in Figure 11.24.
3. For each of these components, when energized reciprocally, a homogeneous and linear *electric* field is established in the region of the volume source (see Fig. 11.25). Each of these reciprocal electric fields forms a similar current field, which is called the electric lead field $\bar{J}_{LE}$. (Note the similarity of Fig. 11.25, illustrating the reciprocal electric field $\bar{E}_{LE}$ of an electric lead, and Fig. 12.7, illustrating the reciprocal magnetic field $\bar{B}_{LM}$ of a magnetic lead.)

12.7.2 The Bipolar Lead System for Detecting the Magnetic Dipole Moment

1. The lead system consists of three components.
2. In the spherically symmetric case, each of

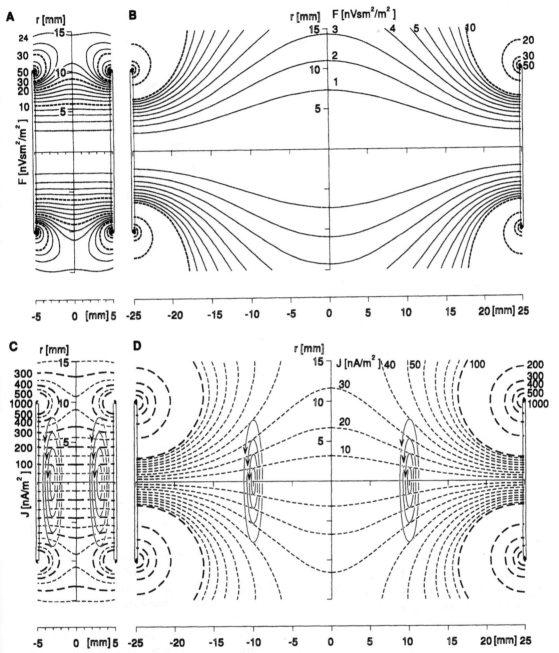

Fig. 12.7 Flux tubes of the reciprocal magnetic field of (A) the Helmholtz coils having a coil separation of r, and (B) bipolar lead with a coil separation of $5r$. The isosensitivity lines for (C) the Helmholtz coils having a coil separation of r, and (D) bipolar lead with a coil separation of $5r$. (Note that the isosensitivity lines are not the same as the flux tubes of the reciprocal magnetic field.)

them is formed by a pair of magnetometers (or gradiometers) located in the direction of the coordinate axes on opposite sides of the source, as illustrated in Figure 12.6C (or 12.8).

3. For each of these components, when ener-

gized reciprocally, a homogeneous and linear *magnetic* field is established in the region of the volume source, as shown in Figure 12.4.

4. Each of these reciprocal magnetic fields forms an electric field, necessarily *tangen-*

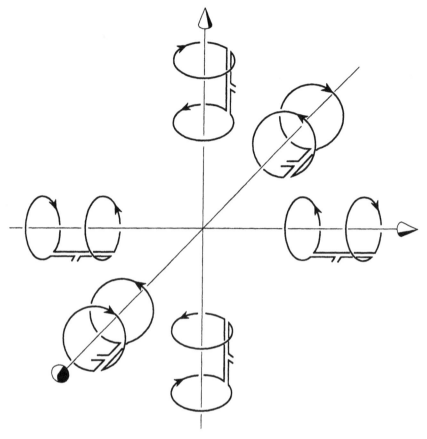

Fig. 12.8   Bipolar lead system for detecting the magnetic dipole moment of a volume source realized with gradiometers.

tial to the boundaries. These reciprocal electric fields give rise to a similar electric current field, which is called the magnetic lead field $\bar{J}_{LM}$, as described in Figure 12.5.

Superimposing Figures 12.8, 12.4, and 12.5 allows one more easily to visualize the generation and shape of the lead fields of magnetic leads.

12.8   THE RADIAL AND TANGENTIAL SENSITIVITIES OF THE LEAD SYSTEMS DETECTING THE ELECTRIC AND MAGNETIC DIPOLE MOMENTS OF A VOLUME SOURCE

PRECONDITIONS:

Source: *Electric and magnetic dipole moments of a volume source*

Conductor: *Infinite, homogeneous*

12.8.1   Sensitivity of the Electric Lead

The radial and tangential sensitivities of the lead system detecting the electric dipole moment of a volume source may be easily estimated for the case where an ideal lead field has been established.

Figure 12.9 describes the cross section of a spherical volume source in an infinite homogeneous volume conductor and two components of the lead field for detecting the electric dipole moment. Let ϕ denote the angle between the horizontal electric lead field flow line and a radius vector $\bar{r}$ from the center of the spherical source to the point at which the radial and tangential source elements $\bar{J}_r^i$ and $\bar{J}_t^i$, respectively, lie. According to Equation 11.30, the lead voltage V_{LE} is proportional to the projection of the impressed current density $\bar{J}^i$ on the lead field flow line. The sensitivity of the total electric

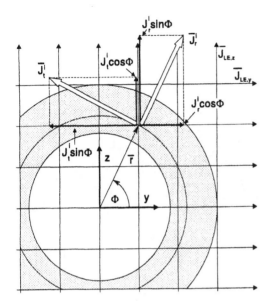

Fig. 12.9 Relative sensitivity of the electric lead system to radial and tangential current dipoles $\bar{J}_r^i$ and $\bar{J}_t^i$.

lead is the sum of the sensitivities of the two component leads; hence for the radial component J_r^i we obtain:

$$V_{LE}(J_r^i) = J_r^i(\sin \phi + \cos \phi) \qquad (12.26)$$

whereas for the tangential component J_t^i it is:

$$V_{LE}(J_t^i) = J_t^i(\sin \phi + \cos \phi) \qquad (12.27)$$

In these expressions the component lead fields are assumed uniform and of unit magnitude.

We note from Equations 12.26 and 12.27 that the total sensitivity of these two components *of the electric lead to radial and tangential current source elements* $\bar{J}^i$ *is equal and independent of their location.* The same conclusion also holds in all three dimensions.

12.8.2 Sensitivity of the Magnetic Lead

From Equation 12.13 and from the definition of the magnetic dipole moment of a volume source (see Equation 12.22), it may be seen that the magnetic lead system and its components are sensitive only to *tangential* source elements. The magnitude of the sensitivity is, as noted before, proportional to the distance from the symmetry axis.

12.9 SPECIAL PROPERTIES OF THE MAGNETIC LEAD FIELDS

PRECONDITIONS:

Source: *Volume source*

Conductor: *Finite, inhomogeneous, cylindrically symmetric*

The special properties of electric lead fields, listed in Section 11.6.10, also hold for magnetic lead fields. Magnetic lead fields also have some additional special properties which can be summarized as follows:

1. If the volume conductor is cut or the boundary of an inhomogeneity is inserted along a lead field current flow line, the form of the lead field does not change (Malmivuo, 1976). This explains why with either a cylindrically or spherically symmetric volume conductor, the form of the symmetric magnetic lead field is unaffected. There are two important practical consequences:
   a. Because the heart may be approximated as a sphere, the highly conducting intracardiac blood mass, which may be considered spherical and concentric, does not change the form of the lead field. This means that the Brody effect does not exist in magnetocardiography (see Chapter 18).
   b. The poorly conducting skull does not affect the magnetic detection of brain activity as it does with electric detection (see Fig. 12.10).
2. Magnetic lead fields in volume conductors exhibiting spherical symmetry are always directed tangentially. This means that the sensitivity of such magnetic leads in a spherical conductor to radial electric dipoles is always zero. This fact has special importance in the MEG (see Fig. 12.11).
3. If the electrodes of a symmetric bipolar electric lead are located on the symmetry axis of the bipolar magnetic field detector arranged for a spherical volume conductor, the lead fields of these electric and magnetic leads are normal to each other throughout the volume conductor, as illustrated in Figure 12.12 (Malmivuo, 1980). (The same holds for corresponding unipolar leads as well, though not shown in the figure.)

4. The lead fields of all magnetic leads include at least one zero sensitivity line, where the sensitivity to electric dipoles is zero. This line exists in all volume conductors, unless there is a hole in the conductor in this region (Eskola, 1979, 1983; Eskola and Malmivuo, 1983). The zero sensitivity line itself is one tool in understanding the form of magnetic leads (as demonstrated in Fig. 12.13).

5. The reciprocity theorem also applies to the reciprocal situation. This means that in a tank model it is possible to feed a "reciprocally reciprocal" current to the dipole in the conductor and to measure the signal from the lead. However, the result may be interpreted as having been obtained by feeding the reciprocal current to the lead with the signal measured from the dipole. The benefit of this "reciprocally reciprocal" arrangement is that for technical reasons the signal-to-noise ratio may be improved while we still have the benefit of interpreting the result as the distribution of the lead field current in the volume conductor (Malmivuo, 1976).

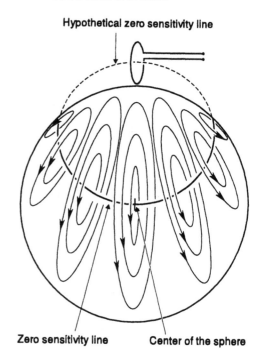

Fig. 12.11 Magnetic lead fields in volume conductors exhibiting spherical symmetry are always directed tangentially. The figure illustrates also the approximate form of the zero sensitivity line in the volume conductor. (The zero sensitivity line may be imagined to continue hypothetically through the magnetometer coil.)

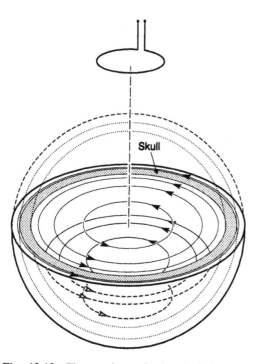

Fig. 12.10 The poorly conducting skull does not affect the magnetic detection of the electric activity of the brain.

12.10   THE INDEPENDENCE OF BIOELECTRIC AND BIOMAGNETIC FIELDS AND MEASUREMENTS

12.10.1   Independence of Flow and Vortex Sources

Helmholtz's theorem (Morse and Feshbach, 1953; Plonsey and Collin, 1961) states:

A general vector field, that vanishes at infinity, can be completely represented as the sum of two independent vector fields; one that is irrotational (zero curl) and another that is solenoidal (zero divergence).

The impressed current density $\bar{J}^i$ is a vector field that vanishes at infinity and, according to the theorem, may be expressed as the sum of two components:

$$\bar{J}^i = \bar{J}^i_F + \bar{J}^i_V \qquad (12.28)$$

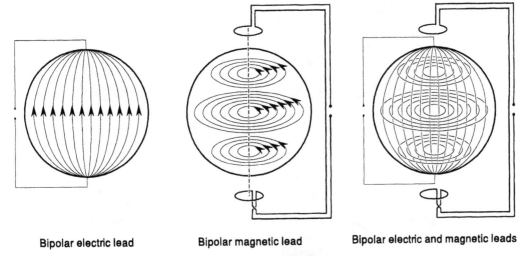

Bipolar electric lead   Bipolar magnetic lead   Bipolar electric and magnetic leads

Fig. 12.12 If the electrodes of a symmetric bipolar electric lead are located on the symmetry axis of the bipolar magnetic field detector arranged for a spherical volume conductor, these lead fields of the electric and magnetic leads are normal to each other throughout the volume conductor.

where F and V denote *flow* and *vortex*, respectively. By definition, these vector fields satisfy $\nabla \times \bar{J}_F^i = 0$ and $\nabla \cdot \bar{J}_V^i = 0$.

We first examine the independence of the electric and magnetic signals in the infinite homogeneous case, when the second term on the right-hand side of Equations 7.10 and 12.6, caused by inhomogeneities, is zero. These equations may be rewritten for the electric potential:

$$4\pi\sigma\Phi = \int_v \nabla\left(\frac{1}{r}\right) \cdot \bar{J}^i dv = \int_v \frac{\nabla \cdot \bar{J}^i}{r}\,dv$$
$$(12.29)$$

and for the magnetic field:

$$4\pi\bar{H} = -\int_v \nabla\left(\frac{1}{r}\right) \times \bar{J}^i dv = -\int_v \frac{\nabla \times \bar{J}^i}{r}\,dv$$
$$(12.30)$$

Substituting Equation 12.28 into Equations 12.29 and 12.30 shows that under homogeneous and unbounded conditions, the bioelectric field arises from $\nabla \cdot \bar{J}_F^i$, which is the *flow source* (Equation 7.5), and the biomagnetic field arises from $\nabla \times \bar{J}_V^i$, which is the *vortex source* (Equation 12.17). Since the detection of the first biomagnetic field, the magnetocardiogram, by Baule and McFee in 1963 (Baule and McFee, 1963), the demonstration discussed above

raised a great deal of optimism among scientists. If this independence were confirmed, the magnetic detection of bioelectric activity could bring much new information not available by electric measurement.

Rush was the first to claim that the independence of the electric and magnetic signals is only a mathematical possibility and that physical constraints operate which require the flow and vortex sources, and, consequently, the electric and magnetic fields, to be fundamentally interdependent in homogeneous volume conductors (Rush, 1975). This may be easily illustrated with an example by noting that, for instance, when the atria of the heart contract, their bioelectric activity produces an electric field recorded as the P-wave in the ECG. At the same time their electric activity produces a magnetic field detected as the P-wave of the MCG. Similarly, the electric and magnetic QRS-complexes and T-waves are interrelated, respectively. Thus, full independence between the ECG and the MCG is impossible.

In a more recent communication, Plonsey (1982) showed that the primary cellular source may be small compared to the secondary cellular source and that the latter may be characterized as a double layer source for both the electric scalar and magnetic vector potentials.

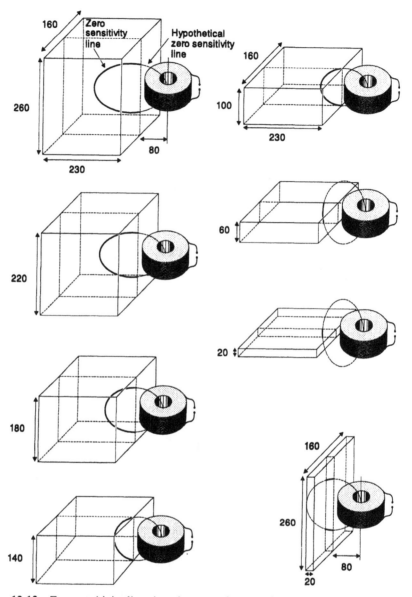

Fig. 12.13 Zero sensitivity lines in volume conductors of various forms. The dimensions are given in millimeters (Eskola, 1979, 1983; Eskola and Malmivuo, 1983). As in Figure 12.11, the zero sensitivity lines are illustrated to continue hypothetically through the magnetometer coils.

12.10.2 Lead Field Theoretic Explanation of the Independence of Bioelectric and Biomagnetic Fields and Measurements

The question of the independence of the electric and magnetic fields of a volume source and the interpretation of Helmholtz's theorem can be better explained using the lead field theory. We discuss this question in connection with the equivalent electric and magnetic dipoles of a volume source. The discussion can, of course, be easily extended to more complex source models as well.

As explained in Section 11.6.6 the electric lead field is given by Equation 11.54. As discussed in Section 11.6.7, the lead system detecting the electric dipole moment of a volume source includes three orthogonal, linear, and homogeneous reciprocal electric fields $\overline{E}_{\mathrm{LE}}$

which raise three orthogonal, linear, and homogeneous electric lead fields $\bar{J}_{LE}$. These three leads are mutually independent and they detect the three orthogonal components of the flow source.

As discussed in Section 12.3 the magnetic lead field is given by Equation 12.11. It was shown in Section 12.5 that the lead system detecting the magnetic dipole moment of a volume source includes three orthogonal, linear, and homogeneous reciprocal magnetic fields $\bar{B}_{LM}$ which raise three orthogonal circular magnetic lead fields $\bar{J}_{LM}$. These three leads are mutually independent and they detect the three orthogonal components of the vortex source.

In the aforementioned example, owing to Helmholtz's theorem, the three independent electric *leads* are independent of the three independent magnetic *leads*. In other words, no one of these six leads is a linear combination of the other five. However, in the case of a physiological volume source, the electric and magnetic *fields* and their three plus three orthogonal components which these six leads detect are not fully independent, because when the source is active, it generates all the three plus three components of the electric and magnetic fields in a way that links them together. Consequently, while all these six leads of a vector-electromagnetic lead system have the capability to sense independent aspects of a source, that capability is not necessarily realized.

It will be shown in Chapter 20 in the discussion of magnetocardiography that when measuring the electric and magnetic dipole moments of a volume source, both methods include three independent leads and include about the same amount of information from the source. The information of these methods is, however, different and therefore the patient groups which are diagnosed correctly with either method are not identical. If in the diagnosis the electric and magnetic signals are used simultaneously, the correctly diagnosed patient groups may be combined and the overall diagnostic performance increases. This may also be explained by noting that in the combined method we have altogether $3 + 3 = 6$ independent leads. This increases the total amount of information obtained from the source.

12.11 SENSITIVITY DISTRIBUTION OF BASIC MAGNETIC LEADS

PRECONDITIONS:

Source: *Volume source*
Conductor: *Finite, inhomogeneous, cylindrically symmetric*

12.11.1 The Equations for Calculating the Sensitivity Distribution of Basic Magnetic Leads

Because in an infinite homogeneous volume conductor the magnetic lead field flow lines encircle the symmetry axis, it is easy to calculate the sensitivity distribution of a magnetic lead in a cylindrically symmetric volume conductor, whose symmetry axis coincides with the magnetometer axis. Then the results may be displayed as a function of the distance from the symmetry axis with the distance from the detector as a parameter (Malmivuo, 1976).

Figure 12.14 illustrates the magnetometer coil L_1 and one coaxially situated lead field current flow line L_2. The magnetic flux F_{21} that links the loop L_2 due to the reciprocally ener-

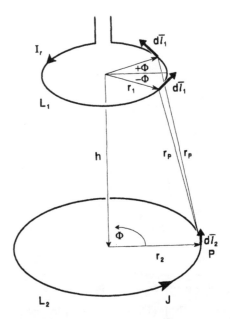

Fig. 12.14 Geometry for calculating the spatial sensitivity of a magnetometer in a cylindrically symmetric situation.

gizing current I_r in the magnetometer coil is most readily calculated using the magnetic vector potential $\bar{A}$ at the loop L_2 (Smythe, 1968, p. 290).

Faraday's law states that a time-varying magnetic field induces electromotive forces whose line integral around a closed loop equals the rate of change of the enclosed flux

$$\oint \bar{E} \cdot d\bar{l} = \frac{dF}{dt} \qquad (12.31)$$

where $F = \int \bar{B} \cdot \bar{n}\, da$ is the magnetic flux evaluated by the integral of the normal component of the magnetic induction $\bar{B}$ across the surface of the loop. For a circular loop the integral on the left-hand side of Equation 12.31 equals $2\pi r E$, where r is the radius of the loop, and we obtain for the current density

$$J = \sigma E = \frac{\sigma}{2\pi r}\frac{dF}{dt} \qquad (12.32)$$

where σ is the conductivity of the medium. The current density is tangentially oriented. Now the problem reduces to the determination of the magnetic flux linking a circular loop in the medium due to a reciprocally energizing current in the coaxially situated magnetometer coil.

The basic equation for calculating the vector potential at point P due to a current I flowing in a thin conductor is

$$\bar{A}_P = \frac{\mu}{4\pi} \oint \frac{I\,d\bar{l}}{r_P} \qquad (12.33)$$

where

μ = magnetic permeability of the medium
r_P = distance from the conductor element to the point P

This equation can be used to calculate the vector potential at the point P in Figure 12.14. From symmetry we know that in spherical coordinates the magnitude of $\bar{A}$ is independent of angle ϕ. Therefore, for simplicity, we choose the point P so that $\phi = 0$. We notice that when equidistant elements of length $d\bar{l}_1$ at $+\phi$ and $-\phi$ are paired, the resultant is normal to hr. Thus $\bar{A}$ has only the single component A_ϕ. If we let dl_ϕ be the component of $d\bar{l}_1$ in this di-

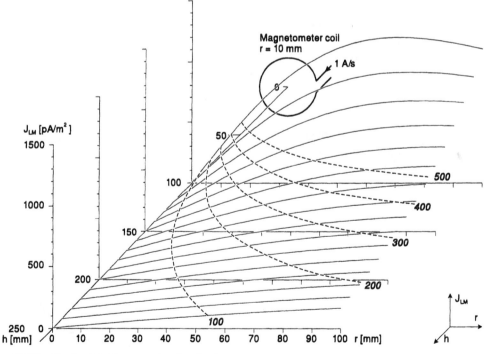

Fig. 12.15 The lead field current density distribution of a unipolar single-coil magnetometer with a 10 mm coil radius in a cylindrically symmetric volume conductor calculated from Equation 12.42. The dashed lines are the *isosensitivity lines,* joining the points where the lead field current density is 100, 200, 300, 400, and 500 pA/m², respectively, as indicated by the numbers in italics.

rection, then Equation 12.33 may be rewritten as

$$A_\phi = \frac{\mu I_R}{4\pi} \oint_{L_1} \frac{dl_\phi}{r_P} = \frac{\mu I_R}{4\pi} \oint_{L_1} \frac{dl_1 \cos\phi}{r_P}$$

$$= \frac{\mu I_R}{2\pi} \int_0^\pi \frac{r_1 \cos\phi \, d\phi}{(r_1^2 + r_2^2 + h^2 - 2r_1 r_2 \cos\phi)^{1/2}}$$

$$(12.34)$$

The magnetic flux F_{21} may be calculated from the vector potential:

$$F_{21} = \oint_{L_2} \bar{A}_2 \cdot d\bar{l}_2 = 2\pi r_2 A_\phi \quad (12.35)$$

With the substitution $\phi = \pi - 2\alpha$, this becomes

$$F_{21} = \mu I_R \sqrt{r_1 r_2} \int_0^{\pi/2} \frac{k(2\sin^2\alpha - 1)}{\sqrt{1 - k^2\sin^2\alpha}} \, d\alpha$$

$$= \mu I_R \sqrt{h^2 + (r_1 + r_2)^2}$$

$$\left[\left(1 - \frac{k^2}{2}\right) K(k) - E(k) \right] \quad (12.36)$$

where

$$k^2 = \frac{4r_1 r_2}{h^2 + (r_1 + r_2)^2} \quad (12.37)$$

and $K(k)$ and $E(k)$ are complete elliptic integrals of the first and second kind, respectively. These are calculated from Equations 12.38A,B. (Abramowitz and Stegun, 1964, p. 590)

$$K\left(k, \frac{\pi}{2}\right) = \int_0^{\pi/2} (1 - k^2\sin^2\phi)^{-1/2} \, d\phi$$

$$(12.38A)$$

$$E\left(k, \frac{\pi}{2}\right) = \int_0^{\pi/2} (1 - k^2\sin^2\phi)^{1/2} \, d\phi$$

$$(12.38B)$$

The values $K(k)$ and $E(k)$ can also be calculated using the series:

$$K\left(k, \frac{\pi}{2}\right) = \frac{\pi}{2} \left[1 + \left[\frac{1}{2}\right]^2 k^2 + \left[\frac{3}{2 \cdot 4}\right]^2 k^4 \right.$$

$$\left. + \left[\frac{3 \cdot 5}{2 \cdot 4 \cdot 6}\right]^2 k^6 + \cdots \right]$$

$$(12.39A)$$

$$E\left(k, \frac{\pi}{3}\right) = \frac{\pi}{2} \left[1 - \left[\frac{1}{2}\right]^2 k^2 - \left[\frac{3}{2 \cdot 4}\right]^2 \frac{k^4}{3} \right.$$

$$\left. - \left[\frac{3 \cdot 5}{2 \cdot 4 \cdot 6}\right]^2 \frac{k^6}{5} - \cdots \right]$$

$$(12.39B)$$

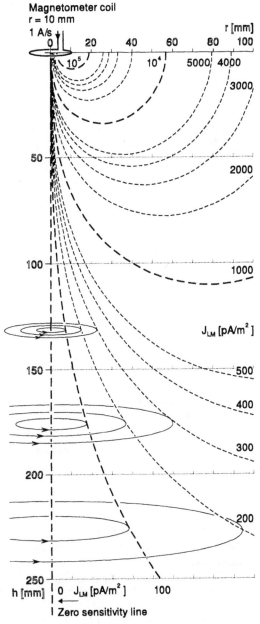

Fig. 12.16 The isosensitivity lines for a unipolar single-coil magnetometer of Figure 12.15; the coil radius is 10 mm, and the volume conductor is cylindrically symmetric. The vertical axis indicates the distance h from the magnetometer and the horizontal axis the radial distance r from the symmetry axis. The symmetry axis, drawn with a thick dashed line, is the *zero sensitivity line*. Thin solid lines represent lead field current flow lines.

The calculation of $K(k)$ and $E(k)$ is faster from the series, but they give inaccurate results at small distances from the coil and therefore the

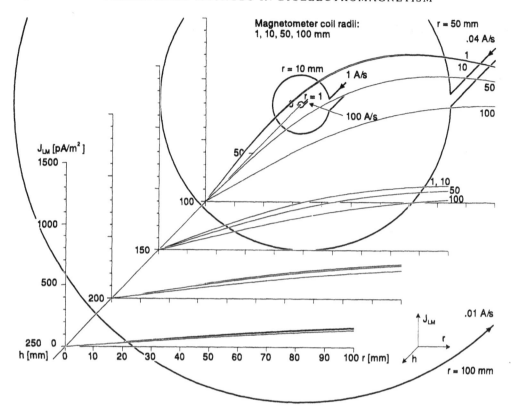

Fig. 12.17 Lead field current density for unipolar leads of coils with 1 mm, 10 mm, 50 mm, and 100 mm radii. The energizing current in the coils is normalized in relation to the coil area to obtain a constant dipole moment.

use of the Equations 12.38A,B is recommended.

Substituting Equation 12.36 into Equation 12.32 gives the lead field current density J_{LM} as a function of the rate of change of the coil current in the reciprocally energized magnetometer:

$$J_{LM} = \frac{\sigma 4\pi \cdot 10^{-7}}{2\pi r_2} \sqrt{h^2 + (r_1 + r_2)^2} \cdot$$
$$\left[\left(1 - \frac{k^2}{2} \right) K(k) - E(k) \right] \frac{dI_r}{dt} \quad (12.40)$$

Because we are interested in the spatial sensitivity distribution and not in the absolute sensitivity with certain frequency or conductivity values, the result of Equation 12.40 can be normalized by defining (similarly as was done in Section 12.3.1 in deriving the equation for magnetic lead field)

$$\frac{dI_r}{dt} = 1$$
$$\sigma = 1 \quad (12.41)$$

and we obtain the equation for calculating the lead field current density for a single-coil magnetometer in an infinite homogeneous volume conductor:

$$J_{LM} = \frac{2 \cdot 10^{-7}}{r_2} \sqrt{h^2 + (r_1 + r_2)^2} \cdot$$
$$\left[\left(1 - \frac{k^2}{2} \right) K(k) - E(k) \right] \quad (12.42)$$

where all distances are measured in meters, and current density in [A/m²].

If the distance h is large compared to the coil radius r_1 and the lead field current flow line radius r_2, the magnetic induction inside the flow line may be considered constant, and Equation 12.42 is greatly simplified. The value of the magnetic flux becomes πr^2. Substituting it into Equation 12.32, we obtain

$$J_{LM} = \frac{\sigma r}{2} \frac{dB}{dt} \quad (12.43)$$

The magnetic induction may be calculated in this situation as for a dipole source. Equation

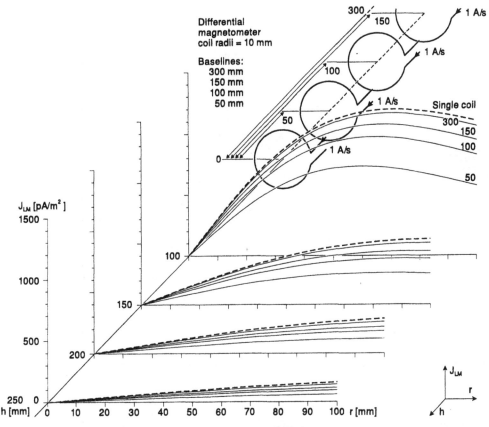

Fig. 12.18 Lead field current density for unipolar leads realized with differential magnetometers of 10 mm coil radius and with 300 mm, 150 mm, 100 mm, and 50 mm baseline.

12.43 shows clearly that in the region of constant magnetic induction and constant conductivity, the lead field current density is proportional to the radial distance from the symmetry axis. Note that this equation is consistent with Equation 12.11.

12.11.2 Lead Field Current Density of a Unipolar Lead of a Single-Coil Magnetometer

Owing to symmetry, the lead field current density is independent of the angle ϕ in Figure 12.14. Therefore, the lead field current density may be plotted as a function of the radial distance r from the symmetry axis with the distance h from the magnetometer as a parameter. Figure 12.15 shows the lead field current density distribution of a unipolar lead created by a single-coil magnetometer with a 10 mm coil radius in a cylindrically symmetric volume conductor calculated from Equation 12.42. The lead field current density is directed in the tangential direction. (With proper scaling, the figure may be used for studying different measurement distances.)

Figure 12.15 shows that in a unipolar lead the lead field current density is strongly dependent on the magnetometer coil distance. It also shows the small size of the region where the lead field current density increases approximately linearly as a function of the radial distance from the symmetry axis, especially in the vicinity of the coil.

The dashed lines in Figure 12.15 are the *isosensitivity lines*; these join the points where the lead field current density is 100, 200, 300, 400, and 500 pA/m² respectively, as indicated by the numbers in italics.

Figure 12.16 illustrates the isosensitivity lines for a unipolar single-coil magnetometer of Figure 12.15; the coil radius is 10 mm, and

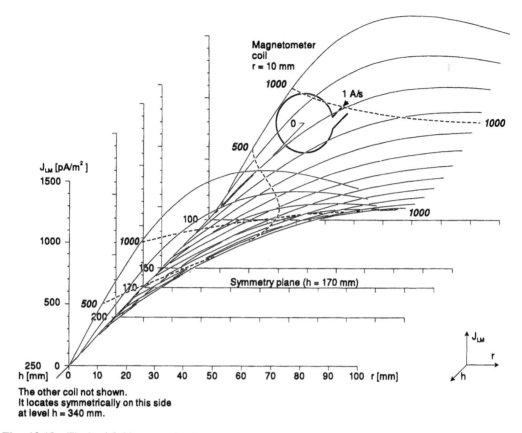

The other coil not shown.
It locates symmetrically on this side
at level h = 340 mm.

Fig. 12.19 The lead field current density distribution of a bipolar lead in a cylindrically symmetric volume conductor realized with two coaxial single-coil magnetometers with 10 mm coil radius. The distance between the coils is 340 mm. The dashed lines are the *isosensitivity lines,* joining the points where the lead field current density is 500 and 1000 pA/m², respectively, as indicated with the numbers in italics.

the volume conductor is cylindrically symmetric. The vertical axis indicates the distance h from the magnetometer and the horizontal axis the radial distance r from the symmetry axis. The symmetry axis, drawn with thick dashed line, is the *zero sensitivity line.* The lead field current flow lines are concentric circles around the symmetry axis. To illustrate this, the figure shows three flow lines representing the current densities 100, 200, and 300 pA/m² at the levels h = 125 mm, 175 mm, and 225 mm. As in the previous figure, the lead field current density values are calculated for a reciprocal current of I_R = 1 A/s.

The effect of the coil radius in a unipolar lead on the lead field current density is shown in Figure 12.17. In this figure, the lead field current density is illustrated for coils with 1 mm, 10 mm, 50 mm, and 100 mm radii. The energizing current in the coils is normalized in

relation to the coil area to obtain a constant dipole moment. The 10 mm radius coil is energized with a current of dI/dt = 1 [A/s].

12.11.3   The Effect of the Distal Coil to the Lead Field of a Unipolar Lead

Because of the small signal-to-noise ratio of the biomagnetic signals, measurements are usually made with a first- or second-order gradiometer. The first-order gradiometer is a magnetometer including two coaxial coils separated by a certain distance, called *baseline.* The coils are wound in opposite directions. Because the magnetic fields of distant (noise) sources are equal in both coils, they are canceled. The magnetic field of a source close to one of the coils produces a stronger signal in the proximal coil (i.e., the coil closer to the source) than in the distal coil (farther from the source), and the difference of these fields is detected. The magnetometer sensitivity to the source is diminished by the distal coil by an amount that is greater the shorter the baseline. The distal coil also increases the *proximity effect*—that is, the sensitivity of the differential magnetometer as a function of the distance to the source decreases faster than that of a single-coil magnetometer.

Figure 12.18 illustrates the lead field current density for unipolar leads realized with differential magnetometers (i.e., gradiometers). Lead field current density *J is illustrated with various baselines* as a function of radial distance *r* from the symmetry axis with the magnetometer distance *h* as a parameter. The differential magnetometers have a 10 mm coil radius and a 300 mm, 150 mm, 100 mm, and 50 mm baseline.

12.11.4 Lead Field Current Density of a Bipolar Lead

As discussed in Section 12.7 and illustrated in Figure 12.5, when detecting the dipole moment of a volume source with dimensions which are large compared to the measurement distance, the lead field within the source area is much more ideal if a bipolar lead instead of a unipolar one is used. Figure 12.19 shows the lead field current density distribution of a bipolar lead in a cylindrically symmetric volume conductor realized with two coaxial single-coil magnetometers with 10 mm coil radius. The distance between the coils is 340 mm. Note that in the bipolar lead arrangement the coils are wound in the same direction and the source is located between the coils. The lead field current density as the function of radial distance is lowest on the symmetry plane, that is, on the plane located in the middle of the two coils. Because the two coils compensate each other's proximity effect, the lead field current density does not change very much as a function of distance from the coils in the vicinity of the symmetry plane. This is illustrated with the isosensitivity line of 500 pA/m². Therefore, the bipolar lead forms a very ideal lead field for detecting the dipole moment of a volume source.

Figure 12.20 illustrates the lead field current density for the bipolar lead of Figure 12.19 with isosensitivity lines. This figure shows still more clearly than the previous one the compensating

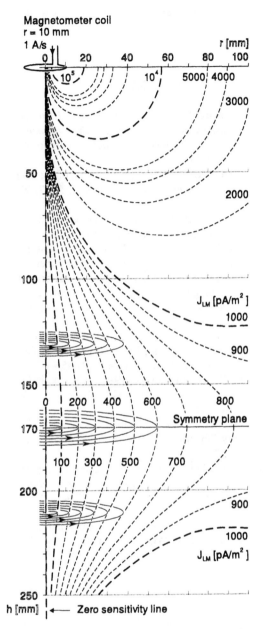

Fig. 12.20 The isosensitivity lines for the bipolar lead of Figure 12.19. The coil radii are 10 mm and the distance between the coils is 340 mm. The vertical axis indicates the distance *h* from the first magnetometer and the horizontal axis the radial distance *r* from the symmetry axis. The symmetry axis, drawn with thick dashed line, is the *zero sensitivity line*. Lead field current flow lines encircle the symmetry axis and are illustrated with thin solid lines.

effect of the two coils in the vicinity of the symmetry plane, especially with short radial distances. The lead field current flows tangentially around the symmetry axis. The flow lines are represented in the figure with thin solid lines.

REFERENCES

Abramowitz M, Stegun IA (eds.) (1964): *Handbook of Mathematical Functions with Formulas, Graphs, and Mathematical Tables*, 1046 pp. Wiley, New York.

Baule GM, McFee R (1963): Detection of the magnetic field of the heart. *Am. Heart J.* 55:(7) 95–6.

Eskola H (1979): Properties of the unipositional lead system in the measurement of the vector magnetocardiogram. *Tampere Univ. Tech., Tampere, Finland*, pp. 72. (In Finnish) (Master's thesis)

Eskola H (1983): On the properties of vector magnetocardiographic leads. *Tampere Univ. Tech., Tampere, Finland*, Thesis, pp. 154. (Dr. tech. thesis)

Eskola HJ, Malmivuo JA (1983): Optimizing vector magnetocardiographic lead fields by using physical torso model. *Nuovo Cim.* 2:(2) 356–67.

Estola K-P, Malmivuo JA (1982): Air-Core induction coil magnetometer design. *J. Phys. E.: Sci. Instrum.* 15: 1110–3.

Faraday M (1834): Experimental researches on electricity, 7th series. *Phil. Trans. R. Soc. (Lond.)* 124: 77–122.

Geselowitz DB (1970): On the magnetic field generated outside an inhomogeneous volume conductor by internal current sources. *IEEE Trans. Magn.* MAG-6:(2) 346–7.

Jackson JD (1975): *Classical Electrodynamics*, 2nd ed., 84 pp. John Wiley, New York.

Malmivuo JA (1976): On the detection of the magnetic heart vector—An application of the reciprocity theorem. *Helsinki Univ. Tech.*, Acta Polytechn. Scand., El. Eng. Series. Vol. 39., pp. 112. (Dr. tech. thesis)

Malmivuo JA (1980): Distribution of MEG detector sensitivity: An application of reciprocity. *Med. & Biol. Eng. & Comput.* 18:(3) 365–70.

Malmivuo JA, Lekkala JO, Kontro P, Suomaa L, Vihinen H (1987): Improvement of the properties of an eddy current magnetic shield with active compensation. *J. Phys. E.: Sci. Instrum.* 20:(1) 151–64.

Morse PM, Feshbach H (1953): *Methods of Theoretical Physics. Part I*, 997 pp. McGraw-Hill, New York.

Plonsey R (1972): Capability and limitations of electrocardiography and magnetocardiography. *IEEE Trans. Biomed. Eng.* BME-19:(3) 239–44.

Plonsey R (1982): The nature of sources of bioelectric and biomagnetic fields. *Biophys. J.* 39: 309–19.

Plonsey R, Collin RE (1961): *Principles and Applications of Electromagnetic Fields*, 554 pp. McGraw-Hill, New York.

Rush S (1975): On the interdependence of magnetic and electric body surface recordings. *IEEE Trans. Biomed. Eng.* BME-22: 157–67.

Smythe WR (1968): *Static and Dynamic Electricity*, 3rd ed., 623 pp. McGraw-Hill, New York.

Stratton JA (1941): *Electromagnetic Theory*, McGraw-Hill, New York.

Williamson SJ, Romani G-L, Kaufman L, Modena I (eds.) (1983): *Biomagnetism: An Interdisciplinary Approach. NATO ASI Series, Series A: Life Sciences*, Vol. 66, 706 pp. Plenum Press, New York.

IV

Electric and Magnetic Measurement of the Electric Activity of Neural Tissue

The remainder of this book focuses on clinical applications. Parts IV and V discuss the detection of bioelectric and biomagnetic signals, classified on an anatomical basis, as having neural and cardiac tissues as their sources, respectively. Within these parts the discussion is then further divided between bioelectricity and biomagnetism to point out the parallelism between them.

A wide variety of applications for bioelectric measurements are utilized in neurophysiology. These include measurements on both peripheral nerves and on the central nervous system as well as neuromuscular studies. The basic bioelectromagnetic theory underlying them all is, however, the same. For this reason, and because it is not the purpose of this book to serve as a clinical reference, the aforementioned applications are included in but not discussed here systematically.

Theoretically, especially with respect to volume conductors, the measurement principle of *electroencephalography (EEG)* is most interesting in the clinical applications of bioelectricity in neurology. Therefore, only this method is discussed in Chapter 13.

Similarly, in Chapter 14, in order to show the relationship between electric and magnetic measurements of the bioelectric activity of the brain, the *magnetoencephalogram (MEG)* is cited as an example of biomagnetic measurements in neurology.

13

Electroencephalography

13.1 INTRODUCTION

The first recording of the electric field of the human brain was made by the German psychiatrist Hans Berger in 1924 in Jena. He gave this recording the name *electroencephalogram* *(EEG)* (Berger, 1929). (From 1929 to 1938 he published 20 scientific papers on the EEG under the same title "Über das Elektroenkephalogram des Menschen.")

The electric activity of the brain is usually divided into three categories:

1. spontaneous activity,
2. evoked potentials, and
3. bioelectric events produced by single neurons.

Spontaneous activity is measured on the scalp or on the brain and is called the electroencephalogram. The amplitude of the EEG is about 100 μV when measured on the scalp, and about 1–2 mV when measured on the surface of the brain. The bandwidth of this signal is from under 1 Hz to about 50 Hz, as demonstrated in Figure 13.1. As the phrase "spontaneous activity" implies, this activity goes on continuously in the living individual.

Evoked potentials are those components of the EEG that arise in response to a stimulus (which may be electric, auditory, visual, etc.).

Such signals are usually below the noise level and thus not readily distinguished, and one must use a train of stimuli and signal averaging to improve the signal-to-noise ratio.

Single-neuron behavior can be examined through the use of microelectrodes which impale the cells of interest. Through studies of the single cell, one hopes to build models of cell networks that will reflect actual tissue properties.

13.2 THE BRAIN AS A BIOELECTRIC GENERATOR

PRECONDITIONS:

Source: *Distribution of impressed current source elements $\bar{J}^i$ (volume source)*

Conductor: *Finite, inhomogeneous*

The number of nerve cells in the brain has been estimated to be on the order of 10^{11}. Cortical neurons are strongly interconnected. Here the surface of a single neuron may be covered with 1,000–100,000 synapses (Nunez, 1981). The electric behavior of the neuron corresponds to the description of excitable cells introduced in the earlier chapters. The resting voltage is around −70 mV, and the peak of the action

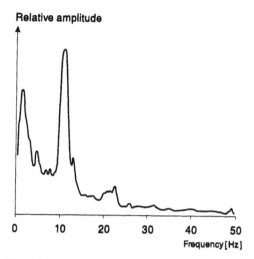

Relative amplitude

0   10   20   30   40   50

Frequency [Hz]

Fig. 13.1   Frequency spectrum of normal EEG.

potential is positive. The amplitude of the nerve impulse is about 100 mV; it lasts about 1 ms.

The bioelectric impressed current density $\bar{J}^i$ associated with neuronal activation produces an electric field, which can be measured on the surface of the head or directly on the brain tissue. The electric field was described by Equation 7.10 for a finite inhomogeneous model. This equation is repeated here:

$$4\pi\sigma\Phi(r) = \int_v \bar{J}^i \cdot \nabla\left(\frac{1}{r}\right)dv$$
$$+ \sum_j \int_{S_j} (\sigma_j'' - \sigma_j')\Phi\nabla\left(\frac{1}{r}\right) \cdot d\bar{S}_j$$
$$(7.10)$$

While for most excitable tissue the basis for the impressed current density $\bar{J}^i$ is the propagating action potential, for the EEG it appears to arise from the action of a chemical transmitter on postsynaptic cortical neurons. The action causes localized depolarization—that is, an excitatory postsynaptic potential (EPSP)—or hyperpolarization—that is, an inhibitory postsynaptic potential (IPSP). The result in either case is a spatially distributed discontinuity in the function $\sigma\Phi$ (i.e., $\sigma_o\Phi_o - \sigma_i\Phi_i$) which, as pointed out in Equation 8.28, evaluates a double-layer source in the membranes of all cells. This will be zero for resting cells; however, when a cell is active by any of the aforementioned processes (in which case $\Phi_o - \Phi_i = V_m$ varies over a cell surface), a nonzero primary source will result.

For distant field points the double layer can be summed up vectorially, yielding a net dipole for each active cell. Since neural tissue is generally composed of a very large number of small, densely packed cells, the discussion in Section 8.5 applies, leading to the identification of a continuous volume source distribution $\bar{J}^i$ which appears in Equations 7.6 and 7.10.

Although in principle the EEG can be found from the evaluation of Equation 7.10, the complexity of brain structure and its electrophysiological behavior have thus far precluded the evaluation of the source function $\bar{J}^i$. Consequently, the quantitative study of the EEG differs from that of the ECG or EMG, in which it is possible to evaluate the source function. Under these conditions the quantitative EEG is based on a statistical treatment, whereas the clinical EEG is largely empirical.

13.3   EEG LEAD SYSTEMS

The internationally standardized *10–20 system* is usually employed to record the spontaneous EEG. In this system 21 electrodes are located on the surface of the scalp, as shown in Figure 13.2A and B. The positions are determined as follows: Reference points are *nasion*, which is the delve at the top of the nose, level with the eyes; and *inion*, which is the bony lump at the base of the skull on the midline at the back of the head. From these points, the skull perimeters are measured in the transverse and median planes. Electrode locations are determined by dividing these perimeters into 10% and 20% intervals. Three other electrodes are placed on each side equidistant from the neighboring points, as shown in Figure 13.2B (Jasper, 1958; Cooper, Osselton, and Shaw, 1969).

In addition to the 21 electrodes of the international 10–20 system, intermediate 10% electrode positions are also used. The locations and nomenclature of these electrodes are standardized by the American Electroencephalographic Society (Sharbrough et al., 1991; see Fig. 13.2C). In this recommendation, four electrodes have different names compared to the 10–20 system; these are T_7, T_8, P_7, and P_8. These electrodes are drawn black with white text in the figure.

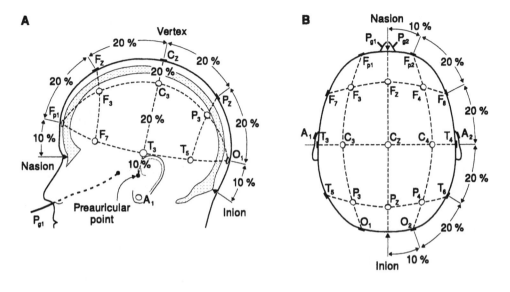

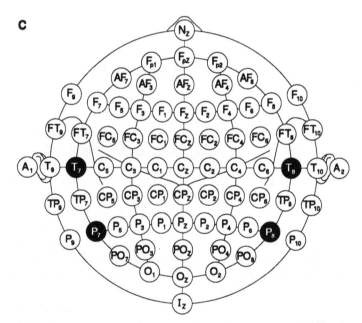

Fig. 13.2 The international 10–20 system seen from (A) left and (B) above the head. A = Ear lobe, C = central, Pg = nasopharyngeal, P = parietal, F = frontal, Fp = frontal polar, and O = occipital.

(C) Location and nomenclature of the intermediate 10% electrodes, as standardized by the American Electroencephalographic Society. (Redrawn from Sharbrough, 1991.)

Besides the international 10–20 system, many other electrode systems exist for recording electric potentials on the scalp. The *Queen Square system* of electrode placement has been proposed as a standard in recording the pattern

of evoked potentials in clinical testings (Blumhardt et al., 1977).

Bipolar or unipolar electrodes can be used in the EEG measurement. In the first method the potential difference between a pair of elec-

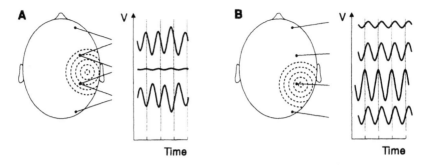

Fig. 13.3 (A) Bipolar and (B) unipolar measurements. Note that the waveform of the EEG depends on the measurement location.

trodes is measured. In the latter method the potential of each electrode is compared either to a neutral electrode or to the average of all electrodes (see Fig. 13.3). The most recent guidelines for EEG-recording are published in Gilmore (1994).

13.4 SENSITIVITY DISTRIBUTION OF EEG ELECTRODES

Rush and Driscoll (1969) calculated the sensitivity distribution of bipolar surface electrodes on the scalp based on a concentric spherical head model. They published the results in the form of lead field isopotential lines. The direction of the lead field current density—that is, the direction of the sensitivity—is a negative gradient of the potential field. This is not immediately evident from such a display.

Puikkonen and Malmivuo (1987) recalculated the sensitivity distribution of EEG electrodes with the same model as Rush and Driscoll, but they presented the results with the lead field current flow lines instead of the isopotential lines of the lead field. This display is illustrative since it is easy to find the direction of the sensitivity from the lead field current flow

lines. Also the magnitude of the sensitivity can be seen from the density of the flow lines. A minor problem in this display is that because the lead field current distributes both in the plane of the illustration as well as in the plane normal to it, part of the flow lines must break in order to illustrate correctly the current density with the flow line density in a three-dimensional problem. Suihko, Malmivuo, and Eskola (1993) calculated further the isosensitivity lines and the *half-sensitivity* volume for the electric leads. As discussed in Section 11.6.1, the concept of half-sensitivity volume denotes the region where the lead field current density is at least one half of its maximum value. Thus this concept is a figure of merit to describe how concentrated the sensitivity distribution of the lead is. As discussed in Section 11.6.6, when the conductivity is isotropic, as it is in this head model, the isosensitivity lines follow the isofield lines of the (reciprocal) electric field. If the lead would exhibit such a symmetry that adjacent isopotential surfaces would be a constant distance apart, the isosensitivity lines would coincide with the isopotential lines. That is not the case in the leads of Figure 13.4.

Figure 13.4 displays the lead field current flow lines, isosensitivity lines and half-sensitivity volumes for the spherical head model with

Fig. 13.4 Sensitivity distribution of EEG electrodes in the spherical head model. The figure illustrates the lead field current flow line (thin solid lines), isosensitivity lines (dotted lines) and the half-sensitivity volumes (shaded region). The sensitivity distribution is in the direction of the flow lines, and

its magnitude is proportional to the density of the flow lines. The lead pair are designated by small arrows at the surface of the scalp and are separated by an angle of 180°, 120°, 60°, 40°, and 20° shown at the top of each figure.

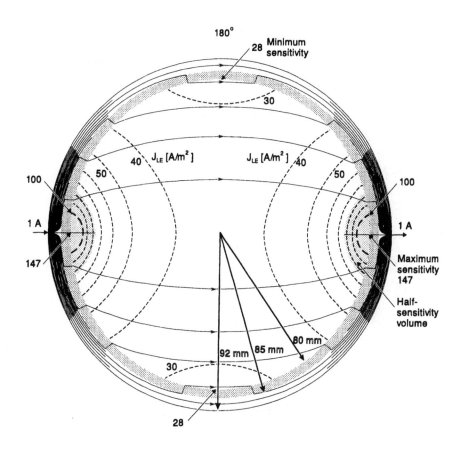

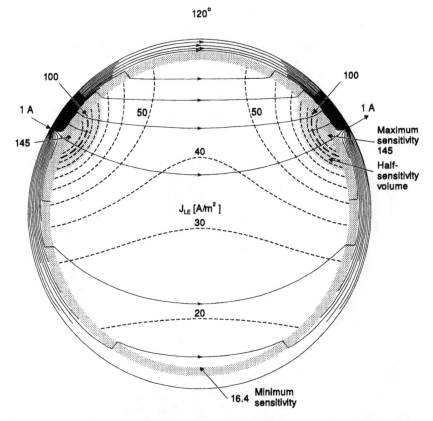

261

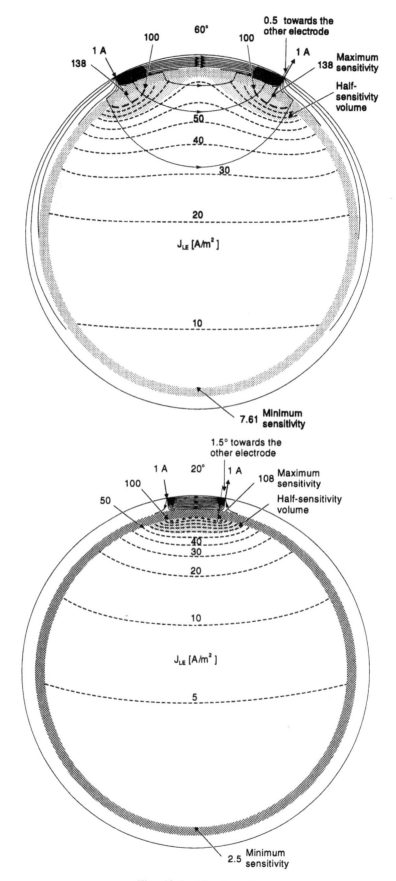

Fig. 13.4 (*Continued*)

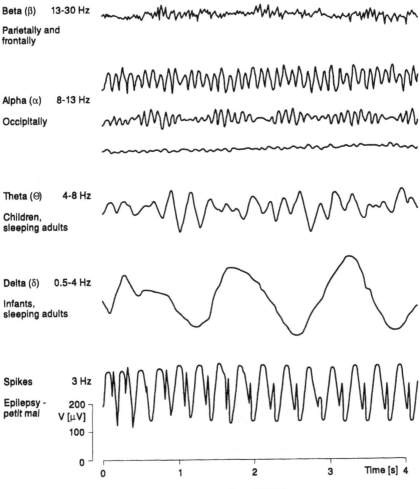

Fig. 13.5 Some examples of EEG waves.

the electrodes located within 180°, 120°, 60°, and 20° angles. Note that in each case the two electrodes are connected by 10 continuous lead field flow lines. Between them are three flow lines shown broken prior to the center, indicating that the lead field current also distributes in the plane normal to the paper. The figure shows clearly the strong effect of the poorly conducting skull to the lead field. Though in a homogeneous model the sensitivity would be highly concentrated at the electrodes, in the 180° case the skull allows the sensitivity to be more homogeneously distributed throughout the brain region. The closer the electrodes are to each other, the smaller the part of the sensitivity that locates within the brain region. Locating the electrodes closer and closer to each

other causes the lead field current to flow more and more within the scalp region, decreasing the sensitivity in the brain region and increasing the noise.

13.5 THE BEHAVIOR OF THE EEG SIGNAL

From the EEG signal it is possible to differentiate alpha (α), beta (β), delta (δ), and theta (Θ) waves as well as spikes associated with epilepsy. An example of each waveform is given in Figure 13.5.

The alpha waves have the frequency spectrum of 8–13 Hz and can be measured from the occipital region in an awake person when the

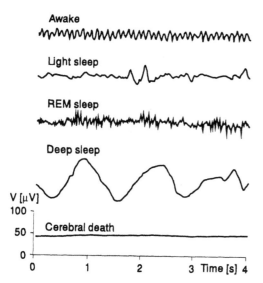

Fig. 13.6 EEG activity is dependent on the level of consciousness.

a characteristic EEG signal. In deep sleep, the EEG has large and slow deflections called delta waves. No cerebral activity can be detected from a patient with complete cerebral death. Examples of the above-mentioned waveforms are given in Figure 13.6.

REFERENCES

Berger H (1929): Über das Elektroenkephalogram des Menschen. *Arch. f. Psychiat.* 87: 527–70.

Blumhardt LD, Barrett G, Halliday AM, Kriss A (1977): The asymmetrical visual evoked potential to pattern reversal in one half field and its significance for the analysis of visual field effects. *Br. J. Ophthalmol.* 61: 454–61.

Cooper R, Osselton JW, Shaw JC (1969): *EEG Technology*, 2nd ed., 275 pp. Butterworths, London.

Gilmore RL (1994): American Electroencephalographic Society guidelines in electroencephalography, evoked potentials, and polysomnography. *J. Clin. Neurophysiol.* 11:(1, January) 147 pp.

Jasper HH (1958): Report of the Committee on Methods of Clinical Examination in Electroencephalography. *Electroenceph. Clin. Neurophysiol.* 10: 370–1.

Nunez PL (1981): *Electric Fields of the Brain: The Neurophysics of EEG*, 484 pp. Oxford University Press, New York.

Puikkonen J, Malmivuo JA (1987): Theoretical investigation of the sensitivity distribution of point EEG-electrodes on the three concentric spheres model of a human head—An application of the reciprocity theorem. *Tampere Univ. Techn., Inst. Biomed. Eng., Reports* 1:(5) 71.

Rush S, Driscoll DA (1969): EEG-electrode sensitivity—An application of reciprocity. *IEEE Trans. Biomed. Eng.* BME-16:(1) 15–22.

Sharbrough F, Chatrian Gian-E, Lesser RP, Lüders H, Nuwer M, Picton TW (1991): American Electroencephalographic Society Guidelines for Standard Electrode Position Nomenclature. *J. Clin. Neurophysiol* 8: 200–2.

Suihko V, Malmivuo JA, Eskola H (1993): Distribution of sensitivity of electric leads in an inhomogeneous spherical head model. *Tampere Univ. Techn., Ragnar Granit Inst., Rep.* 7:(2).

eyes are closed. The frequency band of the beta waves is 13–30 Hz; these are detectable over the parietal and frontal lobes. The delta waves have the frequency range of 0.5–4 Hz and are detectable in infants and sleeping adults. The theta waves have the frequency range of 4–8 Hz and are obtained from children and sleeping adults.

13.6   THE BASIC PRINCIPLES OF EEG DIAGNOSIS

The EEG signal is closely related to the level of consciousness of the person. As the activity increases, the EEG shifts to higher dominating frequency and lower amplitude. When the eyes are closed, the alpha waves begin to dominate the EEG. When the person falls asleep, the dominant EEG frequency decreases. In a certain phase of sleep, rapid eye movement called (REM) sleep, the person dreams and has active movements of the eyes, which can be seen as

14

Magnetoencephalography

14.1 THE BRAIN AS A BIOMAGNETIC GENERATOR

PRECONDITIONS:

Source: *Distribution of impressed current source elements $\bar{J}^i$ (volume source)*

Conductor: *Finite, inhomogeneous with spherical symmetry*

The bioelectric impressed current density $\bar{J}^i$ associated with brain activity produces an electric and a magnetic field. The magnetic field is given by Equation 12.6.

$$4\pi\bar{H}(r) = \int_v \bar{J}^i \times \nabla\left(\frac{1}{r}\right) dv$$
$$+ \sum_j \int_{S_j} (\sigma_j'' - \sigma_j')\Phi \nabla\left(\frac{1}{r}\right) \times d\bar{S}_j \quad (12.6)$$

This signal is called the *magnetoencephalogram* (MEG). David Cohen was the first to succeed in detecting the magnetic alpha rhythm. In this first successful experiment he used an induction coil magnetometer in a magnetically shielded room (Cohen, 1968). David Cohen was also the first scientist to detect the MEG with a point contact rf-SQUID in 1970 (Cohen, 1972). The amplitude of the MEG is less than 0.5 picotesla (pT) and its frequency range is similar to that of the EEG. Because the source

of the magnetic field as well as that of the electric field of the brain is the impressed current $\bar{J}^i$, these fields have a very similar appearance.

It should be noted again that the first term on the right side of Equation 12.6 represents the contribution of the bioelectric sources, whereas the second term represents the contribution of the inhomogeneities of the volume conductor. The reader can easily verify this fact by realizing that in a homogeneous conductor, the conductivities are equal on both sides of each interface of the piecewise homogeneous region described in Equation 12.6, and the difference $(\sigma_j'' - \sigma_j')$ is equal to zero.

In the cylindrically symmetric situation, the lead field flow lines do not cross the interfaces of the homogeneous regions in the piecewise homogeneous volume conductor and are therefore not affected by the inhomogeneities. (The spherically symmetric situation is a special case of cylindrical symmetry.) In the mathematical formula this is indicated by the fact that the second expression on the right side of Equation 12.6 does not contribute to the lead voltage V_{LM}. The reason for that is that in evaluating Equation 12.12 we must form the dot product *of the secondary source (which is in the radial direction) with the lead field (which is in the circumferential direction) and the result is equal to zero.*

The source of the MEG signal, as well as that of the EEG signal, is the electric activity of the brain. But as discussed in Chapter 12, the sensitivity distribution of the magnetic measurements differs essentially from the electric because the lead field current densities $\bar{J}_{LM}$ and $\bar{J}_{LE}$ have an essentially different form.

As discussed in Chapter 12, if the electrodes of an electric lead are placed on a spherical volume conductor (the head) and lie on the axis of symmetry of a magnetic lead, the electric and magnetic lead fields are normal to each other everywhere in the volume conductor, (Malmivuo, 1980; see also Fig. 12.2). In this special case, the MEG consequently allows detection of source components that are not sensed with the EEG. It is important to note that since the sensitivity of the magnetic leads are directed tangentially, the poor conductivity of the skull has no effect on the shape of the lead field.

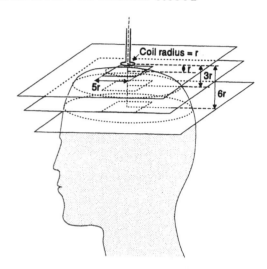

Fig. 14.1 Location of the planes for evaluating the sensitivity distribution of MEG lead systems.

14.2 SENSITIVITY DISTRIBUTION OF MEG LEADS

14.2.1 Sensitivity Calculation Method

In electroencephalography the head is modeled with concentric spheres. As discussed above, this model is valid and important also in magnetoencephalography. Because of the low signal level of MEG, the measurements are usually made as close to the head as possible. Since sensitivity decreases rapidly with distance, and since the detector coil radius is small compared to the dimensions of the head, the head can be successfully modeled as a half-space. This holds also for multichannel MEG-detectors, because the detectors are usually placed on a spherical surface, concentric with the head.

There are two different ways to construct the detector coils. One approach is to construct the detector channels from first- or second-order gradiometers, where the two or three gradiometer coils are located concentrically with a baseline on the order of centimeters. The other approach utilizes *planar gradiometers*; two adjoining detector coils, located on the same

plane, are connected together with the shape of a figure 8.

As explained in Section 12.11 the sensitivity distribution of MEG leads is calculated with a half-space model. In multichannel cases the total sensitivity is easily obtained by superimposing the sensitivities of each channel. The sensitivity distributions are illustrated on planes, oriented parallel to the outer surface of the head, and located at different distances, as illustrated in Figure 14.1. The detector coil is oriented parallel to the surface and has a radius r. It is assumed that all the coils are located in the same plane. This means that in the single-coil case the detector is a single-coil magnetometer. In the double-coil case the detector corresponds to a first-order planar gradiometer.

The lead fields are illustrated as vector fields (Malmivuo and Puikkonen, 1987, 1988). The illustrations are normalized so that the distances of the planes are $1r$, $3r$, and $6r$, where r is the radius of the magnetometer coil(s). (The most distant of these planes ($6r$) is relevant when evaluating the lead fields for small MEG detector coils and the closest one ($1r$) when applying magnetic stimulation with a large coil.) The lead field is shown on each plane within a square having a side dimension of $6r$. In each figure the vector fields are normalized so that the maximum vector has approximately unity magnitude. The normalization coefficient *nc* is given in each figure in relation to Figure 14.2A, which illustrates the lead field of a single coil on a plane at the distance of 1*r* from the coil.

The lead fields are illustrated both with lead vector fields and with isosensitivity lines. In the isosensitivity line illustrations, a *half-sensitivity* volume is also shown. This concept describes the space where the sensitivity is equal or larger than one half of the maximum sensitivity. The smaller the half-sensitivity volume, the more accurately it is possible to detect signals from different areas of the volume source.

14.2.2 Single-Coil Magnetometer

PRECONDITIONS:

Source: *Single-coil magnetometer*

Conductor: *Finite, inhomogeneous with spherical symmetry along the magnetometer axis*

The sensitivity distribution of a single-coil magnetometer is illustrated in Figure 14.2. The sensitivity distribution has the form of concentric circles throughout the spherical volume conductor. At the distance of 1*r* the magnitude

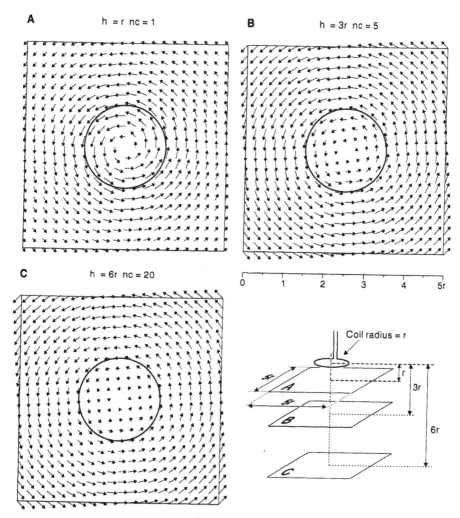

Fig. 14.2 Sensitivity distribution of a single-coil magnetometer having the radius *r*. The sensitivity distribution is given on three parallel planes at dis- tances (A) 1*r*, (B) 3*r*, and (C) 6*r*. Note that the lengths of the vectors in B and C are multiplied by the nor- malization coefficients *nc*.

of the sensitivity increases as a function of the distance from the axis to a peak at about r. On the two more distant planes the maximum sensitivity as a function of the radius is not achieved within the area of the illustration.

It is interesting to compare Figures 14.2 and 12.15. As noted in Chapter 12, these figures represent the same sensitivity distribution illustrated with different methods. The reader will recognize, that the curves in Figure 12.15 correspond to the variation of the length of the vectors in Figure 14.2, and thus they represent the lead field as a function of the radius.

As noted before, the length of the vectors in Figures 14.2B and 14.2C are multiplied by a normalization coefficient nc so that in each figure the maximum length of the vectors is approximately the same.

Figures 14.3A and B illustrate the sensitivity distribution with isosensitivity lines for single coil magnetometers with 10 mm and 5 mm radii, respectively. The isosensitivity lines join the points in the space where the lead field current density has the same value. The isosensitivity lines are illustrated with dashed lines. The figure also illustrates some lead field current flow lines with thin solid lines. Because the lead field of a single coil magnetometer exhibits cylindrical symmetry, the spherical head model can be directly superimposed on this figure. It is supposed that the minimum distance from the coil to the scalp is 20 mm. The sensitivity distribution for a coil with 50 mm radius is presented later (Fig. 24.4) in connection with magnetic stimulation.

The areas of the maximum sensitivity and the half-sensitivity volume are marked with shading. The location of the maximum sensitivity region and the size of the half-sensitivity volume depend on the measurement distance and the coil radius, though this relationship is not very strong.

14.2.3 Planar Gradiometer

PRECONDITIONS:

Source: *Planar gradiometer*
Conductor: *Conducting half-space*

The sensitivity distribution of a planar gradiometer is illustrated in Figure 14.4. From the two adjoining coils, the one on the left is wound in a "positive" direction, and the one on the right in a correspondingly "negative" direction (the latter is drawn with a dashed line). This construction is called the planar gradiometer. This measurement situation may also be achieved by subtracting the measurement signals from two adjoining magnetometers or (axial) gradiometers.

The sensitivity distribution of a planar gradiometer is no longer mainly circular but has a *linear form* within the target region. The more distant the measurement plane is from the detector coil, the more uniform is the sensitivity distribution. The magnitude of the sensitivity of a planar gradiometer decreases faster as a function of distance than does that of a single-coil magnetometer. Therefore, the detected signal originates from sources located mainly in the region closest to the detector.

It should be noted that the sensitivity distribution of a bipolar electric measurement is also linear, as was shown in Figure 13.4. Thus the sensitivity distribution of a planar gradiometer MEG is very similar to that of bipolar EEG measurement.

The isosensitivity lines of a planar gradiometer are illustrated in Figure 14.5. Because this magnetometer arrangement and the lead field it produces are not cylindrically symmetric, the results are accurate only in an infinite, homogeneous volume conductor or in a homogeneous half-space. Therefore a spherical head model cannot be superimposed on these illustrations and a conducting half-space model is used. The distance of the half-space is selected the same as that of the spherical head model directly under the coil. Figure 14.5.A illustrates the isosensitivity lines in the xz-plane, which is the plane including the axes of the coils. This plane includes also the zero sensitivity line. It approaches a line which makes a 35.27° angle with respect to the z-axis. Figure 14.5.B illustrates the isosensitivity lines in the yz-plane. In this plane the isosensitivity lines are concentric circles at distances which are large compared to the coil dimensions. At distances of $10r$ and $100r$ they differ within 1% and 0.1% from a circle, respectively. The thin solid lines illustrate the lead field current flow lines. These are not accurate solutions.

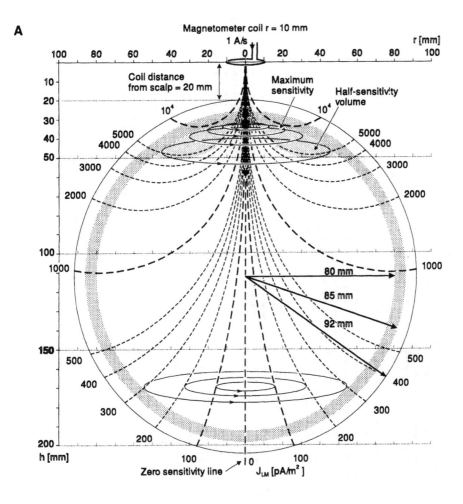

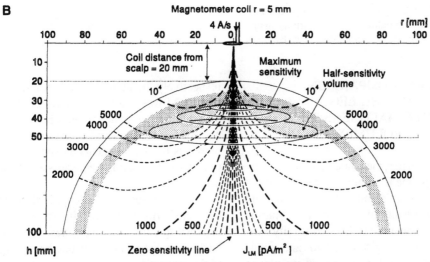

Fig. 14.3 Isosensitivity lines in MEG measurement in a spherical head model with a single coil magnetometer having the radii of (A) 10 mm and (B) 5 mm. The sensitivity is everywhere oriented tangential to the symmetry axis which is the line of zero sensitivity. Within the brain area the maximum sensitivity is located at the surface of the brain and it is indicated with shading.

269

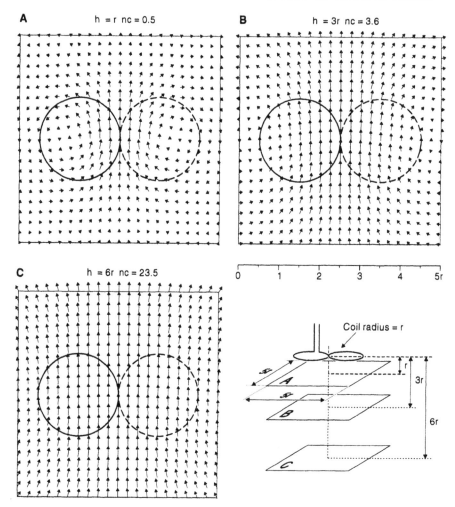

Fig. 14.4 Sensitivity distribution of a planar gradiometer having the radius r. The sensitivity distribution is given on three parallel planes at distances (A) $1r$, (B) $3r$, and (C) $6r$. The lengths of the vectors in A, B, and C are multiplied by the normalization coefficients nc.

14.3 COMPARISON OF THE EEG AND MEG HALF-SENSITIVITY VOLUMES

As discussed earlier, the evaluation of the half-sensitivity volume is a figure-of-merit describing the lead system's ability to concentrate its measurement sensitivity. Suihko and Malmivuo (1993) compared the half-sensitivity volumes (in the brain region) for two- and three-electrode electric leads and for axial and planar gradiometer magnetic leads as a function of electrode distance/gradiometer baseline. The electric and magnetic leads are those described in Figure 13.4 and in Figures 14.3 and 14.5,

respectively. In addition to those, a three-electrode lead was evaluated where all electrodes are equidistant, the lateral ones being interconnected to serve as the other terminal. The head model is the inhomogeneous spherical model of Rush and Driscoll. The results are illustrated in Figure 14.6.

All these leads have, as expected, minimum half-sensitivity volumes with small electrode distances/gradiometer baselines. The electric leads have the smallest values being superior to the magnetic leads. The half-sensitivity volume of the three-electrode lead at 1° separation is 0.2 cm^3 and that of the two-electrode lead is 1.2 cm^3. The half-sensitivity volume of the two-electrode lead is only 30% of that of

A

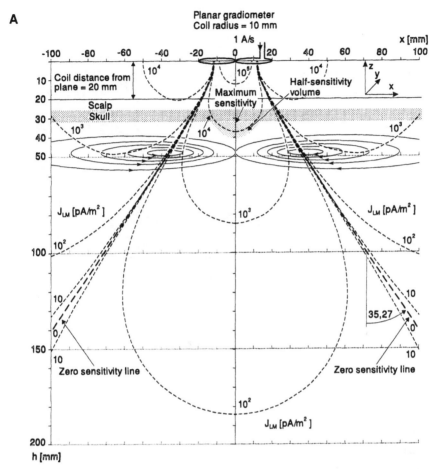

Fig. 14.5 Isosensitivity lines (dashed lines) and half-sensitivity volume for a planar gradiometer calculated for a conducting half-space. Lead field current flow lines are drawn with thin solid lines. They are not accurate solutions. A) In the xz-plane the zero sensitivity line approaches asymptotically the line which makes a 35.27° angle with respect to the z-axis. B) In the yz-plane the isosensitivity lines approach concentric circles at long distance.

the planar gradiometer (3.4 cm³), while that of the axial gradiometer is as large as 21.8 cm³. The gradiometer results are calculated at 20 mm coil distance from scalp.

The 20 mm coil distance and 10 mm coil radius are realistic for the helmetlike whole head MEG detector. There exist, however, MEG devices for recording at a limited region where the coil distance and the coil radius are of the order of 1 mm. Therefore it is illustrated in Figure 14.6 the half-sensitivity volume for planar gradiometers with 1 mm coil radius at 0–20 mm recording distance. These curves show that when the recording distance is about 12 mm, such a planar gradiometer has about the same half-sensitivity volume as the two-electrode EEG.

Another aspect in the comparison of the electric and magnetic leads is the form of the sensitivity distribution. With a short electrode distance/gradiometer baseline the lead fields of the two-electrode and planar gradiometer leads are mainly tangential to the head, as illustrated in Figure 13.4 (at 20° and 40° electrode distances) and in Figure 14.4, respectively. The three-electrode lead has primarily a radial sensitivity distribution (not illustrated in this book) and the axial gradiometer has a sensitivity distribution which is that of a vortex (tangential to the symmetry axis of the gradiometer), see Figures 14.2 and 14.3.

In summary, under practical measurement conditions the differences between the two-electrode EEG lead and the planar gradiometer

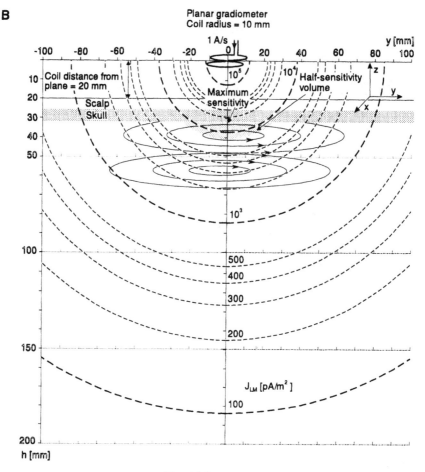

Fig. 14.5 (*Continued*)

MEG lead in the size of the half-sensitivity volumes and the form of the sensitivity distributions are very small. This result is important because it is generally believed that the high resistivity of the skull forces the electric leads to record the signal from a larger region. However, this is not the case since the two-electrode EEG and the planar gradiometer MEG are about equally effective in concentrating their sensitivities while the three-electrode electric lead is still more effective.

14.4   SUMMARY

In this chapter the sensitivity distribution was calculated for single and multichannel MEG detectors. The method used in this chapter is valid under cylindrically symmetric conditions. This is a relevant approximation in practical

MEG measurement situations. Other methods exist for calculating the sensitivity distribution of MEG detectors which give accurate results in situations having less symmetry; they are therefore more complicated and, unfortunately, less illustrative (Eaton, 1992; Esselle and Stuchly, 1992).

If two adjoining coils are connected together either directly or by summing up the detected signals so that the coils detect the magnetic field in different directions, the combination of these coils form a planar gradiometer. The sensitivity distribution of such a construction is no longer circular (vortex) but linear and resembles very much that of an electric lead. The maximum of the sensitivity and, therefore, the most probable location of the signal source for such a construction are located directly under the coils (on the symmetry axis).

There are various multichannel MEG detec-

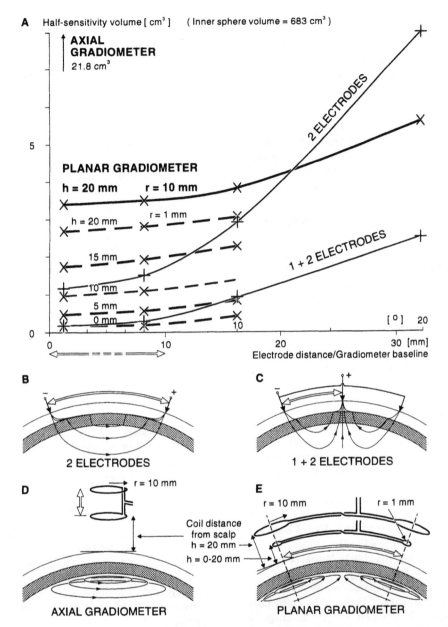

Fig. 14.6 (A) Half-sensitivity volumes for two- and three-electrode electric leads (thin lines), planar gradiometers of 10 mm coil radius (thick line), and 1 mm coil radius (dashed lines) as a function of electrode distance/gradiometer baseline. (The half-sensitivity volume of the axial gradiometer falls out- side the figure.) The measurement situations are shown for the two-electrode (B) and three-electrode (C) electric leads, and for the axial (D), planar (E) gradiometers. The head model is the inhomogeneous spherical model of Rush and Driscoll (Suihko and Malmivuo, 1993).

tors. The number of channels has increased from 7 (Knuutila et al., 1987) to 24 (Kajola et al., 1990) and 32 (Hoenig et al., 1989) to 124 (Knuutila et al., 1991). The detector coils are usually located on a spherical surface concentric with the head. On this surface the coils are usually placed as close to each other as possible, forming a honeycomb-like pattern. In the 124-channel construction the dewar covers the head in a helmetlike construction.

Though the magnetic field is a vector quantity (unlike the electric potential field which is a scalar quantity) the majority of the MEG detectors record only one component of the magnetic field. There exist, however, some works where all the three components of the magnetic field are recorded. Early on, in his pioneering work, David Cohen illustrated the vectorial form of the magnetic field of the brain (Cohen, 1972). As an example of modern MEG research with a vector gradiometer the work of Yoshinori Uchikawa and his colleagues should be mentioned (Uchikawa et al., 1992, 1993).

In MEG we are mainly interested in the electric activity at the surface of the brain, the cortex. Therefore, unipolar measurements are relevant when measuring the MEG. As will be discussed later in Chapter 20, in MCG we are interested in the electric activity of the whole cardiac muscle. Therefore bipolar (symmetric) measurements are more relevant in measuring the MCG.

REFERENCES

Cohen D (1968): Magnetoencephalography, evidence of magnetic fields produced by alpharhythm currents. *Science* 161: 784–6.

Cohen D (1972): Magnetoencephalography: Detection of brain's electric activity with a superconducting magnetometer. *Science* 175:(4022) 664–6.

Eaton H (1992): Electric field induced in spherical conductor from arbitrary coils: Application to magnetic stimulation and MEG. *Med. & Biol. Eng. & Comput.* 30:(July) 433–40.

Esselle KP, Stuchly MA (1992): Neural stimulation with magnetic fields: Analyis of induced electric fields. *IEEE Trans. Biomed. Eng.* 39:(7) 693–700.

Hoenig HE, Daalmans G, Folberth W, Reichenberger H, Schneider S, Seifert H (1989): Biomagnetic multichannel system with integrated squids and first order gradiometers operating in a shielded room. *Cryogenics* 29:(8) 809–13.

Kajola M, Ahlfors S, Ehnholm GJ, Hällström J, Hämäläinen MS, Ilmoniemi RJ, Kiviranta M, Knuutila J, Lounasmaa OV, Tesche CD, Vilkman V (1990): A 24-channel magnetometer for brain research. In *Advances in Biomagnetism*, ed. SJ Williamson, L Kaufman, pp. 673–6, Plenum Press, New York.

Knuutila J, Ahlfors S, Ahonen A, Hällström J, Kajola
M, Lounasmaa OV, Tesche C, Vilkman V (1987): A large-area low-noise seven-channel dc-squid magnetometer for brain research. *Rev. Sci. Instrum.* 58: 2145–56.

Knuutila J, Ahonen A, Hämäläinen M, Kajola M, Lounasmaa OV, Simola J, Tesche C, Vilkman V (1991): Design of a 122-channel neuromagnetometer covering the whole head. In *Abst. 8th Internat. Conf. Biomagnetism*, ed. M Hoke, pp. 109–10, Westfälische Wilhelms-Universität, Münster.

Malmivuo JA (1980): Distribution of MEG detector sensitivity: An application of reciprocity. *Med. & Biol. Eng. & Comput.* 18:(3) 365–70.

Malmivuo JA, Puikkonen J (1987): Sensitivity distribution of multichannel MEG detectors. In *Abst. 6th Internat. Conf. Biomagnetism, Tokyo, 27–30 August*, ed. K Atsumi, M Kotani, S Ueno, T Katila, SJ Williamson, pp. 112–3, Tokyo Denki University Press, Tokyo.

Malmivuo JA, Puikkonen J (1988): Qualitative properties of the sensitivity distribution of planar gradiometers. *Tampere Univ. Techn., Inst. Biomed. Eng., Reports* 2:(1) pp. 35.

REFERENCES, BOOKS

Hoke M, Grandori F, Romani G-L (eds.) (1990): *Auditory Evoked Magnetic Fields and Electric Potentials*, 362 pp. S. Karger, Basel.

Regan D (1989): *Human Brain. Electrophysiology, Evoked Potentials and Evoked Magnetic Fields in Science and Medicine*, 672 pp. Elsevier, Amsterdam.

Suihko V, Malmivuo J (1993): Sensitivity distributions of EEG and MEG measurements. In *EEG and MEG Signal Analysis and Interpretation, Proceedings of the Second Ragnar Granit Symposium*, ed. J Hyttinen, J Malmivuo, pp. 11–20, Tampere University of Technology, Ragnar Granit Institute, Tampere.

Swithenby SJ (1987): Biomagnetism and the biomagnetic inverse problem. *Phys. Med. Biol.* MJ Day (ed.): The Biomagnetic Inverse Problem, 32:(1) 146. (Papers from a conference at the Open University, April 1986).

Uchikawa Y, Matsumura F, Kobayashi K, Kotani M (1993): Discrimination and identification of multiple sources of the magnetoencephalogram using a three-dimensional second-order gradiometer. *J. Jpn. Biomagn. Bioelectromagn. Soc.* 6:12–5.

V

Electric and Magnetic Measurement of the Electric Activity of the Heart

Part V deals with the application of bioelectromagnetism to cardiology. This subject is discussed in more detail than the application of bioelectromagnetism to neurophysiology because the historical development of the theory of bioelectromagnetism is strongly associated with developments in electrocardiology.

The 12-lead system, discussed in Chapter 15, was an early clinical application of bioelectromagnetism. Theoretically, it is very primitive. Vectorcardiographic lead systems, discussed in Chapter 16, are based upon more advanced theory of volume conductors than the 12-lead system. Chapter 17 includes a further theoretical development of more complicated lead systems which, however, are not in clinical use. Chapter 18 explains briefly the various distortion effects of the real thorax.

The short introduction to clinical ECG diagnosis in Chapter 19 is included in this book, not to serve as an introduction to clinical studies but to give the reader an impression of what kind of changes in the clinical ECG signal are found owing to various pathological conditions in the heart. This permits, for instance, the clinical engineer to understand the basis of the technical requirements for an ECG amplifier and recorder.

Like Part IV, Part V also includes (in Chapter 20) a discussion of the detection of the magnetic field due to the electric activity of the heart muscle.

15

12-Lead ECG System

15.1 LIMB LEADS

PRECONDITIONS:

Source: *Two-dimensional dipole (in the frontal plane) in a fixed location*

Conductor: *Infinite, homogeneous volume conductor or homogeneous sphere with the dipole in its center (the trivial solution)*

Augustus Désiré Waller measured the human electrocardiogram in 1887 using Lippmann's *capillary electrometer* (Waller, 1887). He selected five electrode locations: the four extremities and the mouth (Waller, 1889). In this way, it became possible to achieve a sufficiently low contact impedance and thus to maximize the ECG signal. Furthermore, the electrode location is unmistakably defined and the attachment of electrodes facilitated at the limb positions. The five measurement points produce altogether 10 different leads (see Fig. 15.1A). From these 10 possibilities he selected five—designated *cardinal leads*. Two of these are identical to the *Einthoven leads I* and *III* described below.

Willem Einthoven also used the capillary electrometer in his first ECG recordings. His essential contribution to ECG-recording technology was the development and application of the *string galvanometer*. Its sensitivity greatly exceeded the previously used capillary

electrometer. The string galvanometer itself was invented by Clément Ader (Ader, 1897). In 1908 Willem Einthoven published a description of the first clinically important ECG measuring system (Einthoven, 1908). The above-mentioned practical considerations rather than bioelectric ones determined the Einthoven lead system, which is an application of the 10 leads of Waller. The Einthoven lead system is illustrated in Figure 15.1B.

The Einthoven *limb leads* (standard leads) are defined in the following way:

$$
\begin{aligned}
\text{Lead I:} \quad & V_I = \Phi_L - \Phi_R \\
\text{Lead II:} \quad & V_I = \Phi_F - \Phi_R \qquad (15.1) \\
\text{Lead III:} \quad & V_{III} = \Phi_F - \Phi_L
\end{aligned}
$$

where

V_I = the voltage of lead I
V_{II} = the voltage of lead II
V_{III} = the voltage of lead III
Φ_L = potential at the left arm
Φ_R = potential at the right arm
Φ_F = potential at the left foot

(The left arm, right arm, and left leg (foot) are also represented with symbols LA, RA, and LL, respectively.)

According to Kirchhoff's law these lead voltages have the following relationship:

$$
V_I + V_{III} = V_{II} \qquad (15.2)
$$

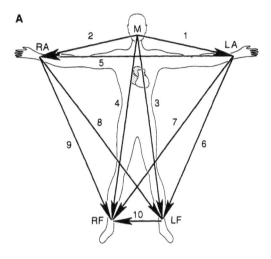

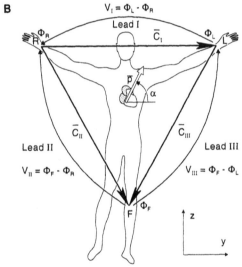

Fig. 15.1 (A) The 10 ECG leads of Waller. (B) Einthoven limb leads and Einthoven triangle. The Einthoven triangle is an approximate description of the lead vectors associated with the limb leads. Lead I is shown as $\overline{C}_{\text{I}}$ in the above figure, etc.

the cardiac sources are represented by a dipole located at the center of a sphere representing the torso, hence at the center of the equilateral triangle. With these assumptions, the voltages measured by the three limb leads are proportional to the projections of the electric heart vector on the sides of the lead vector triangle, as described in Figure 15.1B. These ideas are a recapitulation of those discussed in Section 11.4.3, where it was shown that the sides of this triangle are, in fact, formed by the corresponding lead vectors.

The voltages of the limb leads are obtained from Equation 11.19, which is duplicated below (Einthoven, Fahr, and de Waart, 1913, 1950). (Please note that the equations are written using the coordinate system of Appendix A.)

$$V_{\text{I}} = p \cos \alpha = p_y$$

$$V_{\text{II}} = \frac{p}{2} \cos \alpha - \frac{\sqrt{3}}{2} p \sin \alpha$$

$$= \frac{1}{2} p_y - \frac{\sqrt{3}}{2} p_z$$

$$= 0.5 p_y - 0.87 p_z$$

$$V_{\text{III}} = -\frac{p}{2} \cos \alpha - \frac{\sqrt{3}}{2} p \sin \alpha$$

$$= -\frac{1}{2} p_y - \frac{\sqrt{3}}{2} p_z$$

$$= -0.5 p_y - 0.87 p_z \qquad (11.19)$$

If one substitutes Equation 11.19 into Equation, 15.2, one can again demonstrate that Kirchhoff's law—that is, Equation 15.2—is satisfied, since we obtain

$$V_{\text{I}} + V_{\text{III}} = \frac{p}{2} \cos \alpha - \frac{\sqrt{3}}{2} p \sin \alpha = V_{\text{II}} \quad (15.3)$$

hence only two of these three leads are independent.

The lead vectors associated with Einthoven's lead system are conventionally found based on the assumption that the heart is located in an infinite, homogeneous volume conductor (or at the center of a homogeneous sphere representing the torso). One can show that if the position of the right arm, left arm, and left leg are at the vertices of an equilateral triangle, having the heart located at its center, then the lead vectors also form an equilateral triangle.

A simple model results from assuming that

15.2 ECG SIGNAL

15.2.1 The Signal Produced by the Activation Front

Before we discuss the generation of the ECG signal in detail, we consider a simple example explaining what kind of signal a propagating activation front produces in a volume conductor.

Figure 15.2 presents a volume conductor and a pair of electrodes on its opposite surfaces. The figure is divided into four cases, where both

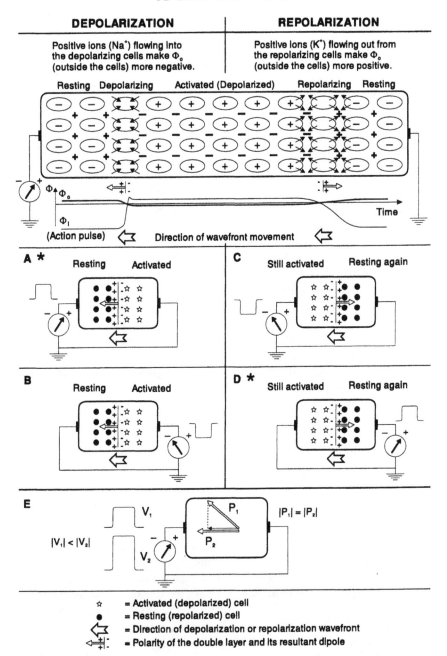

Fig. 15.2 The signal produced by the propagating activation front between a pair of extracellular electrodes.

the depolarization and repolarization fronts propagate toward both positive and negative electrodes. In various cases the detected signals have the following polarities:

Case A: When the depolarization front propagates toward a positive electrode, it produces a positive signal (see the detailed description below).

Case B: When the propagation of activation is away from the positive electrode, the signal has the corresponding negative polarity.

Case C: It is easy to understand that when the repolarization front propagates toward a positive electrode, the signal is negative (see the detailed description below).

Although it is known that repolarization does not actually propagate, a boundary between repolarized and still active regions can be defined as a function of time. It is "propagation" in this sense that is described here.

Case D: When the direction of propagation of a repolarization front is away from the positive electrode, a positive signal is produced.

The positive polarity of the signal in case A can be confirmed in the following way. First we note that the transmembrane voltage ahead of the wave is negative since this region is still at rest. (This condition is described in Fig. 15.2 by the appearance of the minus signs.) Behind the wavefront, the transmembrane voltage is in the plateau stage; hence it is positive (indicated by the positive signs in Fig. 15.2). If Equation 8.25 is applied to evaluate the double-layer sources associated with this arrangement, as discussed in Section 8.2.4, and if the transmembrane voltage under resting or plateau conditions is recognized as being uniform, then a double-layer source arises only at the wavefront.

What is important here is that the orientation of the double layer, given by the negative spatial derivative of V_m, is entirely to the left (which corresponds to the direction of propagation). Because the dipoles are directed toward the positive electrode, the signal is positive. (The actual time-varying signal depends on the evolving geometry of the source double layer and its relationship to the volume conductor and the leads. In this example we describe only the gross behavior.)

The negative polarity of the signal in case C can be confirmed in the following way. In this case the direction of repolarization allows us to designate in which regions V_m is negative (where repolarization is complete and the membrane is again at rest) and positive (where repolarization has not yet begun, and the membrane is still in the plateau stage). These are designated in Figure 15.2 by the corresponding minus $(-)$ and plus $(+)$ markings. In this highly idealized example, we show repolarization as occurring instantly at the $-$ to $+$ interface (repolarization wavefront). But the source asso-

ciated with this spatial distribution of V_m is still found from Equation 8.25. Application of that equation shows that the double layer, given by the negative spatial derivative, is zero everywhere except at the repolarization wavefront, where it is oriented to the right (in this case opposite to the direction of repolarization velocity). Since the source dipoles are directed away from the positive electrode, a negative signal will be measured.

For the case that activation does not propagate directly toward an electrode, the signal is proportional to the component of the velocity in the direction of the electrode, as shown in Figure 15.2E. This conclusion follows from the association of a double layer with the activation front and application of Equation 11.4 (where we assume the direction of the lead vector to be approximated by a line connecting the leads). Note that we are ignoring the possible influence of a changing extent of the wave of activation with a change in direction. Special attention should be given to cases A and D, marked with an asterisk (*), since these reflect the fundamental relationships.

15.2.2 Formation of the ECG Signal

The cells that constitute the ventricular myocardium are coupled together by gap junctions which, for the normal healthy heart, have a very low resistance. As a consequence, activity in one cell is readily propagated to neighboring cells. It is said that the heart behaves as a *syncytium*; a propagating wave once initiated continues to propagate uniformly into the region that is still at rest. We have quantitatively examined the electrophysiological behavior of a uniform fiber. Now we can apply these results to the heart if we consider it to be composed of uniform fibers. These equivalent fibers are a valid representation because they are consistent with the syncytial nature of the heart. In fact, because the syncytium reflects connectivity in all directions, we may choose the fiber orientation at our convenience (so long as the quantitative values of conductivity assigned to the fibers correspond to those that are actually measured).

Much of what we know about the activation

sequence in the heart comes from canine studies. The earliest comprehensive study in this area was performed by Scher and Young (1957). More recently, such studies were performed on the human heart, and a seminal paper describing the results was published by Durrer et al. (1970). These studies show that activation wavefronts proceed relatively uniformly, from endocardium to epicardium and from apex to base.

One way of describing cardiac activation is to plot the sequence of instantaneous depolarization wavefronts. Since these surfaces connect all points in the same temporal phase, the wavefront surfaces are also referred to as *isochrones* (i.e., they are *isochronous*). An evaluation of dipole sources can be achieved by applying generalized Equation 8.25 to each equivalent fiber. This process involves taking the spatial gradient of V_m. If we assume that on one side cells are entirely at rest, while on the other cells are entirely in the plateau phase, then the source is zero everywhere except at the wavefront. Consequently, the wavefront or isochrone not only describes the activation surface but also shows the location of the double-layer sources.

From the above it should be possible to examine the actual generation of the ECG by taking into account a realistic progression of activation double layers. Such a description is contained in Figure 15.3. After the electric activation of the heart has begun at the sinus node, it spreads along the atrial walls. The resultant vector of the atrial electric activity is illustrated with a thick arrow. The projections of this resultant vector on each of the three Einthoven limb leads is positive, and therefore, the measured signals are also positive.

After the depolarization has propagated over the atrial walls, it reaches the AV node. The propagation through the AV junction is very slow and involves negligible amount of tissue; it results in a delay in the progress of activation. (This is a desirable pause which allows completion of ventricular filling.)

Once activation has reached the ventricles, propagation proceeds along the Purkinje fibers to the inner walls of the ventricles. The ventricular depolarization starts first from the left side of the interventricular septum, and therefore, the resultant dipole from this septal activation points to the right. Figure 15.3 shows that this causes a negative signal in leads I and II.

In the next phase, depolarization waves occur on both sides of the septum, and their electric forces cancel. However, early apical activation is also occurring, so the resultant vector points to the apex.

After a while the depolarization front has propagated through the wall of the right ventricle; when it first arrives at the epicardial surface of the right-ventricular free wall, the event is called *breakthrough*. Because the left ventricular wall is thicker, activation of the left ventricular free wall continues even after depolarization of a large part of the right ventricle. Because there are no compensating electric forces on the right, the resultant vector reaches its maximum in this phase, and it points leftward. The depolarization front continues propagation along the left ventricular wall toward the back. Because its surface area now continuously decreases, the magnitude of the resultant vector also decreases until the whole ventricular muscle is depolarized. The last to depolarize are basal regions of both left and right ventricles. Because there is no longer a propagating activation front, there is no signal either.

Ventricular repolarization begins from the outer side of the ventricles and the repolarization front "propagates" inward. This seems paradoxical, but even though the epicardium is the last to depolarize, its action potential durations are relatively short, and it is the first to recover. Although recovery of one cell does not propagate to neighboring cells, one notices that recovery generally does move from the epicardium toward the endocardium. The inward spread of the repolarization front generates a signal with the same sign as the outward depolarization front, as pointed out in Figure 15.2 (recall that both the direction of repolarization and orientation of dipole sources are opposite). Because of the diffuse form of the repolarization, the amplitude of the signal is much smaller than that of the depolarization wave and it lasts longer.

The normal electrocardiogram is illustrated in Figure 15.4. The figure also includes definitions for various segments and intervals in the ECG. The deflections in this signal are denoted

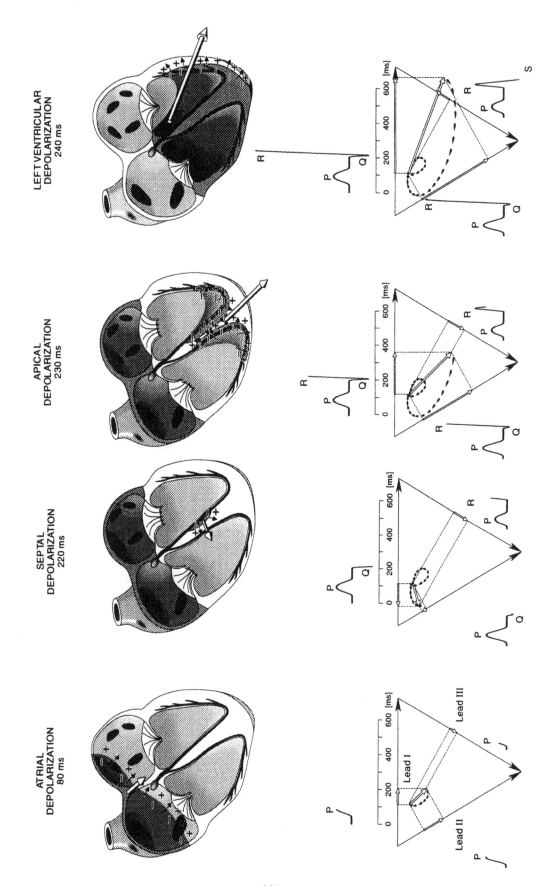

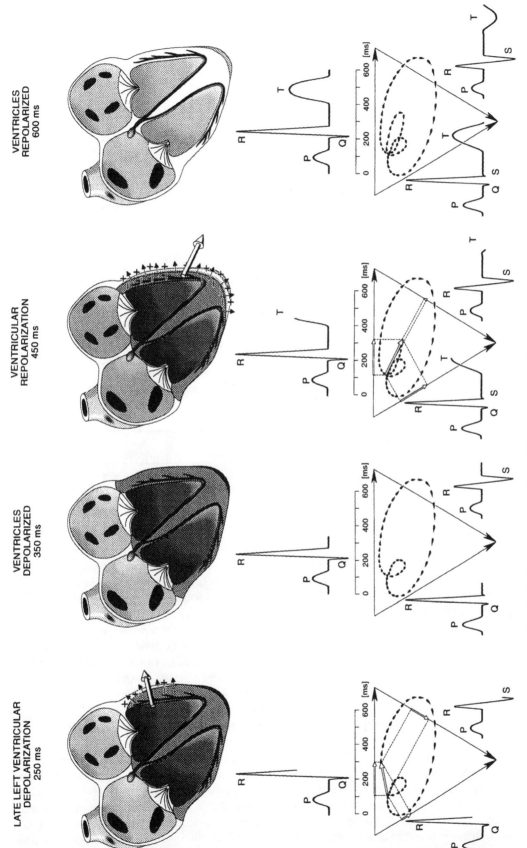

Fig. 15.3 The generation of the ECG signal in the Einthoven limb leads.

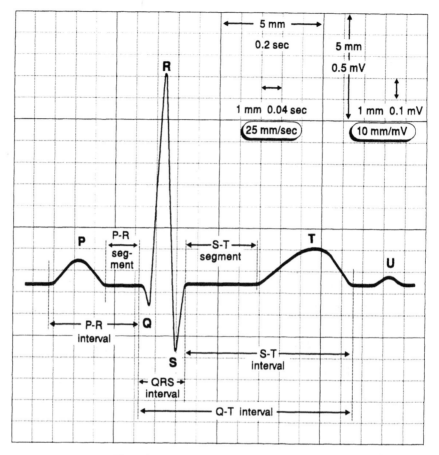

Fig. 15.4 The normal electrocardiogram.

in alphabetic order starting with the letter *P*, which represents atrial depolarization. The ventricular depolarization causes the QRS complex, and repolarization is responsible for the T wave. Atrial repolarization occurs during the QRS complex and produces such a low signal amplitude that it cannot be seen apart from the normal ECG.

15.3   WILSON CENTRAL TERMINAL

Frank Norman Wilson (1890–1952) investigated how electrocardiographic *unipolar* potentials could be defined. Ideally, those are measured with respect to a remote reference (infinity). But how is one to achieve this in the

volume conductor of the size of the human body with electrodes already placed at the extremities? In several articles on the subject, Wilson and colleagues (Wilson, Macleod, and Barker, 1931; Wilson et al., 1934) suggested the use of the *central terminal* as this reference. This was formed by connecting a 5 kΩ resistor from each terminal of the limb leads to a common point called the central terminal, as shown in Figure 15.5. Wilson suggested that unipolar potentials should be measured with respect to this terminal which approximates the potential at infinity.

Actually, the Wilson central terminal is not independent of but, rather, is the average of the limb potentials. This is easily demonstrated by noting that in an ideal voltmeter there is no lead current. Consequently, the total current into the central terminal from the limb leads must add

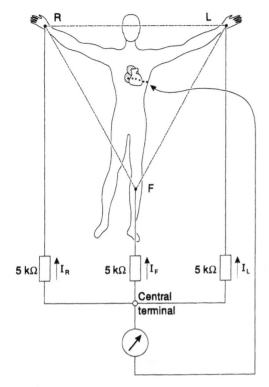

Fig. 15.5 The Wilson central terminal (CT) is formed by connecting a 5 kΩ resistance to each limb electrode and interconnecting the free wires; the CT is the common point. The Wilson central terminal represents the average of the limb potentials. Because no current flows through a high-impedance voltmeter, Kirchhoff's law requires that $I_R + I_L + I_F = 0$.

to zero to satisfy the conservation of current (see Fig. 15.5). Accordingly, we require that

$$I_R \quad + \quad I_L \quad + \quad I_F \quad =$$
$$\frac{\Phi_{CT} - \Phi_R}{5000} + \frac{\Phi_{CT} - \Phi_L}{5000} + \frac{\Phi_{CT} - \Phi_F}{5000} = 0$$
$$(15.4)$$

from which it follows that

$$\Phi_{CT} = \frac{\Phi_R + \Phi_L + \Phi_F}{3} \qquad (15.5)$$

Since the central terminal potential is the average of the extremity potentials it can be argued that it is then somewhat independent of any one in particular and therefore a satisfactory reference. In clinical practice good reproducibility of the measurement system is vital.

Results appear to be quite consistent in clinical applications.

Wilson advocated 5 kΩ resistances; these are still widely used, though at present the high-input impedance of the ECG amplifiers would allow much higher resistances. A higher resistance increases the CMRR and diminishes the size of the artifact introduced by the electrode/skin resistance.

It is easy to show that in the image space the Wilson central terminal is found at the center of the Einthoven triangle, as shown in Figure 15.6.

15.4 GOLDBERGER AUGMENTED LEADS

Three additional limb leads, V_R, V_L, and V_F are obtained by measuring the potential between each limb electrode and the Wilson central terminal. (Note that V denotes a lead and V a lead voltage.) For instance, the measurement from the left leg (foot) gives

$$V_F = \Phi_F - \Phi_{CT} = \frac{2\Phi_F - \Phi_R - \Phi_L}{3} \quad (15.6)$$

In 1942 E. Goldberger observed that these signals can be augmented by omitting that resistance from the Wilson central terminal, which is connected to the measurement electrode (Goldberger, 1942a,b). In this way, the aforementioned three leads may be replaced with a new set of leads that are called *augmented* leads because of the augmentation of the signal (see Fig. 15.7). As an example, the equation for the augmented lead aV$_F$ is:

$$V_{aV_F} = \Phi_F - \Phi_{CT/aV_F}$$
$$= \Phi_F - \frac{\Phi_L + \Phi_R}{2} = \frac{2 \cdot \Phi_F - \Phi_L - \Phi_R}{2}$$
$$(15.7)$$

A comparison of Equation 15.7 with Equation 15.6 shows the augmented signal to be 50% larger than the signal with the Wilson central terminal chosen as reference. It is important to note that the three augmented leads, aV$_R$, aV$_L$, and aV$_F$, are fully redundant with respect to the limb leads I, II, and III. (This holds also for the three unipolar limb leads V$_R$, V$_L$, and V$_F$.)

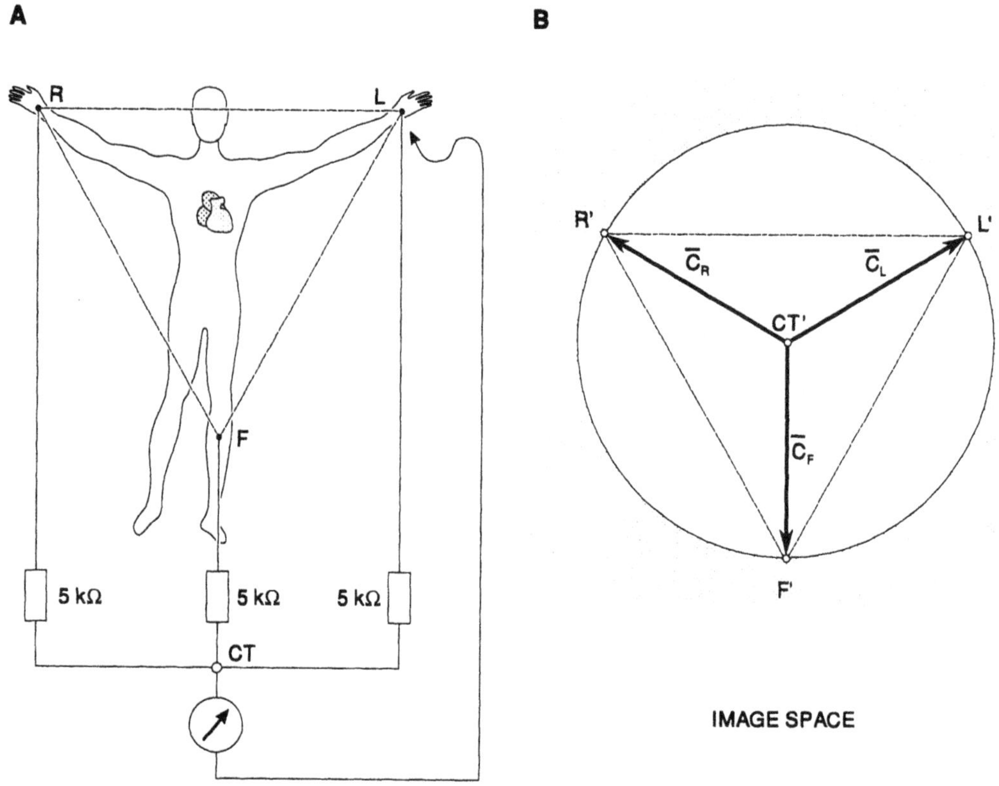

A

B

IMAGE SPACE

Fig. 15.6 (A) The circuit of the Wilson central terminal (CT). (B) The location of the Wilson central terminal in the image space (CT′). It is located in the center of the Einthoven triangle.

15.5 PRECORDIAL LEADS

PRECONDITIONS:

Source: *Dipole in a fixed location*

Conductor: *Infinite, homogeneous volume conductor or homogeneous sphere with the dipole in its center (the trivial solution)*

For measuring the potentials close to the heart, Wilson introduced the *precordial leads* (chest leads) in 1944 (Wilson et al., 1944). These leads, $V_1 - V_6$ are located over the left chest as described in Figure 15.8. The points V_1 and V_2 are located at the fourth intercostal space on the right and left side of the sternum; V_4 is located in the fifth intercostal space at the midclavicular line; V_3 is located between the points V_2 and V_4; V_5 is at the same horizontal level as V_4 but on the anterior axillary line; V_6

is at the same horizontal level as V_4 but at the midline. The location of the precordial leads is illustrated in Figure 15.8.

15.6 MODIFICATIONS OF THE 12-LEAD SYSTEM

The 12-lead system as described here is the one with the greatest clinical use. There are also some other modifications of the 12-lead system for particular applications.

In exercise ECG, the signal is distorted because of muscular activity, respiration, and electrode artifacts due to perspiration and electrode movements. The distortion due to muscular activation can be minimized by placing the electrodes on the shoulders and on the hip instead of the arms and the leg, as suggested by R. E. Mason and I. Likar (1966). The Mason-

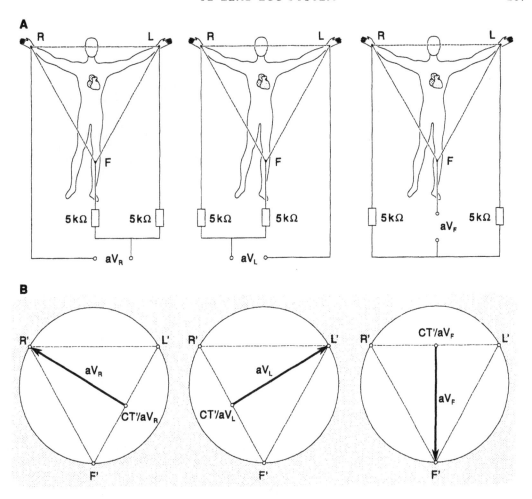

Fig. 15.7 (A) The circuit of the Goldberger augmented leads. (B) The location of the Goldberger augmented lead vectors in the image space.

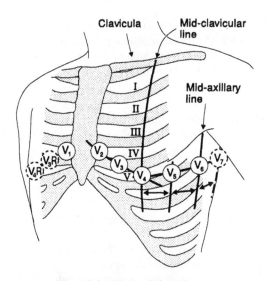

Fig. 15.8 Precordial leads.

Likar modification is the most important modification of the 12-lead system used in exercise ECG.

The accurate location for the right arm electrode in the Mason-Likar modification is a point in the infraclavicular fossa medial to the border of the deltoid muscle and 2 cm below the lower border of the clavicle. The left arm electrode is located similarly on the left side. The left leg electrode is placed at the left iliac crest. The right leg electrode is placed in the region of the right iliac fossa. The precordial leads are located in the Mason-Likar modification in the standard places of the 12-lead system.

In ambulatory monitoring of the ECG, as in the Holter recording, the electrodes are also placed on the surface of the thorax instead of the extremities.

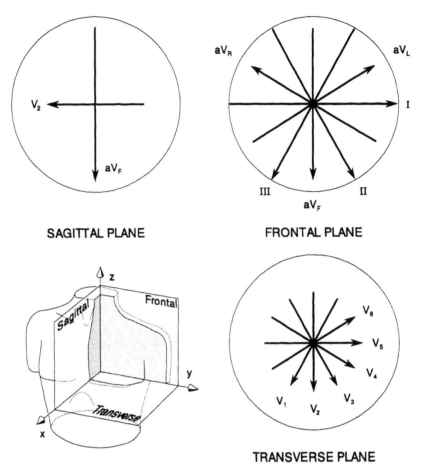

Fig. 15.9 The projections of the lead vectors of the 12-lead ECG system in three orthogonal planes when one assumes the volume conductor to be spherical homogeneous and the cardiac source centrally located.

15.7 THE INFORMATION CONTENT OF THE 12-LEAD SYSTEM

The most commonly used clinical ECG-system, the 12-lead ECG system, consists of the following 12 leads, which are:

I, II, III

aV$_R$, aV$_L$, aV$_F$

V$_1$, V$_2$, V$_3$, V$_4$, V$_5$, V$_6$

Of these 12 leads, the first six are derived from the same three measurement points. Therefore, any two of these six leads include exactly the same information as the other four.

Over 90% of the heart's electric activity can be explained with a dipole source model (Ge-selowitz, 1964). To evaluate this dipole, it is sufficient to measure its three independent components. In principle, two of the limb leads (I, II, III) could reflect the frontal plane components, whereas one precordial lead could be chosen for the anterior-posterior component. The combination should be sufficient to describe completely the electric heart vector. (The lead V$_2$ would be a very good precordial lead choice since it is directed closest to the x axis. It is roughly orthogonal to the standard limb plane, which is close to the frontal plane.) To the extent that the cardiac source can be described as a dipole, the 12-lead ECG system could be thought to have three independent leads and nine redundant leads.

However, in fact, the precordial leads detect

also nondipolar components, which have diagnostic significance because they are located close to the frontal part of the heart. Therefore, the 12-lead ECG system has eight truly independent and four redundant leads. The lead vectors for each lead based on an idealized (spherical) volume conductor are shown in Figure 15.9. These figures are assumed to apply in clinical electrocardiography.

The main reason for recording all 12 leads is that it enhances pattern recognition. This combination of leads gives the clinician an opportunity to compare the projections of the resultant vectors in two orthogonal planes and at different angles. This is further facilitated when the polarity of the lead aV_R can be changed; the lead $-aV_R$ is included in many ECG recorders.

In summary, for the approximation of cardiac electric activity by a single fixed-location dipole, nine leads are redundant in the 12-lead system, as noted above. If we take into account the distributed character of cardiac sources and the effect of the thoracic surface and internal inhomogeneities, we can consider only the four (of six) limb leads as truly redundant.

REFERENCES

Ader C (1897): Sur un nouvel appareil enregistreur pour cables sousmarins. *Compt. rend. Acad. Sci. (Paris)* 124: 1440–2.

Durrer D, van Dam RT, Freud GE, Janse MJ, Meijler FL, Arzbaecher RC (1970): Total excitation of the isolated human heart. *Circulation* 41:(6) 899–912.

Einthoven W (1908): Weiteres über das Elektrokardiogram. *Pflüger Arch. ges. Physiol.* 122: 517–48.

Einthoven W, Fahr G, de Waart A (1913): Über die Richtung und die Manifeste Grösse der Potentialschwankungen im mennschlichen Herzen und über den Einfluss der Herzlage auf die form des Elektrokardiogramms. *Pflüger Arch. ges. Physiol.* 150: 275–315.

Einthoven W, Fahr G, de Waart A (1950): On the direction and manifest size of the variations of potential in the human heart and on the influence of the position of the heart on the form of the electrocardiogram. *Am. Heart J.* 40:(2) 163–211.

(Reprint 1913, translated by HE Hoff, P Sekelj).

Geselowitz DB (1964): Dipole theory in electrocardiography. *Am. J. Cardiol.* 14:(9) 301–6.

Goldberger E (1942a): The aVL, aVR, and aVF leads; A simplification of standard lead electrocardiography. *Am. Heart J.* 24: 378–96.

Goldberger E (1942b): A simple indifferent electrocardiographic electrode of zero potential and a technique of obtaining augmented, unipolar extremity leads. *Am. Heart J.* 23: 483–92.

Mason R, Likar L (1966): A new system of multiple leads exercise electrocardiography. *Am. Heart J.* 71:(2) 196–205.

Netter FH (1971): *Heart*, Vol. 5, 293 pp. The Ciba Collection of Medical Illustrations, Ciba Pharmaceutical Company, Summit, N.J.

Scher AM, Young AC (1957): Ventricular depolarization and the genesis of the QRS. *Ann. N.Y. Acad. Sci.* 65: 768–78.

Waller AD (1887): A demonstration on man of electromotive changes accompanying the heart's beat. *J. Physiol. (Lond.)* 8: 229–34.

Waller AD (1889): On the electromotive changes connected with the beat of the mammalian heart, and on the human heart in particular. *Phil. Trans. R. Soc. (Lond.)* 180: 169–94.

Wilson FN, Johnston FD, Macleod AG, Barker PS (1934): Electrocardiograms that represent the potential variations of a single electrode. *Am. Heart J.* 9: 447–71.

Wilson FN, Johnston FD, Rosenbaum FF, Erlanger H, Kossmann CE, Hecht H, Cotrim N, Menezes de Olivieira R, Scarsi R, Barker PS (1944): The precordial electrocardiogram. *Am. Heart J.* 27: 19–85.

Wilson FN, Macleod AG, Barker PS (1931): Potential variations produced by the heart beat at the apices of Einthoven's triangle. *Am. Heart J.* 7: 207–11.

REFERENCES, BOOKS

Macfarlane PW, Lawrie TDV (eds.) (1989): *Comprehensive Electrocardiology: Theory and Practice in Health and Disease*, 1st ed., Vol. 1, 2, and 3, 1785 pp. Pergamon Press, New York.

Nelson CV, Geselowitz DB (eds.) (1976): *The Theoretical Basis of Electrocardiology*, 544 pp. Oxford University Press, Oxford.

Pilkington TC, Plonsey R (1982): *Engineering Contributions to Biophysical Electrocardiography*, 248 pp. IEEE Press, John Wiley, New York.

16

Vectorcardiographic Lead Systems

16.1 INTRODUCTION

In the first article concerning the human electrocardiogram published in 1887, Augustus D. Waller pointed out the dipolar nature of the cardiac electric generator (Waller, 1887; see Fig. 1.17). Because it is possible to describe the electric generator of the heart reasonably accurately with an equivalent dipole, called the *electric heart vector* (EHV), it is natural to display it in vector form. The measurement and display of the electric heart vector is called *vectorcardiography* (VCG), or *vectorelectrocardiography* (VECG) to separate it from vectormagnetocardiography.

Theoretically, an obvious way to display the behavior of the dipole is with an oscilloscope that follows the trajectory of the end point of the vector projected on to principal planes. This display is called *spatial* vectorcardiography. This is illustrated in Figure 16.1. The rectangular coordinate system is a natural selection. These coordinate axes may be either the *body axes* or the *cardiac axes.*

One can display the temporal information (the time scale) by modulating the intensity of the oscilloscope beam so that the trace is periodically interrupted (possibly at 2 ms intervals). By modulating the oscilloscope intensity with a triangular waveform, each 2 ms segment has

a teardrop shape which indicates the direction of the trajectory.

The signal may also be displayed by showing the three vector components as functions of time. This display is called *scalar* vectorcardiography. This display is not used very often in vectorcardiography, because it provides no information that is not in the scalar display of the 12-lead ECG signal.

There are both *uncorrected* and *corrected* VCG lead systems. The uncorrected VCG systems do not consider the distortions caused by the boundary and internal inhomogeneities of the body. The uncorrected lead systems assume that the direction of the spatial line connecting an electrode pair yields the orientation of the corresponding lead vector. Currently it is known that this assumption is inaccurate, as is discussed later. In any event, these uncorrected lead systems are no longer in clinical use.

The goal of the corrected lead system is to perform an *orthonormal* measurement of the electric heart vector. In an orthonormal measurement both of the following requirements are fulfilled:

1. The three measured components of the electric heart vector are *orthogonal* and in the direction of the coordinate axes (i.e., the lead vectors are parallel to the coordinate axes,

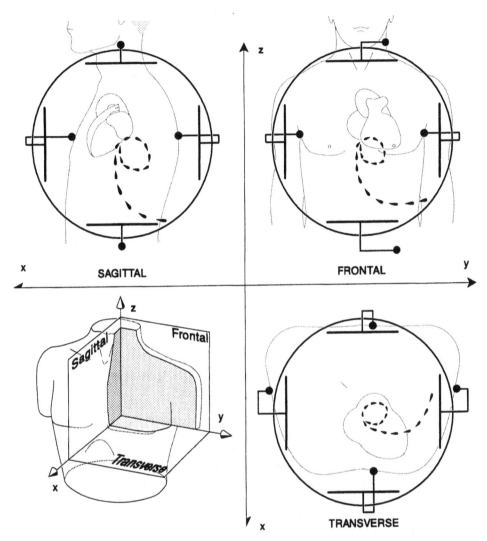

Fig. 16.1 The basic principle of vectorcardiography is illustrated based on ideal uniform lead fields which are mutually orthogonal being set up by parallel electrodes on opposite sides of the torso (bipolar configuration).

which are usually the body axes). Furthermore, each lead field is uniform throughout the heart.

2. Each of the three components of the electric heart vector are detected with the same sensitivity; that is, the measurements are *normalized*.

In the corrected vectorcardiographic lead systems the accuracy of the orthonormal measurement is limited by the applied theoretical method. The theoretical methods for analyzing volume sources and volume conductors were discussed earlier in Chapter 9. Each of them has allowed for a VCG system to be orthonormal within the limits of the performed correction. These lead systems are discussed in detail later in this chapter.

What is the clinical importance of vectorcardiography? The answer is that the information content of the VCG is the same, roughly, as that of the leads V_2, V_6 and aV_F in the 12-lead system, though it is obtained in corrected (orthonormal) form. It is true that the information content in the VCG signal is not greater than in the scalar ECG. However, the display system provides an opportunity to analyze the progress of the activation front in a different way, especially its initial and terminal parts. It is also much easier to observe the direction of the heart vector from the VCG loops. Additionally, the area of the loops, which is not easy to observe from a scalar display, may have clinical importance.

In this chapter we introduce representative examples of the large number of uncorrected and corrected vectorcardiographic lead systems.

16.2 UNCORRECTED VECTORCARDIOGRAPHIC LEAD SYSTEMS

PRECONDITIONS:

Source: *Dipole in a fixed location*

Conductor: *Infinite, homogeneous volume conductor or homogeneous sphere with the dipole in its center (the trivial solution)*

16.2.1 Monocardiogram by Mann

Though Waller was the first to record a set of three nearly orthogonal leads, namely mouth-to-left arm, mouth-to-left leg and back-to-front, he did not display them in vector form. It was Hubert Mann who in 1920 first suggested the concept of vectorcardiography by publishing a *monocardiogram,* which he constructed manually from the limb leads of Einthoven, as shown in Figure 1.18 (Mann, 1920). The monocardiogram of Mann is the projection of the vector loop in the frontal plane, assuming the validity of the Einthoven triangle lead vectors which it uses to interpret the limb lead voltages. Therefore, it is only two-dimensional, and it excludes the back-to-front information from the sagittal and transverse planes. (Note that Mann placed the signals of the leads I, II, and III to the lead vectors in opposite polarity. Therefore, the vector loop is oriented upward and right, though it actually should be oriented downward and left.)

Mann also constructed a special mirror galvanometer that allowed the display of the monocardiogram directly from ECG signals; see Figure 16.2 (Mann, 1938a). This mirror galvanometer included three coils arranged in

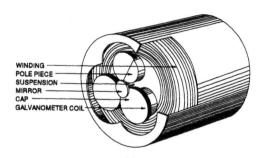

Fig. 16.2 The mirror vectorcardiograph constructed by Hubert Mann was the first instrument to produce a vectorcardiogram. It has three coils symmetrically placed at 120° intervals around a mirror. Thus it produces a vectorcardiogram in the frontal plane from the three limb leads of Einthoven (Mann, 1938a).

one plane and located symmetrically in 120° intervals around a mirror. They were situated in a constant magnetic field produced by a large coil. When the three coils were driven by amplified ECG signals from leads I, II, and III, the net torque of this coil assembly produced a deflection of the mirror, and a ray of light it reflected, proportional to the electric heart vector. Thus Mann's mirror galvanometer was actually an analog computer calculating the monocardiogram from the three limb leads. The work of Mann was largely ignored for more than 15 years. It had to await the invention of the cathode ray tube in the 1930s when it was possible to apply electronic devices to display the projections of the vector loop (Mann, 1931, 1938b).

An interesting invention in the vectorcardiography instrumentation was the cathode ray tube of W. Hollman and H. E. Hollman (1937). They used three pairs of deflection plates arranged at 60° angles with respect to one another corresponding to the directions of the three edges of the Einthoven triangle (see Fig. 16.3). When these deflection plates were driven with amplified leads I, II, and III, the tube produced on the screen a monocardiogram similar to Mann's mirror galvanometer on a film.

16.2.2 Lead Systems Based on Rectangular Body Axes

Most of the uncorrected and corrected vector-cardiographic lead systems are based on the rectangular body axes. From the large number of such uncorrected VCG lead systems, we briefly mention the following ones in this section.

After inventing the central terminal in 1932, Frank Norman Wilson logically progressed to the development of a lead system for vectorcardiography. Wilson and his co-workers published a lead system that added to the Einthoven limb leads an electrode located on the back (about 2.5 cm to the left from the seventh dorsal vertebra) (Wilson and Johnston, 1938, Wilson, Johnston, and Kossmann 1947). The four electrodes formed the corners of a tetrahedron, as shown in Figure 16.4, and consequently permitted the back-to-front component of the heart vector to be recognized. The three components of the electric heart vector were measured as follows (expressed in the consistent coordinate system described in Appendix A): The x-component was measured between the electrode on the back and the Wilson central terminal. The y-component was lead I, and the z-component was lead $-V_F$. This lead system, called the *Wilson tetrahedron*, was the first to display the three components of the electric heart vector.

The lead system of F. Schellong, S. Heller, and G. Schwingel (1937) is two-dimensional,

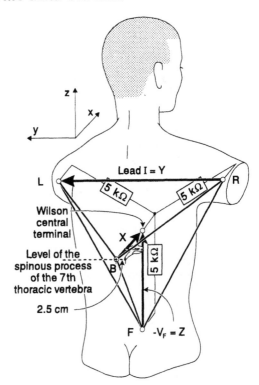

Fig. 16.4 The electrodes of the Wilson tetrahedron lead system.

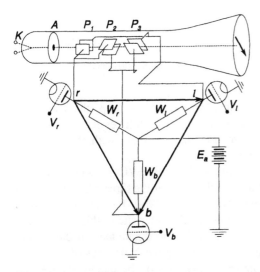

Fig. 16.3 The cathode ray tube of W. Hollman and H. E. Hollman has three pairs of deflection plates oriented in the directions of the edges of the Einthoven triangle. Thus it produces the vectorcardiogram in the frontal plane from the Einthoven limb leads. (Hollman and Hollman, 1937.)

presenting the vector loop only in the frontal plane. The other lead systems—those of Noboru Kimura (1939), Pierre Duchosal and R. Sulzer (1949), A. Grishman and L. Scherlis (1952), and William Milnor, S. Talbot, and E. Newman (1953)—also include the third dimension. These lead systems are illustrated in Figure 16.5. Because of their geometry, the lead system of Grishman and Scherlis was called the "Grishman cube" and the lead system of Duchosal and Schultzer the "double cube."

16.2.3 Akulinichev VCG Lead Systems

I. T. Akulinichev developed two uncorrected VCG-lead systems, one applying five display planes (Akulinichev, 1956) and another one applying three planes (Akulinichev, 1960). In the five-plane system, which he proposed in 1951, the electrodes are located in the corners of a pyramid so that four electrodes are on the anterior side of the thorax and the fifth is on the back, left from the spine on the level of the inferior angle of the scapula.

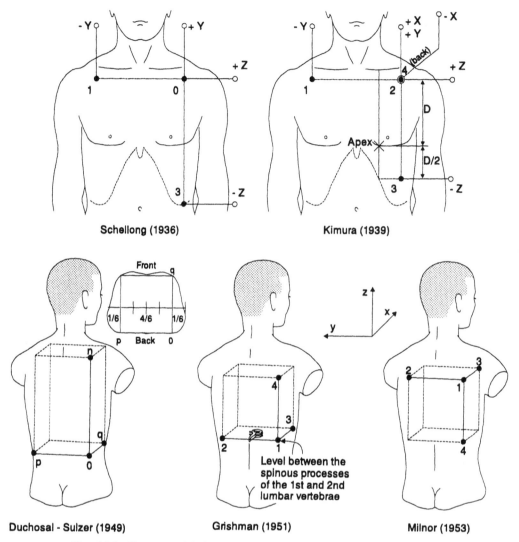

Fig. 16.5 Uncorrected VCG lead systems based on rectangular body axes.

In the five-plane Akulinichev system projection I is the frontal plane. The other four projections have different posterior views (Fig. 16.6A). Projection II examines the left ventricle in a left-superior-posterior view. Projections III and IV are right-inferior-posterior and left-inferior-posterior views, respectively. Projection V examines the atria in a right-superior-posterior view. Note that in the frontal plane the measurement between the electrodes 1 and 3 is oriented approximately along the main axis of the heart. The five projections of the electric heart vector recorded with the Akulinichev system are shown in Figure 16.6B. Because two projections are necessary and sufficient for dis-

playing a spatial vector loop, the five-plane Akulinichev system includes more redundant information than systems with three projections.

From the five-plane VCG system, Akulinichev developed later the three-plane VCG system (Akulinichev, 1960; Pawlov, 1966; Wenger, 1969). A characteristic of this lead system is that the main coordinate axes of the system are oriented along the main axes of the heart. The exact locations of the electrodes are (see Fig. 16.7) as follows: 1 = right arm, 2 = left arm, 4 = V_2, 5 = V_5, 6 = on the right side of xiphoid, 7 = V_9 (at the left side of the spine on the level of V_4 and V_5). The three projections

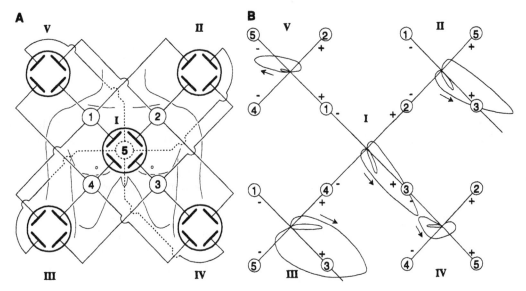

Fig. 16.6 Five-plane Akulinichev VCG system. (A) Location of the electrodes on the thorax and their five connections to the oscilloscope. (B) The five projections of the electric heart vector.

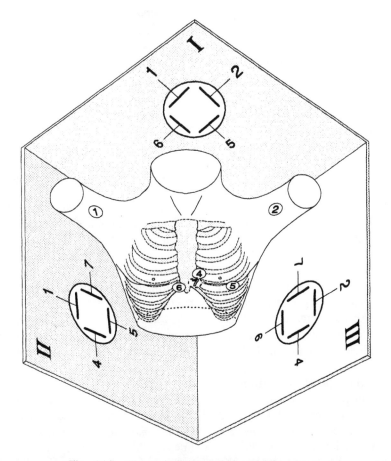

Fig. 16.7 Three-plane Akulinichev VCG system.

are formed as follows: projection I = electrodes 1, 2, 5, and 6 (i.e., the frontal plane); projection II = electrodes 1, 7, 5, and 4 (i.e., parallel to the longitudinal axis of the heart); projection III = electrodes 6, 7, 2, and 4 (i.e., the cross-sectional plane of the heart).

The Akulinichev lead systems have been applied in the (former) Soviet Union and Bulgaria since the 1960s and they are virtually the only clinical vectorcardiographic systems used there to date.

16.3 CORRECTED VECTORCARDIOGRAPHIC LEAD SYSTEMS

16.3.1 Frank Lead System

PRECONDITIONS:

Source: *Dipole in a fixed location*
Conductor: *Finite, homogeneous*

In 1956 Ernest Frank (Frank, 1956) published a vectorcardiographic lead system that was based on his previously published data of image surface (Frank, 1954). Because the image surface was measured for a finite, homogeneous thorax model, the volume conductor model for the Frank VCG-lead system was also the same. In the following, we first discuss the design principles of the Frank lead system. Then we discuss the construction of each orthogonal component of the measurement system. Though we refer here to the original publication of Frank, we use the consistent coordinate system described in Appendix A.

Electrode Location Requirements

To measure the three dipole components, at least four electrodes (one being a reference) are needed. Frank decided to increase the number of electrodes to seven, in order to decrease the error due to interindividual variation in the heart location and body shape.

It is important that the electrode location can be easily found to increase the reproducibility of the measurement. The reproducibility of the limb electrodes is very good. However, the arm electrodes have the problem that the lead fields change remarkably if the patient touches the

sides with the arms, because the electric current flows through the wet skin directly to the thorax. This problem has a special importance to the left arm, the since heart is closer.

Determination of the Electrode Location

Based on the above requirements Frank devised a lead system, now bearing his name, which yields corrected orthogonal leads. Electrode numbers and positions were chosen very deliberately, and were based upon his image surface model (Fig. 11.14). He selected level 6 for electrode placement, because the lead vectors are largest on this level. Specifically, he chose the points designated A, E, I, and M on the left, front, right, and back, respectively. He also chose point C between points A and E because it is close to the heart. In addition, a point on the neck and one on the left foot were included.

Right-to-Left Component (y-Component)

We begin with the right-to-left component (*y*-component) because its construction is the simplest and easy to understand. The lead vector in this direction is determined by applying previously mentioned methods to Figure 16.8. This figure shows the anatomic view of level 6 as well as its image surface as measured by Frank. The image space locations of electrodes A, C, and I are also shown since these were chosen to sense the *y*-component of the heart vector.

The basic principle in the design of the *y*-component of the lead system is to synthesize in image space, with the available electrode points, a lead vector that is oriented in the *y*-direction. This is the only requirement that must be fulfilled for the lead to record the *y*-component.

Additionally, it is advantageous to select from among all those lead vectors that are in the *y*-direction the one that is the largest. This ensures a signal-to-noise ratio that is as high as possible.

If we designate image space point I′ as one end point of the selected lead vector parallel to the *y*-axis, its other end point is found on line A′-C′, and is labeled point a′. Point a′ divides A′-C′ in the proportion 1:3.59. By con-

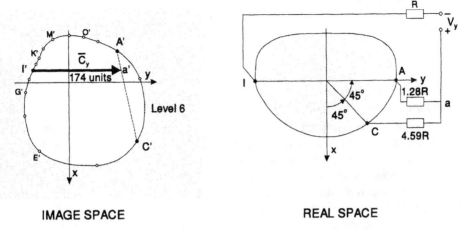

Fig. 16.8 Determination of the right-to-left component (*y*-component) in the Frank lead system. The image space shown on the left corresponds to the actual transverse plane on the right.

necting two resistors having values in this ratio between the points A and C in real space, the point a is realized at their intersection.

From a practical point of view it is important that the impedance the amplifier sees in each lead be equal. A good balance ensures cancellation of common mode noise signals. If we designate this impedance as *R*, we have to add such a resistor to the lead in electrode I and to multiply the parallel resistors of electrodes A and C by the factor 1.28. This yields resistor values 1.28*R* and 4.59*R*, respectively. (Note that now the parallel resistance of these two

resistors is *R*.) From a measurement in image space we determine the length of the lead vector $\bar{c}_y$ to be 174 relative units.

Foot-to-Head Component (*z*-Component)

From the image space in Figure 16.9, we can verify that if we select for one end of the image vector the point H′ on level 1 (i.e., on the neck), there exists a point k′ on line F′-M′ such that K′-H′ forms a lead vector parallel to the *z*-axis. The point k′ divides the axis in proportion 1:1.9. Again the lead is balanced by placing a resistor

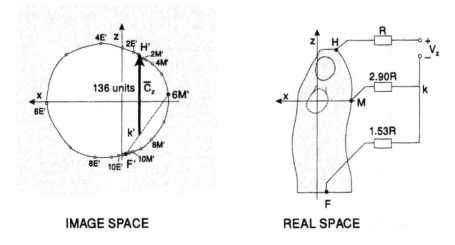

Fig. 16.9 Determination of the foot-to-head component (*z*-component) in the Frank lead system. The image space shown on the left corresponds to the actual sagittal plane on the right.

R in series with electrode H and by multiplying the resistors in electrodes F and M by a factor 1.53 which leads to values of 1.53R and 2.90R, respectively. The length of the lead vector $\bar{c}_z$ is 136 units.

Back-to-Front Component (x-Component)

In the design of the x-component Frank wanted, in addition to the previous requirements, to select such a weighing for the electrodes that the lead vector variation throughout the heart would be as uniform as possible. Consequently, Frank used all the five electrodes on level 6. The transverse plane projection of the image surface is shown again in Figure 16.10, and electrodes A, C, E, I, and M are described in both real and image space.

Frank drew the lines A'-M', E'-C' and g'-I' in the image space, from which the point g' was located on the line E'-C'. Between the lines A'-M' and g'-I' he drew a line segment f'-h' parallel to the x-axis. This is the lead vector corresponding to the x-lead and fully meets the requirements discussed above.

The physical realization of the lead that corresponds to the chosen lead vector is found as follows: From the image space, it is possible to ascertain that the point f' divides the segment of line A'-M' in the proportion 5.56:1. Multiplying these with 1.18, we obtain values 6.56:1.18 having a parallel resistance value of

1. By connecting two resistors of similar proportions in series, between the electrodes A and M, we find that their point of connection in real space is f.

Similarly the point g' divides the image space segment of line C'-E' in the proportion 1.61:1. The parallel value of these is 0.62. The point h' divides the segment of line g'-I' in the proportion 1:2.29. If we multiply this by 0.62, we get 0.62:1.41. Now we have the relative resistor values 1.61, 1, and 1.41 to electrodes C, E, and I, respectively. To adjust their parallel resistances to be equal to 1, we multiply each by 2.32 and we obtain 3.74R, 2.32R, and 3.72R. Now we have synthesized the lead vector $\bar{c}_x$; relative to the assumed image space scale, it has a magnitude of 156 units.

Frank Lead Matrix

We have now determined all three lead vectors that form an orthogonal lead system. This system must still be normalized. Therefore, resistors 13.3R and 7.15R are connected between the leads of the x- and y-components to attenuate these signals to the same level as the z-lead signal. Now the Frank lead system is orthonormal.

It should be noted once again that the resistance of the resistor network connected to each lead pair is unity. This choice results in a balanced load and increases the common mode

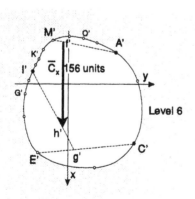

IMAGE SPACE

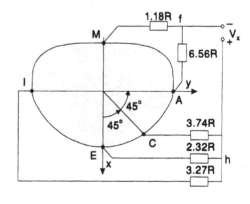

REAL SPACE

Fig. 16.10 Determination of the back-to-front component (x-component) in the Frank lead system. The image space shown on the left corresponds to the actual transverse plane on the right.

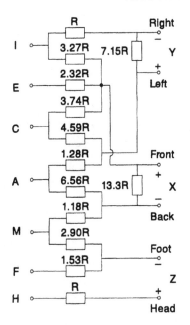

Fig. 16.11 The lead matrix of the Frank VCG system. The electrodes are marked I, E, C, A, M, F, and H, and their anatomical positions are shown. The resistor matrix results in the establishment of normalized x-, y-, and z-component lead vectors, as described in the text.

rejection ratio of the system. The absolute value of the lead matrix resistances may be determined once the value of R is specified. For this factor Frank recommended that it should be at least 25 kΩ, and preferably 100 kΩ. Nowadays the lead signals are usually detected with a high-impedance preamplifier, and the lead matrix function is performed by operational amplifiers or digitally thereafter. Figure 16.11 illustrates the complete Frank lead matrix.

It is worth mentioning that the Frank system is presently the most common of all clinical VCG systems throughout the world.

16.3.2 McFee-Parungao Lead System

PRECONDITIONS:

Source: *Dipole moment of a volume source*

Conductor: *Finite, homogeneous*

McFee and Parungao (1961) published a simple VCG lead system called the *axial* system, based on a lead field theoretic approach. In addition, the heart was modeled with a volume source and the thorax was assumed to be homogeneous.

The three uniform lead fields were designed according to the principle discussed in Section 11.6.10. To detect the three orthogonal components of the electric heart vector, three pairs of (single or multiple) electrodes must be used on each coordinate axis, one on either side of the heart. McFee and Parungao recognized that the closer to the heart the electrodes are placed the more electrodes must be used to achieve a homogeneous lead field within the heart's area.

Back-to-Front Component (x-Component)

McFee and Parungao felt that three anterior electrodes should be assigned to the measurement of the back-to-front component of the VCG. This would generate a lead field with sufficient homogeneity even though the heart is close to the anterior wall of the thorax. They followed the method of synthesizing ideal lead fields as discussed in Section 11.5.8. By connecting 100 kΩ resistances to each electrode, the net lead impedance is 33 kΩ.

The accurate location of the chest electrodes is found as follows: The electrodes form an equilateral triangle so oriented that its base is nearest to the subject's feet. The electrodes are at a distance of 6 cm from the center of the triangle. The center of the triangle is in the fifth intercostal space, 2 cm to the left of the sternal margin. This position should ensure that the chest electrodes are located directly above the center of gravity of the ventricles. (This is illustrated in Fig. 16.12.)

Because the posterior wall of the thorax is more distant from the heart, only one electrode is needed there. The back electrode lies directly behind the center of the chest triangle. McFee and Parungao did not balance the lead system against common mode noise. The authors suggest that if a 33 kΩ resistor were connected to the back electrode, the balancing requirement, discussed earlier, would be fulfilled.

Right-to-Left Component (y-Component)

For the y-component the same procedure as described above was followed. McFee and Parungao placed two electrodes with 66 kΩ resistances on the left side and one electrode on the right side of the thorax. The right electrode is located on the same level as the center of the electrode triangle on the chest. It is placed on the right side, one third of the way from the chest to the back. The electrodes on the left side are also located one third of the way toward the back at longitudinal levels 5.5 cm over and below the level of the center of the chest triangle. The electrode spacing is therefore 11 cm. These produce reasonably uniform right-to-left lead fields in the region of the heart.

McFee and Parungao did not balance the y-lead either. The authors suggest that adding a 33 kΩ resistor to the electrode on the right balances the lead against common mode noise.

Foot-to-Head Component (z-Component)

The electrodes designed to measure the z-component of the VCG are so distant from the heart that McFee and Parungao used only one electrode on the neck and one on the left foot. These electrodes may be equipped with a 33 kΩ re-

sistor for the whole lead system to be balanced. The complete McFee-Parungao VCG lead system is shown in Figure 16.12.

16.3.3 SVEC III Lead System

PRECONDITIONS:

Source: *Dipole moment of a volume source*
Conductor: *Finite, homogeneous*

Otto H. Schmitt and Ernst Simonson developed many versions of vectorcardiographic lead systems, calling them *stereovectorelectrocardiography* (SVEC). The third version, SVEC III, was published in 1955 (Schmitt and Simonson, 1955). It requires a total of 14 electrodes and creates a lead field in the thorax which is very symmetric in relation to the sagittal plane. The lead system is described in Figure 16.13.

In the SVEC III lead system, the electrodes are located on the thorax in the following way: The torso is divided angularly into 30° symmetric sectors about a central vertical axis so that, starting with 1 at the front, Arabic numerals up to 12 divide the torso vertically. Roman numerals refer to interspaces at the sternum and are carried around horizontally on a flat panel so that a grid is established on which a location such as V 7 would mean a location at the vertical level of the fifth interspace and at the middle of the back.

Back-to-Front Component (x-Component)

The back-to-front component, the x-component, is formed from four electrodes on the back and four electrodes on the chest. The back electrodes are located at the grid points III 6, III 8, VI 6, and VI 8. Each of these electrodes is connected with a 100 kΩ resistor to the common back terminal $(-X)$. The chest electrodes are located at grid points III 12, III 2, VI 2, and VI 12. A 70 kΩ resistor is connected from the first one (III 12), and 100 kΩ resistors are connected from the others to the common chest terminal $(+X)$.

Right-to-Left Component (y-Component)

The right terminal $(-Y)$ is obtained by connecting 100 kΩ resistors to the right arm and

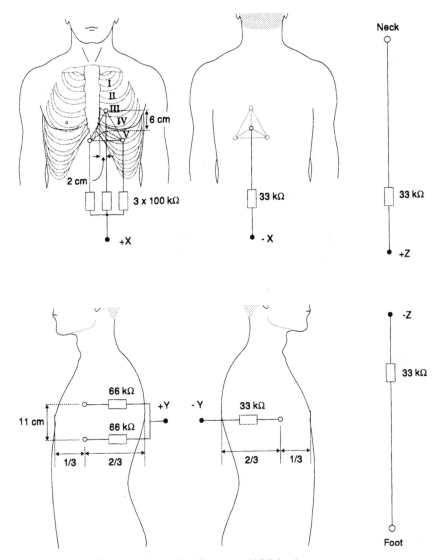

Fig. 16.12 McFee-Parungao VCG lead system.

to the grid point V 11. The left terminal $(+Y)$ is formed similarly by connecting 100 kΩ resistors to the left arm and to the grid point V 3. To normalize the lead, the gain is adjusted to the 75% level.

Foot-to-Head Component (z-Component)

The z-component is obtained simply by placing electrodes to the left foot and to the head. Again, to normalize the lead, the gain is adjusted to the 71% level.

16.3.4 Fischmann-Barber-Weiss Lead System

PRECONDITIONS:

Source: *Dipole moment of a volume source with moving (optimal) location*

Conductor: *Finite, homogeneous*

E. J. Fischmann, M. R. Barber, and G. H. Weiss (1971) constructed a VCG lead system that measures the equivalent electric dipole according to the Gabor-Nelson theorem.

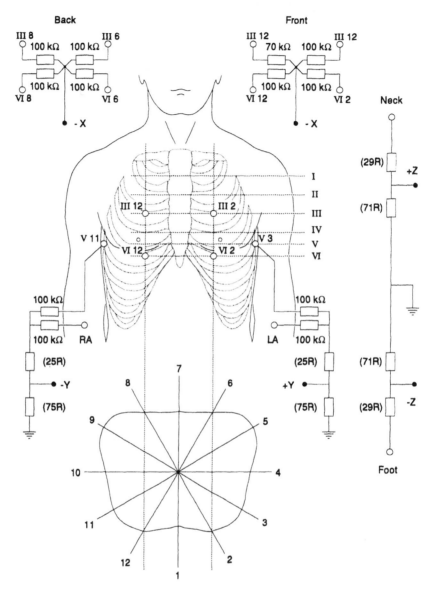

Fig. 16.13 SVEC III VCG lead system.

Their equipment consisted of a matrix of 7 × 8 electrodes on the back of the patient and 11 × 12 on the chest. The latter were fixed on rods that could move along their axes. Similar electrode matrices with 7 × 7 electrodes were also placed on the sides of the patient. When the moving-rod electrodes are pressed against the surface of the thorax, their movement gives information about the thorax shape. This information is needed in the solution of the Gabor-Nelson equation.

This lead system was not intended for clinical use but rather for the demonstration of the Gabor-Nelson theory in the measurement of the vectorcardiogram.

16.3.5 Nelson Lead System

PRECONDITIONS:

Source: *Dipole moment of a volume source with moving (optimal) location*
Conductor: *Finite, homogeneous*

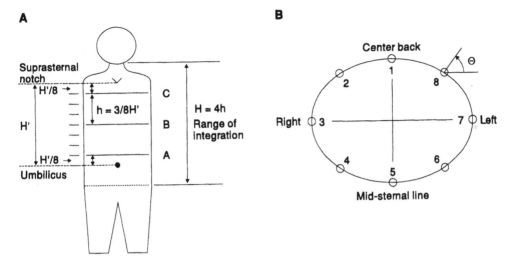

Fig. 16.14 The electrode locations in the Nelson lead system.

In 1971 Clifford V. Nelson and his collaborators published a lead system suitable for clinical use based on the Gabor-Nelson theorem (Nelson et al., 1971). The lead system includes electrodes placed on three levels of the thorax with eight on each level, one electrode on the head, and one on the left leg. The electrode rows are designated A, B, and C, as shown in Figure 16.14. The levels are determined by measuring the distance H' between the suprasternal notch and umbilicus. This distance is divided by 8, and the rows are placed at $\frac{1}{8} H'$, $\frac{4}{8} H'$, and $\frac{7}{8} H'$ from either notch or umbilicus.

As shown in Figure 16.14, electrodes 1 and 5 are placed at center-back and midsternal line, respectively. Electrodes 2, 3, and 4 are equally spaced on the right side, and electrodes 6, 7, and 8 are equally spaced on the left side. If the arms intervene on level C, electrodes 3 and 7 are placed on the right arm and left arm, respectively. The angle θ is the angle between the surface of the thorax and the frontal plane.

Resistors of 500 kΩ (R) are connected to the electrodes on rows A, B, and C (see Fig. 16.15). From these resistors, on each three levels four (R_x and R_y) are variable and are adjusted according to the shape of the thorax of the patient to obey the Gabor-Nelson theory. The adjustment is made so that

$$R_x/R = \sin \theta \qquad (16.1)$$
$$R_y/R = \cos \theta$$

where θ = the angle between the surface normal and the sagittal plane.

Nelson and co-workers claim that on the basis of their measurements this VCG lead system is much more accurate than the McFee or Frank lead systems. Furthermore, this system should be very insensitive to electrode misplacement.

16.4 DISCUSSION OF VECTORCARDIOGRAPHIC LEADS

16.4.1 Interchangeability of Vectorcardiographic Systems

The purpose of the vectorcardiographic systems is to detect the equivalent dipole of the heart. If various systems make this measurement accurately, the measurement results should be identical. This is, however, not the case. In practice, each vectorcardiographic system gives a little different measurement result.

There have been attempts to develop transformation coefficients from one system to another in order to make the various systems commensurable. If the various systems are orthogonal, these transformations should, in principle, also be orthogonal.

Horan, Flowers, and Brody (1965) made a careful study on the transformation coefficients

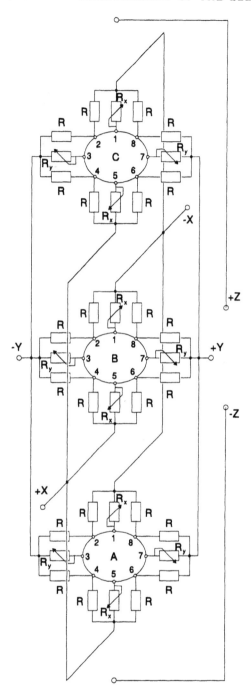

vectorcardiographic systems are not truly orthogonal. They also came to the conclusion that the practical interchangeability of quantitative information obtained from one lead system into that obtained by another is seriously limited because of the wide range of biologic variation in transformation characteristics.

16.4.2 Properties of Various Vectorcardiographic Lead Systems

The previously discussed lead systems have been examined using computer models of the thorax to determine the extent to which they satisfy the fundamental conditions for corrected orthogonal leads.

Under uniform, homogeneous, and bounded conditions, Brody and Arzbaecher (1964) evaluated the lead fields for several VCG systems and compared the degree of uniformity. They found that the Frank, SVEC III, and McFee-Parungao lead systems introduced a degree of distortion. However, the Grishman cube and Wilson tetrahedron lead systems were considerably worse. The McFee-Parungao system was found to have the best orthogonality of all systems, but the strength of the leads was found to be unequal. Macfarlane (1969) introduced a modification that equalized the lead strengths.

The effect of inhomogeneities on the lead vector field has been considered by Milan Horáček (1989). This examination was conducted by a computer simulation in which the influence of inhomogeneities on the image surface was evaluated.

The effect of the intracavitary blood mass tends to counteract that of the lungs. The blood mass decreases tangential dipoles and enhances normal dipoles. The effect of lung conductivity on lead vectors was studied by Stanley, Pilkington, and Morrow (1986). Using a realistic canine torso model, they showed that the z (foot-to-head) dipole moment decreased monotonically as the lung conductivity increased. On the other hand, the y (right-to-left) and x (back-to-front) dipole moment have a bellshaped behavior, with low values for both high and low lung conductivities. They found that the lung conductivity, nevertheless, has relatively little effect on the overall torso volume conductor properties. The inhomogeneity that, in their study, has a significant effect is

Fig. 16.15 Electrode matrix in the Nelson VCG lead system.

between Frank, McFee-Parungao (axial-), and SVEC III lead systems for 35 normal young men. In this study it was found that the transformations between these lead systems were not orthogonal, indicating that at least two of the

the skeletal muscle layer. These results are reasonably consistent with those of Gulrajani and Mailloux (1983) and Rudy and Plonsey (1980).

Jari Hyttinen analyzed the properties of Frank, axial, and SVEC III lead systems with his computer model called the hybrid model (Hyttinen, 1989). He analyzed the magnitude and the direction of the lead vectors in various regions of the heart in an inhomogeneous thorax model. He also conducted studies on the sensitivities of the leads to sources in radial and tangential directions (in relation to the heart), which has certain clinical implications.

In his study of the ideal VCG lead, Hyttinen found that in all of the studied lead systems, the lead vectors of the x-leads are directed downward in the upper posterior part of the heart. The blood masses in and above the heart in the great vessels are mainly responsible for this behavior of the lead vectors. The x-lead, which is closest to ideal, is in the axial system. The total sensitivity in the x-direction is a little lower than that of the SVEC III x-lead, but the homogeneity of the lead is much better. The locations of the chest electrodes are good and the proximity effect is weaker in the axial x-lead compared to the other lead systems.

For the y-leads, the SVEC III y-lead has the best properties. The SVEC III and the axial y-leads have equal sensitivity in the y-direction, but the differences in the spatial sensitivity distribution—that is, the homogeneity of the sensitivity—is better in the SVEC III system. The proximity effect is not so pronounced because of the use of lead I as a part of the SVEC III y-lead.

In the z-leads, the inhomogeneities are the main reasons for distortion of the spatial sensitivity. This can be seen especially in the septal area. The leads are, however, very similar with the Frank z-lead, having slightly better spatial sensitivity properties than the other lead systems.

REFERENCES

Akulinichev IT (1956): Vectorelectrocardioscope. *Voenno-Med. Zh.* 1: 79. (In Russian).

Akulinichev IT (1960): *Practical Questions in Vectorcardioscopy,* Medgiz, Moscow. (In Russian)

Brody DA, Arzbaecher RC (1964): A comparative analysis of several corrected vector-cardiographic leads. *Circulation* 29:(4, Suppl.) 533–45.

Duchosal PW, Sulzer R (1949): *La Vectorcardiographie,* S. Karger, New York, N.Y.

Fischmann EJ, Barber MR, Weiss GH (1971): Multielectrode grids which measure torso area and resistivity and yield dipole moments calibrated for these variables. In *Proc. XIth Internat. Symp. On Vectorcardiography, New York, 1970,* ed. I Hoffman, pp. 30–41, North-Holland Publishing Co., Amsterdam.

Frank E (1954): The image surface of a homogeneous torso. *Am. Heart J.* 47: 757–68.

Frank E (1956): An accurate, clinically practical system for spatial vectorcardiography. *Circulation* 13:(5) 737–49.

Grishman A, Scherlis L (1952): *Spatial Vectorcardiography,* 217 pp. Saunders, Philadelphia.

Gulrajani RM, Mailloux GE (1983): A simulation study of the effects of torso inhomogeneities on electrocardiographic potentials using realistic heart and torso models. *Circ. Res.* 52: 45–56.

Hollman W, Hollman HE (1937): Neue electrocardiographische Untersuchungsmethode. *Z. Kreislaufforsch.* 29: 546–558.

Horáček BM (1989): Lead theory. In *Comprehensive Electrocardiology. Theory and Practice in Health and Disease,* 1st ed. Vol. 1, ed. PW Macfarlane, TDV Lawrie, pp. 291–314, Pergamon Press, New York.

Horan LG, Flowers NC, Brody DA (1965): The interchangeability of vectorcardiographic systems. *Am. Heart J.* 70:(3) 365–76.

Hyttinen J (1989): Development of aimed ECG-leads. *Tampere Univ. Tech., Tampere, Finland,* Thesis, pp. 138. (Lic. Tech. thesis)

Kimura N (1939): Study on heart function by vectorcardiography of three-dimensional projection. *Jpn. Circ. J.* 5: 93.

Macfarlane PW (1969): A modified axial lead system for orthogonal lead electrocardiography. *Cardiovasc. Res.* 3:(10) 510–5.

Mann H (1920): A method for analyzing the electrocardiogram. *Arch. Int. Med.* 25: 283–94.

Mann H (1931): Interpretation of bundle-branch block by means of the monocardiogram. *Am. Heart J.* 6: 447–57.

Mann H (1938a): The monocardiogram. *Stud. Rockefeller Inst. Med. Res.* 109: 409–32.

Mann H (1938b): The monocardiograph. *Am. Heart J.* 15: 681–99.

McFee R, Parungao A (1961): An orthogonal lead system for clinical electrocardiography. *Am. Heart J.* 62: 93–100.

Milnor MR, Talbot SA, Newman EV (1953): A study of the relationship between unipolar leads and spatial vectorcardiograms, using the panoramic vectorcardiograph. *Circulation* 7: 545.

Nelson CV, Gastongay PR, Wilkinson AF, Voukydis PC (1971): A lead system for direction and magnitude of the heart vector. In *Vectorcardiography 2. Proc. XIth Internat. Symp. On Vectorcardiography, New York, 1970*, ed. I Hoffman, IR Hamby, E Glassman, pp. 85–97, North-Holland Publishing Co., Amsterdam.

Pawlov Z (1966): Über einige Fragen des Vektorkardiographischen Dreiflächensystems von Akulinitschev. In *Neue Ergebnisse Der Elektrokardiologie,* ed. E Schubert (Proceedings of the 6th International Colloquium of Vectorcardiography, Leipzig, 1965), VEB Gustav Fischer Verlag, Jena.

Rudy Y, Plonsey R (1980): A comparison of volume conductor and source geometry effects on body surface and epicardial potentials. *Circ. Res.* 46:(2) 283–91.

Schellong F, Heller S, Schwingel G (1937): Das Vectorcardiogram; Eine Untersuchungsmethode des Herzens. *Z. Kreislaufforsch.* 29: 497–509.

Schmitt OH, Simonson E (1955): The present status of vectorcardiography. *A.M.A. Arch. Internal Med.* 96: 574–90.

Stanley PC, Pilkington TC, Morrow MN (1986): The effects of thoracic inhomogeneities on the relationship between epicardial and torso potentials. *IEEE Trans. Biomed. Eng.* BME-33:(3) 273–84.

Waller AD (1887): A demonstration on man of electromotive changes accompanying the heart's beat. *J. Physiol. (Lond.)* 8: 229–34.

Wenger R (1969): *Klinische Vektorkardiographie,* 2nd ed., Dr. Dietrich Steinkopff Verlag, Darmstadt.

Wilson FN, Johnston FD (1938): The vectorcardiogram. *Am. Heart J.* 16: 14–28.

Wilson FN, Johnston FD, Kossmann CE (1947): The substitution of a tetrahedron for the Einthoven triangle. *Am. Heart J.* 33: 594–603.

REFERENCES, BOOKS

Macfarlane PW, Lawrie TDV (eds.) (1989): *Comprehensive Electrocardiology: Theory and Practice in Health and Disease.* 1st ed. Vols. 1, 2, and 3. Pergamon Press, New York. 1785 pp.

17

Other ECG Lead Systems

17.1 MOVING DIPOLE

We have noted that the source associated with cardiac activation is a double layer, which lies at the activation surface. This double layer can be approximated by a single resultant dipole. As the activation front in the ventricular wall progresses, the dipole which is at the center of gravity of the cover that closes the cup-like activation front, also moves. Consequently, the location of the equivalent electric dipole of the heart tracks this movement. However, if there is more than one simultaneous activation wave, this movement will be a complex function of the movement of the individual resultant dipoles. When one is trying to develop an improved model for the cardiac electric generator, the moving dipole is a logical target of interest.

R. M. Arthur conducted experiments to evaluate the moving dipole (Arthur et al., 1971). In these experiments he used a finite homogeneous model for the torso. It appeared that the path of the moving electric center of the cardiac activation is within the heart border throughout the cardiac cycle, in the atria during the P wave and in the ventricles during the QRS and T waves.

Additional insight into the moving dipole model was gained through more recent work by Pierre Savard and colleagues (Savard et al.,

1980). These investigators used an animal model so that the computed trajectory could be compared with actual intramural cardiac data. They obtained their best results when there was only a single confined activation surface, a result that is not unexpected. For this reason, some recent investigators have been examining a two moving dipole model.

17.2 MULTIPLE DIPOLES

The first suggestion for a multiple dipole model of the heart was made by E. J. Fischmann and M. R. Barber (1963). Based on this idea Ronald Selvester constructed a computer model consisting of 20 dipoles (Selvester, Collier, and Pearson, 1965). In this first model the effect of the thorax boundary and internal inhomogeneities were omitted. Selvester later constructed another model in which these effects were included (Selvester et al., 1966; see Fig. 17.1).

J. H. Holt and his colleagues formulated a model consisting of 12 dipoles, whose locations and directions in the myocardium were fixed (Holt et al., 1969a). To evaluate these dipoles, he recorded ECG signals from an 126-electrode array on the surface of the thorax. The number of the electrodes was intentionally selected to be an order of magnitude larger than the number

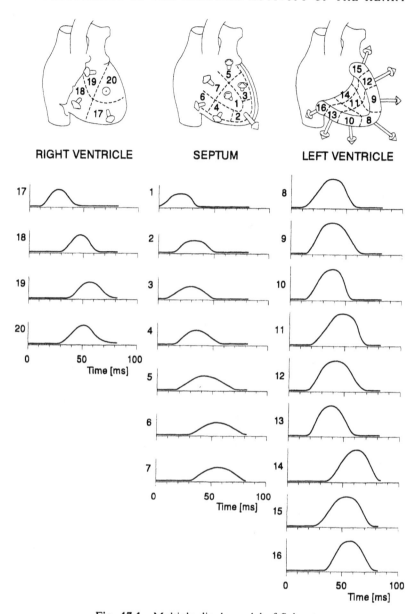

Fig. 17.1 Multiple-dipole model of Selvester.

of variables in the multiple-dipole model. This step provided an opportunity to improve accuracy based on the redundancy, and could compensate for missing signals and for the presence of noise (Lynn et al., 1967).

17.3 MULTIPOLE

The multipole model is based on a spherical harmonic expansion of the volume source and its components are dipole, quadrupole, octapole, and so on. These components of the multipole model have the following number of independent variables: 3 for dipole, 5 for quadrupole, 7 for octapole, and so on. The first scientists to apply the multipole model to cardiac modeling were G. Yeh and colleagues (1958). Research with multipole models has been further extended by David Geselowitz (Geselowitz, 1960) and Daniel Brody (Brody, Bradshaw, and Evans, 1961).

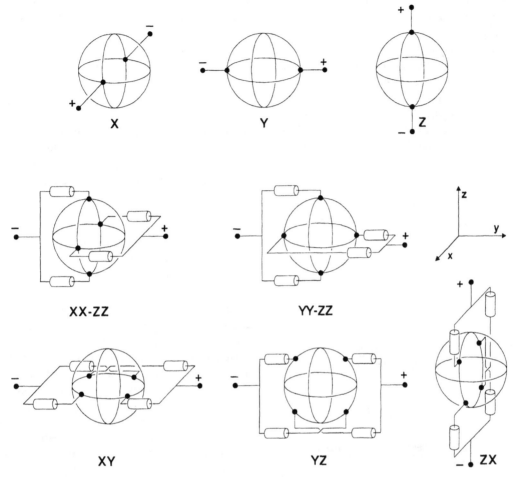

Fig. 17.2 The principle of the measurement of dipole and quadrupole components in a spherical volume conductor.

Figure 17.2 illustrates the basic principle involved in measuring the dipole and quadrupole components of a source lying in a spherical conductor. In actuality, instead of resistor weighing, many electrodes are used and the multipole components are evaluated numerically. The procedure is discussed in Pilkington and Plonsey (1982).

In his research, R. M. Arthur (Arthur et al., 1972), when trying to fit the dipole model to potentials measured at 284 points on the thorax surface, found that the best fit showed an error of 23%. When the quadrupole component was added to the model, the best fit showed an error of 14%. Therefore, the inclusion of the quadrupole component decreased the error by 9%.

A more detailed description of the cardiac models presented here and a critical evaluation of their strengths and weaknesses may be found in Pilkington and Plonsey (1982) and in Gulrajani (1989). As noted, there is growing interest in using multiple body-surface electrodes (25–250) and employing the displayed output to produce a sequence of equipotential surface maps.

17.4 SUMMARY OF THE ECG LEAD SYSTEMS

We briefly discuss the possibilities of evaluating the diagnostic performance of the ECG by improving the model of the source and conductor in light of the investigations discussed above. For this purpose we define the clinical concepts of sensitivity, specificity, and diagnostic performance.

Sensitivity denotes the relative number of abnormals that are detected by the system. *Specificity* denotes the relative number of normals that are classified as normals. The concept of *diagnostic performance* is defined as the average of the sensitivity and specificity of the method (Macfarlane and Lawrie, 1989). We summarize these definitions below:

$$\text{SENSITIVITY} = \frac{\text{number of abnormals that are classified correctly as abnormal}}{\text{total number of abnormals}} 100\%$$

$$= \frac{TP}{TP + FN} 100\% \qquad (17.1)$$

$$\text{SPECIFICITY} = \frac{\text{number of normals that are classified correctly as normal}}{\text{total number of normals}} 100\%$$

$$= \frac{TN}{TN + FP} 100\% \qquad (17.2)$$

$$\text{DIAGNOSTIC PERFORMANCE} = \frac{\text{SENSITIVITY} + \text{SPECIFICITY}}{2} \qquad (17.3)$$

where

FN = false negatives
FP = false positives
TN = true negatives and
TP = true positives

The investigation of Holt, based on the multiple dipole model, gave remarkably good results (Holt et al., 1969b,c). In the diagnosis of hypertrophy the diagnostic performance was about 90%. However, for the diagnosis of myocardial infarction the Holt et al. method gave a diagnostic performance of about 80%. Thus, in spite of being much more sophisticated, it did not achieve better results than the simpler conventional approaches.

Table 17.1 summarizes the volume source and volume conductor models used as the basis for various ECG systems and ECG research. It would be natural to select the most accurate

model for the volume source as well as for the volume conductor when trying to solve the inverse problem most accurately. Hence the choice of modeling approaches should be located on the right side and on one of the lowest rows in Table 17.1.

In Section 7.5.4, it was noted that any model should have good correspondence with the physiological preparation it represents, to have clinical importance. Application of this principle would lead to the choice of the multiple dipole model, since it simulates each region of the myocardium.

The components of the multipole model are orthogonal and can be shown to have a unique solution; however, it is difficult to conceptualize the physiological meaning of this solution. On the other hand, one can show that the evaluation of a multiple dipole model beyond three or four dipoles becomes very sensitive to noise and errors in geometry. The problem is ill-defined. Furthermore, the interpretation of an inverse dipole in terms of underlying cellular behavior is unclear and probably also not unique. Fundamentally, the inverse problem in regard to intramural sources is not unique; this is, in a nutshell, the underlying problem of the inverse solution in ECG. For this reason, it is evident that the single dipole model remains central in clinical electrocardiology.

In recent years a number of sophisticated mathematical techniques have been applied to the inverse problem in electrocardiography. These now concentrate data from lead systems composed of large numbers of electrodes (100–200). In addition, the goal, rather than a search for intramural information, is limited to a determination of epicardial surface potentials. In principle, these are uniquely determined by the body surface potentials, and they additionally provide enhanced regional information. The various approaches utilize different ways to stabilize what is an ill-conditioned problem (involving inversion of ill-conditioned matrices). Such methods depend on a priori physiological constraints such as the outward propagation of activity or the spectral properties and the amplitude of the noise, smoothness of potential distributions, or smoothness of their gradients/Laplacians.

The reader is referred to three publications

Table 17.1 Summary of models used in various ECG systems

		Volume source		Volume conductor (thorax model)		
		Electric heart model	Number of variables	Infinite homogeneous (spherical)	Finite homogeneous	Finite inhomogeneous
			2	I, II, III		
+ +	+	dipole	3	12-lead ECG, VCG (cube, tetrahedron)	VCG (Frank, McFee, SVEC, Gabor-Nelson)	Burger-van Milaan
+	(+)	moving dipole	6		Gabor-Nelson Arthur	
− +	+	multiple dipole	3 n (n)	Selvester	Selvester	Selvester Holt
+	−	multipole dipole quadrupole octapole	3 5 7			

correspondence between the model and the heart

solvability of the heart model

that review and summarize the current status of inverse electrocardiography, namely Pilkington and Plonsey (1982), Gulrajani (1988, 1989), and Rudy and Messinger-Rapport (1988).

REFERENCES

Arthur RM, Geselowitz DB, Briller SA, Trost RF (1971): The path of the electrical center of the human heart determined from surface electrocardiograms. *J. Electrocardiol.* 4:(1) 29–33.

Arthur RM, Geselowitz DB, Briller SA, Trost RF (1972): Quadrupole components of the human surface electrocardiogram. *Am. Heart J.* 83:(5) 663–7.

Brody DA, Bradshaw JC, Evans JW (1961): A theoretical basis for determining heart-lead relationships of the equivalent cardiac multipole. *IRE Trans. Biomed. Electron.* BME-8:(4) 139–43.

Fischmann EJ, Barber MR (1963): 'Aimed' electrocardiography. Model studies, using a heart consisting of 6 electrically isolated areas. *Am. Heart J.* 65:(5) 628–37.

Geselowitz DB (1960): Multipole representation for an equivalent cardiac generator. *Proc. IRE* 48:(1) 75–9.

Gulrajani RM (1989): The inverse problem of electrocardiography. In *Comprehensive Electrocardiology. Theory and Practice in Health and Disease,* 1st ed. Vol. 1, ed. PW Macfarlane, TDV Lawrie, pp. 237–88, Pergamon Press, New York.

Gulrajani RM, Savard P, Roberge FA (1988): The inverse problem in electrocardiography: Solution in terms of equivalent sources. *CRC Crit. Rev. Biomed. Eng.* 16: 171–214.

Holt JH, Barnard ACL, Lynn MS, Svendsen P (1969a): A study of the human heart as a multiple dipole electrical source. I. Normal adult male subjects. *Circulation* 40:(Nov) 687–96.

Holt JH, Barnard CL, Lynn MS (1969b): A study of the human heart as a multiple dipole electrical source. II. Diagnosis and quantitation of left ventricular hypertrophy. *Circulation* 40:(Nov) 697–710.

Holt JH, Barnard CL, Lynn MS, Kramer JO (1969c): A study of the human heart as a multiple dipole electrical source. III. Diagnosis and quantitation of right ventricular hypertrophy. *Circulation* 40:(Nov) 711–8.

Lynn MS, Barnard ACL, Holt JH, Sheffield LT (1967): A proposed method for the inverse problem in electrocardiology. *Biophys. J.* 7:(6) 925–45.

Macfarlane PW, Lawrie TDV (1989): The normal electrocardiogram and vectorcardiogram. In *Comprehensive Electrocardiology: Theory and Practice in Health and Disease,* 1st ed. Vol. 1, ed. PW Macfarlane, TDV Lawrie, pp. 407–57, Pergamon Press, New York.

Pilkington TC, Plonsey R (1982): *Engineering Contributions to Biophysical Electrocardiography,* 248 pp. IEEE Press, John Wiley, New York.

Rudy Y, Messinger-Rapport B (1988): The inverse problem of electrocardiography. Solutions in terms of epicardial potentials. *CRC Crit. Rev. Biomed. Eng.* 16: 215–68.

Savard P, Roberge FA, Perry J-B, Nadeau RA (1980): Representation of cardiac electrical activity by a moving dipole for normal ectopic beats in the intact dog. *Circ. Res.* 46:(3) 415–25.

Selvester RH, Collier CR, Pearson RB (1965): Analog computer model of the vectorcardiogram. *Circulation* 31:(1) 45–53.

Selvester RH, Kalaba R, Collier CR, Bellman R, Kagiwada H (1966): A mathematical model of the electric field of the heart with distance and boundary effects. In *Proc. Long Island Jewish Hosp. Symposium: Vectorcardiography 1965,* ed. I Hoffman, pp. 403–10, North-Holland Publishing, Amsterdam.

Yeh GCK, Martinek J, Beaumont H (1958): Multipole representation of current generators in a volume conductor. *Bull. Math. Biophys.* 20:(1) 203–14.

REFERENCES, BOOKS

Macfarlane PW, Lawrie TDV (eds.) (1989): *Comprehensive Electrocardiology: Theory and Practice in Health and Disease.* 1st ed. Vols. 1, 2, and 3. Pergamon Press, New York. 1785 p.

18

Distortion Factors in the ECG

18.1 INTRODUCTION

The background and realization of various ECG and VCG lead systems were discussed in Chapters 15, 16, and 17. It was pointed out that uncorrected lead systems evince a considerable amount of distortion affecting the quality of the ECG signal. In the corrected lead systems many of these factors are compensated for by various design methods. Distortion factors arise, generally, because the preconditions are not satisfied. For instance, the Frank system VCG signal will be undistorted provided that

1. the sources in the heart can be well described as a single fixed-location dipole;
2. the dipole is located at the position assumed by Frank;
3. the thorax has the same shape as Frank's model; and
4. the thorax is homogeneous.

None of these assumptions are met clinically, and therefore, the VCG signal deviates from the ideal. In addition, there are errors due to incorrect placement of the electrodes, poor electrode-skin contact, other sources of noise, and finally instrumentation error. The character and magnitude of these inaccuracies are discussed in the following sections.

18.2 EFFECT OF THE INHOMOGENEITY OF THE THORAX

As discussed earlier, it is assumed that in the standard 12-lead ECG system the source is a dipole in a fixed location and the volume conductor is either infinite homogeneous or spherical homogeneous. If this is the case, the lead vectors of the 12 leads form a symmetric star model, as illustrated in Figure 15.9. However, this is not the case; rather, the thorax includes several inhomogeneities, and the shape of the thorax is not spherical. These facts have a considerable effect on the directions and magnitudes of the lead vectors.

This effect has been discussed in many publications. In the following, part of the data from a study of Jari Hyttinen (1989, 1993a,b) is presented. Hyttinen constructed a computer model from the transfer impedance data of a physical torso model constructed by Stanley Rush (1975). The computer model used a cubic spline fitting of the data to interpolate the lead vectors for all points of the thorax surface in relation to all points within the heart area. The real values of the 12 lead vectors of the standard 12-lead system were calculated with this model. The result is illustrated in Figure 18.1. It is apparent that the biggest errors are the very high

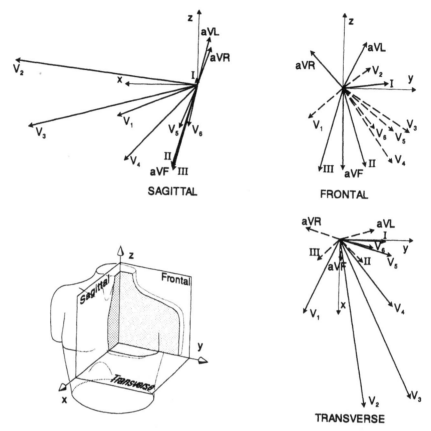

Fig. 18.1 The lead vectors of the standard 12-lead ECG in a finite, homogeneous torso model calculated from the model of Hyttinen (1989, 1993a,b). Compare with the idealized lead vectors shown in Figure 15.9.

sensitivities of the leads V_2 and V_3 as well as the form of the enhancement of the vertical forces in the frontal plane. The frontal plane is also tilted backwards. These effects are similar to those obtained from the image surface of the finite, homogeneous torso model of Frank.

18.3 BRODY EFFECT

18.3.1 Description of the Brody Effect

Daniel Brody investigated the effect of the intracardiac blood mass on the ECG lead field (Brody, 1956). The resistivity of the intracardiac blood is about 1.6 Ωm and that of the cardiac muscle averaging about 5.6 Ωm. The heart is surrounded almost everywhere by the lungs whose resistivity is about 10–20 Ωm.

From the above data one notes that the conductivity increases about 10-fold from the lungs

to the intracardiac blood mass. Therefore, the lead field current path tends to include the well-conducting intracardiac blood mass. Consequently, the lead field bends from the linear direction of the homogeneous model to the radial direction, as illustrated in Figure 18.2. As a consequence, the ECG lead is more sensitive to radial than tangential dipole elements, in contrast to the homogeneous model which predicts that the sensitivity is uniform and unrelated to gross myocardial anatomy. This phenomenon is called the *Brody effect*. The Brody effect is, in fact, more complicated than described above, as reported by van Oosterom and Plonsey (1991).

18.3.2 Effect of the Ventricular Volume

R. W. Millard performed an interesting series of experiments to show the Brody effect on the ECG signal (Voukydis, 1974). He recorded the

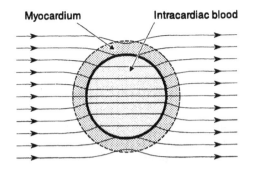

Fig. 18.2 The Brody effect. The spherical volume represents the more highly conducting intracavitary blood mass. Its effect on an applied uniform lead field shows an increased sensitivity to radial and decreased sensitivity to tangential dipoles in the heart muscle region.

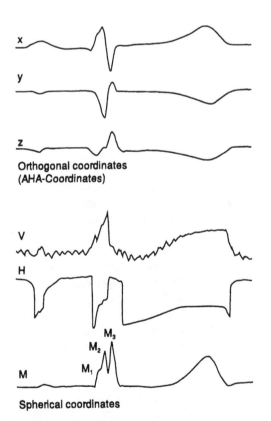

Fig. 18.3 The electric heart vector of a dog in the consistent orthogonal and spherical coordinates of Appendix A. (M = magnitude, V = elevation angle, H = azimuth angle.)

x, y, and z signals from a dog using the Nelson lead system and calculated the magnitude and the two angles of the electric heart vector in spherical coordinates. The result is shown in Figure 18.3.

These investigators noted that during the QRS complex the electric heart vector exhibits three different peaks, which they named M_1, M_2, and M_3. It is known that from these, the peaks M_1 and M_2 arise mainly from radial electric forces and the peak M_3 arises mainly from tangential forces (though, unfortunately, they did not confirm this interpretation with intramural source measurements).

Millard modified the extent of the Brody effect by changing the volume of the left ventricle during the QRS complex by venesection—that is, by removing blood with a catheter. As a consequence, the M_2 peak decreased and the M_3 peak increased. The effect was stronger as more blood was removed from the ventricle, as can be seen in Figure 18.4.

These experimental results are easy to explain. As mentioned, the M_2 peak is formed from radial electric forces, which are enhanced by the Brody effect. If this effect is attenuated by venesection, the corresponding peak is attenuated. The peak M_3 is formed from tan-

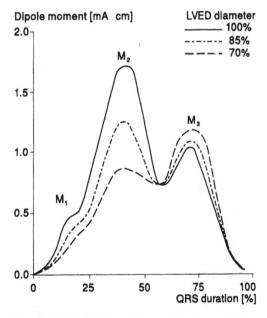

Fig. 18.4 The effect of decreasing the ventricular volume on the electric heart vector amplitude. LVED = left ventricular end-diastolic.

gential forces, which are attenuated by the Brody effect. If the Brody effect is reduced by venesection, the corresponding M_3 signal will be less attenuated (i.e., increased in magnitude).

18.3.3 Effect of the Blood Resistivity

Nelson et al. investigated the Brody effect yet in another way (Nelson et al., 1972). They changed the resistivity of blood by changing its hematocrit. In this way they were able to vary the resistivity from half normal to four times normal. The latter corresponds to the average resistivity of heart muscle.

When the blood resistivity was decreased to half-normal value, the Brody effect increased and consequently the M_2 peak, which is believed to correspond to the radial part of the activation, also increased. The M_3 peak, corresponding to the tangential part of the activation, decreased. When the resistivity was increased fourfold, the opposite effect was produced on the electric heart vector, as expected (see Fig. 18.5). Note that in the latter case the Brody effect should not arise, and the lead fields should be less distorted since the nominal intracavitary and muscle resistivities are equal. However, since the cardiac muscle is anisotropic, these ideas are only approximate.

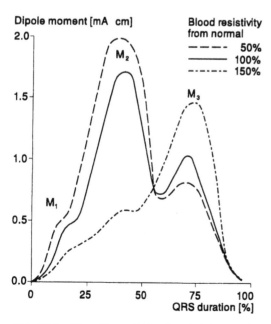

Fig. 18.5 The effect of blood resistivity on the magnitude of the electric heart vector.

18.3.4 Integrated Effects (Model Studies)

More recent investigations of the effect of inhomogeneities have been based on model investigations. Rudy (Rudy, Plonsey, and Liebman, 1979) used an eccentric spheres model of the heart and thorax in which the lungs, pericardium, body surface muscle and fat, as well as intracavitary blood could be represented. Some conclusions reached from this study include the following:

1. Although the Brody effect of the intracavitary blood is clearly demonstrated, the effect is diminished, when the remaining inhomogeneities are included.
2. Both abnormally low and high lung conductivities reduce the magnitude of surface potentials.
3. Low skeletal muscle conductivity enhances the surface potentials.
4. Increasing heart conductivity results in an increase in body surface potentials.

Other investigators have used realistic models of torso, lungs, heart, etc. to determine the effect of inhomogeneities. Gulrajani and Mailloux (1983) showed that the introduction of inhomogeneities in their model simulation of body surface potentials results in a smoothing of the contours without a large change in the pattern. Because of the predominant endocardial to epicardial activation, they noted a very significant Brody effect. In addition to the spatial filtering noted above, these investigations also reported temporal filtering of the ECG signal.

We have already mentioed the work of Horáček (1974), who investigated the effect of the blood mass and the lungs in a realistic torso model through the changes seen in the image surface. A review of the current status of understanding of the effect of inhomogeneities in electrocardiology is found in Gulrajani, Roberge, and Mailloux (1989).

18.4 EFFECT OF RESPIRATION

Both the resistivity and position of the lungs change during respiration. The orientation and location of the heart also change during the res-

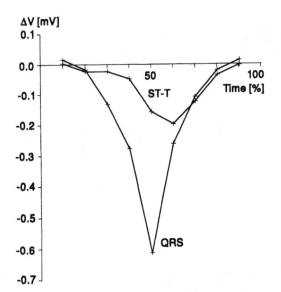

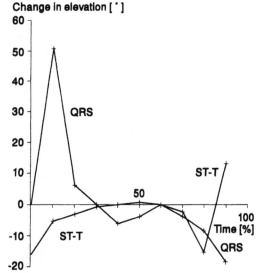

Fig. 18.6 The effect of inspiration on the electric heart vector during the QRS complex and ST-T wave. The ordinate plots the difference in magnitude [mV] between heart vector magnitude determined in midrespiration and full inspiration. The abscissa shows the QRS or ST-T interval divided into 10 equal points (so that the corresponding waveforms are time-normalized).

Fig. 18.7 Effect of inspiration on the elevation angle of the time normalized heart vector for the QRS complex and T-wave (top and bottom, respectively) shown in the consistent coordinate system of Appendix A. The change in angle between midrespiration and full inspiration is shown.

piratory cycle. Ruttkay-Nedecký described certain cyclic changes in the measured electric heart vector to be the consequence of respiration (Ruttkay-Nedecký, 1971). Figure 18.6 illustrates the change of the QRS- and T-vector magnitudes between midrespiration and full inspiration. Data was pooled from seven healthy male subjects using McFee-Parungao

(axial) leads. Statistically significant changes ($p > .05$) exist only in the mid-part of the QRS complex.

Figure 18.7 shows the effect of inspiration on the electric heart vector elevation compared to the midrespiration state. The effect is statistically significant only at 1/10 the normalized QRS-complex duration. The effect of inspiration on the azimuth angle of the QRS and T vectors is illustrated in Figure 18.8.

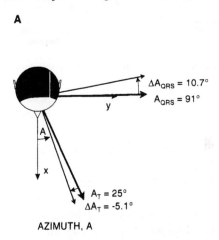

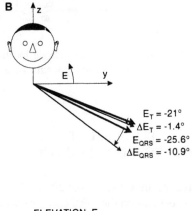

Fig. 18.8 Effect of inspiration on azimuth and elevation angles of QRS and T vectors shown in the consistent coordinate system of Appendix A. The thick line is for the midrespiration condition, whereas the thin line is for full inspiration.

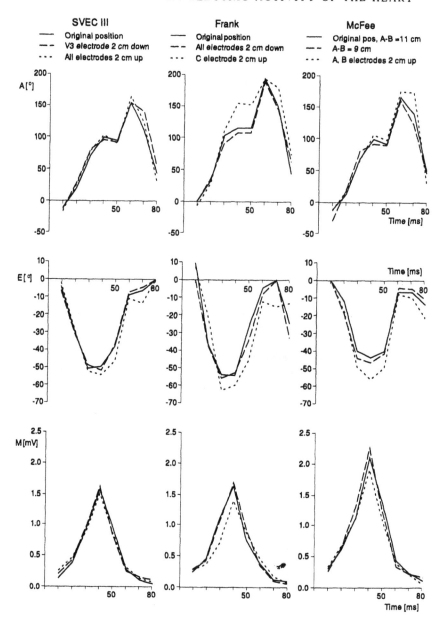

Fig. 18.9 Effect of electrode location on the VCG signal shown in the consistent coordinate system of Appendix A.

18.5 EFFECT OF ELECTRODE LOCATION

Simonson et al. investigated the effect of electrode displacement on the QRS complex when recorded by SVEC III, Frank, and McFee vectorcardiographic systems (Simonson et al., 1966). The electrodes were displaced 2 cm higher and lower from their correct locations in the first two systems and 9 cm in the McFee system. The results are shown in Figure 18.9. The authors concluded that SVEC III was least sensitive and Frank most sensitive to electrode displacement. In addition, the displacement error depended on the body shape.

REFERENCES

Brody DA (1956): A theoretical analysis of intracavitary blood mass influence on the heart-lead relationship. *Circ. Res.* 4:(Nov.) 731–8.

Gulrajani RM, Mailloux GE (1983): A simulation study of the effects of torso inhomogeneities on electrocardiographic potentials using realistic heart and torso models. *Circ. Res.* 52: 45–56.

Gulrajani RM, Roberge FA, Mailloux GE (1989): The forward problem of electrocardiography. In *Comprehensive Electrocardiology: Theory and Practice in Health and Disease,* 1st ed. Vol. 1, ed. PW Macfarlane, TDV Lawrie, pp. 237–88, Pergamon Press, New York.

Horáček BM (1974): Numerical model of an inhomogeneous human torso. In *Advances in Cardiology,* Vol. 10, ed. S Rush, E Lepeshkin, pp. 51–7, S. Karger, Basel.

Woo EJ (1990): Finite element method and reconstruction algorithms in electrical impedance tomography. *Dept. of Electrical and Computer Eng., Univ. of Wisconsin, Madison,* (Ph.D. thesis)

Hyttinen J (1989): Development of aimed ECG-leads. *Tampere Univ. Tech., Tampere, Finland,* Thesis, pp. 138. (Lic. Tech. thesis)

Hyttinen J, Eskola H, Malmivuo J (1993a): Sensitivity properties of the 12-lead ECG—A realistic thorax model study. (To be published).

Hyttinen JAK, Malmivuo JAV, Walker SJ (1993b): Lead field of ECG leads calculated with a computer thorax model—An application of reciprocity. In *Proc. 1993 Computers in Cardiology Meeting,* ed. A Murray, Imperial College, London.

Nelson CV, Rand PW, Angelakos TE, Hugenholtz PG (1972): Effect of intracardiac blood on the spatial vectorcardiogram. *Circ. Res.* 31:(7) 95–104.

van Oosterom A, Plonsey R (1991): The Brody effect revisited. *J. Electrocardiol.* 24:(4) 339–48.

Rudy Y, Plonsey R, Liebman J (1979): The effects of variations in conductivity and geometrical parameters on the electrocardiogram, using an eccentric spheres model. *Circ. Res.* 44: 104–11.

Rush S (1975): *An Atlas of Heart-Lead Transfer Coefficients,* 211 pp. University Press of New England, Hanover, New Hampshire.

Ruttkay-Nedecký I (1971): Respiratory changes of instantaneous spatial cardiac vectors. In *Vectorcardiography 2. Proc. XIth Internat. Symp. Vectorcardiography, New York 1970,* ed. I Hoffman, RI Hamby, E Glassman, pp. 115–8, North-Holland Publishing, Amsterdam.

Simonson E, Horibe H, Okamoto N, Schmitt OH (1966): Effect of electrode displacement on orthogonal leads. In *Proc. Long Island Jewish Hosp. Symposium on Vectorcardiography,* ed. I Hoffman, p. 424, North-Holland Publishing, Amsterdam.

Voukydis PC (1974): Effect of intracardiac blood on the electrocardiogram. *N. Engl. J. Med.* 9: 612–6.

Woo EJ (1990): Finite element method and reconstruction algorithms in electrical impedance tomography. *Dept. of Electrical and Computer Eng., Univ. of Wisconsin, Madison,* (Ph.D. thesis)

REFERENCES, BOOKS

Macfarlane PW, Lawrie TDV (eds.) (1989): *Comprehensive Electrocardiology: Theory and Practice in Health and Disease.* 1st ed. Vols. 1, 2, and 3. Pergamon Press, New York. 1785 p.

19

THE BASIS OF ECG DIAGNOSIS

19.1 PRINCIPLE OF THE ECG DIAGNOSIS

19.1.1 About the Possibilities of Solving the Cardiac Inverse Problem

As discussed in Chapter 7, no unique solution exists for the inverse problem. From clinical practice it is possible to make accurate ECG diagnoses in some diseases and to estimate other diseases with an acceptable probability. How can this discrepancy between theory and practice be explained?

It was said in Chapter 7 that the inverse solution is impossible if measurements cannot be made inside the source and if no additional information about the nature of the source is available. There is, however, much knowledge of the electrophysiological behavior of the heart. This limits the degrees of freedom of the source and reduces the degree of uncertainty in reaching a diagnosis. The following are examples of these helpful constraints:

1. The size, location, and orientation of the heart are well known and their variabilities are limited.
2. The action impulse of individual muscle cells can be approximated as having

only two electrophysiological states: (re)polarization and depolarization.
3. Each muscle cell exhibits a specific form of activation; depolarization is followed by repolarization after approximately 0.2–0.4 seconds.
4. The atria and the ventricles form temporarily separate regions of activation.
5. The propagation velocity of the activation front in various parts of the heart muscle is known.
6. The conduction system has a dominant effect on initiation of the activation front.
7. The relationship between muscle load and muscle hypertrophy is well understood.
8. There are a limited number of causes of muscular overload.
9. The electrophysiological effect of ischemia on heart muscle is known.
10. The location of ischemia or infarction is governed by the anatomy of the coronary arteries.
11. There are a limited number of congenital cardiac abnormalities.

These anatomical and physiological constraints limit the degrees of freedom of the inverse solution and usually make it possible to obtain solutions. However, in most cases the cardiac diagnosis must be made more accurately. The diagnosis often needs to be verified or completely made with other diagnostic methods like auscultation, x-ray, coronary angiography, radiocardiographic imaging, clinical chemistry, ultrasound, and so on.

19.1.2 Bioelectric Principles in ECG Diagnosis

This discussion of ECG diagnosis is based on the following three principles:

First, the propagating activation front is characterized by its resultant vector. This signal can be detected and estimated through the lead vector according to Equation 11.16 and Figure 11.6 in Chapter 11.

$$V = \bar{c} \cdot \bar{p} \qquad (11.16)$$

When the heart's electric activity is considered a vector, it is usually easier first to examine the path (trajectory) of the vector's tip (the vectorcardiogram). Then the signals in the 12-lead ECG may be regarded as projections of the electric heart vector on the respective lead vectors as a function of time (multiplied by the absolute value of the lead vector).

Second, the sensitivity of the lead may be considered distributed according to lead field theory. In this case the propagating activation front contributes to the ECG signal of the lead according to Equation 11.30, namely

$$V_E = \int \frac{1}{\sigma} \bar{J}_L \cdot \bar{J}^i \, dv \qquad (11.30)$$

In this formulation the dipole sources are not reduced to a single resultant dipole, but are considered as spatially distributed. Furthermore, the volume conductor inhomogeneities are taken into account.

Third, the solid angle theorem offers substantial help for understanding the formation of the ECG signal, especially in the diagnosis of myocardial infarction (see Equation 11.7):

$$V = \frac{1}{4\pi} p\, (-\Omega) \qquad (11.7)$$

In arriving at Equation 11.7, one assumes the double layer sources to be uniform, but otherwise takes into account their spatial distribution. However, the volume conductor is assumed to be infinite in extent and uniform.

In this chapter, the forward problem of ECG diagnosis is discussed. This leads to the solution of the inverse problem through the empirical approach, as mentioned in Section 7.5.4. The empirical approach is acceptable in this case, because the purpose of this chapter is to be illustrative only.

19.2 APPLICATION AREAS OF ECG DIAGNOSIS

The main applications of the ECG to cardiological diagnosis include the following (see also Fig. 19.1):

1. The electric axis of the heart
2. Heart rate monitoring
3. Arrhythmias
    a. Supraventricular arrhythmias
    b. Ventricular arrhythmias
4. Disorders in the activation sequence
    a. Atrioventricular conduction defects (blocks)
    b. Bundle-branch block
    c. Wolff-Parkinson-White syndrome
5. Increase in wall thickness or size of the atria and ventricles
    a. Atrial enlargement (hypertrophy)
    b. Ventricular enlargement (hypertrophy)
6. Myocardial ischemia and infarction
    a. Ischemia
    b. Infarction
7. Drug effect
    a. Digitalis
    b. Quinidine
8. Electrolyte imbalance
    a. Potassium
    b. Calcium
9. Carditis
    a. Pericarditis
    b. Myocarditis
10. Pacemaker monitoring

Most of these application areas of ECG diagnosis are discussed in this chapter. Items 7, 8, and 9—drug effect, electrolyte imbalance, and carditis—are not included in this discussion because their effects on the ECG signal cannot readily be explained with the methods included in this textbook.

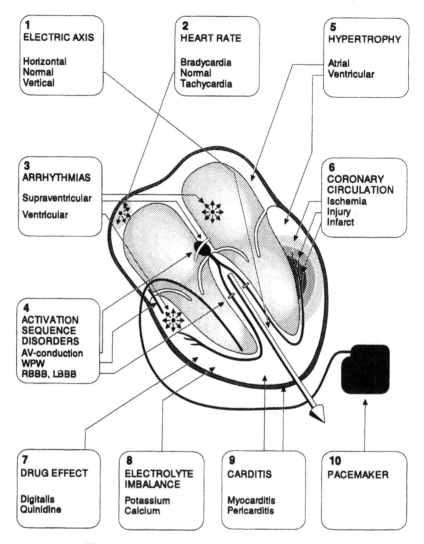

Fig. 19.1   Application areas of ECG diagnosis.

19.3 DETERMINATION OF THE ELECTRIC AXIS OF THE HEART

The concept of the electric axis of the heart usually denotes the average direction of the electric activity throughout ventricular (or sometimes atrial) activation. The term mean vector is frequently used instead of "electric axis." The direction of the electric axis may also denote the instantaneous direction of the electric heart vector. This is shown in vector-cardiography as a function of time.

The normal range of the electric axis lies between $+30°$ and $-110°$ in the frontal plane and between $+30°$ and $-30°$ in the transverse

plane. (Note that the angles are given in the consistent coordinate system of Appendix A.)

The direction of the electric axis may be approximated from the 12-lead ECG by finding the lead in the frontal plane, where the QRS complex has largest positive deflection. The direction of the electric axis is in the direction of this lead vector. The result can be checked by observing that the QRS complex is symmetrically biphasic in the lead that is normal to the electric axis. The directions of the leads were summarized in Figure 15.9. (In the evaluation of the ECG it is beneficial to use the lead $-aV_R$ instead of the lead aV_R, as noted in Section 15.7.)

Deviation of the electric axis to the right is

an indication of increased electric activity in the right ventricle due to increased right ventricular mass. This is usually a consequence of chronic obstructive lung disease, pulmonary emboli, certain types of congenital heart disease, or other disorders causing severe pulmonary hypertension and cor pulmonale.

Deviation of the electric axis to the left is an indication of increased electric activity in the left ventricle due to increased left ventricular mass. This is usually a consequence of hypertension, aortic stenosis, ischemic heart disease, or some intraventricular conduction defect.

The clinical meaning of the deviation of the heart's electric axis is discussed in greater detail in connection with ventricular hypertrophy.

19.4 CARDIAC RHYTHM DIAGNOSIS

19.4.1 Differentiating the P, QRS, and T Waves

Because of the anatomical difference of the atria and the ventricles, their sequential activation, depolarization, and repolarization produce clearly differentiable deflections. This may be possible even when they do not follow one another in the correct sequence: P-QRS-T.

Identification of the normal QRS-complex from the P- and T-waves does not create difficulties because it has a characteristic waveform and dominating amplitude. This amplitude is about 1 mV in a normal heart and can be much greater in ventricular hypertrophy. The normal duration of the QRS is 0.08–0.09 s.

If the heart does not exhibit atrial hypertrophy, the P wave has an amplitude of about 0.1 mV and duration of 0.1 s. For the T wave both of these numbers are about double. The T wave can be differentiated from the P wave by observing that the T-wave follows the QRS complex after about 0.2 s.

19.4.2 Supraventricular Rhythms

Definition

Cardiac rhythms may be divided into two categories: supraventricular (above the ventricles) and ventricular rhythms.

The origin of supraventricular rhythms (a single pulse or a continuous rhythm) is in the atria or AV junction, and the activation proceeds to the ventricles along the conduction system in a normal way. Supraventricular rhythms are illustrated in Figure 19.2.

Normal Sinus Rhythm

Normal sinus rhythm is the rhythm of a healthy normal heart, where the sinus node triggers the cardiac activation. This is easily diagnosed by noting that the three deflections, P-QRS-T, follow in this order and are differentiable. The sinus rhythm is normal if its frequency is between 60 and 100/min.

Sinus Bradycardia

A sinus rhythm of less than 60/min is called sinus bradycardia. This may be a consequence of increased vagal or parasympathetic tone.

Sinus Tachycardia

A sinus rhythm of higher than 100/min is called sinus tachycardia. It occurs most often as a physiological response to physical exercise or psychical stress, but may also result from congestive heart failure.

Sinus Arrhythmia

If the sinus rhythm is irregular such that the longest PP or RR interval exceeds the shortest interval by 0.16 s, the situation is called sinus arrhythmia. This situation is very common in all age groups. This arrhythmia is so common in young people that it is not considered a heart disease. One origin for the sinus arrhythmia may be the vagus nerve which mediates respiration as well as heart rhythm. The nerve is active during respiration and, through its effect on the sinus node, causes an increase in heart rate during inspiration and a decrease during expiration. The effect is particularly pronounced in children.

Note, that in all of the preceding rhythms the length of the cardiac activation cycle (the P-QRS-T waves together) is less than directly proportional to the PP time. The main time interval change is between the T wave and the next P wave. This is easy to understand since the pulse rate of the sinus node is controlled mainly by factors external to the heart while the cardiac conduction velocity is controlled by conditions internal to the heart.

NORMAL SINUS RHYTHM
Impulses originate at S-A node at normal rate

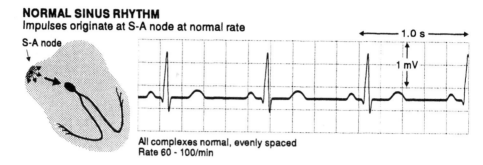

All complexes normal, evenly spaced
Rate 60 - 100/min

SINUS BRADYCARDIA
Impulses originate at S-A node at slow rate

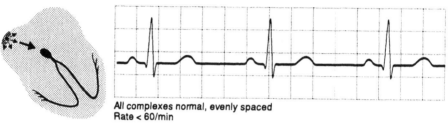

All complexes normal, evenly spaced
Rate < 60/min

SINUS TACHYCARDIA
Impulses originate at S-A node at rapid rate

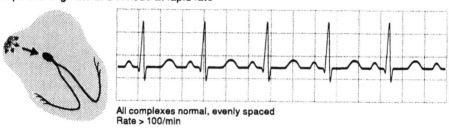

All complexes normal, evenly spaced
Rate > 100/min

SINUS ARRHYTHMIA
Impulses originate at S-A node at varying rate

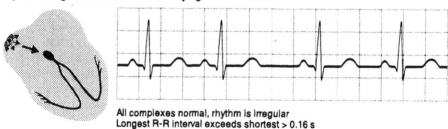

All complexes normal, rhythm is irregular
Longest R-R interval exceeds shortest > 0.16 s

Fig. 19.2 Supraventricular rhythms.

Nonsinus Atrial Rhythm

The origin of atrial contraction may be located somewhere else in the atria other than the sinus node. If it is located close to the AV node, the atrial depolarization occurs in a direction that is opposite the normal one. An obvious conse- quence is that in the ECG the P wave has op- posite polarity.

Wandering Pacemaker

The origin of the atrial contraction may also vary or *wander*. Consequently, the P waves will

WANDERING PACEMAKER
Impulses originate from varying points in atria

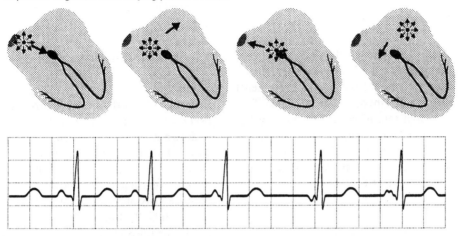

Variation in P-wave contour, P-R and P-P interval
and therefore in R-R intervals

ATRIAL FLUTTER
Impulses travel in circular course in atria

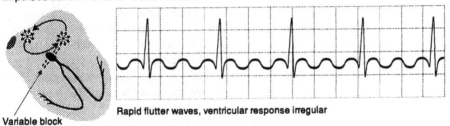

Variable block

Rapid flutter waves, ventricular response irregular

ATRIAL FIBRILLATION
Impulses have chaotic, random pathways in atria

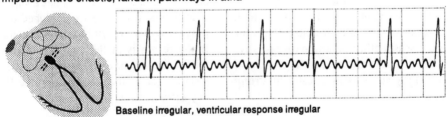

Baseline irregular, ventricular response irregular

JUNCTIONAL RHYTHM
Impulses originate at AV node
with retrograde and antegrade direction

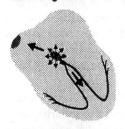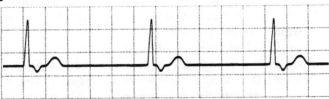

P-wave is often inverted, may be under or after QRS complex
Heart rate is slow

Fig. 19.2 *(Continued)*

vary in polarity, and the PQ interval will also vary.

Paroxysmal Atrial Tachycardia (PAT)

Paroxysmal atrial tachycardia (PAT) describes the condition when the P waves are a result of a reentrant activation front (circus movement) in the atria, usually involving the AV node. This leads to a high rate of activation, usually between 160 and 220/min. In the ECG the P wave is regularly followed by the QRS complex. The isoelectric baseline may be seen between the T wave and the next P wave.

Atrial Flutter

When the heart rate is sufficiently elevated so that the isoelectric interval between the end of T and beginning of P disappears, the arrhythmia is called atrial flutter. The origin is also believed to involve a reentrant atrial pathway. The frequency of these fluctuations is between 220 and 300/min. The AV node and, thereafter, the ventricles are generally activated by every second or every third atrial impulse (2:1 or 3:1 heart block).

Atrial Fibrillation

The activation in the atria may also be fully irregular and chaotic, producing irregular fluctuations in the baseline. A consequence is that the ventricular rate is rapid and irregular, though the QRS contour is usually normal. Atrial fibrillation occurs as a consequence of rheumatic disease, atherosclerotic disease, hyperthyroidism, and pericarditis. (It may also occur in healthy subjects as a result of strong sympathetic activation.)

Junctional Rhythm

If the heart rate is slow (40–55/min), the QRS complex is normal, the P waves are possibly not seen, then the origin of the cardiac rhythm is in the AV node. Because the origin is in the junction between atria and ventricles, this is called *junctional rhythm*. Therefore, the activation of the atria occurs retrograde (i.e., in the opposite direction). Depending on whether the AV-nodal impulse reaches the atria before, simultaneously, or after the ventricles, an opposite polarity P wave will be produced before,

during, or after the QRS complex, respectively. In the second case the P wave will be superimposed on the QRS complex and will not be seen.

19.4.3   Ventricular Arrhythmias

Definition

In ventricular arrhythmias ventricular activation does not originate from the AV node and/ or does not proceed in the ventricles in a normal way. If the activation proceeds to the ventricles along the conduction system, the inner walls of the ventricles are activated almost simultaneously and the activation front proceeds mainly radially toward the outer walls. As a result, the QRS complex is of relatively short duration. If the ventricular conduction system is broken or the ventricular activation starts far from the AV node, it takes a longer time for the activation front to proceed throughout the ventricular mass.

The criterion for normal ventricular activation is a QRS-interval shorter than 0.1 s. A QRS interval lasting longer than 0.1 s indicates abnormal ventricular activation. Ventricular arrhythmias are presented in Figure 19.3.

Premature Ventricular Contraction

A premature ventricular contraction is one that occurs abnormally early. If its origin is in the atrium or in the AV node, it has a supraventricular origin. The complex produced by this supraventricular arrhythmia lasts less than 0.1 s. If the origin is in the ventricular muscle, the QRS complex has a very abnormal form and lasts longer than 0.1 s. Usually the P wave is not associated with it.

Idioventricular Rhythm

If the ventricles are continuously activated by a ventricular focus whose rhythm is under 40/ min, the rhythm is called idioventricular rhythm. The ventricular activity may also be formed from short (less than 20 s) bursts of ventricular activity at higher rates (between 40 and 120/min). This situation is called accelerated idioventricular rhythm.

The origin of the ventricular rhythm may be located by observing the polarity in various leads. The direction of the activation front is,

PREMATURE VENTRICULAR CONTRACTION
A single impulse originates at right ventricle

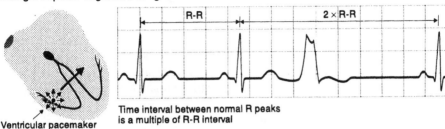

Ventricular pacemaker

Time interval between normal R peaks
is a multiple of R-R interval

VENTRICULAR TACHYCARDIA
Impulses originate at ventricular pacemaker

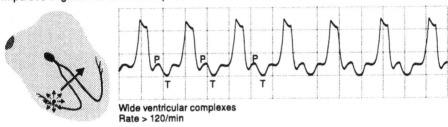

Wide ventricular complexes
Rate > 120/min

VENTRICULAR FIBRILLATION
Chaotic ventricular depolarization

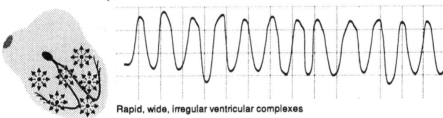

Rapid, wide, irregular ventricular complexes

PACER RHYTHM
Impulses originate at transvenous pacemaker

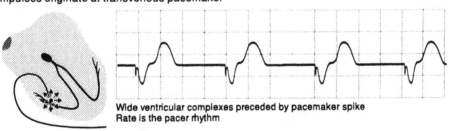

Wide ventricular complexes preceded by pacemaker spike
Rate is the pacer rhythm

Fig. 19.3   Ventricular arrhythmias.

of course, the direction of the lead vector in that lead where the deflection is most positive. The origin of the activation is, of course, on the opposite side of the heart when one is looking from this electrode.

Ventricular Tachycardia

A rhythm of ventricular origin may also be a consequence of a slower conduction in ischemic ventricular muscle that leads to circular activation (reentry). The result is activation of the ventricular muscle at a high rate (over 120/min), causing rapid, bizarre, and wide QRS complexes; the arrythmia is called ventricular tachycardia. As noted, ventricular tachycardia is often a consequence of ischemia and myocardial infarction.

Ventricular Fibrillation

When ventricular depolarization occurs chaotically, the situation is called ventricular fibrillation. This is reflected in the ECG, which demonstrates coarse irregular undulations without QRS-complexes. The cause of fibrillation is the establishment of multiple reentry loops usually involving diseased heart muscle. In this arrhythmia the contraction of the ventricular muscle is also irregular and is ineffective at pumping blood. The lack of blood circulation leads to almost immediate loss of consciousness and death within minutes. The ventricular fibrillation may be stopped with an external defibrillator pulse and appropriate medication.

Pacer Rhythm

A ventricular rhythm originating from a cardiac pacemaker is associated with wide QRS complexes because the pacing electrode is (usually) located in the right ventricle and activation does not involve the conduction system. In pacer rhythm the ventricular contraction is usually preceded by a clearly visible pacer impulse spike. The pacer rhythm is usually set to 72/min.

19.5 DISORDERS IN THE ACTIVATION SEQUENCE

19.5.1 Atrioventricular Conduction Variations

Definition

As discussed earlier, if the P-waves always precede the QRS complex with a PR interval of 0.12–0.2 s, the AV conduction is normal and a sinus rhythm is diagnosed. If the PR interval is fixed but shorter than normal, either the origin of the impulse is closer to the ventricles (see

Section 19.4.2) or the atrioventricular conduction is utilizing an (abnormal) bypass tract leading to pre-excitation of the ventricles. The latter is called the Wolff-Parkinson-White syndrome and is discussed below. The PR interval may also be variable, such as in a wandering atrial pacemaker and multifocal atrial tachycardia. Atrioventricular blocks are illustrated in Figure 19.4.

First-Degree Atrioventricular Block

When the P wave always precedes the QRS complex but the PR-interval is prolonged over 0.2 s, first-degree atrioventricular block is diagnosed.

Second-Degree Atrioventricular Block

If the PQ interval is longer than normal and the QRS-complex sometimes does not follow the P-wave, the atrioventricular block is of *second-degree*. If the PR interval progressively lengthens, leading finally to the dropout of a QRS-complex, the second degree block is called a *Wenkebach phenomenon*.

Third-Degree Atrioventricular Block

Complete lack of synchronism between the P wave and the QRS complex is diagnosed as third-degree (or total) atrioventricular block. The conduction system defect in third degree AV-block may arise at different locations such as:

Over the AV node

In the bundle of His

Bilaterally in the upper part of both bundle branches

Trifascicularly, located still lower, so that it exists in the right bundle-branch and in the two fascicles of the left bundle-branch

19.5.2 Bundle-Branch Block

Definition

Bundle-branch block denotes a conduction defect in either of the bundle-branches or in either fascicle of the left bundle-branch. If the two

A-V BLOCK, FIRST DEGREE
Atrio-ventricular conduction lengthened

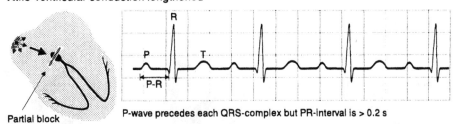

Partial block

P-wave precedes each QRS-complex but PR-interval is > 0.2 s

A-V BLOCK, SECOND DEGREE
Sudden dropped QRS-complex

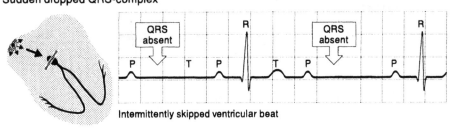

Intermittently skipped ventricular beat

A-V BLOCK, THIRD DEGREE
Impulses originate at AV node and proceed to ventricles
Atrial and ventricular activities are not synchronous

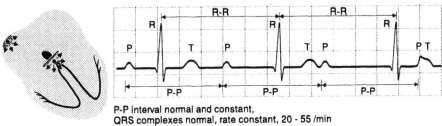

P-P interval normal and constant,
QRS complexes normal, rate constant, 20 - 55 /min

Fig. 19.4   Atrioventricular blocks.

bundle-branches exhibit a block simultaneously, the progress of activation from the atria to the ventricles is completely inhibited; this is regarded as third-degree atrioventricular block (see the previous section). The consequence of left or right bundle-branch block is that activation of the ventricle must await initiation by the opposite ventricle. After this, activation proceeds entirely on a cell-to-cell basis. The absence of involvement of the conduction system, which initiates early activity of many sites, results in a much slower activation process along normal pathways. The consequence

is manifest in bizarre shaped QRS complexes of abnormally long duration. The ECG changes in connection with bundle-branch blocks are illustrated in Figure 19.5.

Right Bundle-Branch Block

If the right bundle-branch is defective so that the electrical impulse cannot travel through it to the right ventricle, activation reaches the right ventricle by proceeding from the left ventricle. It then travels through the septal and right ventricular muscle mass. This progress is, of course, slower than that through the conduction

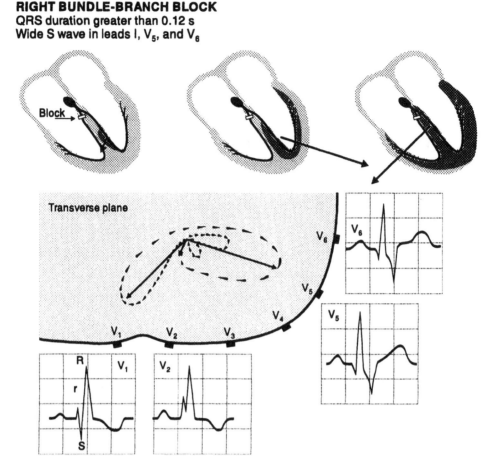

RIGHT BUNDLE-BRANCH BLOCK
QRS duration greater than 0.12 s
Wide S wave in leads I, V_5, and V_6

Fig. 19.5 Bundle branch blocks.

system and leads to a QRS complex wider than 0.1 s. Usually the duration criterion for the QRS complex in right bundle-branch block (RBBB) as well as for the left bundle-branch block (LBBB) is >0.12 s.

With normal activation the electrical forces of the right ventricle are partially concealed by the larger sources arising from the activation of the left ventricle. In right bundle-branch block (RBBB), activation of the right ventricle is so much delayed, that it can be seen following the activation of the left ventricle. (Activation of the left ventricle takes place normally.)

RBBB causes an abnormal terminal QRS-vector that is directed to the right ventricle (i.e., rightward and anterior). This is seen in the ECG as a broad terminal S wave in lead I. Another typical manifestation is seen in lead V_1 as a double R wave. This is named an RSR′ complex.

Left Bundle-Branch Block

The situation in left bundle-branch block (LBBB) is similar, but activation proceeds in a direction opposite to RBBB. Again the duration criterion for complete block is 0.12 s or more for the QRS complex. Because the activation wavefront travels in more or less the normal direction in LBBB, the signals' polarities are generally normal. However, because of the abnormal sites of initiation of the left ventricular activation front and the presence of

LEFT BUNDLE-BRANCH BLOCK
QRS duration greater than 0.12 s
Wide S wave in leads V_1 and V_2, wide R wave in V_5, and V_6

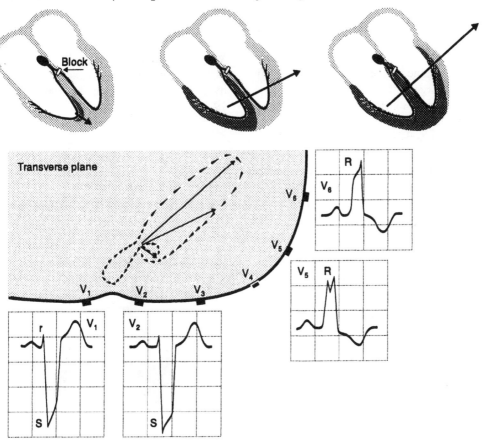

Fig. 19.5 (*Continued*)

normal right ventricular activation the outcome is complex and the electric heart vector makes a slower and larger loop to the left and is seen as a broad and tall R wave, usually in leads I, aV_L, V_5, or V_6.

19.5.3 Wolff-Parkinson-White Syndrome

One cause for a broad QRS complex that exceeds over 0.12s, may be the Wolff-Parkinson-White syndrome (WPW syndrome). In the WPW syndrome the QRS complex initially exhibits an early upstroke called the *delta wave*.

The interval from the P wave to the R spike is normal, but the early ventricular excitation forming the delta wave shortens the PQ time.

The cause of the WPW syndrome is the passage of activation from the atrium directly to the ventricular muscle via an abnormal route, called the *bundle of Kent,* which bypasses the AV junctions. This activates part of the ventricular muscle before normal activation reaches it via the conduction system (after a delay in the AV junction). The process is called preexcitation, and the resulting ECG depends on the specific location of the accessory pathway.

19.6   INCREASE IN WALL THICKNESS OR SIZE OF ATRIA AND VENTRICLES

19.6.1   Definition

Atrial and ventricular muscles react to physical stress in the same way as skeletal muscles: The muscles enlarge with increased amount of exercise. The extra tension may arise as a result of increased pressure load or volume load.

Pressure overload is a consequence of increased resistance in the outflow tract of the particular compartment concerned (e.g., aortic stenosis). *Volume overload* means that either the outflow valve or the inflow valve of the compartment is incompetent, thus necessitating a larger stroke volume as compensation for the regurgitant backflow.

The increase in the atrial or ventricular size is called *atrial* or *ventricular enlargement*. The increase of the atrial or ventricular wall thickness is called *atrial* or *ventricular hypertrophy*. Very often they both are called hypertrophy, as in this presentation. Atrial and ventricular hypertrophies are illustrated in Figures 19.6 and 19.7, respectively.

19.6.2   Atrial Hypertrophy

Right Atrial Hypertrophy

Right atrial hypertrophy is a consequence of right atrial overload. This may be a result of

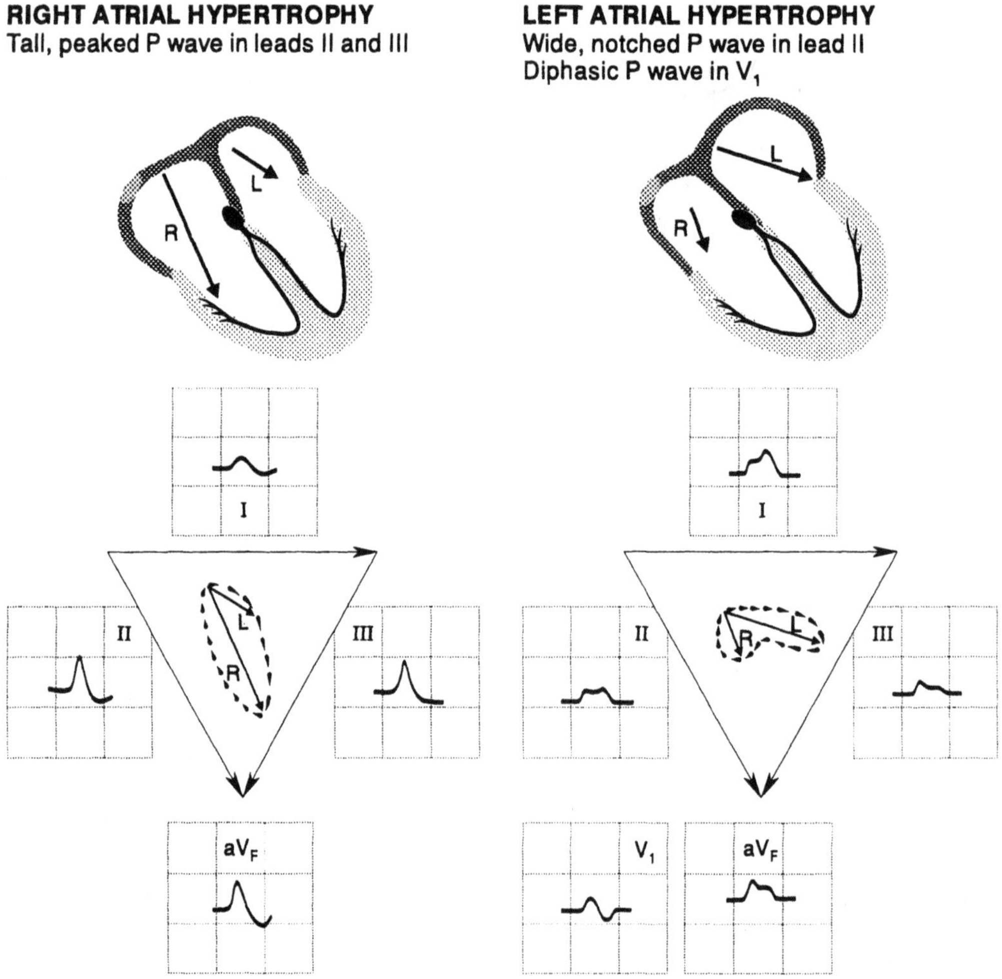

Fig. 19.6   Atrial hypertrophy.

tricuspid valve disease (stenosis or insufficiency), pulmonary valve disease, or pulmonary hypertension (increased pulmonary blood pressure). The latter is most commonly a consequence of chronic obstructive pulmonary disease or pulmonary emboli.

In right atrial hypertrophy the electrical force due to the enlarged right atrium is larger. This electrical force is oriented mainly in the direction of lead II but also in leads aV_F and III. In all of these leads an unusually large (i.e., ≥ 0.25 mV) P wave is seen.

Left Atrial Hypertrophy

Left atrial hypertrophy is a consequence of left atrial overload. This may be a result of mitral valve disease (stenosis or insufficiency), aortic valve disease, or hypertension in the systemic circulation.

In left atrial hypertrophy the electrical impulse due to the enlarged left atrium is strengthened. This electrical impulse is directed mainly along lead I or opposite to the direction of lead V_1. Because the atrial activation starts from the right atrium, the aforementioned left atrial activation is seen later, and therefore, the P wave includes two phases. In lead I these phases have the same polarities and in lead V_1 the opposite polarities. This typical P wave form is called the *mitral P wave*. The specific diagnostic criterion for left atrial hypertrophy is the terminal portion of the P wave in V_1, having a duration ≥ 0.04 s and negative amplitude ≥ 0.1 mV.

RIGHT VENTRICULAR HYPERTROPHY
Large R wave in leads V_1 and V_2,
large S wave in leads V_5 and V_6

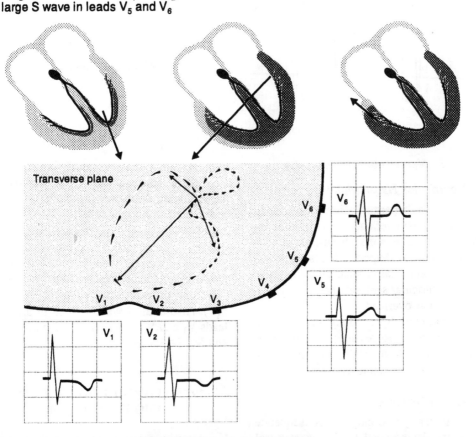

Fig. 19.7 Ventricular hypertrophy.

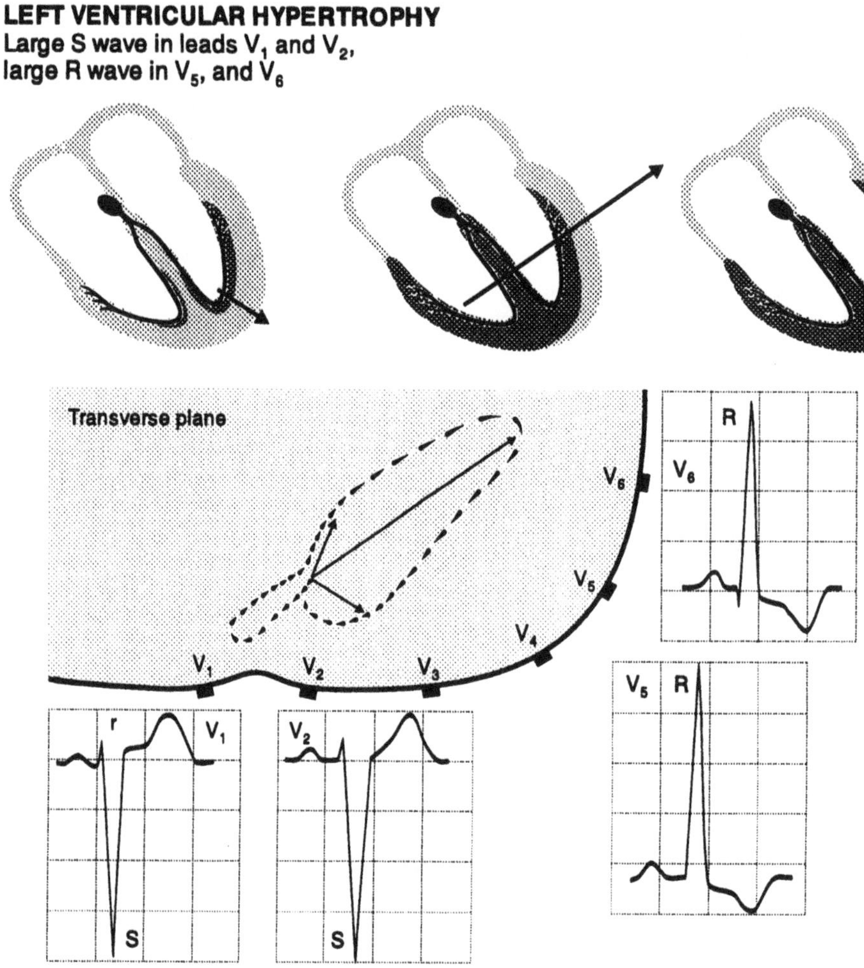

LEFT VENTRICULAR HYPERTROPHY
Large S wave in leads V_1 and V_2,
large R wave in V_5, and V_6

Fig. 19.7 (*Continued*)

19.6.3 Ventricular Hypertrophy

Right Ventricular Hypertrophy

Right ventricular hypertrophy is a consequence of right ventricular overload. This is caused by pulmonary valve stenosis, tricuspid insufficiency, or pulmonary hypertension (see above). Also many congenital cardiac abnormalities, such as a ventricular septal defect, may cause right ventricular overload.

Right ventricular hypertrophy increases the ventricular electrical forces directed to the right ventricle—that is, to the right and front. This is seen in lead V_1 as a tall R wave of ≥ 0.7 mV.

Left Ventricular Hypertrophy

Left ventricular hypertrophy is a consequence of left ventricular overload. It arises from mitral valve disease, aortic valve disease, or systemic hypertension. Left ventricular hypertrophy may also be a consequence of obstructive hypertrophic cardiomyopathy, which is a sickness of the cardiac muscle cells.

Left ventricular hypertrophy increases the ventricular electric forces directed to the left ventricle—that is, to the left and posteriorly. Evidence of this is seen in lead I as a tall R wave and in lead III as a tall S wave (≥ 2.5 mV). Also a tall S wave is seen in precordial leads V_1 and V_2 and a tall R wave in leads V_5 and V_6, (≥ 3.5 mV).

19.7 MYOCARDIAL ISCHEMIA AND INFARCTION

If a coronary artery is occluded, the transport of oxygen to the cardiac muscle is decreased,

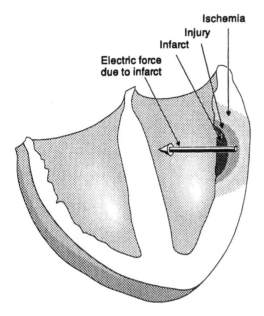

Electric force
due to infarct

Infarct

Injury

Ischemia

Fig. 19.8 Myocardial ischemia and infarction.

An infarct area is electrically silent since it has lost its excitability. According to the solid angle theorem (Section 11.2.2) the loss of this outward dipole is equivalent to an electrical force pointing inward. With this principle it is possible to locate the infarction. (Of course, the infarct region also affects the activation sequence and the volume conductor so the outcome is more complicated.)

causing an oxygen debt in the muscle, which is called *ischemia*. Ischemia causes changes in the resting potential and in the repolarization of the muscle cells, which is seen as changes in the T wave. If the oxygen transport is terminated in a certain area, the heart muscle dies in that region. This is called an *infarction*. These are illustrated in Figure 19.8.

REFERENCES

Goldman MJ (1986): *Principles of Clinical Electrocardiography,* 12th ed., 460 pp. Lange Medical Publications, Los Altos, Cal.

Macfarlane PW, Lawrie TDV (eds.) (1989): *Comprehensive Electrocardiology: Theory and Practice in Health and Disease,* 1st ed., Vols. 1, 2, and 3, 1785 pp. Pergamon Press, New York.

Netter FH (1971): *Heart,* Vol. 5, 293 pp. The Ciba Collection of Medical Illustrations, Ciba Pharmaceutical Company, Summit, N.J.

Scheidt S (1983): *Basic Electrocardiography: Leads, Axes, Arrhythmias,* Vol. 2/35, 32 pp. Ciba Pharmaceutical Company, Summit, N.J.

Scheidt S (1984): *Basic Electrocardiography: Abnormalities of Electrocardiographic Patterns,* Vol. 6/36, 32 pp. Ciba Pharmaceutical Company, Summit, N.J.

20

Magnetocardiography

20.1 INTRODUCTION

The first biomagnetic signal to be detected was the magnetocardiogram (MCG) by Baule and McFee (1963). The discovery raised a lot of optimism, as it was believed that MCG would provide as much new information about the heart's electric activity as had the ECG. Though this has been shown theoretically (Rush, 1975) and in practical clinical studies not to be true, there are still many potential clinical applications of the MCG. For instance, as will be discussed in Section 20.7, according to present understanding, with the combined use of the ECG and the MCG, called *electromagneto-cardiogram* (EMCG), in some cardiac diseases the number of incorrectly diagnosed patients can be decreased by one half of that when only the ECG is used.

Since the concept of the *magnetic heart vector* was introduced by Baule and McFee in 1970, studies have been conducted to detect the vectormagnetocardiogram (i.e., in which the heart is considered as a magnetic dipole). Though the detection of the magnetic heart vector is an obvious selection as the first clinical tool, many of the MCG studies of today have been made by mapping the normal component of the magnetic field of the heart around the thorax.

There exist also many other kinds of trials for finding out clinical applications for the MCG—for example, testing the risk for sudden cardiac death and for rejection of an implanted heart. The localization of arrhythmogenic centers has also been a subject of intensive research. An overview of the methods for solving the biomagnetic inverse problem can be found in Swithenby (1987).

The main purpose of this chapter is to discuss the lead systems currently being applied in detecting the equivalent magnetic dipole of the heart, and to discuss briefly the ECG-MCG relationship.

20.2 BASIC METHODS IN MAGNETOCARDIOGRAPHY

20.2.1 Measurement of the Equivalent Magnetic Dipole

PRECONDITIONS:

Source: *Magnetic dipole in a fixed location*

Conductor: *Finite, homogeneous (or possibly inhomogeneous)*

Table 17.1 (Section 17.4) lists several source and conductor models, tacitly assumed in various electrocardiographic lead systems. From

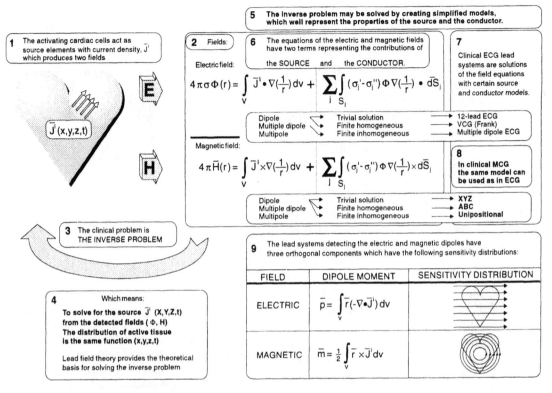

Fig. 20.1 Selection of the magnetic dipole as the basis of the clinical magnetocardiographic measurement system.

that table, one can see that in present clinical electrocardiography (standard 12-lead system and Frank vectorelectrocardiography (VECG)), a dipole with a fixed location is used as the model of the cardiac electric source. The volume conductor is modeled either with the trivial solution (i.e., a homogeneous unbounded or spherical boundary) in the 12-lead ECG or with a finite (realistic), homogeneous conductor in the Frank VECG.

Magnetocardiography was intended, at least initially, to complement the electric measurements of the heart's electric activity, or possibly replace it (e.g., in screening tests). It is therefore natural to select source and conductor models for magnetocardiography that are on the same level of complexity as for electrocardiography. This means that in clinical applications the obvious selection for the source model is the magnetic dipole. The accuracy of the conductor model may vary, but because of the self-centering effect of the well-conducting heart muscle and intracardiac blood mass (Baule and McFee,

1970) none of the extra arrangements required in the finite, inhomogeneous model are needed.

As a consequence, a magnetocardiographic signal includes three components which may be displayed either in scalar form as a function of time, or in the form of vector loops (one lead as a function of another). The selection of the display is of secondary importance (Baule and McFee, 1970; Malmivuo, 1976, 1980, 1981). The selection of the magnetic heart vector as the basis of the clinical MCG system is further explained in Figure 20.1.

20.2.2 The Magnetic Field Mapping Method

PRECONDITIONS:

Source: *Distribution of $\bar{J}^i$*

Conductor: *Infinite, homogeneous*

In electrocardiography, the mapping of the distribution of the electric potential on the surface of the thorax has been applied since the first detection of the human electrocardiogram by Augustus Waller in 1887 (see Fig. 1.16). It has, however, not come into clinical use but has remained primarily as a research tool.

Similarly, in magnetocardiography, the mapping of the magnetic field around the thorax has been a research tool. Though the magnetic field is a vector quantity and has therefore three components at each location in space, the mapping method has usually been applied for registering only one component (the x-component) of the magnetic field around the thorax. The mapping has usually been done on a certain grid. Such grids were first introduced by Cohen and McCaughan (1972). The most popular grid, introduced by Malmivuo, Saarinen, and Siltanen (1973), includes 6×6 measurement locations on the anterior thoracic wall. Later, the anatomic measures of this grid were defined in more detail; this grid became known as the "standard grid" (Karp, 1981).

In lead field theory, it may be shown that lead systems used in mapping often introduce a distortion of the signal that necessarily originates from the inhomogeneities of the volume conductor. (The situation is the same as in mapping the electric potential field.) Some of these magnetic measurements may also be realized with a similar sensitivity distribution by use of electric measurements with a higher signal-to-noise ratio and with easier application (Figure 20.2).

20.2.3   Other Methods of Magnetocardiography

In addition to the analysis of the parameters of the MCG signals, recorded either by determining the equivalent magnetic dipole or by the mapping method, several other techniques have also been applied. Of these the localization of cardiac sources is briefly discussed here.

The localization of cardiac electric sources is a highly desired objective since it may enable the localization of cardiac abnormalities including those of abnormal conduction pathways. These may cause dangerous arrhythmias or contribute to a reduction in cardiac performance. Abnormal conduction pathways, for example, conduct electric activity from the atrial muscle directly to the ventricular muscle, by-

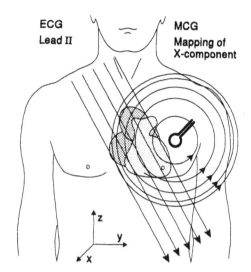

Fig. 20.2   The similarity between the lead fields of certain electric and magnetic leads are illustrated. If the magnetic field is measured in such an orientation (in the x direction in this example) and location, that the symmetry axis is located far from the region of the heart, the magnetic lead field in the heart's region is similar to the electric lead field of a lead (lead II in this example), which is oriented normal to the symmetry axis of the magnetic lead. This similarity may also be verified from the similarity of the corresponding detected signals.

passing the AV junction. This is called the Wolff-Parkinson-White or (WPW) syndrome. If a retrograde conduction pathway also exists from the ventricular mass back to the atrial mass, this reentry path may result in tachycardia. If the symptoms due to this abnormal conduction do not respond to drugs, then the tissue forming the abnormal pathway must be removed surgically, hence requiring prior localization.

In clinical practice the conduction pathways are at present localized invasively with a catheter in an electrophysiological study, which may last several hours. This time may be shortened by first making an initial noninvasive localization of the equivalent source of the conduction pathway from the electric potentials on the surface of the thorax. A review of these methods is published by Gulrajani, Savard, and Roberge (1988).

In magnetocardiographic localization the goal is to introduce an alternative to the electric localization using the magnetic methods. Utilization of this complementary technique may improve the overall localization accuracy. The magnetocardiographic localization is usually made by mapping the x component of the cardiac magnetic field at 30–40 locations on the anterior surface of the thorax with consecutive measurements using a single-channel magnetometer or simultaneously using a multichannel magnetometer. The dipole model is the most obvious to use as a source model for the localization methods. It has been shown that with the addition of the quadrupolar model, the accuracy of localization may be increased (Nenonen et al., 1991b). The accuracy of the magnetocardiographic localization depends to a great extent on the accuracy of the volume conductor model applied (Nenonen et al., 1991a). The accuracy of the magnetocardiographic localization of the origin of an abnormal conduction pathway is of the order of 2–3 cm. Because magnetocardiographic localization has been shown to have greater complexity and costs as compared to the electric method, the magnetic method does not, at present, compete with the electric method in clinical practice.

20.3 METHODS FOR DETECTING THE MAGNETIC HEART VECTOR

20.3.1 The Source and Conductor Models and the Basic Form of the Lead System for Measuring the Magnetic Dipole

PRECONDITIONS:

Source: *Distribution of $\bar{J}^i$ forming a volume source (at the origin)*

Conductor: *Finite, spherical, homogeneous: spherical conducting heart region inside insulating lung region*

In the following discussion we assume that the heart is a spherical conducting region between the insulating lungs. For the XYZ and ABC lead systems it would be enough to assume cylindrical symmetry for each component, which leads to a spherically symmetric volume con-

ductor for the three orthogonal measurements. The y and z components of the unipositional lead system require, however, an assumption of a conducting spherical heart region inside the insulating lungs. This assumption forces the lead fields to flow tangentially within the heart region. This is called a *self-centering* effect (Baule and McFee, 1970). This is also an anatomically realistic assumption.

Earlier, in Section 12.5 it was stated that, by definition, the magnetic dipole moment of a volume current distribution $\bar{J}$ in an infinite, homogeneous volume conductor with respect to an arbitrary origin is defined as (Stratton, 1941):

$$\bar{m} = \tfrac{1}{2} \int \bar{r} \times \bar{J}\, dv \qquad (20.1)$$

Similarly, as stated further in Section 12.5, in an infinite, homogeneous volume conductor, the magnetic dipole moment of an impressed current density distribution $\bar{J}^i$ is represented by the first term on the right side of Equation 12.25:

$$\bar{m} = \tfrac{1}{2} \int \bar{r} \times \bar{J}^i dv \qquad (20.2)$$

Section 12.6 showed that the lead system that detects this magnetic dipole moment has three orthogonal components. Each component produces, when energized with the reciprocal current, a linear, homogeneous, reciprocal magnetic field $\bar{B}_{LM}$ over the source region. These reciprocal magnetic fields induce lead fields $\bar{J}_{LM}$ in which the lead current is directed tangentially, and its density is proportional to the distance from the symmetry axis, as illustrated in Figure 20.3.

Furthermore, Section 12.7 showed that a natural method to realize such a lead system is to make either unipolar or bipolar measurements on the coordinate axes (Malmivuo, 1976), as described in Figure 20.4.

20.3.2 Baule-McFee Lead System

The first description of the concept of the magnetic heart vector and of the principle for its measurement was given by Gerhard M. Baule and Richard McFee in 1970. In the same article (Baule and McFee, 1970) the authors intro-

A

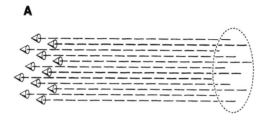

B

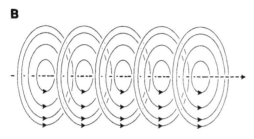

Fig. 20.3 (A) One component of the reciprocal magnetic field $\overline{B}_{LM}$, and (B) one component of the lead field $\overline{J}_{LM}$ of an ideal lead system detecting the magnetic dipole moment of a volume source. Three such orthogonal components form the complete lead system.

duced a device for measuring the magnetic field of the heart. Their system is described in Figure 20.5.

The lead system was designed for induction-coil magnetometers using ferromagnetic cores rather than for magnetometers using the SQUID (which did not exist at that time). The lead system was designed to utilize a combination of ten coils to make bipolar measurements of the three orthogonal components of the magnetic heart vector simultaneously.

Figure 20.5A describes the general construction of the ferromagnetic core system of magnodes. The principle for the measurement of the x component is illustrated in Figure 20.5B. In this measurement the magnodes in the center of the ferromagnetic cores are utilized. This figure shows the generation of the reciprocal magnetic field in the direction of the x axis within the region of the heart. When one replaces the reciprocal current generator with an amplifier, it is, according to the lead field theory, possible to detect the x component of the magnetic heart vector. The principle for the measurement of the y component is illustrated in Figure 20.5C. This figure shows the generation of the reciprocal magnetic field in the direction of the y axis within the region of the heart. The detection of the z component is realized with a similar circuit of coils located with the other two pairs of magnodes in the z direction, as illustrated in Figure 20.5D.

The lead system of Baule and McFee was never realized because it would have been disturbed by ambient magnetic noise to such an extent that it would have been unable to detect the MCG. Its main purpose was to demonstrate

A

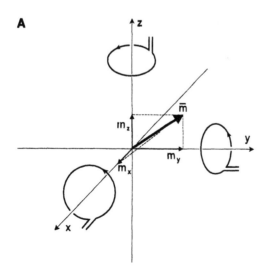

B

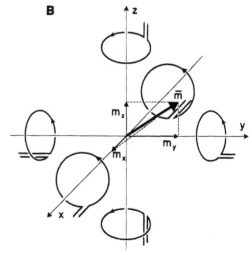

Fig. 20.4 A natural method to measure the magnetic dipole moment of a source locating in the origin is to measure the x-, y-, and z-components of the magnetic field on corresponding coordinate axes. These may be either unipolar (A) or bipolar (B) measurements.

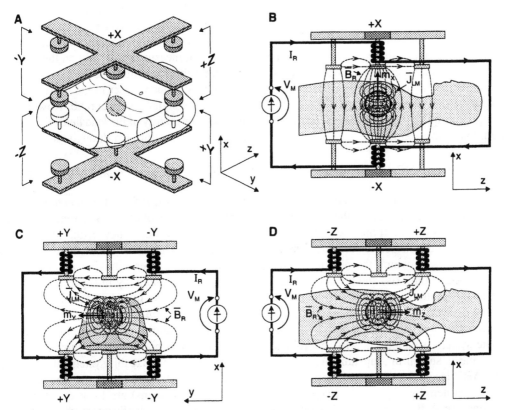

Fig. 20.5 Baule-McFee lead system. (A) The general construction of the measurement system. (B) Measurement of the *x* component of the magnetic heart vector. (C) Measurement of the *y*-component of the magnetic heart vector. (D) Measurement of the *z*-component of the magnetic heart vector. Baule-McFee lead system makes a bipolar measurement of the equivalent magnetic dipole of the heart.

one possible option for detecting the magnetic heart vector.

20.3.3 XYZ Lead System

The magnetic lead system illustrated in Figure 20.4 was first applied to magnetocardiography by Malmivuo (1976). This method, which is called the XYZ lead system, is further described in Figure 20.6. The symmetric bipolar form of the XYZ lead system is shown in this figure. Each of the three components are measured symmetrically (i.e., on both sides of the source). This method has the drawback that measurement of the component along the *z* axis (foot-to-head axis) of the body is very difficult. Also, in the measurement along the *y* axis (right-to-left axis), the detectors must be placed quite far from the source.

The symmetric (bipolar) XYZ lead system requires six magnetometers or six consecutive

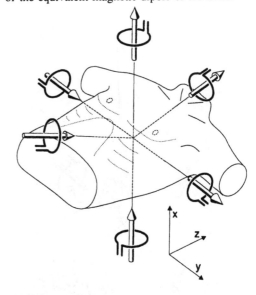

Fig. 20.6 Symmetric XYZ lead system. The bipolar arrangement provides good lead field uniformity. The difficulty arises in locating all magnetometers in their correct position surrounding the body.

measurements with one magnetometer. If the measurements are made nonsymmetrically (unipolarly) on only one side of the body (on positive coordinate axes), three magnetometers or consecutive measurements are needed. The latter arrangement increases the signal amplitude owing to the shorter measurement distance, but decreases the quality of the lead field due to the unipolar measurement.

20.3.4   ABC Lead System

Malmivuo (1976) proposed a method to avoid the difficulties encountered in the application of the XYZ lead system. If the three orthogonal coordinate axes are chosen to coincide with the edges of a cube, in which the diagonal is the x axis (back-to-front axis) and the corner is located in the center of the heart, we obtain a coordinate system that is oriented more symmetrically in relation to the body. This coordinate system is called the ABC coordinate system and is shown in Appendix A.

The ABC lead system is obtained from the XYZ lead system by aligning the magnetometers along the ABC coordinates. Figure 20.7

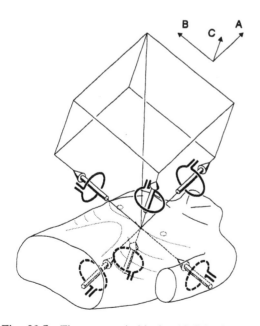

Fig. 20.7   The symmetric bipolar ABC lead system.

illustrates the ABC lead system in its symmetric (bipolar) form. The ABC lead system may also be applied nonsymmetrically (unipolarly) by conducting measurements only on the anterior side of the thorax. In this case the measurements can be made much closer to the heart, thus increasing the signal-to-noise ratio. However, in this case the quality of the lead fields decreases, as they are less uniform throughout the heart.

20.3.5   Unipositional Lead System

In the application of SQUID magnetometry, the separate location of each magnetometer is considered a major deficiency owing to high cost of multiple magnetometers or increased measurement time when applying a single magnetometer consecutively in separate locations. In 1976 Malmivuo introduced a third lead system, called the *unipositional lead system*, which avoids the difficulty of multiple measurement locations. In its nonsymmetric (unipolar) form it is possible to realize this system with a single liquid helium dewar because the three coils (or gradiometer systems) are located at the same position. This is a significant improvement over the XYZ and ABC lead systems (Malmivuo, 1976). The fact that in addition to the x component, the y and z components of the magnetic heart vector may also be measured from the same location as the one where the x component is measured with the XYZ lead system, is based on the following theory (see Fig. 20.8A):

We divide the magnetic dipole $\overline{m}$ into three components, m_x, m_y, and m_z. We consider the three components H_x, H_y, and H_z of the magnetic field $\overline{H}$ on the x axis due to this magnetic dipole $\overline{m}$. From the magnetic field lines we recognize that the x component of the magnetic field (H_x) is in the same direction as the x component of the magnetic dipole (m_x). The y and z components of the magnetic field are, however, parallel but opposite to the directions of the y and z components of the magnetic dipole, respectively. Furthermore, for m_x, m_y, and m_z of equal magnitude, the amplitudes of the components H_y and H_z of the magnetic field are one half that of the component H_x. This is a consequence of the equations of the magnetic field of a magnetic dipole (oriented in the z direction) (see Fig. 20.8B):

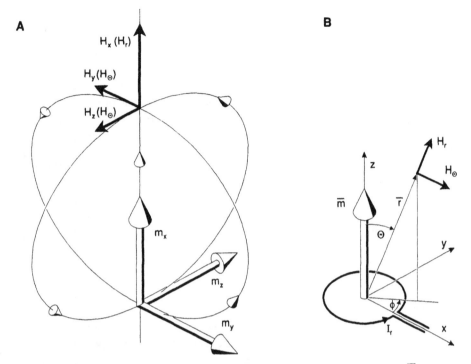

Fig. 20.8 (A) The three components H_x, H_y, and H_z of the magnetic field $\overline{H}$ due to the three components m_x, m_y, and m_z of a magnetic dipole $\overline{m}$. (B) Components of the magnetic field of a dipole.

$$H_r = \frac{2m}{4\pi r^3} \cos\theta$$

$$H_\Theta = \frac{m}{4\pi r^3} \sin\theta \qquad (20.3)$$

$$H_\phi = 0$$

where

m = the moment of the magnetic dipole
r = radius vector (distance)
θ = the angle between the moment (z-axis) and the radius vector (polar or colatitude angle)
ϕ = the angle about the moment (z-axis) (azimuth angle)

In the arrangement of Figure 20.8 the magnetic field component H_x corresponds to H_r, and components H_y and H_z correspond to H_θ of Equation 20.3.

The principle of the unipositional lead system may be similarly considered in terms of the lead field. We consider the reciprocal magnetic field due to feeding a reciprocal current I_r to the magnetometer coil (see Fig. 20.9). The strength of the dipole moment for a single-turn coil can

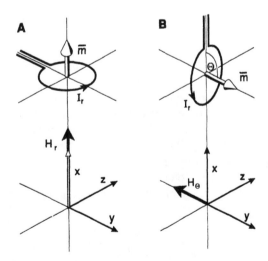

Fig. 20.9 Generation of the reciprocal magnetic field in the heart's region when measuring (A) the x component and (B) the y component of the magnetic heart vector with the unipositional lead system. The situation in the measurement of the z component is similar to that in the measurement of the y component.

be found from Equation 20.4 (higher moments can apparently be ignored, if the field is at a large distance compared to the coil radius a):

$$m = I\pi a^2 \qquad (20.4)$$

where

$$I = \text{coil current}$$
$$a = \text{coil radius}$$

(For N turns, $m = I\pi a^2 N$.) The direction of $\overline{m}$ is normal to the plane of the coil.

In Figure 20.9A the magnetometer coil is oriented ($\theta = 0°, 180°$) so that its axis passes through the heart, whose center is located at the coordinate origin. This corresponds to the arrangement for measuring the x-component of the magnetic heart vector with the XYZ lead system. Now application of Equation 20.3 shows that the (reciprocal) magnetic field in the region of the heart is

$$H_r = \frac{2m}{4\pi r^3}$$
$$H_\theta = 0 \qquad (20.5)$$

Equation 20.3 again demonstrates that a magnetometer on the x-axis is sensitive to the same component of the magnetic heart dipole as corresponds to its own orientation. The aforementioned result is obtained only when the coil is at a sufficiently large distance from the heart compared to the extent of the heart so that, to a satisfactory approximation, all points in the heart (relative to an origin at the coil) are described by $r = r$, $\theta = 0°$.

To measure the y component of the magnetic heart vector, the magnetometer coil is tilted 90°, whereupon points in the heart may be approximated by $\theta = 90°, 270°$, as in Figure 20.9B (assuming, as before, that the distance to the heart is large compared to the extent of the heart). Consequently, the magnetic field in the heart's region is

$$H_r = 0 \qquad (20.6)$$
$$H_\theta = \frac{m}{4\pi r^3}$$

This equation is also obtained from Equation 20.3 based on the assumption that any point in the heart has the coordinate ($r = r$, $\theta = 90°$). It again demonstrates that the magnetometer is sensitive to the magnetic dipole

component of the heart in the same direction as the magnetometer axis (although, in this case, opposite to it). The situation for measuring the z component follows a similar argument.

We note that the intensity of the reciprocal magnetic field in the former case (x component) is exactly twice that in the latter case (y and z component). Furthermore, in the former case, the reciprocal magnetic field orientation is the same as the direction of the dipole moment of the reciprocally energized coil. In the second case, the reciprocal magnetic field direction is opposite to the direction of the dipole moment of the coil. Therefore, when one is using the unipositional lead system, the two nonaxial components (y and z) of the *magnetic heart vector* (MHV) are obtained from the *magnetic field vector* (MFV; the uncorrected lead signal from the mutually perpendicular magnetometer coils) by multiplying by a factor of -2, as shown in Equation 20.7. Figure 20.10 illustrates the realization of the unipositional lead system.

$$\begin{vmatrix} X \\ Y \\ Z \end{vmatrix}_{MHV} = \begin{vmatrix} 1 & 0 & 0 \\ 0 & -2 & 0 \\ 0 & 0 & -2 \end{vmatrix} \begin{vmatrix} X \\ Y \\ Z \end{vmatrix}_{MFV} \qquad (20.7)$$

where

$$MHV = \text{magnetic heart vector}$$
$$MFV = \text{magnetic field vector}$$

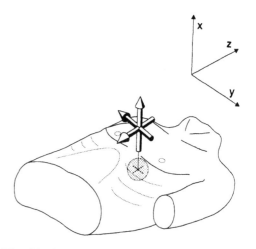

Fig. 20.10 Realization of the unipositional lead system. The arrows indicate the measurement direction. The shaded sphere represents the heart.

Corrected Unipositional Lead System

Eskola and Malmivuo proposed an improved version of the nonsymmetric unipositional lead system in 1983 (Eskola, 1983; Eskola and Malmivuo, 1983). Model experiments showed that in the unipolar measurement situation, a more accurate result is obtained when the factor of -2 in the nonaxial components is replaced by a factor -1 (as illustrated in Equation 20.8). This modification is explained by the proximity effect (see the next section), the boundary at the thorax, and the way in which internal inhomogeneities affect the lead fields in the nonsymmetric measurement situation:

$$\begin{vmatrix} X \\ Y \\ Z \end{vmatrix}_{MHV} = \begin{vmatrix} 1 & 0 & 0 \\ 0 & -1 & 0 \\ 0 & 0 & -1 \end{vmatrix} \begin{vmatrix} X \\ Y \\ Z \end{vmatrix}_{MFV} \quad (20.8)$$

where

MHV = magnetic heart vector
MFV = magnetic field vector

These model experiments also evaluated the optimum location for the measurement. It was found that the distortion of the lead field was smallest when the magnetometer is placed at the fourth left intercostal space at the sternal edge, corresponding to the location of V_2 in the standard 12-lead ECG. This measurement position, shown in Figure 20.11, is also easy to locate.

Symmetric Unipositional Lead System

As in the XYZ and ABC lead systems, the quality of the lead fields of the unipositional lead system can be considerably improved with a symmetric (bipolar) measurement arrangement. In the symmetric unipositional lead system, measurements are made on both sides of the heart, at the same distance from the center of the heart on the line parallel to the x axis, at the same location as shown in Figure 20.11 for the nonsymmetric unipositional system. Then the signals for the x, y, and z components are averaged with correct sign convention as is done in the symmetric XYZ and ABC lead systems as well.

In the symmetric unipositional lead system, Equation 20.7 is valid because the magnetom-

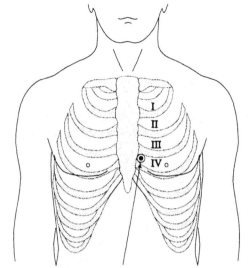

The opening of the fourth intercostal space (Location of ECG Lead V_2)

Fig. 20.11 Measurement location of the unipositional lead system is at the fourth left intercostal space at the sternal edge (the same location as for electrocardiographic precordial lead V_2).

eter on the anterior side is located further from the heart and because the distortion in the lead field is to a high degree compensated by the symmetry (see Figure 20.16). The realization of the symmetric unipositional system is shown in Figure 20.12.

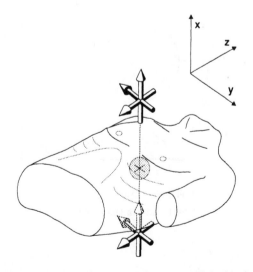

Fig. 20.12 Realization of the symmetric unipositional lead system.

20.4 SENSITIVITY DISTRIBUTION OF BASIC MCG LEADS

20.4.1 Heart and Thorax Models and the Magnetometer

In this section, the sensitivity distribution of a single-coil magnetometer is calculated according to Section 12.11. The sensitivity distribution is calculated for the cylindrically symmetric situation. We assume that the anteroposterior dimension of the thorax is 210 mm and that the radius of the spherical heart model is 56 mm, as shown in Figure 20.13. The center of the heart is located 70 mm behind the anterior chest wall and 140 mm in front of the posterior chest wall. We further assume that the magnetometer coil radius is 10 mm and the distance from its center to the chest wall is 30 mm. Thus, when the magnetometer is located at the an-

terior or posterior side of the thorax, the minimum distance from the center of the magnetometer coil to the center of the heart is 100 mm or 170 mm, respectively (Malmivuo, 1976). These measures correspond to the unipolar and bipolar unipositional measurements. In this section it is assumed that the magnetometer does not have the compensation coils (i.e., the magnetometer is not a gradiometer).

20.4.2 Unipolar Measurement

As noted before in Section 12.11, in the cylindrically symmetric situation the lead field current is tangentially oriented, and its amplitude is independent of the angle ϕ. Therefore, the lead field current distribution may be illustrated as a function of the radial distance r from the symmetry axis, with the distance h from the magnetometer as a parameter. Figure 20.14 illustrates the sensitivity distribution within the

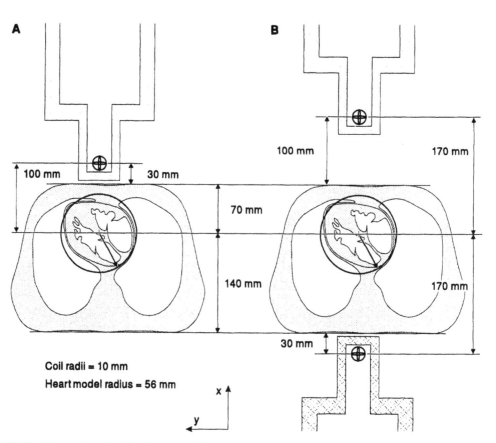

Fig. 20.13 Dimensions for the thorax and heart models and the measurement distances in unipolar and bipolar unipositional measurements. (A) Uni-

polar (nonsymmetric) measurement location on the anterior side. (B) Bipolar (symmetric) measurement locations on the anterior and posterior sides.

A

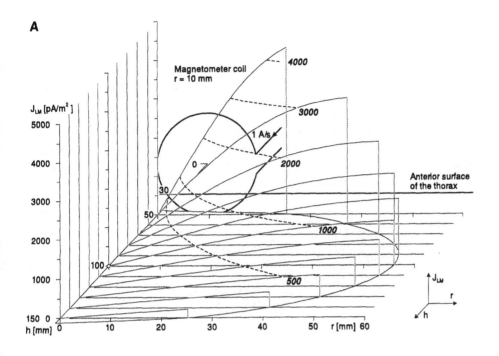

B

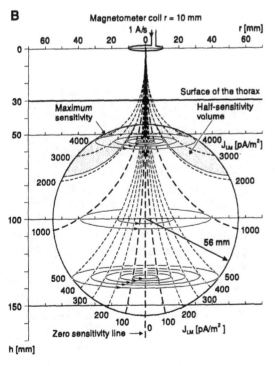

Fig. 20.14 Sensitivity distribution of a unipolar (nonsymmetric) measurement within the region of the spherical heart model for a 100 mm magnetometer-heart center separation. The figure also illustrates the location and size of the magnetometer. This measurement situation corresponds to the measurement of the *x* component of the MHV with the nonsymmetric unipositional lead system at the anterior side of the thorax. (A) Sensitivity distribution in the region of the heart. The magnetometer distance *h* and radial distance *r* are not shown to the same scale. (B) Isosensitivity curves are illustrated with dashed lines. Lead field current flow lines are sketched with thin solid lines. The dimensions of *h* and *r* are to the same scale.

region of the spherical heart model for the measurement distance of 100 mm. This is shown both with a series of curves illustrating the lead field current density as a function of radial distance (Fig. 20.14A) and with isosensitivity curves (Fig. 20.14B). The figure illustrates also the location and size of the magnetometer. This measurement situation corresponds to the measurement of the x component of the MHV with the nonsymmetric (unipolar) unipositional lead system on the anterior side of the thorax as illustrated in Figure 20.10. Figure 20.15 illustrates the same information for the measurement distance of 170 mm. This measurement situation corresponds to the unipolar measurement on the posterior side of the thorax.

As can be seen from Figure 20.14, the sensitivity of the unipolar measurement is concentrated on the anterior region of the heart. This is called the *proximity effect.*

20.4.3 Bipolar Measurement

The proximity effect can be compensated by using bipolar measurements where the two measurements are made symmetrically on opposite sides of the heart. This is the case in Figures 20.6 and 20.7 in the symmetric (bipolar) XYZ and ABC lead systems, respectively. This is also the case in measuring the x component with the symmetric unipositional lead system as shown in Figure 20.12.

Figure 20.16 illustrates the sensitivity distribution in the bipolar measurement of the axial component of the magnetic field. The magnetometer coil radius is again 10 mm. The magnetometer distance is, on both sides, 170 mm from the center of the heart, because this is the minimum distance on the posterior side of the thorax. This measurement situation corresponds to the measurement of the x component of the MHV on both sides of the thorax with the symmetric XYZ lead system or with the symmetric unipositional lead system. (For the symmetric measurement of the y and z components in the XYZ lead system and for all components of the ABC lead system the measurement distances would be larger.) In this figure the lead field current densities of the anterior and posterior measurements are summed. This corresponds to the summing of the cor-

responding MCG signals. Please note that the noise of these measurements is also summed. Therefore, the sensitivity scales of Figures 20.15 and 20.16 are relevant when comparing signal amplitudes but not when comparing signal-to-noise ratios.

In the measurement of the y and z components of the unipositional lead system, the measurement situation is not cylindrically symmetric because the measured fields are not the axial components. Therefore we must assume that the heart model is a conducting sphere surrounded by insulating lung tissue. Figure 20.17 shows the reciprocal magnetic field in the measurement of the y component. It is shown both in the zx and yz planes. In the measurement of the z component the reciprocal magnetic field is, of course, similar. Note that as discussed in Section 20.3.5, the reciprocal magnetic field strength is one half of that in the measurement of the x component. Therefore the coefficient -2 is needed in Equation 20.7.

Figures 20.16 and 20.17 illustrate that the proximity effect can be very accurately compensated by the bipolar (symmetric) measurement. Because the anterior location of the magnetometer coil is further from the torso surface in the bipolar measurement than in the unipolar, its sensitivity is reduced to that of the posterior magnetometer. Nevertheless the symmetric (bipolar) arrangement is recommended because it yields a sensitivity distribution much closer to the ideal.

20.5 GENERATION OF THE MCG SIGNAL FROM THE ELECTRIC ACTIVATION OF THE HEART

As pointed out earlier, the source of the MCG signal is the *electric* activity of the heart muscle. The generation of the MCG signal from the progress of the activation front in the heart can be sketched similarly with the aid of the MCG lead fields, as was done in Section 15.2 for the ECG with the electric lead fields.

In Figure 20.18 the generation of the MCG signal in the x and z leads is sketched. This illustration is only a rough approximation, and its purpose is to give an impression of the prin-

A

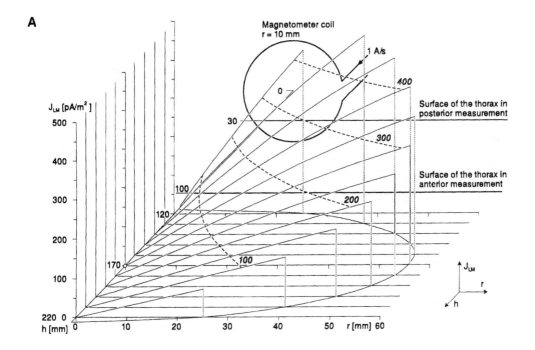

B

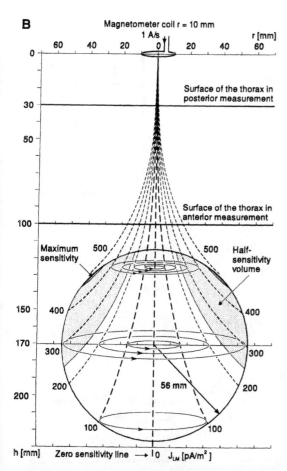

Fig. 20.15 The sensitivity distribution of a unipolar (nonsymmetric) measurement within the region of the spherical heart model for a 170 mm magnetometer-heart center separation. This measurement situation corresponds to the measurement of the x component of the MHV at the posterior side of the thorax. (A) Sensitivity distribution within the heart region. The magnetometer distance h and radial distance r are not shown in the same scale. (B) Isosensitivity curves are illustrated with dashed lines. Lead field current flow lines are sketched with thin solid lines. The dimensions of h and r are in the same scale.

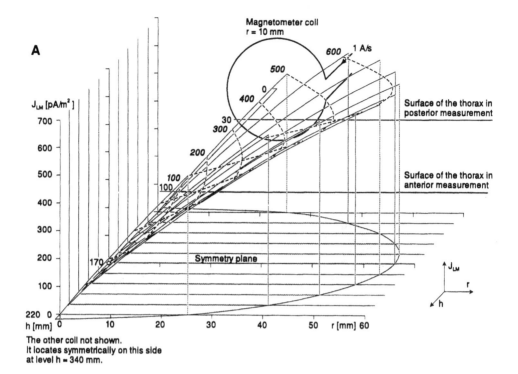

A

J$_{LM}$ [pA/m^2]

Magnetometer coil
r = 10 mm

The other coil not shown.
It locates symmetrically on this side
at level h = 340 mm.

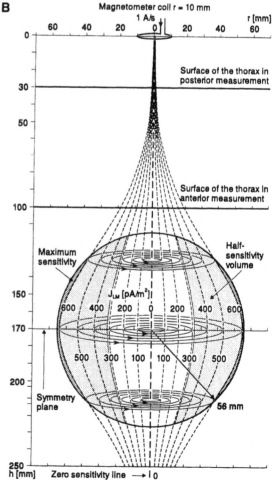

B

Magnetometer coil r = 10 mm

Fig. 20.16 Sensitivity distribution of a bipolar (symmetric) measurement within the region of the spherical heart model. The figure also illustrates the anterior magnetometer. This measurement situation corresponds to the measurement of the *x* component of the MHV with the symmetric XYZ lead system or with the symmetric unipositional lead system with measurements on both sides of the thorax. (A) Sensitivity distribution. The region of the heart is shaded. The magnetometer distance *h* and radial distance *r* are not shown to the same scale. (B) Isosensitivity curves are illustrated with dashed lines. Lead field current flow lines are sketched with thin solid lines. The dimensions of *h* and *r* are in scale.

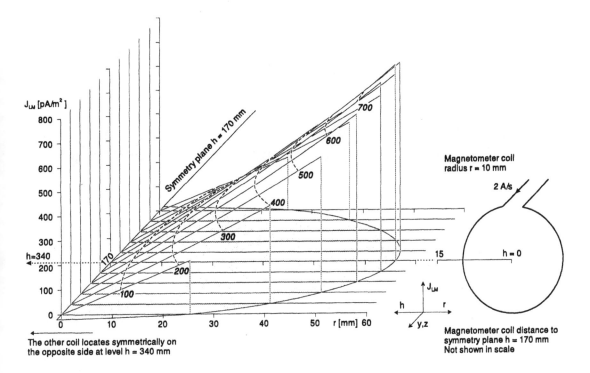

J_{LM} [pA/m²]

800
700
600
500
400
h=340
200
100
0

Symmetry plane h = 170 mm

170
100
200
300
400
500
600
700

0   10   20   30   40   50   r [mm] 60

The other coil locates symmetrically on
the opposite side at level h = 340 mm

Magnetometer coil
radius r = 10 mm

2 A/s

15   h = 0

h   r

J_{LM}

y,z

Magnetometer coil distance to
symmetry plane h = 170 mm
Not shown in scale

B

Magnetometer coil r = 10 mm

I_r = 2 A/s   z [mm]

-60   -40   -20   0   20   40   60

0

30   Surface of the thorax in
            posterior measurement

50

            Surface of the thorax in
            anterior measurement

100

            800   Maximum
                   sensitivity
            700

Symmetry   600   Zero
plane of   500   sensitivity
the coils   400   line
            300
            200
150   100
            0
170   100
            200
            300
            400
200   500   56 mm
            600
Sensitivity 700
is cylindrically 800   Half-
symmetric   J [pA/m²]   sensitivity
around the zero   volume
sensitivity line

250
h [mm]

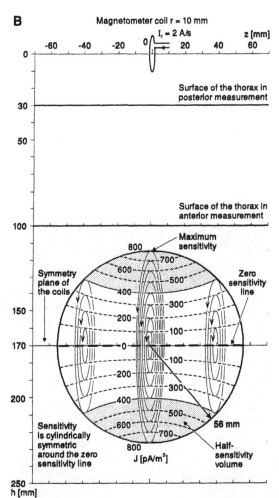

Fig. 20.17 Reciprocal magnetic field in the measurement of the y component with the symmetric
unipositional lead system illustrated (A) in the zx
plane and (B) in the yz plane. Reciprocal magnetic
field lines are illustrated with dashed lines. Lead field
current flow lines are sketched with thin solid lines.

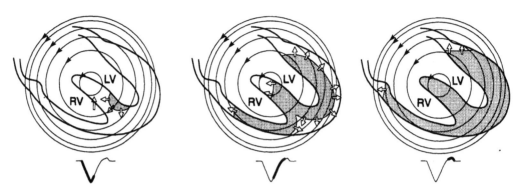

Fig. 20.18   Schematic illustration of the generation of the *x* and *z* components of the MCG signal.

ciple of how the signal is produced. As regards the *x* component, it is assumed that because of the strong proximity effect, the signal is generated mainly from the activation in the anterior part of the heart. As regards the *z* component, it is pointed out that in nonsymmetric unipo-

sitional MCG measurements the zero sensitivity line is located in the posterior side of the heart. Because the sensitivity is proportional to the distance from the zero sensitivity line, the contribution of the anterior part of the heart is again dominating.

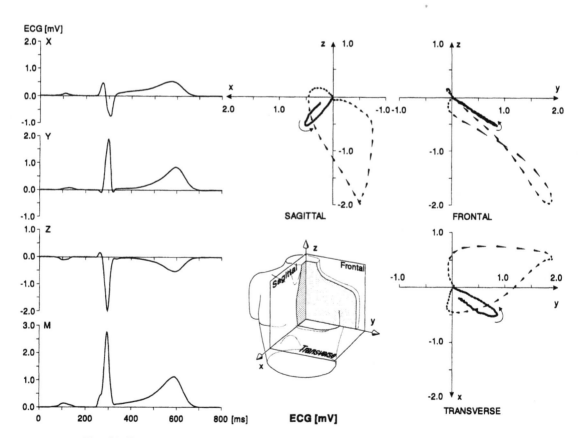

Fig. 20.19   Averaged EHV of a healthy 30 year old man recorded with the Frank lead system.

20.6   ECG–MCG RELATIONSHIP

The relationship between the normal ECG and the normal MCG was discussed theoretically in Sections 12.9 and 12.10. In the following, this relationship is examined using actual signal measurements. Figure 20.19 illustrates the averaged electric heart vector of a healthy 30 year old man recorded with the Frank lead system. The averaged magnetic heart vector of the same subject, recorded with the corrected unipositional lead system, is illustrated in Figure 20.20 (Nousiainen, Lekkala, and Malmivuo, 1986; Nousiainen, 1991).

It may be seen from Figures 20.19 and 20.20 that at the peak of the QRS complex the electric and magnetic heart vectors are very close to being 90° apart. This could also be predicted theoretically (Wikswo et al., 1979). If the angle were always exactly 90°, there would be no new information in the MCG. However, it has been found that this angle varies considerably during the QRS complex, both from patient to patient and in various cardiac disorders. Figure 20.21 shows the variation of this angle as a function of time, and averaged over 17 normal subjects. The arrow indicates the instant of the maximum QRS complex (Nousiainen, Lekkala, and Malmivuo, 1986; Nousiainen, 1991).

Not only does the angle between the EHV and the MHV vary during the QRS but their magnitude ratio also varies. Figure 20.22 illustrates this phenomenon. It is possible to identify three peaks—namely M_1, M_2, and M_3—in the MHV magnitude curve. It was noted in Section 18.3 that M_1 appears to be generated by radial, M_2 by radial and tangential, and M_3 mainly by tangential forces. As pointed out previously, in the ideal case the electric lead is as sensitive to radial as to tangential forces, but the magnetic lead is sensitive only to tangential forces.

Figure 20.22 illustrates clearly how the electric measurement, which is more sensitive to

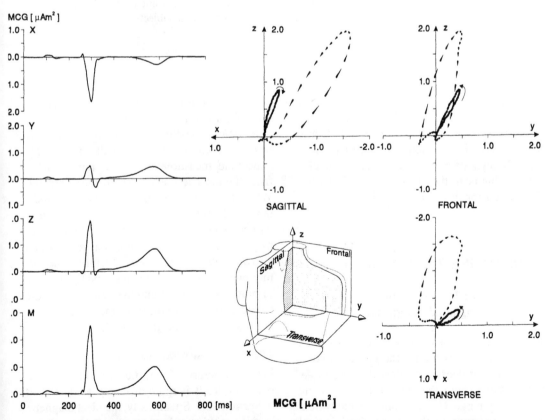

Fig. 20.20 Averaged MHV of the same subject as in the previous figure recorded with the corrected unipositional lead system.

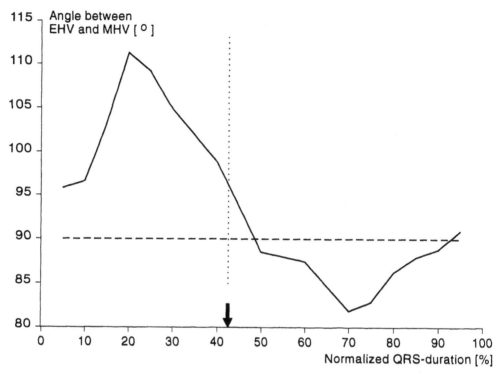

Fig. 20.21 Instantaneous angle between the EHV and the MHV during the normalized duration of the QRS complex. The arrow indicates the maximum value of the MHV. The curve is an average over the QRS complexes of 17 normal subjects.

the radial electric forces, detects the peak M_1 with a relatively higher sensitivity. Peak M_3, which is formed mainly by tangential electric forces, is seen in the magnetic measurement as a clearly separate peak. However, at the beginning of this peak the electric signal is larger. The reason for this is not yet clear.

20.7 CLINICAL APPLICATION OF MAGNETOCARDIOGRAPHY

20.7.1 Advantages of Magnetocardiography

We have noted that the bioelectric activity in the heart is responsible for the generation of a source current density, namely $\bar{J}^i\,(x,y,z,t)$. As stated before, both the electric and magnetic fields are generated by this same source which, in turn, responds to the electrophysiological

phenomenon of depolarization and repolarization of cardiac muscle cells.

A logical question arises as to whether any new information might be provided by the magnetic field measurement that is not available from the electric potential field measurement. While it appears, on certain theoretical grounds, that the electric and magnetic fields are not fully independent, other reasons exist for the use of magnetocardiography. These may be divided into *theoretical* and *technical* features. The former ones are based on the universal properties of biomagnetic fields and the latter ones to the technical features of the instrumentation. These are discussed in the following paragraphs.

Theoretical Advantages

First, the nature of lead fields of electric and magnetic leads is quite different, as described in Section 12.9. Specifically, the ideal magnetic lead is sensitive only to tangential components

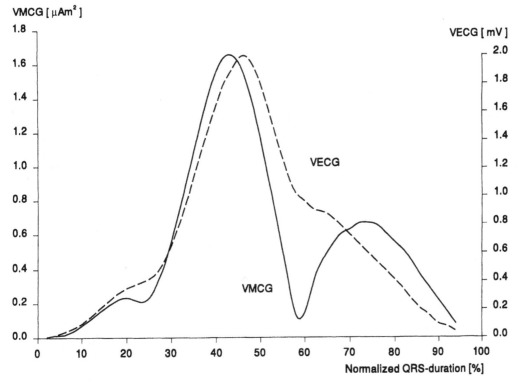

Fig. 20.22 Simultaneous plots of the magnitude curves of the EHV (dashed curve) and the MHV (solid curve) during the QRS complex.

of activation sources and therefore should be particularly responsive to abnormalities in activation (since normal activation sources are primarily radial). Furthermore, the tangential components are attenuated in the ECG because of the Brody effect. Another factor is that the signal-to-noise ratio for the electrical and magnetic recordings are affected by different factors, so there could be a practical advantage in using one over the other despite their similarities in content.

Second, the magnetic permeability of the tissue is that of free space. Therefore the sensitivity of the MCG is not affected by the high electric resistivity of lung tissue. This makes it possible to record with MCG from the posterior side of the thorax the electric activity of the posterior side of the heart. That is difficult to do with surface ECG electrodes, but is possible to do with an esophageal electrode which is, however, inconvenient for the patient. Another important application of this feature is the recording of the fetal MCG. During a certain

phase of pregnancy the fetal ECG is very difficult to record because of the insulating fat layer in the fetus.

Technical Advantages

First, a possibly important distinction is that the magnetic detector is not in contact with the subject. For mass screening, there is an advantage in not requiring skin preparation and attachment of electrodes. (In the case of patients with skin burns this is a crucial advantage.)

Second, the SQUID (Superconducting QUantum Interference Device) magnetometer is readily capable of measuring DC signals. These are associated with the S-T segment shift in myocardial infarction (Cohen et al., 1971; Cohen and Kaufman, 1975). Such signals can be obtained electrically only with great difficulty. Although the clinical value has yet to be demonstrated, it should be noted that because of the difficulty in performing electrical measurements, there have been few investigations of DC potentials.

20.7.2   Disadvantages of Magnetocardiography

There are many reasons for preferring the use of the ECG rather than the MCG. An important consideration is the ease of application. For example, if only the heart rate is desired, then the ECG may prove much simpler. The reason is that the measurement of the MCG, at present, is technologically more complicated and requires complex and expensive equipment. Specifically, this includes a SQUID magnetometer, liquid helium, and a low-noise environment. Because of the development of the SQUID technology, a shielded room is no longer needed in magnetocardiography. (In the near future, it seems possible to operate the SQUIDs at the liquid nitrogen temperature which decreases the operational costs considerably.)

20.7.3   Clinical Application

The clinical application of magnetocardiography may be based on either theoretical (bioelectromagnetic) or technical features of the method. The main technical benefits of MCG are given in Section 20.2.1. The theoretical features include the *different sensitivity distribution* of the MCG to the *bioelectric sources* of the heart.

Several studies on the diagnostic performance of the MCG have been published in the literature. An overview of these can be found in the review article of Siltanen (1989). The patient materials have included most of the main categories of cardiac diseases that are investigated with ECG, including infarction, hypertrophy, and conduction defects. In most studies the MCG has been done with the *mapping method* by recording only the x component of the heart's magnetic field at several recording points on the anterior side of the thorax without utilizing the vectorial nature of the magnetic field (Cohen and McCaughan, 1972; Saarinen et al., 1978). There are also many reports in which the three components of the magnetic vector field of the heart have been recorded with the mapping method (Cohen and Chandler, 1969; Rosen and Inouye, 1975; Seppänen et al., 1983; Shirae, Furukawa, and Katayama, 1988; Sakauchi et al., 1989). In the mapping method, the number of the measurement points is usually 30–40. If the signal is recorded with a single-channel magnetometer (as is usually done because of the large dimensions of the measurement grid) and if we assume 1 minute for positioning the magnetometer and another minute for data collection, this leads to a total recording time of more than 1 hour per patient. Using the mapping method for various cardiac abnormalities, the diagnostic performance of the MCG has been, on average, about the same as that of the ECG.

We briefly summarize here the results of one study, made at the Ragnar Granit Institute in cooperation with the Tampere University Hospital, where the diagnostic performance of magnetocardiography was studied utilizing the unipositional lead system (Oja, 1993). A total of 526 subjects were chosen, of whom 290 were healthy subjects and 236 patients had various cardiac disorders including myocardial infarction, left ventricular hypertrophy, ventricular conduction defects, and Wolf-Parkinson-White syndrome. The statistical analysis to evaluate the diagnostic performance of VECG (Frank lead system) and VMCG was made with a stepwise linear discriminant analysis.

The variation of the VMCG in normal subjects and the effect of constitutional variables were first investigated by Nousiainen and colleagues (Nousiainen, 1991; Nousiainen, Oja, and Malmivuo, 1994ab). This forms the basis for determining the diagnostic performance of the VMCG.

The diagnostic performance of the VECG and the VMCG were first compared in their capacity to distinguish among five groups consisting of (1) normal subjects; and patients with (2) anteroseptal myocardial infarction, (3) inferior myocardial infarction, (4) lateral myocardial infarction, and (5) left ventricular hypertrophy. When the VECG was used, the best results were obtained when a total of 30 parameters from the QRS vector and ST-T segment were used. In the VMCG, the best results were obtained by using 11 parameters from the QRS vector and two from the ST-T segment. Under these conditions the sensitivity (i.e., percentage classified correctly) of the VECG and VMCG were the same, namely 73.7%.

Significant improvements in the classifica-

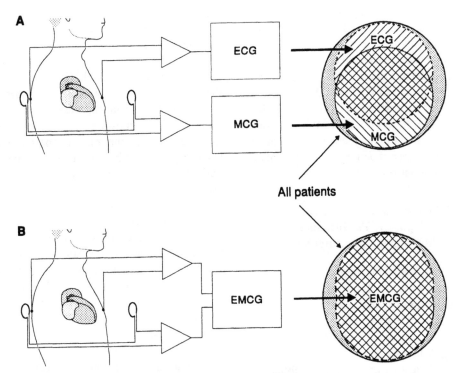

Fig. 20.23 Illustration of the principle by which the diagnostic performance may be increased by use of biomagnetic measurements. (A) If electric and magnetic methods (ECG and MCG) are based on source models having the same number of independent variables, the number of correctly diagnosed patients is about the same with both methods. The more different the sensitivity distributions of these systems, the more clearly differentiated are the populations of correctly diagnosed patients. Because we do not know which individual patients are diagnosed correctly with each method, the overall diagnostic performance cannot be increased by use of separate electric and magnetic methods. (B) If the diagnosis is based on the combination of electric and magnetic data (EMCG), the number of correctly diagnosed patients may be increased to the area bordered with correctly diagnosed patients by both methods.

tion rate in classifying the five aforementioned groups were obtained, when part of the 30 parameters were selected from the ECG and the rest from the MCG. In this combination of ECG and MCG the correct classification rate was 81.4%. The improvement in the diagnostic performance is based on the fact that the MCG leads are independent of the ECG leads. Therefore, though both ECG and MCG have about the same diagnostic performance and the number of the correctly diagnosed patients is about the same, these groups are not identical. In the combination of ECG and MCG, called *electromagnetocardiogram* (EMCG), it is possible to combine the groups of the correctly diagnosed patients, as illustrated in Figure 20.23.

On the basis of this study and the existing literature of other studies, we may draw the following conclusions concerning the diagnostic performance of MCG:

1. Though the unipositional MCG measurement is made at only one location compared to the 30–40 measurement locations of the mapping method, the diagnostic performance of the unipositional VMCG method is at least as good as that of the mapping system.
2. There is no significant difference between the diagnostic performance of the MCG compared to Frank's ECG.
3. The diagnostic classifications of ECG and MCG are dissimilar. (This means that the individual subjects classified in each group

are not the same with both methods even though the number of the correctly diagnosed patients are the same.)

4. The diagnostic performance of the EMCG is better than that of the ECG or MCG alone, even though the EMCG uses the same total number of parameters as in either the ECG or the MCG. At its best, the EMCG, by combining electric and magnetic data, could reduce the number of patients classified incorrectly to about one half.

20.7.4 Basis for the Increase in Diagnostic Performance by Biomagnetic Measurement

The basic idea behind the increase in diagnostic performance when applying electromagnetocardiography (item 4, above) is fundamental to the application of biomagnetic methods to clinical diagnosis in general, and it may be further clarified as follows.

If the MCG leads were a linear combination of the ECG leads (as is the case in Fig. 20.3), the groups of correctly diagnosed patients would be identical in both tests. Such a case has been demonstrated by Willems and Lesaffre (1987) who have shown that the 12-lead ECG and Frank VCG have an equal diagnostic performance. A combination of these lead systems did not improve the diagnostic performance. That is natural, however, because one of these lead systems is a linear combination of the other one.

But, as the Helmholtz theorem states, the ECG and MCG leads are mathematically independent. Therefore the correctly diagnosed patient materials with both methods are about as large, but not identical. Therefore, with a combination of the ECG and MCG signals it is possible to combine the groups of correctly diagnosed patients and to increase the diagnostic performance even without increasing the number of parameters in the diagnostic procedure. This is a consequence of the fact that in the combined method we have $3 + 3 = 6$ independent leads if both ECG and MCG are based on the dipole model.

This principle is illustrated in Figure 20.23, where the whole population is represented with a large circle. Suppose that the patients who

are diagnosed correctly with ECG can be represented with a smaller circle within it, and those patients who can be diagnosed correctly with MCG can be represented with another similar circle. If the ECG and MCG systems include the same number of independent measurements (both are, for instance, based on a dipole model), their diagnostic performances are about as good and thus the areas of the circles representing the number of correctly diagnosed patients with each system have about an equal area.

Because we do not know which are the individual patients who are diagnosed correctly with ECG but incorrectly with MCG, or vice versa, with separate diagnostic systems of ECG and MCG we cannot increase the overall diagnostic performance. (If we could know who are the patients who are diagnosed correctly and who are diagnosed incorrectly, then the diagnostic performance would, of course, be 100%!) The overall diagnostic performance can be increased only if both the electric and the magnetic signals are *simultaneously* included in the diagnostic procedure in the form of *electromagnetocardiography (EMCG)*. The diagnostic performance of the combined system would then equal the surface bordered together by the ECG and MCG circles lying slightly apart.

This is the fundamental principle behind the increase of diagnostic performance which can be achieved with a biomagnetic method in addition to that of a bioelectric method. This principle is not only applicable to magnetocardiography but may also be applied to magnetoencephalography and other areas of biomagnetism as well.

20.7.5 General Conclusions on Magnetocardiography

On the basis of the theory of bioelectromagnetism and the existing literature on MCG research, we may draw the following general conclusions regarding the application of magnetocardiography (Malmivuo, 1976):

1. The MCG measures the *electric* activity of the heart muscle. Therefore, on grounds of cost-effectiveness, if only one of these methods is used when such recordings can be

done electrically, the ECG should be used unless there are *technical* reasons for selecting the MCG (e.g., in screening tests, in patients with skin burns, in recording DC fields, etc.).

2. The ECG measures the electric potential field, which is a *scalar* field. Therefore, one measurement at each measurement location is enough. The MCG measures the magnetic field, which is a *vector* field. Therefore, MCG measurements should provide a vector description—that is, three orthogonal measurements at each measurement location—to get all available information (Malmivuo, 1976; Oostendorp, van Oosterom, and Huiskamp, 1992).

3. In MCG we are interested in the electric activation of the whole cardiac muscle, not only on its anterior surface. Therefore, to compensate the proximity effect, MCG measurements should be done symmetrically both on the anterior and on the posterior side of the thorax. Actually, the posterior measurement of the MCG increases the information especially on the posterior side of the heart, where the sensitivity of all ECG leads is low due to the insulating effect of the lungs. (As noted earlier, in the measurement of the MEG, we are mainly interested in the electric activation of the surface of the brain, the cortex. Therefore a unipolar measurement is more relevant in measuring the MEG.)

4. On the basis of the existing literature on the MCG, nonsymmetric unipositional measurement seems to give the same diagnostic performance as the mapping of the x component of the magnetic field on the anterior side of the thorax.

5. A *combination* of electric and magnetic measurements (i.e., ECG and MCG) gives a better diagnostic performance than either method alone with the same number of diagnostic parameters, because the number of independent measurements doubles.

REFERENCES

Baule GM, McFee R (1963): Detection of the magnetic field of the heart. *Am. Heart J.* 55:(7) 95–6.

Baule GM, McFee R (1970): The magnetic heart vector. *Am. Heart J.* 79:(2) 223–36.

Cohen D, Chandler L (1969): Measurements and simplified interpretation of magnetocardiograms from humans. *Circulation* 39: 395–402.

Cohen D, Kaufman LA (1975): Magnetic determination of the relationship between the S-T segment shift and the injury current produced by coronary artery occlusion. *Circ. Res.* 36: 414.

Cohen D, McCaughan D (1972): Magnetocardiograms and their variation over the chest in normal subjects. *Am. J. Cardiol.* 29:(5) 678–85.

Cohen D, Norman JC, Molokhia F, Hood W (1971): Magnetocardiography of direct currents: S-T segment and baseline shifts during experimental myocardial infarction. *Science* 172:(6) 1329–33.

Eskola H (1983): On the properties of vector magnetocardiographic leads. *Tampere Univ. Tech.*, Tampere, Finland, Thesis, pp. 154. (Dr. tech. thesis)

Eskola HJ, Malmivuo JA (1983): Optimizing vector magnetocardiographic lead fields by using physical torso model. *Nuovo Cim.* 2:(2) 356–67.

Gulrajani RM, Savard P, Roberge FA (1988): The inverse problem in electrocardiography: Solution in terms of equivalent sources. *CRC Crit. Rev. Biomed. Eng.* 16: 171–214.

Karp P (1981): Cardiomagnetism. In *Biomagnetism, Proc. Third Internat. Workshop On Biomagnetism, Berlin (West), May 1980*, ed. SN Erné, H-D Hahlbohm, H Lübbig, pp. 219–58, Walter de Gruyter, Berlin.

Malmivuo JA (1976): On the detection of the magnetic heart vector—An application of the reciprocity theorem. *Helsinki Univ. Tech.*, Acta Polytechn. Scand., El. Eng. Series. Vol. 39., pp. 112. (Dr. tech. thesis)

Malmivuo JA (1980): Distribution of MEG detector sensitivity: An application of reciprocity. *Med. & Biol. Eng. & Comput.* 18:(3) 365–70.

Malmivuo JA (1981): Properties of an ideal MCG-recording system. In *Biomagnetism. Proc. Third Internat. Workshop On Biomagnetism, Berlin (West), May 1980*, ed. SN Erné, H-D Hahlbohm, H Lübbig, pp. 343–9, Walter de Gruyter, Berlin.

Malmivuo JA, Saarinen M, Siltanen P (1973): A clinical method in magnetocardiography. In *Digest X Internat. Conf. Med. Biol. Eng*, Vol. I, ed. A Albert, W Vogt, W Helbig, p. 251,, Dresden.

Nenonen J, Katila T, Leiniö M, Montonen J, Mäkijärvi M, Siltanen P (1991a): Magnetocardiographic functional localization using current multipole models. *IEEE Trans. Biomed. Eng.* BME-38:(7) 648–57.

Nenonen J, Purcell CJ, Horácek BM, Stroink G, Katila T (1991b): Magnetocardiographic functional localization using a current dipole in a realistic torso. *IEEE Trans. Biomed. Eng.* BME-38:(7) 658–64.

Nousiainen JJ (1991): Behavior of the vector magnetocardiogram in normal subjects and in some abnormal cases. *Tampere Univ. Tech., Tampere, Finland,* Thesis, pp. 177. (Dr. tech. thesis)

Nousiainen JJ, Lekkala JO, Malmivuo JA (1986): Comparative study of the normal vector magnetocardiogram and vector electrocardiogram. *J. Electrocardiol.* 19:(3) 275–90.

Nousiainen JJ, Oja OS, Malmivuo JA (1994a): Normal vector magnetocardiogram. I. Correlation with the normal vector ECG *J. Electrocardiol.* 27:(3) 221–31.

Nousiainen JJ, Oja OS, Malmivuo JA (1994b): Normal vector magnetocardiogram. II. Effect of constitutional variables. *J. Electrocardiol.* 27:(3) 233–41.

Oja OS (1993): Vector magnetocardiogram in myocardial disorders. *University of Tampere, Medical Faculty,* 168 pp. (MD thesis).

Oostendorp TF, van Oosterom A, Huiskamp GJ (1992): The activation sequence of the heart as computed from all three magnetic field components. In *Proc. of the XIX International Congress on Electrocardiology,* p. 132, Lisbon.

Rosen A, Inouye GT (1975): A study of the vector magnetocardiographic waveforms. *IEEE Trans. Biomed. Eng.* BME-22: 167–74.

Rush S (1975): On the interdependence of magnetic and electric body surface recordings. *IEEE Trans. Biomed. Eng.* BME-22: 157–67.

Saarinen M, Karp P, Katila T, Siltanen P (1978): The normal magnetocardiogram: I. Morphology. *Ann. Clin. Res.* 10:(S21) 1–43.

Sakauchi Y, Kado H, Awano N, Kasai N, Higuchi M, Chinone K, Nakanishi M, Ohwada K, Kariyone

M (1989): Measurement of cardiac magnetic field vector. In *Advances in Biomagnetism,* ed. SJ Williamson, M Hoke, G Stroink, M Kotani, pp. 425–8, Plenum Press, New York.

Seppänen M, Katila T, Tuomisto T, Varpula T, Duret D, Karp P (1983): Measurement of the biomagnetic fields using multichannel superconducting magnetometer techniques. *Nuovo Cim.* 2 D: 166–74.

Shirae K, Furukawa H, Katayama M (1988): Measurements and characteristics of vector magnetocardiography. In *Biomagnetism '87,* ed. K Atsumi, M Kotani, S Ueno, T Katila, SJ Williamson, pp. 294–7, Tokyo Denki University Press, Tokyo.

Siltanen P (1989): Magnetocardiography. In *Comprehensive Electrocardiology. Theory and Practice in Health and Disease,* Vol. 2, ed. PW Macfarlane, TDV Lawrie, pp. 1405–38, Pergamon Press, New York.

Stratton JA (1941): *Electromagnetic Theory,* McGraw-Hill, New York.

Swithenby SJ (1987): Biomagnetism and the biomagnetic inverse problem. *Phys. Med. Biol.* MJ Day (ed.): The Biomagnetic Inverse Problem, 32:(1) 146. (Papers from a conference at the Open University, April 1986).

Waller AD (1887): A demonstration on man of electromotive changes accompanying the heart's beat. *J. Physiol. (Lond.)* 8: 229–34.

Wikswo JP, Malmivuo JA, Barry WM, Leifer M, Fairbank WM (1979): The theory and application of magnetocardiography. In *Advances in Cardiovascular Physics,* Vol. 2, ed. DN Ghista, pp. 1–67, S. Karger, Basel.

Willems JL, Lesaffre E (1987): Comparison of multigroup logistic and linear discriminant ECG and VCG classification. *J. Electrocardiol.* 20: 83–92.

VI

Electric and Magnetic Stimulation of Neural Tissue

Parts VI and VII focus on the second subdivision of bioelectromagnetism—stimulation and magnetization—also called electro- and magnetobiology. The discussion of electric stimulation is also divided along anatomical lines. Part VI deals with neural tissue and Part VII with cardiac tissue.

Chapter 21 describes the electric stimulation of peripheral nervous tissue, especially in order to produce muscular activity. Therefore it is called *functional* electric stimulation. The electric stimulation of biological tissue is an important topic in clinical applications. This subdivision of bioelectromagnetism was also historically first applied to human subjects. Because of space considerations, we have excluded many very important clinical applications of electric stimulation. The discussion on electric stimulation of the central nervous system is not included because, theoretically, the distribution of the electric current in the brain tissue follows, according to the reciprocity theorem, the sensitivity distribution of the corresponding measurement electrodes. Similarly, other important topics, such as electric treatment of pain, are also excluded because from a theoretical point of view they offer little that is new while the physiological/clinical goals are poorly documented.

Chapter 22 discusses the principle of magnetic stimulation and its neurological applications. At present the widest application of magnetic stimulation is the stimulation of the central nervous system.

Electromagnetic energy can be applied also to nonexcitable tissues. Such applications include, for instance, electrosurgical devices (surgical diathermy) and electrotherapeutic devices. The latter have many applications in physiotherapy. Similarly, we could also list magnetotherapeutic devices. Because these methods and devices do not raise new theoretical concerns that lie within the scope of this book, they are excluded.

21

Functional Electric Stimulation

21.1 INTRODUCTION

There are a growing number of documented scientific therapeutic uses of electricity (Seligman, 1982). In most cases, although the mechanism is not always clearly understood, it appears to arise as a consequence of the depolarization or hyperpolarization of excitable cell membranes resulting from the applied currents. Other mechanisms that appear to be sometimes involved include thermal (heating) and neurohumoral effects.

Functional electric stimulation is a very straightforward application for the therapeutic use of electricity. Another area in which electrotherapy may be applied is in the electric stimulation of cardiac tissue, including cardiac pacemakers and cardiac defibrillation. These topics are discussed in the next two chapters.

Since the electric stimulation of biological tissues requires the use of electrodes, any practical study should include consideration of electrodes and electrode-tissue interaction. The mechanical properties of electrodes are important particularly with respect to implants whose lifetime is measured in years. Since the flow of electricity from the electrode (where electrons carry the charges) into the tissue (where ions carry the charges) may involve an electrochemical reaction, this area must be carefully studied

as well. Consequently, several sections of this chapter are devoted to these electrode characteristics.

21.2 SIMULATION OF EXCITATION OF A MYELINATED FIBER

In this and the following section, we consider the behavior of several models of nerve stimulation based on principles of electrophysiology. As the reader will see, these models are fairly simple; this is both an asset (in the mathematical analysis) and a limitation (since we are actually interested in more complex structures). The results are nevertheless important as they provide a starting point toward the elucidation of more realistic models, and as some of the insights gained have wider applicability.

In the simplest example of nerve stimulation, a point current source of strength I_a is placed near a uniform myelinated fiber, and both source and nerve are considered to lie in a uniform conducting medium of unlimited extent. In this configuration (as described in Fig. 21.1), the source-fiber distance is shown as h, the fiber diameter (i.e., external myelin diameter) d_o, and axon diameter (internal myelin diameter) d_i. The internodal length is designated as l, and

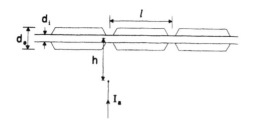

Fig. 21.1 A point current stimulus, I_a, lies at a distance h from a single myelinated nerve fiber. A node of Ranvier is assumed to be aligned with the stimulating monopole. The internodal distance l is related to the outer diameter of the myelin, d_o (i.e., the fiber diameter, as shown) where $l = 100 \cdot d_o$.

the ratio of internodal length to fiber diameter is assumed to be a constant (100). This model has been investigated by McNeal (1976), whose paper is closely followed in this presentation.

The electric model corresponding to Figure 21.1 is described in Figure 21.2. In Figure 21.2 it is assumed that transmembrane current is confined solely to the nodal region. More recent experimental work, summarized by Chu and Ritchie (1984), has shown that in the mammalian nerve fiber the potassium channels are found in the internodal axolemma. This appears to introduce quantitative but not qualitative differences in the simpler amphibian (frog) nerve model of Frankenhauser and Huxley (1964), described by Figure 21.2. We shall continue to utilize the latter for its simplicity and qualitatively adequate character.

Since the node is relatively narrow, the network representing the membrane is essentially described by lumped-parameter elements. These are shown as a parallel RC-structure at all but the central node (node 0). McNeal reasoned that for stimuli up to and including threshold, all nodes (except the central node) respond in a sufficiently linear fashion to require only a passive network representation. Only the central node is described by the Frankenhauser and Huxley (1964) expressions.

The axial intracellular current path introduces the internodal resistance r_i, where

$$r_i = \frac{4\rho_i l}{\pi d_i^2} \qquad (21.1)$$

where

r_i = axial intracellular resistance per internodal length [$k\Omega/l$]

ρ_i = intracellular resistivity [$k\Omega \cdot cm$] (chosen as 0.1 $k\Omega \cdot cm$)

l = internodal length [cm]

d_i = axon diameter (internal myelin diameter) [cm]

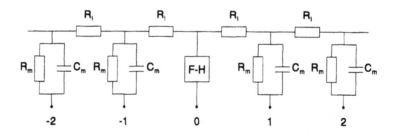

Fig. 21.2 Electric model of a myelinated fiber stimulated by a point current source of strength I_a. The node directly beneath the source is labeled 0 and its membrane is modeled by Frankenhauser-Huxley (F-H) equations. Lateral nodes are assumed to be subthreshold and represented by parallel resistance and capacitance (where R_m, C_m are the total nodal lumped resistance and capacitance per nodal area). The total intracellular internodal resistance is r_i.

McNeal assumed that the potential on the extracellular side of the nodal membrane was fixed by the stimulating field. Since the latter is a point source (i.e., a monopole), the stimulating (applied) potential field Φ_o (see Equation 8.7) is

$$\Phi_o = \frac{I_a}{4\pi\sigma_o r} \tag{21.2}$$

where

Φ_o = stimulating (applied, extracellular) potential field [mV]

I_a = applied current [μA]

σ_o = extracellular conductivity of the medium [kΩ·cm]

r = distance from any node to the point source [cm]

This formulation, in effect, considers the fiber itself to have little influence on the applied field (i.e., the secondary sources at the fiber surface set up a very weak field compared to Φ_o. arising from I_a and described by Equation 21.2). If one notes the very small extracellular fields generated by nerve impulses propagating on isolated fibers (Plonsey, 1974), then the extracellular potentials from the secondary sources (which are smaller than action potential sources) should certainly be negligible.

On the basis of the network described in Figure 21.2 and the applied field of Equation 21.2 one can determine the response to step currents of varying strengths (up to that required for excitation at node 0). The equations that must be solved are based on Kirchhoff's laws. Letting subscript i denote intracellular, o extracellular, and n the index denoting a specific node (where the central node is designated 0), we have for the transmembrane current I_m per nodal area at the nth node

$$I_{m,n} = \frac{1}{r_i}(V_{i,n-1} - 2V_{i,n} + V_{i,n+1})$$
$$= C_m \frac{dV_{m,n}}{dt} + I_{i,n} \tag{21.3}$$

where

$I_{m,n}$ = transmembrane current per nodal area at the nth node

$I_{i,n}$ = transmembrane ionic current per nodal area at the nth node

$V_{m,n}$ = transmembrane voltage at the nth node

C_m = membrane capacitance per nodal area at the nth node

r_i = axial intracellular resistance per internodal length

The second term of Equation 21.3 expresses the difference of the intracellular axial current entering the nth node (i.e., $(V_{i,n-1} - V_{i,n})/r_i$) minus that leaving this node (i.e., $(V_{i,n} - V_{i,n+1})/r_i$); this difference has been set equal to the (outward) transmembrane current of the nth node (right-hand side of Equation 21.3), which correctly satisfies the conservation of current. Except at $n = 0$ (the central node governed by the Frankenhauser-Huxley equations) we assume that subthreshold conditions are elsewhere in effect and the ionic current is given by

$$I_{i,n} = \frac{V_n}{R_m} \tag{21.4}$$

where

R_m = transmembrane resistance per nodal area (constant)

Using the definition of transmembrane voltage $V_n = V_{i,n} - V_{o,n}$ in Equation 21.3 gives

$$\frac{dV_{m,n}}{dt} = \frac{1}{C_m}\left[\frac{1}{r_i}(V_{m,n-1} - 2V_{m,n} + V_{m,n+1}\right.$$
$$\left. + V_{o,n-1} - 2V_{o,n} + V_{o,n+1}) - \frac{V_{m,n}}{R_m}\right] n \neq 0 \tag{2.15}$$

where Equation 21.4 has been substituted for $I_{i,n}$. When $n = 0$, however, one gets

$$\frac{dV_{m,0}}{dt} = \frac{1}{C_m}\left[\frac{1}{r_i}(V_{m,-1} - 2V_{m,0} + V_{m,1} + V_{o,-1}\right.$$
$$\left. - 2V_{o,0} + V_{o,1}) - \pi d_i \nu(i_{Na} + i_K + i_l + i_p)\right] \tag{21.6}$$

where ν is the nodal width, and the ionic currents are found from the Frankenhauser-Huxley equations. The extracellular nodal potentials in Equations 21.5 and 21.6 are found from Equation 21.2, and constitute the forcing function. We assume that the stimulating current is switched on at $t = 0$ so that $V_{m,n} = 0$ for all n at $t = 0$; the stimulating current is assumed to remain on for a specified time interval. For stimuli that are subthreshold at all nodes (including the central node), Equation 21.5 alone

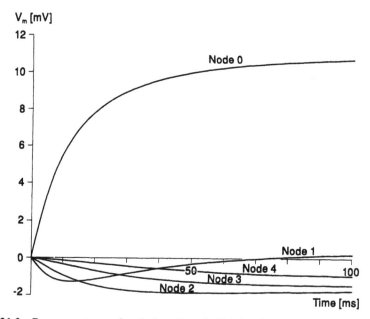

Fig. 21.3 Response at central node ($n = 0$) and adjoining four nodes to a point current source located 1 mm from the fiber and excited with a current step of 0.1 mA. The geometry is describe–d in Figure 21.1. The fiber diameter is 20 μm, and the internodal spacing is 2 mm. Other parameters are given in Table 21.1.

is sufficient to describe the response and may be applied also at $n = 0$.

The solution of Equation 21.5 (for sub-threshold conditions) or Equation 21.5 and 21.6 (for near-threshold conditions) at $n = 0$ requires temporal discretization and the solution of the resulting system of equations by iteration or by matrix techniques. The steady-state response to the stimulus diminishes rapidly with increasing values of n so that only a finite number of nodes (i.e., equations) need to be considered. One wishes to use the smallest number; McNeal (1976) explored the use of a total of 11, 21,

and 31 nodes and found that the response to a 1ms pulse was within 0.2 % accuracy with only 11 nodes.

The response to a subthreshold (at all nodes) current step evaluated at the central node and its four neighbors is described in Figure 21.3. These were calculated from a total of 31 nodes using the same parameters as were chosen by McNeal (see Table 21.1); the results appear to be identical to those obtained by McNeal with 11 nodes. Since the stimulus monopole was assumed to be cathodal, current must leave from the closest node(s) while, to conserve current,

Table 21.1 Electric properties of myelinated nerve fibers

Symbol	Parameter	Value
ρ_i	axoplasm resistivity	0.11 kΩ·cm
ρ_o	extracellular resistivity	0.3 kΩ·cm
C_m	nodal membrane capacitance/unit area	2.0 μF/cm^2
G_m	nodal membrane conductance/unit area	0.4 mS/cm^2
ν	nodal gap width	0.5 μm
l/d_o	ratio of internode spacing to fiber diameter	100
d_i/d_o	ratio of axon diameter (internal myelin) to fiber diameter	0.7
R_{mn}	nodal membrane resistance $= 1/(G_m \pi d_i \nu)$	29.9 MΩ
C_{mn}	nodal membrane capacitance $= C_m \pi d_i \nu$	2.2 pF
r_{il}	internodal resistance $= 4\rho_i l/(\pi d_i^2)$	14.3 MΩ

current must enter lateral nodes. This accounts for hyperpolarization of nodes $\pm 2, \pm 3, \pm 4 \ldots$ and depolarization of the central node. The behavior of node ± 1 changes as the membrane capacitances charge up. Initially it is hyperpolarized, but its steady-state potential (response to a pulse of very long duration) is a depolarization. If the stimulus were anodal, then the signs of all responses in Figure 21.3 would be reversed; the initial largest depolarization occurs at node ± 1, but after around 15 ms the largest depolarization is at ± 2. Thus excitation resulting from a stimulus duration of $t \leq 15$ ms and that for $t > 15$ ms occur at different nodes!

Returning to the case of cathodal stimulation, it is clear that for a transthreshold stimulus, activation occurs at node 0. A determination of the quantitative values of current strength and duration to achieve activation requires (at least) the use of Equation 21.6 to describe the central node. McNeal was able to calculate that for a 100 ms pulse the threshold current is 0.23 mA. By determinination of the corresponding threshold current for a series of different pulse durations, an experimental *strength-duration* curve (reproduced in Fig. 21.4) was constructed. This curve describes conditions under which excitation is just achieved for the specific case of a 20 μm fiber with a point source at a distance of 1 mm. Under the idealized con-

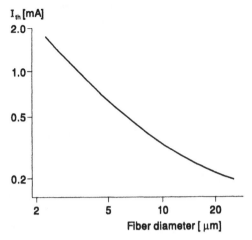

Fig. 21.5 Log-log plot of the relationship between threshold current and myelinated fiber diameter for a point current source 1 mm from the fiber. The geometry is described in Figure 21.1, and the fiber electrical properties are given in Table 21.1. (From McNeal, 1976.)

ditions described in Chapter 3, we expect this curve to have a slope of -1 for small pulse duration, but this is not the case in an experimental curve. The reason for this discrepancy is that the experiment is affected by accommodation, distributed fiber structure, and source geometry.

The dependence of excitability on the fiber diameter of a nerve is important since it describes how a nerve bundle (consisting of fibers of different diameter) will respond to a stimulus (monopole in this case). An examination of Equations 21.5 and 21.6 shows that changes in fiber diameter d_o affect the solution only through its link with the internodal spacing, l. Figure 21.5 gives the threshold current for a monopole at a distance of 1 mm from a fiber whose diameter d_o satisfies (2 μm $\leq d_o \leq$ 25 μm) where the pulse duration is 100 μs. A 10-fold decrease in diameter (from 20 to 2 μm) affects r_i and R_m proportionately (each increases by 10). As a rough approximation the induced transmembrane voltage at node 0 is the same fraction of the applied potential difference between nodes zero and 1. This potential decreases quite considerably for the 2 μm diameter nerve versus the 20 μm diameter one since l is 10 times greater in the latter case. Accordingly the excitability is expected to decrease for the nerve of lower diameter. Figure 21.5

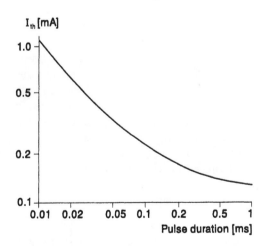

Fig. 21.4 Log-log plot of a strength duration that just produces activation of 20 μm diameter myelinated fiber from a point source of current 1 mm distant. The geometry is described in Figure 21.1, and the fiber electrical properties are tabulated in Table 21.1. (From McNeal, 1976.)

confirms this effect through the simulation. Note that at the larger diameters the slope is around $-\frac{1}{2}$, meaning that the threshold is approximately inversely proportional to the square root of the fiber diameter.

21.3 STIMULATION OF AN UNMYELINATED AXON

The response of a single unmyelinated fiber to a stimulating field can be found through the same type of simulation described for the myelinated fiber. In fact, to obtain numerical solutions it is necessary to discretize the axial coordinate (x) into elements Δx and a network somewhat similar to that considered in Figure 21.2 results. One obtains an expression for the transmembrane current at the nth element, from the cable equations, as

$$i_m \Delta x = \frac{1}{r_i} \frac{\partial^2 V_i}{\partial x^2} \Delta x \qquad (21.7)$$

where

r_i = the intracellular axial resistance per unit length.

Approximating the second derivative in Equation 21.7 by second differences gives us

$$(i_m \Delta x)_n = \frac{1}{r_i \Delta x} (V_{i,n-1} - 2V_{i,n} + V_{i,n+1}) \qquad (21.8)$$

where

$V_{i,n}$ = intracellular potential at the nth element, etc.

The desired equation is found by equating the transmembrane current evaluated from Equation 21.8 (which is determined by the fiber *structure*) with that demanded by the intrinsic nonlinear membrane properties:

$$\frac{1}{r_i \Delta x} (V_{i,n-1} - 2V_{i,n} + V_{i,n+1})$$
$$= \left[c_m \frac{\partial V_{m,n}}{\partial t} + i_{mI} \right] \Delta x \qquad (21.9)$$

where

c_m = membrane capacitance per unit length
i_{mI} = ionic component of the membrane current per unit length

The ionic currents are those of sodium, potassium, and chloride ions, as found from Hodgkin and Huxley (1952) and so on.

(Note that had we assumed steady-state conditions, the capacitive term could be set equal to zero, whereas if linear conditions could be assumed, then $i_{mI} = V_{m,n}/R_m$.) If, now, we replace $V_{i,n}$ by $V_{m,n} + V_{o,n}$ and reorganize, we have

$$\frac{dV_{m,n}}{dt} = \frac{1}{c_m} \left[\frac{1}{r_i (\Delta x)^2} (V_{m,n-1} - 2V_{m,n} + V_{m,n+1} \right.$$
$$\left. + V_{o,n-1} - 2V_{o,n} + V_{o,n+1}) - i_{mI} \right] \qquad (21.10)$$

which is essentially the same as Equation 21.6 except that the spacing between elements in Equation 21.10, namely Δx, may be much smaller than the spacing in Equation 21.6, namely l. Of course, the internodal spacing is set by the myelinated histology while Δx is at our disposal.

The forcing function in Equation 21.10 is essentially $\partial^2 V_o/\partial x^2$. Depending on the spatial behavior of V_o and the length l, the forcing function in Equation 21.6 is also given approximately by $\partial^2 V_o/\partial x^2$. We have noted that V_o is normally the field of the stimulating electrodes in the absence of the stimulated fiber. That is, for a single isolated fiber its (secondary) effect on the axial field in which it is placed is, ordinarily, negligible, as discussed earlier. So $\partial^2 V_o/\partial x^2$ can be evaluated from the field of the stimulating electrodes alone. Clearly, the response to a stimulating field is contained in this second-derivative behavior, designated the "activating function" by Rattay (1986). In fact, for the linear behavior that necessarily precedes excitation, Equation 21.10 may be replaced by the following equation (an approximation that improves as $\Delta x \rightarrow 0$, hence less satisfactory for myelinated fibers where $\Delta x = l$)

$$\frac{dV_{m,n}}{dt} \approx \frac{1}{c_m} \left[\frac{1}{r_i} \frac{\partial^2 V_{m,n}}{\partial x^2} \right.$$
$$\left. + \frac{1}{r_i} \frac{\partial^2 V_o}{\partial x^2} - \frac{V_{m,n}}{r_m} \right] \qquad (21.11)$$

where

r_m = membrane resistance per unit length (resistance times length)
r_i = intracellular axial resistance per unit length

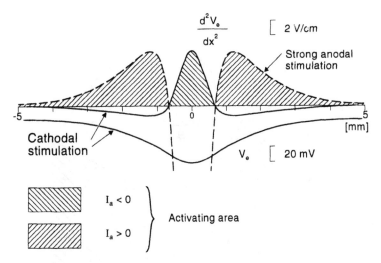

Fig. 21.6 The cathodal applied field $V_o(x)$ along a fiber oriented along x due to a point source, and $\partial^2 V_o(x)/\partial x^2$ for both cathodal and anodal stimuli. The cathodal threshold current of -290 μA initiates activation at $x = 0$ which corresponds to the peak of the "activating function" $\partial^2 V_o(x)/\partial x^2$. For anodal conditions the stimulus for threshold activation is 1450 μA and the corresponding activating function is shown. The fivefold increase in current is required to bring the corresponding (anodal) positive peak of $\partial^2 V_o/\partial x^2$ to the same level it has under threshold cathodal conditions. Note that excitation takes place at x lateral to the point 0. (From Rattay, 1986.)

We consider the response, $V_{m,n}$, to a stimulating field, V_o, which is turned on at $t = 0$ (i.e., a step function). Activation is possible if $\partial V_{m,n}/\partial t > 0$, and this condition in turn seems to depend on $\partial^2 V_o/\partial x^2 > 0$. Rattay assumed this relationship to be valid and designated $\partial^2 V_o/\partial x^2$ as an "activating function." An application, given by Rattay, is described below. However, the reader should note that $V_{m,n}$ is not directly dependent on $\partial^2 V_o/\partial x^2$ but, rather, arises from it only through the solution of Equation 21.11. But this solution also depends on the homogeneous solution plus the boundary conditions. That the outcome of the same forcing function can vary in this way suggests that the interpretation of $\partial^2 V_o/\partial x^2$ as an activating function is not assured.

Figure 21.6 shows the applied field $V_o(x)$ along an unmyelinated fiber for a point source that is 1 mm distant, and the corresponding activating function for both an anodal and a cathodal condition. For a negative (cathodal) current of -290 μA, threshold conditions are just reached at the fiber element lying at the foot of the perpendicular from the monopole (which is at the location of the positive peak of the plotted d^2V_o/dx^2 curve). For a positive (anodal) current source, 1450 μA is required just to reach excitation; this is seen in the curve of the corresponding activating function (d^2V_o/dx^2) that results. The fivefold increase in current compensates for the lateral peaks in the activating function, being only one-fifth of the central peak. The location of the excitation region can be found from Equation 21.2 written as

$$V_o = \frac{I_a}{4\pi\sigma_o \sqrt{h^2 + x^{2pmu3}}} \qquad (21.12)$$

where

$h =$ distance from the point source to the fiber
$x =$ axial distance along fiber
$\sigma_o =$ conductance of the extracellular medium

We examine the lateral behavior of

$$\frac{\partial^2 V_o}{\partial x^2} = \frac{I_a}{4\pi\sigma_o}\left[\frac{2x^2 - h^2}{(h^2 + x^2)^{5/2}}\right] \qquad (21.13)$$

and note that for anodal excitation, depolarization results only for $|x| \geq h/\sqrt{2}$ (hyperpolarization is produced for $|x| \leq h/\sqrt{2}$). Conversely, activation from cathodal stimulation is confined to the region $|x| \leq h/\sqrt{2}$, while hyperpolarization is produced laterally.

For cathodal stimulation and for increasing stimulus intensity, a threshold level is reached that results in activation. A continued increase in stimulus intensity is followed by little change

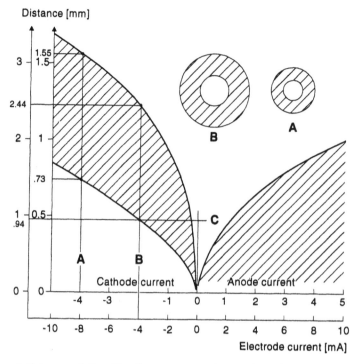

Fig. 21.7 Current-distance relationship for unmyelinated fibers. Excitation occurs for points lying in the shaded region. For cathodal stimulation, a minimum distance arises at the point where anodal block prevents the escape of the action impulse. For anodal stimulation, block does not occur; thus there is no lower limit on the source-fiber distance. The inner scales are for a fiber diameter of 9.6 μm, and the outer for a diameter of 38.4 μm. (An examination of Equations 21.10 and 21.13 shows that scaling the excitation with respect to both current strength, source-fiber distance, and fiber diameter leaves the solution unchanged.) (From Rattay, 1987.)

in behavior until a level some eight times threshold is reached. At this point the hyperpolarization lateral to the active region can block the emerging propagating impulse. Rattay (1987) investigated this behavior quantitatively by solving Equation 21.10 with the ionic currents evaluated from the Hodgkin-Huxley equations and with the point source field of Equation 21.12. The results are plotted in Figure 21.7 for an unmyelinated fiber of 9.6 μm diameter (inner scales) and 38.4 μm diameter (outer scales).

Figure 21.7 may be explained as follows. For a cathodal stimulus of −4 mA and the smaller-diameter fiber (use inner coordinate scale), excitation occurs (cross-hatched region) if the source-field distance rages from 0.73 to 1.55 mm (following line (A)) whereas for the larger fiber, excitation requires the source-field distance to lie between 0.94 and 2.44 mm (follow-

ing line (B)). The spherical insets describe the relative minimum and maximum radii for excitation of the smaller fiber (A) and larger fiber (B). Consistent with the results obtained with myelinated fibers, we note the greater excitability of the larger fiber, where excitation can be initiated at a maximum distance of 2.44 mm compared with 1.55 mm for a fiber with one-fourth the diameter. For a bundle of fibers of different diameters and radial position, with no fiber interaction (i.e., each fiber behaves as if isolated), Figure 21.7 could describe the selective effect of any given level of stimulation of a fiber at a specified position.

21.4 MUSCLE RECRUITMENT

If a muscle fiber is electrically stimulated, it responds with a twitch, as shown in Figure 21.8.

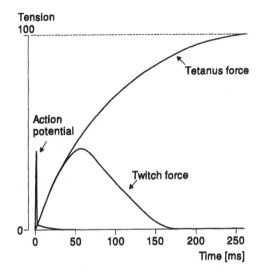

Fig. 21.8 The twitch response (tension vs. time) for a single muscle fiber. The stimulus is described by the initial impulse.

If a train of stimuli is applied whose time interval is shorter than the twitch duration, then temporal summation will occur and a larger tensile force will be developed. For a high enough frequency a smooth (rather than bumpy) tension response is observed (this is the fusion frequency), leading to a maximum (tetanus) contraction.

The magnitude and duration of the twitch response differ depending on the muscle fiber type. One can separate skeletal muscle into three general groups according to their physiological and metabolic properties (Mortimer, 1981):

1. *Fast twitch, glycolytic* (FG): These fibers depend mainly on glycolytic metabolism with little oxidative. When stimulated, the twitch contraction is of short duration and the response to repeated stimulation shows a rapid fatigue and slow recovery. In a mixed muscle this fiber tends to be found near the periphery. The fiber diameter is relatively large, as is the relative strength of its peak force (for cat gastrocnemius a peak force of 1.5–2.0 kg/cm^2 of muscle cross-sectional area is reached).
2. *Fast twitch, oxidative* (FO): Distinct from the FG group are the fast twitch oxidative,

which utilize both oxidative as well as glycolytic metabolism. The response to repeated stimulation is slower to fatigue and quicker to recover than for the FG fiber type. The diameter of the FO fiber is smaller than the FG while its peak force is on the order of 2.6–2.9 kg/cm^2 of muscle cross-sectional area for cat gastrocnemius.

3. *Slow twitch, oxidative* (SO): These fibers have the smallest cross-sectional area of the three groups. They have a low capacity for glycolytic metabolism. Their twitch response is longest in duration and lowest in magnitude (the fusion frequency is the lowest) of the three groups. Repeated stimulation causes less fatigue, and recovery is rapid. These fiber tend to lie in the central region of a muscle bundle. In the cat gastrocnemius, they generate a peak force of around 0.6 kg/cm^2.

Each fiber in a bundle is innervated by a single motor neuron, but each motor neuron activates several fibers. The group of fibers activated by a single motor neuron is called a motor unit. All fibers in a motor unit are of a similar type. Not surprisingly large-diameter muscle fibers are innervated by large-diameter neurons. Consequently, motor units producing the largest forces are those innervated by axons of large diameter; conversely, small forces are produced by small-diameter axons. The natural order of recruitment is the development of small forces from SO fibers followed, ultimately, by the largest forces due to recruitment of the FG motor units. The FO fibers contribute in the midrange. Thus the modest forces needed to maintain posture for a long period are derived from the SO type fiber, whereas the baseball batter's swing describes the momentary recruitment of FG fibers (for a large force of short duration whose fatigue and slow recovery is of less consequence). Other more conventional physiological tasks have this same character, as seen in baseball.

The strength-duration curves for the stimulation of a motor nerve and the direct stimulation of muscle are shown in Figure 21.9. We note the very great difference in excitability so that, for the most part, all functional electric stimulation (FES) systems concentrate on the

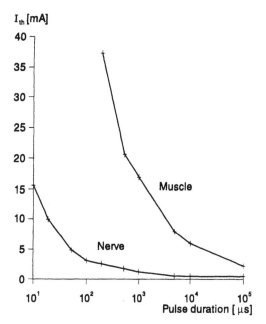

Fig. 21.9 Experimentally determined strength-duration relationship for motor nerve stimulation and for direct stimulation of the muscle. In each case the muscle response was held at the same constant value (a relatively low level of force). (From Mortimer, 1981.)

stimulation of the motor neuron which, in turn, activates the associated muscle. One may stimulate the nerve centrally or peripherally (in the vicinity of the neuromuscular junction). The latter has the advantage, usually, of greater selectivity.

Figures 21.5 and 21.7 show that with point-source stimulation the excitability increases with increasing fiber diameter. This relationship is true in general regardless of the type of electrode system or placement relative to the target nerve. But this means that the large-diameter neurons,—hence large-diameter muscle fibers (i.e., FG)—are recruited first. This is inverse to the natural order and results in the excitation of a fiber type with rapid fatigue for ordinary tasks. This result is a serious limitation to the applicability of FES.

Several approaches have been taken to deal with the problem noted above. The first is to devise a technique that will result in the electric stimulation of the smaller-diameter nerve fiber before the larger-diameter one. For example, one can first stimulate all fibers with a supramaximal pulse and then at a point closer to the muscle place a hyperpolarizing block. One adjusts the strength of the block to be inversely proportional to the desired control signal. Since larger-diameter fibers are most easily blocked, a low control signal—hence a large block—will block all but the smallest fibers, whereas increasing force requirements will result in reduced block (permitting the FO and finally the FG to escape block). Consequently, the behavior follows more closely the natural recruitment order (Zhou, Baratta, and Solomonow, 1987), though there are still a number of practical difficulties with the application of this method. An alternate application of the technique, which depends on the use of a quasi-trapezoidal stimulus current, appears to achieve a natural order of recruitment (Fang and Mortimer, 1987).

A second approach is to implant several electrodes each in a different part of the muscle and to excite them sequentially. In this way, the actual stimulus frequency of each subunit is reduced by a factor equal to the number of electrodes. Since spatial summation results, the behavior of the whole muscle is characterized by the higher frequency which is chosen to exceed the fusion frequency. The lower actual frequency results in reduced fatigue of the muscle. The method is referred to as "roundabout stimulation" (Holle et al., 1984).

A third approach has been to convert FG muscle into SO muscle by a period of electrical stimulation. The results of a daily regimen of "exercise" over a 4-week period include a decrease in fusion frequency from 40 to 10 Hz and an improved ability to maintain force. In fact, analysis of such stimulated muscle shows histochemical changes consistent with a transition from fast twitch to slow twitch. In addition, one also sees a marked increase in the number of capillaries per fiber consistent with an increased capacity for oxidative metabolism (Mortimer, 1981).

21.5 ELECTRODE-TISSUE INTERFACE

A discussion of electric stimulation of tissue would be clearly incomplete without a consideration of electrodes and their behavior. In this context since a replacement of the charge carrier from conduction electron in the metal electrode to ion in the tissue must occur at the electrode-

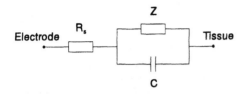

Fig. 21.10 The electrode-tissue interface includes a series ohmic resistance R_s, a series capacitance C_s, and a faradaic impedance Z. The capacitance represents a double layer that arises at the metal-electrolyte interface, whereas the faradaic impedance includes several physical and chemical processes that may occur.

tissue interface, a consideration of the electrochemistry and its relationship to electrode material and shape is important. In addition, we need to touch upon the mechanical properties of electrodes, as they too are influenced by material and shape.

There is extensive literature on the electrochemistry at the metal-electrolyte interface (Conway, 1965). For our purposes, here, we call attention to the equivalent electric circuit depicted in Figure 21.10 which summarizes the electrode tissue behavior (Dymond, 1976). The capacitance reflects the double layer of charge that arises at the metal-electrolyte interface; the single layer in the metal arises because of its connection to the battery, whereas that in the electrolyte is due to the attraction of ions in the electric field. These layers are separated by the molecular dimensions of the water molecule so the effective capacitance (being inversely proportional to charge separation) is quite high.

At sufficiently low levels the current will be primarily capacitive with little or no flow through the pathway represented by the faradic impedance Z in Figure 21.10. But for high currents that exceed the capabilities of the capacitance channel, irreversible chemical reactions will take place, and these are reflected in Figure 21.10 by a much reduced impedance Z. The consequences of these chemical reactions are undesirable since they are detrimental to the tissue or electrode or both.

In general, the goal is to operate stimulating electrodes to utilize exclusively their capacitance and thereby to keep within their operating (linear) range. Under these conditions the electrode current is, essentially capacitive and reversible; in this way one can avoid detrimental

chemical reactions. For example, if a stainless steel electrode is excessively anodic one gets

$$Fe \rightarrow Fe^{2+} + 2e^- \qquad (21.14)$$

and the dissolution of the electrode results. For an excessively cathodic condition the result is

$$2H_2O + 2e^- \rightarrow H_2 + 2OH^- \qquad (21.15)$$

An increasingly negative electrode may result in

$$O_2 + H_2O + 2e^- \rightarrow OH^- + O_2H^- \qquad (21.16)$$

In either case a consequent rise in pH results which can produce tissue damage.

Operating an electrode in its linear (capacitive) range is desirable since it is entirely reversible and results in neither tissue damage or electrode dissolution. To do so requires that the electrode be positioned as close as possible to the target nerve (so that the maximum required current will be minimal) and, if possible, to have a large area for a low current density. Finally the electrode material should be chosen to have maximum capacitance (other things being the same). A roughened surface appears to result in a decrease in microscopic current density without affecting the overall size of the electrode. The values of charge storage appears to increase from 0.5 to 2.0 $\mu C/mm^2$, yet remain in the reversible region for platinum and stainless steel materials.

If the stimulating current is unipolar, then even though one pulse causes the storage of charge within the reversible range, subsequent pulses will eventually cause the operating point to move out of the reversible region. The reasons are that under the usual operating conditions accumulation of charge takes place but there is inadequate time for the charge to leak away. Thus practical stimulation conditions require the use of biphasic pulses. In fact, these must be carefully balanced to avoid an otherwise slow buildup of charge. A series capacitance will ensure the absence of DC components (Talonen et al., 1983).

21.6 ELECTRODE MATERIALS AND SHAPES

For the most part FES utilizes electrodes that are implanted into the body since transcutaneous stimulation requires high current levels and may result in local tissue damage and unwanted nerve excitation. The electrode materials are therefore confined to those that are essentially inert such as platinum, platinum-iridium, and 316 stainless steel.

Less trauma results from electrodes that are flexible; consequently, small-diameter wires are preferred. Rather than transverse bending of a straight wire, these may often be coiled into a helix since bending is converted into torsional rotation, hence reducing stress. In fact, the use of stranded wires represents a further useful step to reduce breakage (or to afford some redundancy if some wires should fail).

In the stimulation of the brain, of particular concern is preventing breakdown of the blood-brain barrier. Low values of charge density storage ($<0.3 \ \mu C/mm^2$) are suggested; that is, electrodes are generally surface electrodes. For nerve stimulation circular (ring) electrodes are placed within an insulating cuff; consequently, smaller amounts of current are required because the field is greatly confined. Also lower current tends to minimize unwanted excitation of surrounding tissue. Finally, intramuscular electrodes, because of the flexing that must be withstood, are usually of the coiled-wire variety discussed above.

REFERENCES

Chu SY, Ritchie JM (1984): On the physiological role of internodal potassium channels and the security of conduction in myelinated nerve fibers. *Proc. R. Soc. (Lond.)* B220: 415–22.

Conway BE (1965): *Theory and Principles of Electrode Processes*, 303 pp. Ronald, New York.

Dymond AM (1976): Characteristics of the metal-tissue interface of stimulation electrodes. *IEEE Trans. Biomed. Eng.* BME-23:(4) 274–80.

Fang ZB, Mortimer JT (1987): A method for attaining natural recruitment order in artificially activated muscles. In *Proc. Ninth Annual Conf. IEEE Eng. In Med. And Biol. Society*, Vol. 2, pp. 657–8, IEEE Press, New York.

Frankenhauser B, Huxley AF (1964): The action potential in the myelinated nerve fibre of Xenopus Laevis as computed on the basis of voltage clamp data. *J. Physiol. (Lond.)* 171: 302–15.

Hodgkin AL, Huxley AF (1952): A quantitative description of membrane current and its application to conduction and excitation in nerve. *J. Physiol. (Lond.)* 117: 500–44.

Holle J, Frey M, Gruber H, Kern H, Stöhr H, Thoma H (1984): Functional electrostimulation of paraplegics. *Orthop.* 7: 1145–55.

McNeal DR (1976): Analysis of a model for excitation of myelinated nerve. *IEEE Trans. Biomed. Eng.* BME-23:(4) 329–37.

Mortimer JT (1981): Motor prostheses. In *Handbook of Physiology, Section 1: The Nervous System. Motor Control Part I*, Vol. II, ., pp. 155–87, American Physiological Society, Bethesda, Md.

Plonsey R (1974): The active fiber in a volume conductor. *IEEE Trans. Biomed. Eng.* BME-21:(5) 371–81.

Rattay F (1986): Analysis of models for external stimulation of axons. *IEEE Trans. Biomed. Eng.* BME-33:(10) 974–7.

Rattay F (1987): Ways to approximate current-distance relations for electrically stimulated fibers. *J. Theor. Biol.* 125: 339–49.

Seligman LJ (1982): Physiological stimulators: From electric fish to programmable implants. *IEEE Trans. Biomed. Eng.* BME-29:(4) 270–84.

Talonen P, Malmivuo JA, Baer G, Markkula H, Häkkinen V (1983): Transcutaneous, dual channel phrenic nerve stimulator for diaphragm pacing. *Med. & Biol. Eng. & Comput.* 21:(1) 21–30.

Zhou B-H, Baratta R, Solomonow M (1987): Manipulation of muscle force with various firing rate and recruitment control strategies. *IEEE Trans. Biomed. Eng.* BME-34:(2) 128–39.

REFERENCES, BOOKS

Eccles JC, Dimitrijevic MR (eds.) (1985): *Upper Motor Neuron Functions and Dysfunctions*, 345 pp. S. Karger, Basel.

Hambrecht FT, Reswick JB (eds.) (1977): *Functional Electrical Stimulation. Application in Neural Prosthesis*, Vol. 3, 543 pp. Marcel Dekker, N.Y.

Lazorthes Y, Upton ARM (eds.) (1985): *Neurostimulation: An Overview*, 320 pp. Futura, Mount Kisco, N.Y.

Mannheimer JS, Lampe GN (1987): *Clinical Transcutaneous Electrical Nerve Stimulation*, 636 pp. F.A. Davis, Philadelphia.

Myklebust JB, Cusick JF, Sances AJ, Larson SJ (eds.) (1985): *Neural Stimulation*, Vol. I and II, 158+160 pp. CRC Press, Boca Raton, Fla.

Reilly JP (1992): *Electrical Stimulation & Electropathology*, 504 pp. Cambridge University Press, Cambridge.

Wolf SL (ed.) (1981): *Electrotherapy*, 204 pp. Churchill Livingstone, New York.

22

Magnetic Stimulation of Neural Tissue

22.1 INTRODUCTION

In Chapter 12 it was pointed out that the origin of the biomagnetic field is the electric activity of biological tissue. This bioelectric activity produces an electric current in the volume conductor which induces the biomagnetic field. This correlation between the bioelectric and biomagnetic phenomena is, of course, not limited to the generation of the bioelectric and biomagnetic fields by the same bioelectric sources. This correlation also arises in the stimulation of biological tissue.

Magnetic stimulation is a method for stimulating excitable tissue with an electric current induced by an external time-varying magnetic field. It is important to note here that, as in the electric and magnetic detection of the bioelectric activity of excitable tissues, both the electric and the magnetic stimulation methods excite the membrane with *electric current*. The former does that directly, but the latter does it with the electric current which is induced within the volume conductor by the time-varying applied magnetic field.

The reason for using a time-varying magnetic field to induce the stimulating current is, on the one hand, the different distribution of stimulating current and, on the other hand, the fact that the magnetic field penetrates unattenuated through such regions as the electrically insulating skull. This makes it possible to avoid a high density of stimulating current at the scalp in stimulating the central nervous system and thus avoid pain sensation. Also, no physical contact of the stimulating coil and the target tissue is required, unlike with electric stimulation.

The first documents on magnetic stimulation described the stimulation of the retina by Jacques d'Arsonval (1896) and Silvanus P. Thompson (1910). The retina is known to be very sensitive to stimulation by induced currents, and field strengths as low as 10 mT rms at 20 Hz will cause a stimulation (Lövsund, Öberg, and Nilsson, 1980).

From the pioneering works of d'Arsonval and Thompson it took some time before the magnetic method was applied to neuromuscular stimulation. Bickford and Fremming (1965) used a damped 500 Hz sinusoidal magnetic field and demonstrated muscular stimulation in animals and humans. Magnetic stimulation of nerve tissue was also demonstrated by Öberg (1973). The first successful magnetic stimulation of superficial nerves was reported by Polson et al. in 1982 (Polson, Barker, and Freeston, 1982).

Transcranial stimulation of the motor cortex is the most interesting application of magnetic stimulation because the magnetic field (unlike the electric current) penetrates through the skull without attenuation. The first transcranial stimulation of the central nervous system was achieved in 1985 (Barker and Freeston, 1985; Barker, Freeston, Jalinous, Merton, and Morton, 1985; Barker, Jalinous, and Freeston, 1985). A more complete history of magnetic stimulation may be found from a review article of Geddes (1991).

22.2 THE DESIGN OF STIMULATOR COILS

A magnetic stimulator includes a coil that is placed on the surface of the skin. To induce a current into the underlying tissue, a strong and rapidly changing magnetic field must be generated by the coil. In practice, this is generated by first charging a large capacitor to a high voltage and then discharging it with a thyristor switch through a coil. The principle of a magnetic stimulator is illustrated in Figure 22.1.

The Faraday-Henry law states that if an electric conductor, which forms a closed circuit, is linked by a time-varying magnetic flux F, a current is observed in the circuit. This current is due to the electromotive force (emf) induced by the time-varying flux. The magnitude of emf depends on the rate of change of the magnetic flux dF/dt. The direction of emf is such that

the time-varying magnetic field that results from it is always opposite to that of dF/dt; therefore,

$$\mathscr{E} = -\frac{dF}{dt} \qquad (22.1)$$

where

$\mathscr{E}$ = electromotive force (emf) [V]
F = magnetic flux [Wb = Vs]
t = time [s]

Corresponding to a magnetic field $\bar{B}$ the flux $\bar{F}$, linking the circuit is given by $\bar{F} = \int \bar{B} \cdot d\bar{S}$, where the integral is taken over any surface whose periphery is the circuit loop.

If the flux is due to a coil's own current I, the flux is defined as: $F = LI$, where L is the inductance of the coil and the emf can be written

$$\mathscr{E} = -\frac{dF}{dt} = -L\frac{dI}{dt} \qquad (22.2)$$

where

L = inductance of the coil [H = Wb/A = Vs/A]
I = current in the coil [A]

and other variables are as in Equation 22.1.

The magnitude of induced emf is proportional to the rate of change of current, dI/dt. The coefficient of proportionality is the inductance L. The term dI/dt depends on the speed with which the capacitors are discharged; the latter is increased by use of a fast solid-state

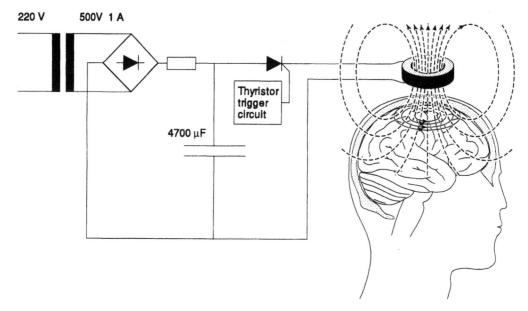

Fig. 22.1   The principle of the magnetic stimulator.

switch (i.e., fast thyristor) and minimal wiring length. Inductance L is determined by the geometry and constitutive property of the medium. The principal factors for the coil system are the shape of the coil, the number of turns on the coil, and the permeability of the core. For typical coils used in physiological magnetic stimulation, the inductance may be calculated from the following equations.

Multiple-Layer Cylinder Coil

The inductance of a multiple-layer cylinder coil (Fig. 22.2A) is:

$$L \approx \mu N^2 \left(\frac{\pi r^2}{l + 0.9r} - \frac{0.3rs}{l} \right) \qquad (22.3)$$

where

  L = inductance of the coil [H]
  μ = permeability of the coil core [Vs/Am]
  N = number of turns on the coil
  r = coil radius [m]
  l = coil length [m]
  s = coil width [m]

The following example is given of the electric parameters of a multiple-layer cylinder coil (Rossi et al., 1987): A coil having 19 turns of 2.5 mm² copper wound in three layers has physical dimensions of $r = 18$ mm, $l = 22$ mm, and $s = 6$ mm. The resistance and the inductance of the coil were measured to be 14 mΩ and 169 μH, respectively.

Flat Multiple-Layer Disk Coil

The inductance of a flat multiple-layer disk coil (Fig. 22.2B) is

$$L \approx \mu N^2 \frac{\pi r^2}{0.8r + 1.1s} \qquad (22.4)$$

where N, r, and s are the same as in the equation above.

A coil having 10 turns of 2.5 mm² copper wire in one layer has physical dimensions of $r = 14 \ldots 36$ mm. The resistance and the inductance of the coil had the measured values of 10 mΩ and 9.67 μH, respectively.

Long Single-Layer Cylinder Coil

The inductance of a long single-layer cylinder coil (Fig. 22.2C) is

$$L \approx \mu N^2 \frac{\pi r^2}{l} \qquad (22.5)$$

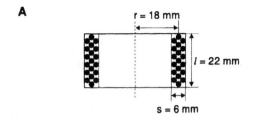

A

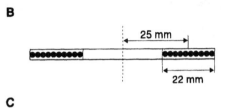

B

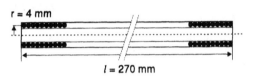

C

Fig. 22.2 Dimensions of coils of different configuration. (A) Multiple-layer cylinder coil. (B) Flat multiple-layer disk coil. (C) Long single-layer cylinder coil. Expressions for inductance of these coils are given in Equations 22.3–22.5.

where N, r, and l are again the same as in the equation above.

22.3 CURRENT DISTRIBUTION IN MAGNETIC STIMULATION

The magnetic permeability of biological tissue is approximately that of a vacuum. Therefore the tissue does not have any noticeable effect on the magnetic field itself. The rapidly changing field of the magnetic impulse induces electric current in the tissue, which produces the stimulation.

Owing to the *reciprocity theorem*, the current density distribution of a magnetic stimulator is the same as the sensitivity distribution of such a magnetic detector having a similar construction. (Similarly, this is, of course, true for electric stimulators and detectors as well (Malmivuo, 1992a,b).) Note that in the lead field theory, the reciprocal energization equals the application of stimulating energy. The distribution of the current density in magnetic stimulation may be calculated using the method introduced by Malmivuo (1976) and later applied for the MEG (Malmivuo, 1980). As mentioned in Section 14.3, there are also other methods for calculating the sensitivity distribution of MEG detectors. They give accurate results in situations having less symmetry and are therefore more complicated and, unfortunately, less illustrative (Durand, Ferguson, and Dalbasti, 1992; Eaton, 1992; Esselle and Stuchly, 1992).

Single Coil

The current distribution of a single coil, producing a dipolar field, was presented earlier in this book in Sections 12.11 and 14.2. The stimulation energy distribution can be readily seen in the form of vector fields from Figure 14.2 and is not repeated here. Figure 22.3 illustrates the isointensity lines and half-intensity volume

for a coil with a 50 mm radius. The concepts of isointensity line and half-intensity volume are reciprocal to the isosensitivity line and half-sensitivity volume, discussed in Section 11.6.1. As discussed in Section 12.3.3, because of cylindrical symmetry the isointensity lines coincide with the magnetic field lines. The reader may again compare the effect of the coil radius on the distribution of the stimulus current by comparing Figures 22.3 and 14.3.

Quadrupolar Coil Configuration

The coils can be equipped with cores of highly permeable material. One advantage of this arrangement is that the magnetic field that is produced is better focused in the desired location. Constructing the permeable core in the form of the letter U results in the establishment of a quadrupolar magnetic field source. With a

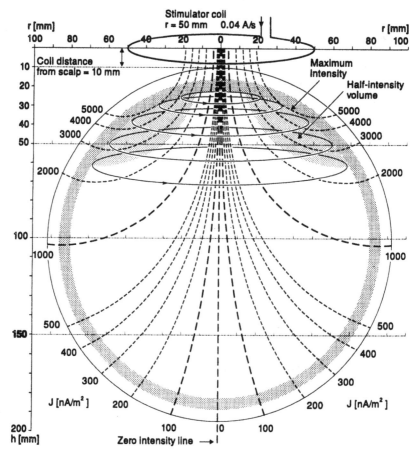

Fig. 22.3 Isointensity lines and half-intensity volume for a stimulation coil with 50 mm radius. The distance of the coil plane from the scalp is 10 mm.

quadrupolar magnetic field, the stimulating electric current field in the tissue has a linear instead of circular form. In some applications the result is more effective stimulation. On the other hand, a quadrupolar field decreases as a function of distance faster than that of a dipolar coil. Therefore, the dipolar coil is more effective in stimulating objects that are located deeper within the tissue.

The first experiments with the quadrupolar magnetic field were made by Rossi et al. (1987). The distribution of the stimulating electric current field of a figure-of-eight coil system was calculated by Malmivuo and Puikkonen (1987). This method has subsequently been applied to magnetic stimulation by many scientists (Ueno, Tashiro, and Harada, 1988).

The sensitivity distributions of dipolar and quadrupolar magnetometer coils were discussed in detail in Section 14.2. The sensitivity distributions shown in Figures 14.4 and 14.5 are similarly applicable to magnetic stimulation as well and are therefore not reproduced here.

22.4 STIMULUS PULSE

The experimental stimulator examined by Irwin et al. (1970) had a multicapacitor construction equaling a capacitance of 4760 μF. This was charged to 90–260 V and then discharged with a bank of eight thyristors through the stimulating coil. The result was a magnetic field pulse of 0.1–0.2 T, 5 mm away from the coil. The length of the magnetic field pulse was of the order of 150–300 μs. Today's commercial magnetic stimulators generate magnetic energies of some 500 J and use typically 3–5 kV to drive the coil. Peak fields are typically 2 T, risetimes of order 100 μs, and peak values of $dB/dt = 5 \times 10^4$ T/s.

The energy required to stimulate tissue is proportional to the square of the corresponding magnetic field. According to Faraday's induction law, this magnetic field is in turn approximately proportional to the product of the electric field magnitude and the pulse duration (Irwin et al., 1970):

$$W \propto B^2 \propto E^2 t^2 \qquad (22.6)$$

Thus

$$E \propto \frac{\sqrt{W}}{t} \qquad (22.7)$$

where

W = energy required to stimulate tissue
B = magnetic flux density
E = electric field
t = pulse duration

The effectiveness of the stimulator with respect to energy transfer is proportional to the square root of the magnetic energy stored in the coil when the current in the coil reaches its maximum value. A simple model of a nerve fiber is to regard each node as a leaky capacitor that has to be charged. Measurements with electrical stimulation indicate that the time constant of this leaky capacitor is of the order of 150–300 μs. Therefore, for effective stimulation the current pulse into the node should be shorter than this (Hess, Mills, and Murray, 1987). For a short pulse in the coil less energy is required, but obviously there is a lower limit too.

22.5 ACTIVATION OF EXCITABLE TISSUE BY TIME-VARYING MAGNETIC FIELDS

The actual stimulation of excitable tissue by a time-varying magnetic field results from the flow of induced current across membranes. Without such flow a depolarization is not produced and excitation cannot result. Unfortunately, one cannot examine this question in a general sense but rather must look at specific geometries and structures. To date this has been done only for a single nerve fiber in a uniform conducting medium with a stimulating coil whose plane is parallel to the fiber (Roth and Basser, 1990).

In the model examined by Roth and Basser, the nerve is assumed to be unmyelinated, infinite in extent, and lying in a uniform unbounded conducting medium, the membrane described by Hodgkin-Huxley equations. The transmembrane voltage V_m is shown to satisfy the equation

$$\lambda^2 \frac{\partial^2 V_m}{\partial x^2} - V_m = \tau \frac{\partial V_m}{\partial t} + \lambda^2 \frac{\partial E_x}{\partial x} \qquad (22.8)$$

where

V_m = transmembrane voltage
λ = membrane space constant
τ = membrane time constant
x = orientation of the fiber
E_x = x component of the magnetically induced electric field (proportional to the x component of induced current density)

It is interesting that it is the axial derivative of this field that is the driving force for an induced voltage. For a uniform system in which end effects can be ignored, excitation will arise near the site of maximum *changing* current and not maximum current itself.

In the example considered by Roth and Basser the coil lies in the xy plane with its center at $x = 0$, $y = 0$, while the fiber is parallel to the x axis and at $y = 2.5$ cm and $z = 1.0$ cm. They consider a coil with radius of 2.5 cm wound from 30 turns of wire of 1.0 mm radius. The coil, located at a distance of 1.0 cm from the fiber, is a constituent of an *RLC* circuit; and the time variation is that resulting from a voltage step input. Assuming $C = 200$ μF and $R = 3.0$ Ω, an overdamped current waveform results. From the resulting stimulation it is found that excitation results at $x = 2.0$ cm (or -2.0 cm, depending on the direction of the magnetic field) which corresponds to the position of maximum $\partial E_x/\partial x$. The threshold applied voltage for excitation is determined to be 30 V. (This results in a peak coil current of around 10 A.) These design conditions could be readily realized.

The effect of field risetime on efficiency of stimulation has been quantified (Barker, Freeston, and Garnham, 1990; Barker, Garnham, Freeston, 1991). Stimulators with short risetimes (< 60 μs) need only half the stored energy of those with longer risetimes (> 180 μs). The use of a variable field risetime also enables membrane time constant to be measured and this may contain useful diagnostic information.

22.6 APPLICATION AREAS OF MAGNETIC STIMULATION OF NEURAL TISSUE

Magnetic stimulation can be applied to nervous stimulation either centrally or peripherally.

The main benefit of magnetic stimulation is that the stimulating current density is not concentrated at the skin, as in electric stimulation, but is more equally distributed within the tissue. This is true especially in transcranial magnetic stimulation of the brain, where the high electric resistivity of the skull does not have any effect on the distribution of the stimulating current. Therefore, magnetic stimulation does not produce painful sensations at the skin, unlike stimulation of the motor cortex with electrodes on the scalp (Mills, Murray, and Hess, 1987; Rimpiläinen et al., 1990, 1991).

Another benefit of the magnetic stimulation method is that the stimulator does not have direct skin contact. This is a benefit in the sterile operation theater environment.

As mentioned at the beginning of this chapter, the first papers introducing the clinical application of magnetic stimulation were published in 1985. Now magnetic stimulators for clinical applications are produced by several manufacturers. It may be predicted that the magnetic stimulation will be applied particularly to the stimulation of cortical areas, because in electric stimulation it is difficult to produce concentrated stimulating current density distributions in the cortical region and to avoid high current densities on the scalp.

REFERENCES

Barker AT, Freeston IL (1985): Medical applications of electric and magnetic fields. *Electron. Power* 31:(10) 757–60.

Barker AT, Freeston IL, Garnham CW (1990): Measurement of cortical and peripheral neural membrane time constant in man using magnetic nerve stimulation. *J. Physiol. (Lond.)* 423: 66.

Barker AT, Freeston IL, Jalinous R, Merton PA, Morton HB (1985): Magnetic stimulation of the human brain. *J. Physiol. (Lond.)* 369: 3P.

Barker AT, Garnham CW, Freeston IL (1991): Magnetic nerve stimulation—the effect of waveform on efficiency, determination of neural membrane time constants and the measurement of stimulator output. *EEG & Clin. Neurophysiol.* 43(Suppl.).

Barker AT, Jalinous R, Freeston IL (1985): Noninvasive magnetic stimulation of human motor cortex. *Lancet* 1:(8437) 1106–7.

Bickford RG, Fremming BD (1965): Neuronal stimulation by pulsed magnetic fields in animals and man. In *Digest of the 6th Internat. Conf. Medical Electronics and Biological Engineering*, p. 112, IFMBE.

d'Arsonval JA (1896): Dispositifs pour la mésure des courants alternatifs de toutes fréquences. *C. R. Soc. Biol. (Paris)* 2: 450–1.

Durand D, Ferguson AS, Dalbasti T (1992): Effect of surface boundary on neuronal magnetic stimulation. *IEEE Trans. Biomed. Eng.* 39:(1) 58–64.

Eaton H (1992): Electric field induced in spherical conductor from arbitrary coils: Application to magnetic stimulation and MEG. *Med. & Biol. Eng. & Comput.* 30:(July) 433–40.

Esselle KP, Stuchly MA (1992): Neural stimulation with magnetic fields: Analysis of induced electric fields. *IEEE Trans. Biomed. Eng.* 39:(7) 693–700.

Geddes LA (1991): History of magnetic stimulation of the nervous system. *J. Clin. Neurophysiol* 8: 3–9.

Hess CW, Mills KR, Murray NMF (1986): Methodological considerations on the determination of central motor conduction time. In *Proc. of the Third Internat. Evoked Potential Symposium*, ed. AB Person, CD Person, Berlin-West.

Hess CW, Mills KR, Murray NFM (1987): Magnetic brain stimulation: Central motor conduction studies in multiple sclerosis. *Ann. Neurol.* 22: 744–52.

Irwin DD, Rush S, Evering R, Lepeshkin E, Montgomery DB, Weggel RJ (1970): Stimulation of cardiac muscle by a time-varying magnetic field. *IEEE Trans. Magn.* MAG-6:(2) 321–2.

Lövsund P, Öberg PÅ, Nilsson SEG (1980): Magnetophosphenes: A quantitative analysis of thresholds. *Med. & Biol. Eng. & Comput.* 18: 326–34.

Malmivuo JA (1976): On the detection of the magnetic heart vector–An application of the reciprocity theorem. *Helsinki Univ. Tech.*, Acta Polytechn. Scand., El. Eng. Series. Vol. 39, pp. 112. (Dr. tech. thesis)

Malmivuo JA (1980): Distribution of MEG detector sensitivity: An application of reciprocity. *Med. & Biol. Eng. & Comput.* 18:(3) 365–70.

Malmivuo JA (1992a): Distribution of electric current in inhomogeneous volume conductors. In *Proceedings of the 8th Internat. Conference on Electrical Bio-Impedance*, ed. T Lahtinen, pp. 18–20, University of Kuopio, Center for Training and Development, Kuopio, Finland.

Malmivuo JA (1992b): Distribution of stimulation fields in the tissue. In *Proceedings of the First Ragnar Granit Symposium*, ed. V Suihko, H Eskola, pp. 5–29, Tampere University of Technology, Ragnar Granit Institute, Tampere.

Malmivuo JA, Puikkonen J (1987): Sensitivity distribution of multichannel MEG detectors. In *Abst. 6th Internat. Conf. Biomagnetism, Tokyo, 27–30 August*, ed. K Atsumi, M Kotani, S Ueno, T Katila, SJ Williamson, pp. 112–3, Tokyo Denki University Press, Tokyo.

Mills KR, Murray NMF, Hess CW (1987): Magnetic and electrical transcranial brain stimulation: Physiological mechanisms and clinical applications. *Neurosurg.* 20: 164–8.

Öberg PÅ (1973): Magnetic stimulation of nerve tissue. *Med. & Biol. Eng. & Comput.* 11: 55–64.

Polson MJ, Barker AT, Freeston IL (1982): Stimulation of nerve trunks with time-varying magnetic fields. *Med. & Biol. Eng. & Comput.* 20:(2) 243–4.

Porter R (1982): Neural events associated with movement performance. *Proc. Aust. Physiol. Pharmacol. Soc.* 13:(2) 31–46.

Rimpiläinen I, Eskola HJ, Häkkinen V, Karma P (1991): Transcranial facial nerve stimulation by magnetic stimulator in normal subjects. *Electromyogr. Clin. Neurophysiol.* 31: 259–63.

Rimpiläinen I, Laranne J, Eskola HJ, Häkkinen VK, Karma P (1990): Transcranial magnetic stimulation of the facial nerve in patients with Bell's palsy. *Neurophysiol. Clin.* 20: 85–7.

Rossi R, Puikkonen J, Malmivuo JA, Eskola HJ, Häkkinen V (1987): Magnetic stimulation - Design of a prototype and preliminary clinical experiments. *Tampere Univ. Techn., Inst. Biomed. Eng., Reports* 1:(6) 25.

Roth BJ, Basser PJ (1990): A model of the stimulation of a nerve fiber by electromagnetic induction. *IEEE Trans. Biomed. Eng.* BME-37:(6) 588–97.

Thompson SP (1910): A physiological effect of an alternating magnetic field. *Proc. R. Soc. (Biol.)* 82: 396–8.

Ueno S, Tashiro T, Harada K (1988): Localized stimulation of neural tissue in the brain by means of a paired configuration of time-varying magnetic fields. *J. Appl. Phys.* 64: 5862–4.

York DH (1987): Review of descending motor pathways involved with transcranial stimulation. *Neurosurg.* 20:(1) 70–3.

VII

Electric and Magnetic Stimulation of the Heart

Part VII continues the discussion on the second subdivision of bioelectromagnetism (i.e., electro- and magnetobiology), with applications to cardiology. The electric stimulation of cardiac tissue has two very important clinical applications: *cardiac pacing* and *cardiac defibrillation*.

The purpose of cardiac pacing is to maintain the heart rate at a sufficient level even though the activity of the sinus node may not reach the ventricular muscle because of an interrupt in the conduction system. Too low a heart rate cannot provide a high enough blood pressure to maintain the body with sufficient oxygen concentration.

The purpose of cardiac defibrillation is to stop continuous and uncontrolled multiple reentrant activation circuits causing fibrillating muscular contractions. Fibrillation of the ventricular muscle causes a total loss of the blood pumping action and thus leads to a dramatically decreased blood pressure, lack of oxygen in the brain tissue, and death, unless the fibrillation can be stopped with a defibrillator within a few minutes.

In clinical practice, both cardiac pacing and cardiac defibrillation are achieved solely with electric methods. Some experiments in accomplishing these with magnetic stimulation have been performed. They are, however, so limited that a separate chapter on magnetic stimulation of the heart muscle is not included but these experiments are referred to in the appropriate chapters on (electric) cardiac pacing and defibrillation.

23

Cardiac Pacing

23.1 STIMULATION
OF CARDIAC MUSCLE

In Chapter 4 we described the behavior of excitable membranes both qualitatively and quantitatively through the Hodgkin-Huxley formalism. This lay the groundwork for Chapter 21 in which the response of nerve to electric stimulation was considered. This chapter considers the response of cardiac muscle to electric stimulation. It draws on these same fundamentals, but considers its particular application to the pacing and defibrillating of the heart (Greatbatch and Seligman, 1988; Tacker, 1988; El-Sherif and Samet, 1991).

There are a number of significant differences that distinguish cardiac activation from the stimulation of nerve arising in FES (Chapter 22), and these are listed in Table 23.1. They come about first because of the size differences in these two cases. For stimulation of a nerve the target region is of the order of a few cubic millimeters, while the target region in the heart is in the order of a few cubic centimeters. For FES it is often necessary to achieve a finely graded response, entailing recruitment of fibers from small to large diameter. FES thus contrasts sharply with electric stimulation of cardiac tissue where a stimulus activates either the entire heart or none of it as a consequence of the syn-

cytial structure. The large size of the heart usually means that excitable tissue whose excitation must be avoided can be excluded based on good spatial separation. In view of the cardiac syncytium the physical arrangement of stimulating electrodes is not in any way critical or demanding. One of the great challenges in FES is to devise ways to deal with fatigue; fortunately, heart muscle does not fatigue. However, all the advantages do not lie with cardiac muscle. We mention that care must be exercised that a pacemaker stimulus is not inadvertently delivered during the vulnerable period, or the serious consequence of fibrillation could result. This hazard does not arise in striated muscle.

23.2 INDICATIONS
FOR CARDIAC PACING

In Chapter 7 we described the normal cardiac conduction system. The heart's own pacemaker is located in the atrium and is responsible for initiation of the heartbeat. The heartbeat begins with activation of atrial tissue in the pacemaker region (i.e., the SA node), followed by cell-to-cell spread of excitation throughout the atrium. The only normal link of excitable tissue connecting the atria to the ventricles is the AV conduction system. Propagation takes place at

Table 23.1 Comparison in stimulating cardiac and striated muscle

Heart muscle	Striated muscle
Target region is large	Limited target region
Easy to avoid excitation of unwanted nerve	Excitable tissue to be avoided is close to target tissue
In effect, all cells are similar in size and excitability	Fibers vary in diameter, questions there are concerning recruitment, order of recruitment, and order that can differ from normal
Does not fatigue	Fatigue must be considered
Pulse-on-T	Does not fibrillate

a slow velocity, but at the ventricular end the bundles of His carry the excitation to many sites in the right and left ventricle at a relatively high velocity of 1–2 m/s. The slow conduction in the AV junction results in a delay of around 0.1 s between atrial and ventricular excitation; this timing facilitates terminal filling of the ventricles from atrial contraction prior to ventricular contraction. (Without a proper atrial contraction preceding the ventricular cardiac output may be reduced by 15%.)

Disease affecting the AV junction may result in interference with normal AV conduction. This is described by different degrees of block. In first-degree block the effect is simply slowed conduction, in second-degree block there is a periodic dropped beat, but in third-degree block no signal reaches the ventricles. This latter condition is also referred to as complete heart block. In this case the ventricles are completely decoupled from the atria. Whereas the atrial heart rate is still determined at the AV node, the ventricles are paced by ectopic ventricular sites. Since under normal conditions the ventricles are driven by the atria, the latent ventricular pacemakers must have a lower rate. Consequently, in complete heart block the ventricles beat at a low rate (bradycardia). Even this condition may not require medical attention, but if the heart rate is too low, a condition known as *Stokes-Adams syndrome*, the situation becomes life-threatening. The prognosis in the case of complete heart block and Stokes-Adams is 50% mortality within one year. In this case

the implantation of an artificial pacemaker is mandatory.

Another condition, known as the *sick sinus syndrome*, is also one for which the artificial pacemaker is the treatment of choice. Here the bradycardia results from the atrial rate itself being abnormally low. Thus, even though the AV junction is normal, the ventricles are driven at too low a rate.

23.3 CARDIAC PACEMAKER

23.3.1 Pacemaker Principles

We have noted previously the differences in stimulation of cardiac tissue in contrast to that of nervous tissue. Basically since the heart is an electric syncytium, excitation in any suitable region readily spreads throughout the entire heart. Furthermore, since the heart is a very large organ, the stimulating electrodes require no special design. And since there is a good separation from other excitable tissue, whatever necessary stimulation thresholds are required (times a safety factor), they can normally be fulfilled without excitation of other organs. The engineering challenges thus lie primarily in areas other than the classical electrophysiology described in previous chapters. These critical areas have to do, mainly, with logical decisions to provide or withhold pulses and/or to adjust their timing to make them as physiological as possible.

The following sections are devoted to a description of the various practical aspects of pacemaker design and an elucidation of the points raised above. We consider the following topics:

Control of impulses

Site of stimulation

Excitation parameters and configuration

Implantable energy sources

Electrodes

23.3.2 Control of Impulses

The earliest implantable pacemakers were designed to control the Stokes-Adams syndrome and for this purpose the simplest design is one where the ventricle is continuously stimulated at a safe rate. The pulse generator design required simply the generation of transthreshold pulses at the desired fixed heart rate. A pulse of about 2 ms duration, amplitude (essentially the battery voltage) of 5–8 V, and a frequency of 72 beats per minute were typically used. In general, the electrodes were sutured to the ventricle, and both electrodes and generator were implanted following a thoracotomy.

This system has a number of shortcomings. First, it does not respond to the physiological needs for a variable heart rate depending on the body's oxygen requirements. (For example, these increase during exercise). Second, the patient may have only sporadic periods of Stokes-Adams syndrome. By pacing during regular ventricular activation, not only is there an unnecessary drain on implanted batteries but there is no coordination between the artificial stimulus and the naturally occurring one (in fact, this type of stimulation is called asynchronous). One potentially dangerous consequence is that the artificial stimulus might fall into the naturally occurring T-wave vulnerable period initiating tachycardia or fibrillation.

Particularly with the advent of integrated circuits it became possible to implant electronics that could sense the presence of an atrial and/or ventricular signal and to respond in an appropriate physiological way. For example, if the pathology is solely complete heart block, then the atrial pulse can be normal. An improved pacemaker design is one that senses the atrial excitation and delivers a ventricular pacing stimuli after a suitable delay (around 0.1 ms).

An alternative was to sense the ectopic ventricular excitation, when it occurred. In its presence, an artificial stimulus was inhibited (or timed to coincide with the R wave). In the absence of a ventricular pulse, after a maximum acceptable delay, an artificial ventricular pulse was generated. Such pacemakers were termed a "demand" type.

In the mid-1970s pacemakers were being developed with programmable logic of this kind. A nomenclature code was developed to describe the particular logical pacemaker design implemented; this is reproduced in Table 23.2. (Although this code has been superseded by a more sophisticated one, it is still referred to in some current literature, and for this reason is included here.) The code consists of three letters: the first, giving the chamber paced (A = atrial, V = ventricular, and D = both, i.e., dual); the second, the chamber sensed; and the third, the type of response. Thus the asynchronous, fixed-rate, early type with ventricular pacing is simply V00. VVI describes the situation where a ventricular stimulus is inhibited if an acceptable intrinsic ventricular beat is sensed. In VAT, the atrial electrophysiology is normal; thus the atria is sensed and the ventricle triggered (after a suitable delay).

23.3.3 Dual Chamber Multiprogrammable

The continued improvement in technology has made possible the implantation of microprocessors. This, coupled with improved technology, has permitted the placement of sensing/pacing leads routinely in both atria and ventri-

Table 23.2 ICHD nomenclature code for implantable cardiac pacemaker

Chamber paced	Chamber sensed	Response	Description of mechanism
V	0	0	Fixed-rate ventricular pacing
A	0	0	Fixed-rate atrial pacing
D	0	0	Fixed-rate AV pacing
V	V	I	Ventricular sensing and pacing, inhibited mode
V	V	T	Ventricular sensing and pacing, triggered mode
A	A	I	Atrial sensing and pacing, inhibited mode
A	A	T	Atrial sensing and pacing, triggered mode
V	A	T	Atrial sensing, ventricular pacing, triggered mode
D	V	I	Ventricular sensing, AV pacing, inhibited

Source: Parsonnet, Furman, and Smyth (1974).

Table 23.3 Fourth and fifth letter of NASPE/BPEG pacemaker code

Fourth letter: rate modulation	Fifth letter: antiarrhythmia function
0 = none	0 = none
P = Simple programmable	P = Pacing (anti-tachyarrhythmia)
M = Multiprogrammable	S = Shock
C = Communicating	D = Dual (i.e., P and S)
R = Rate modulation	

Note: First, second, third letters as in Table 23.2.
Source: Bernstein et al. (1987).

cles. An important aspect of this improvement is in the power source, mainly the lithium battery, which significantly improves the available energy. The result is a much greater repertoire of electrophysiological behavior. An indication of this increased sophistication is the current pacemaker code. This consists of five letters. The first three are similar to the original ICHD code described in Table 23.2. The fourth and fifth letters are described in Table 23.3. These describe two additional functions of implantable pacemakers that have become possible with present technology.

23.3.4 Rate Modulation

The natural heart rate is modulated by the sympathetic and parasympathetic central nervous systems. These respond to baroreceptor activity in the cardiovascular system, hypoxia, exercise, circulating catecholamines, and so on. Although it is impossible to devise a system that could respond to all of these, physiological control signals have been introduced that are believed significantly to evaluate the desired cardiac output. These include oxygen saturation (using optical methods), physical body movement, respiration rate, temperature, and so on. The introduction of *rate modulation* is, in effect, adaptive pacing to achieve more realistic physiological behavior and represents a higher level of sophistication than heretofore available. The goal is to keep the system as a whole in a reasonable physiological state.

The fourth position in the NASPE/BPEG code (Table 23.3) shows R if the system is capable of rate modulation, as described in the previous paragraph. When this feature is not present, this position describes the extent to which the pulse generator's operating values can be modified noninvasively. S (= Simple programmable) refers to the capability of adjusting the rate, output, or both; M (= Multiprogrammable) describes more extensive program capability; and C (= Communicating) the presence of some degree of telemetry. This degree of sophistication implies a multiprogrammable system. Similarly R (= Rate modulation) normally implies some degree of telemetry.

23.3.5 Anti-Tachycardia/Fibrillation

As we have seen, the pacemaker was originally devised to benefit patients with Stokes-Adams syndrome. The design requirements were simple and could be met with a fixed-rate pulse generator (mode V00). With the advent of increasingly sophisticated technology, the pacemaker functions were broadened and extended to patients with such conditions as sick sinus syndrome. An important additional category is patients with malignant tachycardia. These patients have occasional periods of tachycardia which can, if not treated, lead to fibrillation and death. Two main approaches are available. One consists of a set of rapid pacemaker pulses (approximately 20–30% faster than the tachycardia) delivered to the atria or ventricles. This may terminate the arrhythmia. The second approach entails the application of a shock of high energy with cardiac currents comparable to that present with external defibrillation. (A description of defibrillation systems, including implantable defibrillators, constitutes the material of Chapter 24).

In the fifth position of the NASPE/BPEG code (Table 23.3), the anti-tachyarrhythmia function of the pacemaker is described. With P (= Pacing), low-energy stimulation (noted above), which is in the form of bursts, is present. S (= Shock) reflects the existence of a high-energy anti-tachyarrhythmia intervention capability for cardioversion or defibrillation. D (= Dual) describes both high- and low-energy intervention. Many believe that permanent pacing for ventricular tachycardia is too hazardous since it can lead to unstable ventricular tachycardia or even ventricular fibrillation. For these possibilities a shock backup presence is deemed essential. (An exception is physician-activated pacing which, in the presence of the physician, is used as an adjunctive therapy for sustained ventricular tachycardia.) For this purpose non-invasive activation is achieved by a magnet or rf telemetry.

23.4 SITE OF STIMULATION

In the early pacemaker models, electrodes were sutured directly to the heart and the wires led to the pulse generators which were placed in a thoracic or abdominal pocket. But to avoid the trauma of a thoracotomy electrodes were increasingly placed in the heart cavities through a transvenous route. (The term transvenous while very popular, is a misnomer since it actually refers to the threading of electrodes *through* a vein into the right atria and/or ventricle). At present, around 95% of pacemaker electrodes are *endocardial*. Several veins are and have been used, including, typically, the subclavian, cephalic, and external jugular. The electrodes are manipulated by a stiff stylet wire from the distal end under fluoroscopic visualization. The right atrial electrode is hooked into the right atrial appendage, whereas the right ventricular electrode lies at the right ventricular apex position. The electrode tips are fabricated with tines that lodge in the right ventricular trabeculation and the right atrial appendage for stabilization. (Also, after removal of the stylet wire, the atrial lead curves into a J shape that adds additional stabilization.) The pulse generator is usually placed in a prepectoral location.

From an electrophysiological standpoint, the actual location of the ventricular myocardial or endocardial electrode is not important. From the right heart position the activation wave must resemble that in left bundle branch block and reflect mainly cell-to-cell conduction. The hemodynamic consequence is that a satisfactory cardiac output is achieved. Experiments also show that the threshold stimulating currents do not vary widely, suggesting a certain symmetry between current source and depolarization achieved. One can in fact set up a very sim-

plified ideal model based on the bidomain model of Chapter 9, and this is done in the following section.

23.5 EXCITATION PARAMETERS AND CONFIGURATION

In Section 9.5 we considered the induced transmembrane potential from a point current source in a homogeneous isotropic bidomain. This result can be readily modified to the present case where the electrode has a finite radius a. Because of the spherical symmetry the fields vary with r only. At $r = a$ we require that

$$-\left.\frac{\partial \Phi_i}{\partial r}\right|_{r=a} = 0 \qquad (23.1)$$

since the current leaving the electrode enters the interstitial space only. In fact, the boundary condition in the interstitial space is that the total current entering this space at $r = a$ is the total applied current I_a. In view of Equation 23.1 and the definition of V_m then at $r = a$ we have

$$\left.\frac{\partial \Phi_o}{\partial r}\right|_{r=a} = -\left.\frac{\partial V_m}{\partial r}\right|_{r=a} \qquad (23.2)$$

Consequently, the aforementioned boundary condition is

$$\left.\frac{4\pi r^2 \sigma_o^b \partial V_m}{\partial r}\right|_{r=a} = -I_a \qquad (23.3)$$

where

σ_o^b = interstitial bidomain conductivity, as described in Equation 9.17

I_a = applied current, assumed to be cathodal (hence the minus sign)

Now Equation 9.28 describes the behavior of V_m in the region $r \geq a$ under steady-state conditions (namely $V_m = K_A e^{-r/\lambda}/r$). If this is substituted into Equation 23.3 and solved for the coefficient K_A we obtain

$$K_A = \frac{I_a e^{a/\lambda}}{4\pi\sigma_o^b(1 + a/\lambda)} \qquad (23.4)$$

Substituting this back into Equation 9.28 gives an expression for V_m, namely

$$V_m = \frac{I_o e^{a/\lambda}}{4\pi\sigma_o^b(1 + a/\lambda)} \frac{e^{-r/\lambda}}{r} \qquad (23.5)$$

The maximum induced voltage is at $r = a$; in this case, Equation 23.5 reduces to $V_{m \text{ max}}$ or

$$V_{m \text{ max}} = \frac{I_a}{4\pi\sigma_o^b a(1 + a/\lambda)} \qquad (23.6)$$

One notes from Equation 23.6 that the smaller the electrode the larger the induced voltage. For electrodes that are large compared with the space constant, the induced voltage varies inversely as the square of the electrode radius; but when the radius is much smaller than the space constant, the voltage varies only as the first power of the inverse radius.

With an endocardial lead the electrode is surrounded by cardiac tissue on one side and blood on the other. Since the blood conductivity is about three times greater than cardiac tissue, in our very simple isotropic model the applied current should possibly be reduced by some factor over what it would be in the assumed uniform model developed in Chapter 9 and extended above. We have chosen this factor to be around 35%. For a 1 ms stimulus pulse the membrane should come close to the assumed steady-state value (Cartee, 1992). Equation 23.6 gives the maximum steady-state induced voltage if we identify a as the equivalent radius of the (spherical) electrode. A fairly typical electrode has an area of 8.8 mm^2 (Breivik, Hoff, and Ohm, 1985). This is converted into a sphericalized radius of 1.2 mm as described in Miller et al. (1985). We also choose the space constant as $\lambda = 0.5$ mm (Plonsey and Barr, 1982), and assign σ_o^b (the interstitial conductivity as defined in Eq. 9.17) the value of 0.002 S/cm. Then

$$V_{m \text{ max}} = 34 \cdot I_a \qquad (23.7)$$

where

I_a = applied cathodal current [mA]
$V_{m \text{ max}}$ = maximum membrane voltage [mV]

If I_a is 0.44 mA, then V_m is 15.0 mV, which is not an unreasonable threshold voltage, considering the many approximations in this simple, homogeneous, isotropic model. The result is in the range of published measurements (Breivik, Hoff, and Ohm, 1985) and the empirical current threshold value of 0.05 mA/mm^2 (Tarjan, 1991). Based on Equation 23.6 the use of a smaller-sized electrode will diminish the required current for a given threshold transmembrane voltage, as noted above. There is a limit to the amount by which the electrode size can be decreased. The reason is that one has to reach the required threshold current with a fixed battery voltage, and this limits the maximum allowable circuit impedance. The latter, however, is mainly the electrode-tissue impedance, which increases inversely with the electrode radius. In a practical design one should also include the possible effect of growth of fibrous tissue around the electrode since this will increase the size of the effective radius a in Equation 23.6 (see Section 23.7). We note that in Equation 23.6, V_m is positive (depolarization) for an assumed cathodal (monopolar) electrode.

When the electrode is monopolar, the reference electrode is invariably chosen as the case of the pulse generator unit. The main advantage of the monopolar system is that only a single electrode wire (per chamber) has to be implanted. For endocardial leads this smaller size compared to a bipolar lead is clearly desirable. In addition, it also represents a smaller wire lying in the tricuspid valve, through which the catheter electrode must run. One of the disadvantages, though, is the presence of stimulating current throughout a large part of the thorax; thus striated muscles lying in this region may be stimulated, giving rise to annoying muscle twitch. Both the phrenic and diaphragmatic nerves have also been known to be affected.

The bipolar electrode has an electric field that varies as $1/r^3$ rather than $1/r^2$ and, consequently, is less likely to affect excitable tissues remote from the site at which the electrodes have been placed. In addition, when these electrodes are used in the sensing mode, the bipolar configuration is less sensitive to interference from distant extraneous signals. Such electromagnetic interference may at times be mistaken for a cardiac signal and incorrect logical inferences drawn by a multiprogrammable pacemaker. With present technology the advantage of handling a single versus double wire per chamber is no longer very great. For more historical reasons unipolar systems are favored in the United States, whereas European systems favor bipolar.

23.6   IMPLANTABLE ENERGY SOURCES

At the time of the development of the early pacemakers the battery with longest life was the zinc-mercury battery. This was adopted for pacemaker use, but even as late as 1970 the best that could be achieved, on average, was a 2 year life-span. A second problem with the zinc-mercury cell is liberation of hydrogen gas at high pressure (300 psi). A consequence is the inability to create a hermetical seal of the cell. By 1970 the limiting step in pacemaker longevity was this power source.

A very wide range of power sources for pacemakers have been proposed and investigated. These include schemes that utilize the body's own chemistry and energy. For example, the energy from the beating heart itself was investigated. Various types of fuel cells were considered. None have been actually used clinically. In addition, rechargeable systems using external power sources coupled through the body tissue have been tried, but very few have actually been used.

A major breakthrough was the introduction of the lithium battery, which is now used in virtually all new pacemaker systems. The reaction involves lithium and iodine:

$$2Li + I_2 \rightarrow 2LiI \qquad (23.8)$$

Since no gas is produced, the lithium cell can be hermetically sealed. Furthermore the serious problem of breakdown of the separator in the zinc-mercury battery does not arise in the lithium-iodine cell since, in the latter, the separator forms spontaneously and is self-healing. The lithium battery also has a reliable end-of-life decay characteristic which fails slowly enough to permit its detection in a normal checkup and the scheduling of a timely replacement. In addition to these attractive features, the approximate 50% survival of the lithium-iodine battery is 12 years (Bernstein, 1991).

23.7   ELECTRODES

The pacemaker system consists of a package containing the pulse generator and pulse-sensing elements along with the associated logic circuits and the battery; this package is connected by leads to the electrodes themselves. The leads carry heart signals from the heart to the electronics and current stimuli to the heart. While simple in function, the latter components have posed challenging engineering problems.

The leads are insulated wires that must carry current with low resistance and be capable of reliable operation for many years in spite of repeated flexing. The use of hard flexible metals is required. Early leads were twisted or braided strands placed in a hollow catheter. At present, in the United States a helical coiled lead is favored, which is put into position by a stylet wire. This shape converts the various types of body and heart movement into torsion, which the metal can easily tolerate. The coil may be made of stainless steel, Eigiloy, or MP35N, all of which are alloys with excellent strength. The insulating materials that have proven best are silicone rubber and polyurethane.

The electrodes themselves are also, usually, an alloy. Surface preparation is important since microcracks can become a site of local currents and corrosion. A series capacitance is always used to eliminate any DC-current flow and achieve the balanced biphasic condition discussed in Chapter 21. The use of porous electrodes has also been suggested to improve ingrowth of tissue and stabilization of the electrode. The endocardial electrode generally becomes encased in collagen. Using Equation 23.6 we can consider that this increases the effective electrode radius, hence decreasing the stimulating voltage, for a given current source. A typical capsule thickness of 0.6 mm (Miller et al., 1985) increases a from 1.2 to 1.8 mm in the illustrative example leading to Equation 23.7. The result is a change of coefficient in Equation 23.7:

$$V_{m \ max} = 16.8 \cdot I_a \qquad (23.9)$$

This amounts to a reduction in the stimulus strength by 2.0. In fact in experimental studies, one finds that the initial threshold at the time of placement of a ventricular pacing lead increases by factors of 2–4 over the following period (Miller et al., 1985).

23.8 MAGNETIC STIMULATION OF CARDIAC MUSCLE

Several experiments with magnetic stimulation of cardiac muscle have been reported (Bourland et al., 1990; Irwin et al., 1970; Mouchawar et al., 1992).

In their experiments, Mouchawar et al. (1992) used two coplanar stimulation coils placed close to the heart of an anesthetized dog. The coils had an outer radius of 8.5 cm, a thickness of 1.25 cm, and included 30 turns. The distance from the coils to the ventricles within the chest ranged from 2 to 3.5 cm. The magnetic stimulator produced an ectopic beat in the vagal-arrested dogs with an average energy of approximately 12 kJ. This is much higher than the energy needed to stimulate magnetically the human peripheral nervous system, which requires typically 400 J.

REFERENCES

Bernstein AD (1991): Classification of cardiac pacemakers. In *Cardiac Pacing and Electrophysiology,* 3rd ed., ed. N El-Sherif, P Samet, pp. 494–503, W.B. Saunders, Philadelphia.

Bernstein AD, Camm AJ, Fletcher RD, Gold RD, Rickards AF, Smyth NPD, Spielman SR, Sutton R (1987): The NASPE/BPEG generic pacemaker code for antibradyarrhythmia and adaptive-rate pacing and antitachyarrhythmia devices. *PACE, Pacing Clin. Electrophysiol.* 10: 794–9.

Bourland JD, Mouchawar GA, Nyenhuis JA, Geddes LA, Foster KS, Jones JT, Graber GP (1990): Transchest magnetic (eddy-current) stimulation of the dog heart. *Med. & Biol. Eng. & Comput.* 28: 196–8.

Breivik K, Hoff PI, Ohm OJ (1985): In favor of bipolar ventricular leads. In *Pacemaker Leads,* ed. AE Aubert, H Ector, pp. 33–8, Elsevier, Amsterdam.

Cartee LA, Plonsey R (1992): The transient subthreshold response of spherical and cylindrical cell models to extracellular stimulation. *IEEE Trans. Biomed. Eng.* 39: 76–85.

El-Sherif N, Samet P (eds.) (1991): *Cardiac Pacing and Electrophysiology,* 3rd ed., 784 pp. Saunders, Philadelphia.

Greatbatch W, Seligman LJ (1988): Pacemakers. In *Encyclopedia of Medical Devices and Instrumentation,* ed. JG Webster, pp. 2175–203, John Wiley & Sons, New York.

Irwin DD, Rush S, Evering R, Lepeshkin E, Montgomery DB, Weggel RJ (1970): Stimulation of cardiac muscle by a time-varying magnetic field. *IEEE Trans. Magn.* MAG-6:(2) 321–2.

Miller SL, Mac Gregor DC, Margules ES, Bobyn JD, Wilson GJ (1985): Theoretical justification for size reduction of porous-surfaced electrodes. In *Pacemaker Leads,* ed. AE Aubert, H Ector, pp. 57–62, Elsevier, Amsterdam.

Mouchawar GA, Bourland JD, Nyenhuis JA, Geddes LA, Foster KS, Jones JT, Graber GP (1992): Closed-chest cardiac stimulation with a pulsed magnetic field. *Med. & Biol. Eng. & Comput.* 30:(2) 162–8.

Parsonnet V, Furman S, Smyth N (1974): Implantable cardiac pacemakers. *Am. J. Cardiol.* 34: 487–500.

Plonsey R, Barr RC (1982): The four-electrode resistivity technique as applied to cardiac muscle. *IEEE Trans. Biomed. Eng.* BME-29: 541–6.

Tacker WA (1988): Electrical defibrillators. In *Encyclopedia of Medical Devices and Instrumentation,* Vol. 2, ed. JG Webster, pp. 939–44, John Wiley & Sons, New York.

Tarjan PP (1991): Engineering aspects of modern cardiac pacing. In *Cardiac Pacing and Electrophysiology,* 3rd ed., ed. N El-Sherif, P Samet, pp. 484–93, W.B. Saunders, Philadelphia.

24

Cardiac Defibrillation

24.1 INTRODUCTION

In this chapter we explore the use of cardiac stimulation to terminate arrhythmias. Our focus is mainly on *defibrillation*, in which very high energy shocks are applied for the purpose of ending the fibrillation (which is otherwise lethal). The application of biophysical principles and the use of simulation and modeling that characterizes other chapters in this book is greatly limited here. The reason is that the mechanisms of both fibrillation and defibrillation are incompletely understood.

The subject of ventricular fibrillation is the center of much attention from clinical and basic scientists since it is one of the leading causes of death in the Western world (1,200 daily). It has been established that the underlying cause is atherosclerotic coronary artery disease, which results in occlusion of coronary perfusion. In many cases the more recent technique of the implantable defibrillator offers a more successful approach to the control of life-threatening arrhythmia than antiarrhythmic drugs. The subject is therefore of great importance and represents a potential area for application of the electrophysiological principles developed in this book.

24.2 MECHANISMS OF FIBRILLATION

As noted in the introduction, the underlying cause of most cardiac arrhythmias is coronary artery disease involving the development of atherosclerotic plaques. These narrow and occlude the arterial vessels, resulting in ischemia and infarction of cardiac tissue. The electrophysiological properties of ischemic and infarcted tissue in turn provide opportunities for reentrant arrhythmias.

24.2.1 Reentry

Reentry in a ring of cardiac tissue was studied by Mines (1913) whose observations are still appropriate today. In Figure 24.1A, a stimulus at the single site within the ring gives rise to propagation in opposite directions around the ring. These activation waves meet on the opposite side of the diameter from the stimulation site, and collision results. Since at the collision site all neighboring tissue is absolutely refractory, the excitable tissue volume is reduced to zero, and excitation/propagation is terminated. There is no reentry, and this reflects normal cardiac behavior.

A

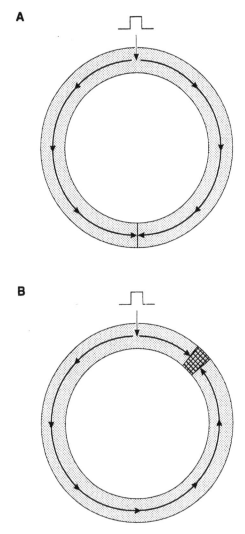

B

Fig. 24.1 Demonstration of conditions that lead to reentry. (A) In the normal tissue collision and annihilation prevent reentry from occurring. (B) The cross-hatched area is functionally a unidirectional block and facilitates a counterclockwise circus movement.

In Figure 24.1B the cross-hatched region is assumed to block propagation which is initiated in the clockwise direction. (The block arises possibly because the cells in this region are still in their refractory period.) Consequently, propagation takes place only counterclockwise, following an "alternate path." When propagation finally reaches the region of block, if it is no longer refractory then activation will continue past this site to the starting point and then continue around a second time. This pattern can

now continue for successive periods; it is a description of reentry. The behavior of the hatched region is described as *unidirectional block* since, as it turned out, propagation was successful in the counterclockwise direction but not in the clockwise direction.

Observation of Figure 24.1 suggests the following conditions for reentry: (1) An area of unidirectional block must be present. (2) Activation, while blocked around one path, must be able to propagate around an alternate path (the counterclockwise direction in Figure 24.1). (3) The propagation time around the alternate path must be greater than the total refractory period of the cells in the unidirectional block. One defines the *wavelength* as the distance traveled during the duration of the refractory period. (It can be calculated as the product of conduction velocity times refractory period duration.) In Figure 24.1B the wavelength must be shorter than the counterclockwise path length in order for reentry to take place. This requirement can be facilitated by a shortened refractory period of the tissue, slow conduction velocity, or both.

In normal activation of the heart propagation ceases when conduction reaches the boundaries of the myocardium. At this point, there is no longer any tissue available that is not in the refractory state. When the next beat is initiated at the SA node, the entire heart is quiescent, and the ensuing process is a repetition of previous ones. The significance of the occurrence of reentry is that the normal pacemaker-initiated process is bypassed. If, as is usual, the activation cycle is very short, then the tissues undergoing reentry serve is a stimulus site for driving the entire heart at a faster rate (tachycardia).

In the example given above, the basis for the unidirectional block was described as due to inhomogeneity of the refractory period. Although this is the most likely cause, there are other mechanisms as well. One arises from the anisotropy of cardiac tissue. The reason is that the axial resistance is much less along than transverse to the fiber direction, and this gives rise to anisotropy in velocity. In addition, there are differences in the organization of intercellular junctions which appears to increase the safety factor for transverse propagation compared to longitudinal (Spach and Dolber, 1985).

Consequently, in the case of a premature excitation, propagation along the fiber direction can be blocked yet take place in the transverse direction, resulting in a reentry loop as in Figure 24.1B.

24.2.2 Reentry With and Without Anatomic Obstacles

In Figure 24.1 we assumed the circular path to be defined by a nonconducting interior obstacle.

In the absence of this obstacle, one would wonder whether the circular path would maintain itself in view of a possible "short-circuiting" by conduction along a diagonal. However, reentry can be demonstrated even in the absence of an obstacle, as can be seen in Figure 24.2 (from the experimental work of Allessie, Bonke, and Schopman, 1976).

Figure 24.2.A describes the activation pattern resulting from regularly paced (500 ms interval) stimuli in an isolated rabbit left atrial prepa-

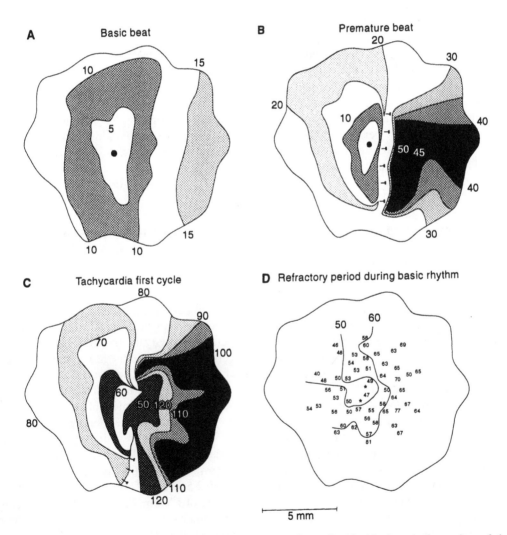

Fig. 24.2 Actual maps of the spread of activation during the onset of tachycardia induced by a premature stimulus in an isolated rabbit heart atrial preparation. (A) Map of the basic beat. (B) Premature beat elicited following a 56 ms delay. (C) First cycle of the tachycardia (double bars indicate sites of the conduction block). (D) Refractory period duration as determined for the corresponding sites. (From Allessie, Bonke, and Schopman, 1976.)

ration. A premature stimulus is applied at the central position (the large dot shown in the figure) after a 56 ms delay. Figure 24.2D describes the length of the refractory period at different points, and this helps explain the response to the premature stimulus shown in Figure 24.2B. One notes propagation to the left into recovered tissue and block to the right (double bars) where the refractory period has not ended. But propagation winds back to this region after a delay so that the region of block is now excitable. Figure 24.2C shows the first cycle of tachycardia; a reentrant circuit (called a *circus movement*), it does not involve a nonconducting obstacle but, rather, is based on the inhomogeneous recovery properties of the preparation.

The smallest path that permits this circular-type propagation (i.e., the wavelength of the circuit) has been called the *leading circle* (Allessie, Bonke, and Schopman, 1977). As before, the wavelength can be evaluated as the product of velocity and refractory period. However, in this type of reentry the refractory period and the conduction velocity are interrelated. The pathway length of a reentrant circuit of the leading circle type is approximately 8 mm.

The reentrant circuit is seen as a consequence of the inhomogeneity in refractoriness in Figure 24.2D. Such conditions (along with short refractory periods, and slow conduction) are found in ischemic myocardium. An examination of successive beats shows the position around which propagation takes place to shift continuously. The reason is that the cells in the region of the vortex during one cycle may show a large action potential (hence be part of the circulating wave) in the following cycle. In spite of this beat-to-beat variation the reentry in the case of tachycardia is relatively orderly and results in a regular rhythm. Random reentry, which characterizes fibrillation, is characterized by pathways whose size and location are continually changing. In addition, several independent wave fronts may be present simultaneously and interact with one another. The resulting rhythm is consequently relatively irregular and chaotic.

Figure 24.3 shows the activation patterns of three successive "beats" during ventricular fibrillation. These illustrate the multiple regions of conduction block which shift continuously.

One can also determinate collision and fusion of wavefronts, and interrupted circus movements. The diameters of such circuits vary between 8 and 30 mm. Because of the complexity of the patterns, maps such as these, which describe behavior only on the bounding surface, leave many of the details hidden from view (in the third dimension).

With very slow conduction (in, say, elevated K^+ at perhaps 5 cm/s), and very short refractory periods (50–100 ms), one can have a very short wavelengths (<1 cm). These give rise to reentrant circuits characterized as *microreentrant*. It has been thought that such circuits might be seen in intact hearts with acute regional ischemia.

In addition to the reentry described above which arises in ischemic and infarcted myocardium, reentry can also occur that utilizes structures of the heart. Clinical examples may be found that demonstrate reentry involving the AV junction, the His-Purkinje system, the SA node, and so on. We omit further details since our goal here is only to develop sufficient background for the subject of defibrillation.

24.3 THEORIES OF DEFIBRILLATION

24.3.1 Introduction

The basic goal in defibrillation is to interfere, electrically, with the reentry circuits to bring this electric activity to a halt. Since the reentrant circuits lie throughout the heart, achieving this goal requires an adequate stimulating field at all points within the heart. This is in contrast to pacemaking, where an adequate stimulus was required only at one site. For pacemaking, an empirical applied current density adequate for stimulation is 5.0 mA/cm^2 which, assuming a tissue resistivity of 500 Ωcm, gives an applied field of 2.5 V/cm. This compares with other estimates of 1 V/cm. But for defibrillation, empirical studies show a need for around 8 V/cm throughout the heart.

One can speculate that with an applied electric field that is 3–6 times normal threshold much of the relatively refractory tissue as well as recovered tissue that is facing the advancing

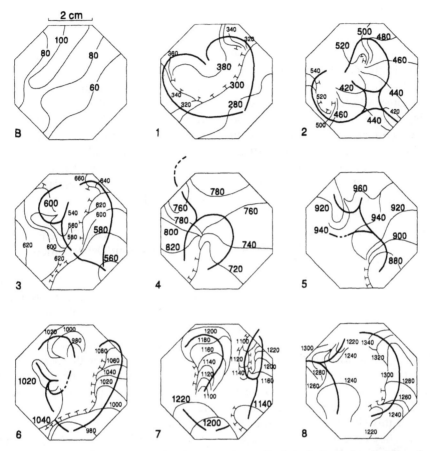

Fig. 24.3 Activation patterns of eight successive activations during ischemia-induced ventricular fibrillation in an isolated perfused pig heart following premature stimulus. Reentry occurs between first and second activation. These patterns demonstrate the presence of multiple wavefronts. and both collision and fusion of wavefronts. Beat 7 shows microcircus movement. (From Janse et al., 1980.)

wavefronts can be activated. This volume is synchronously activated and consequently should greatly modify the activation pattern that would otherwise arise. This, however, is about as close to a defibrillatory mechanism as understood at this time. In spite of this situation, a great deal is known about defibrillation through many animal experiments that have been performed. In the following, we summarize the main ideas.

24.3.2 Critical Mass Hypothesis

In the critical mass hypothesis the basic mechanism of defibrillation is assumed to be the interruption of activation fronts by depolarization of refractory and recovered tissue by the defibrillating field. However, it is further assumed that not all such tissue is necessarily activated to terminate fibrillation; instead, only a critical amount (often suggested to be 75% or more) is required. A comprehensive study of this hypothesis was undertaken by Witkowski and colleagues (Witkowski, Penkoske, and Plonsey, 1990). These authors note that although the interval between activations (ACT-ACT) during fibrillation is irregular, it nevertheless satisfies a definite statistical description. This was used to test whether, following a shock, the electric activity was continuing or fibrillation had been successfully annihilated. This was examined at each of their 120 surface electrode locations.

The shock magnitude (as described by its electric field strength) was also evaluated at each electrode. The authors concluded that with unsuccessful defibrillation at least one ventricular site could be clearly identified where defibrillation had failed. But in the case of successful defibrillation either all sites showed an absence of fibrillating activity in the postshock period or a single site had a self-terminating fibrillation (in one to three activations). The latter single site was located in a region of minimum defibrillatory field strength. From this they concluded that a critical mass less than 100% could lead to successful defibrillation.

An alternative hypothesis, called the *upper limit of vulnerability* hypothesis has been advanced by Chen and colleagues (Chen, Wolf, and Ideker, 1991). In the referenced paper they disputed the conclusions drawn by Witkowski et al. and suggested that the same data (including their own experiments) required a different interpretation. They agreed with Witkowski et al. that following unsuccessful defibrillation the site of earliest activation is at the lowest defibrillatory field strength. However, their statistical analysis showed that the electrophysiological behavior at this site is definitely affected by the shock. They concluded that the shock did, in fact, defibrillate. However, in the absence of a shock intensity great enough, fibrillation was reinitiated.

There is agreement on several important points. First, typical shocks generate field strengths throughout the heart that are quite variable. Placing defibrillating electrodes on the right atrium and left ventricular apex of a dog, Ideker et al. (1987) found the potential field gradient to vary over a 15:1 range on the epicardium. Second the site of earliest measured activity following unsuccessful defibrillation coincided with the region with the lowest shock field strength. These conclusions support the idea that the goal of a defibrillating electrode system is the generation of a uniform field within the heart. (This avoids having damagingly high fields in some spots to ensure an adequate field elsewhere.) The minimum field for successful defibrillation was found by both groups to lie in the range of 3–9 V/cm.

While the aforementioned studies are valuable to the development of an understanding of fibrillation, they do not actually elucidate a *mechanism* in the electrophysiological sense. The only way a shock can influence the behavior of fibrillating cells is through the induced transmembrane potential. The result could be activation of a cell in the resting or relative refractory period. However one has to keep in mind that fibrillating cells do not behave in the same way as normal cells. Furthermore, the question is not simply what happens to individual cells but how the interaction of these cells is modified.

24.3.3 One-Dimensional Activation/Defibrillation Model

As noted above, one would like to know what electrophysiological effect is produced by the application of a stimulating current pulse (shock) on a group of fibrillating cardiac cells. This is a difficult problem to model. For one there is no model of the healthy ventricular membrane, let alone a fibrillating membrane that is satisfactory in all respects. Second it is also not clear what structural model is necessary that adequately reflects the electric interconnection of cells as well as the interstitial spaces necessary to reflect changes in ionic concentration (clefts). And finally there is the problem of handling the large three-dimensional structures (matrices) even with fast modern computers. A very much simpler problem was addressed by Plonsey, Barr, and Witkowski (1991) in which the response of a one-dimensional cardiac strand to a current stimulus was considered. In this it was assumed that the membrane could be considered to be passive and under steady-state conditions. (For shocks with a typical duration of 3–10 ms the steady-state assumption under subthreshold conditions appears to be valid (Cartee, 1991; Cartee and Plonsey, 1992).)

In the aforementioned reference it is assumed that the heart can be considered as consisting of similar parallel fibers running from apex to base and that a uniform applied defibrillating current (also from apex to base) divides equally between such fibers. Consequently, the behavior of the heart can be examined through the

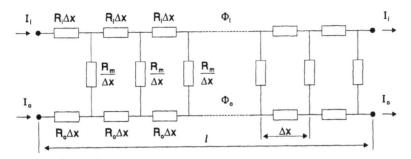

Fig. 24.4 Core-conductor electric network for a single cell that is a component of an equivalent single cardiac fiber. The cell is connected to its neighbors by an intracellular coupling resistance, R_j, at its ends. Steady-state subthreshold conditions are assumed.

behavior of any typical fiber. The response of a single uniform fiber to a current applied at its ends is considered in Section 9.4. Since the length of an equivalent cardiac fiber is perhaps 14 cm and since, for cardiac muscle, $\lambda = 650$ μm (Ideker et al. 1987), then the fiber is 215 λ in length. It is pointed out in Section 9.4 (see, e.g., Equations 9.11 and 10.12) that beyond around 5 λ from the ends ΔV_m is essentially zero and the axial current is uniform and divides in inverse proportion to the axial resistances. That is,

$$\frac{I_o}{I_i} = \frac{r_i}{r_o} \qquad (24.1)$$

where

I_i = axial current inside the cell
I_o = axial current outside the cell
r_i = axial intracellular resistance per unit length
r_o = axial extracellular resistance per unit length

This means that perhaps 95% of the individual cells making up the cardiac fiber are unaffected by the stimulus! But this result depends on the equivalent fiber being uniform and neglects the intercellular junctions. If a single such junction is considered to link the intracellular space of adjoining cells (reflecting the gap-junctional resistance R_j), then each cell behaves identically and as described in Figure 24.4.

In Figure 24.4, since the cell shown is replicated in a chain of around 1,200 such cells making up the total fiber, then voltages and currents must be periodic with a periodicity of one cell.

Thus, for example, I_i entering at the left must equal I_i leaving at the right, since they are exactly one cell length apart. Now if the coupling resistances R_j were equal to zero, then the fiber would be uniform and the transmembrane current variation proportional to the second derivative of V_m as given by Equation 9.10. Consequently, it would also be essentially zero beyond 5 λ of the ends. The effect of a finite R_j is to drive a small amount of current into and out of each cell (exactly the same must leave and enter since I_i must be periodic), and this movement is associated with a nonzero V_m in each cell. In fact, one can see that R_j causes a discontinuity in Φ_i just equal to the voltage drop, namely $I_i R_j$. This also represents a discontinuity in V_m. The presence of R_j forces some of the intracellular current out of the cell on the right half, but for the expected periodicity to be attained this current must enter the cell in the left half. Consequently both i_m and concomitantly V_m must be antisymmetric.

A mathematical description of V_m over the extent of the cell starts with the governing differential Equation 9.4. If we choose the origin at the center of the cell, then the solution to 9.4 should be chosen in terms of $\sinh(x/\lambda)$ to obtain the expected antisymmetry. From Equation 24.1, but including the junctional resistance's contribution to the net intracellular resistance per unit length, we have

$$I_i = I_o \frac{r_o}{r_i + r_o + R_j/l} \qquad (24.2)$$

where

I_i = intracellular axial current
I_o = extracellular axial current
r_i = intracellular axial resistance per unit length
r_o = extracellular axial resistance per unit length
R_j = coupling resistance between cells
l = length of the cell

Consequently since the discontinuity at the ends of each cell requires that $V_m(x = \pm l/2) = I_i R_j$, we get

$$V_m(x) = \frac{I_o R_j r_o}{2(r_i + r_o + R_j/l)} \frac{\sinh(x/\lambda)}{\sinh(l/2\lambda)} \quad (24.3)$$

In Equation 24.3 the factor of 2 takes into account the positive and negative excursion of the expression, whereas the factor $\sinh(l/2\lambda)$ is a constant that is required by the boundary condition. An estimate of the applied current in the equivalent fiber, I_o, can be made by starting with the *total current* applied by the defibrillator. From the model we assume that the fraction associated with the equivalent fiber is the cross section of the fiber and its associated interstitial space divided by the cross section of the entire heart. Using typical physiological values, one obtains cellular depolarizations of $\pm(6-30)$ mV (Plonsey, Barr, and Witkowski, 1991), which is in a range that could certainly affect a cell's electrophysiological behavior.

The above examination of the effect of the intracellular junctional resistance in producing a V_m from a uniform stimulating electric field demonstrates that this effect can arise from any interruption in tissue uniformity. Other histological nonuniformities can also be important in "converting" a uniform applied electric field into an induced transmembrane potential. Recent studies suggest that such a role may be performed by the fiber rotation known to take place in the myocardium.

24.4 DEFIBRILLATOR DEVICES

The high amount of energy that must be delivered is achieved with conventional defibrillators by first charging a large capacitance and then discharging it in a damped *RLC* circuit. In certain designs the pulse is terminated by short-circuiting the capacitance, resulting in a trapezoidal-like wave. Both the damped sine wave and the trapezoidal waveform are generally used, and there is little evidence that one is better than the other (Greatbatch and Seligman, 1988; Kerber, 1990).

Defibrillators are calibrated by the energy discharged into a 50 Ω load. This measure of defibrillation strength competes with the more recent understanding that defibrillation is achieved by the current-flow field, as discussed above. Strength-duration curves are available for applied energy, charge, and current, based on animal studies in which these quantities are varied. For durations greater than 1 ms the current magnitude required for defibrillation remains about the same (suggesting a chronaxie of perhaps 0.5 ms).

Transchest defibrillator electrodes have diameters in the range of 8–13 cm. Electrodes manufactured for direct application to the heart (e.g., during a surgical procedure) are smaller (4–8 cm) in diameter. Large-diameter electrodes are used in an attempt to achieve a uniform field within the heart and also to avoid high current densities that could burn the skin. The total dry transchest impedance is found to be 25–150 Ω, while the transcardiac impedance is typically 20–40 Ω. (The transchest impedance depends on the electrode-skin impedance and, with the use of an appropriate gel, will be about 50 Ω). Transchest defibrillation energy is in the range of 200–360 joules. Assuming a transchest impedance of 50 Ω means that a current of 2–3 A or a voltage of 100–150 V output can be expected from such a device. An inadequate current for defibrillation can result from the selection of a low energy level while being unaware of a high transchest impedance (inadequate skin preparation). Some devices first sense this impedance and then choose the energy level to ensure an adequate current.

Totally implanted defibrillators have been increasingly used, as discussed in the earlier section on cardiac pacemakers. Because they connect directly with the heart, a threshold current of 1–2 A can be achieved at lower voltages and energies. Assuming a transcardiac impedance of 20 Ω requires an applied voltage of around 30 V and an energy of perhaps 30 J.

Experimental work is also in progress for

developing a cardiac defibrillator which uses a magnetic field to stimulate the cardiac muscle (Bourland et al., 1990; Irwin et al., 1970; Kubota et al., 1993; Mouchawar et al., 1992).

REFERENCES

Allessie MA, Bonke FIM, Schopman FJG (1976): Circus movement in rabbit atrial muscle as a mechanism of tachycardia. II. *Circ. Res.* 39: 168–77.

Allessie MA, Bonke FIM, Schopman FJG (1977): Circus movement in rabbit atrial muscle as a mechanism of tachycardia. III The 'leading circle' concept: A new model of circus movement in cardiac tissue without involvement of an anatomical obstacle. *Circ. Res.* 41: 9–18.

Bourland JD, Mouchawar GA, Nyenhuis JA, Geddes LA, Foster KS, Jones JT, Graber GP (1990): Transchest magnetic (eddy-current) stimulation of the dog heart. *Med. & Biol. Eng. & Comput.* 28: 196–8.

Cartee L (1991): The cellular response of excitable tissue models to extracellular stimulation. *Dept. Biomed. Eng., Duke Univ., Durham*, pp. 158. (Ph.D. thesis)

Cartee LA, Plonsey R (1992): Active response of a one-dimensional cardiac model with gap junctions to extracellular stimulation. *Med. & Biol. Eng. & Comput.* 30:(4) 389–98.

Chen Peng-S, Wolf PD, Ideker RE (1991): Mechanism of cardiac defibrillation: A different point of view. *Circulation* 84: 913–9.

Greatbatch W, Seligman LJ (1988): Pacemakers. In *Encyclopedia of Medical Devices and Instrumentation*, ed. JG Webster, pp. 2175–203, John Wiley & Sons, New York.

Ideker RE, Chen P-S, Shibata N, Colavita PG, Wharton JM (1987): Current concepts of the mechanisms of ventricular defibrillation. In *Nonpharmacological Theory of Tachyarrhythmias*, ed. G Breithardt, M Borggrefe, DP Zipes, pp. 449–64, Futura Pub. Co., Mount Kisco, New York.

Irwin DD, Rush S, Evering R, Lepeshkin E, Montgomery DB, Weggel RJ (1970): Stimulation of cardiac muscle by a time-varying magnetic field. *IEEE Trans. Magn.* Mag-6:(2) 321–2.

Janse MJ, Van Capelle FJL, Morsink H, Kléber AG, Wilms-Schopman FJG, Cardinal R, Naumann d'Alnoncourt C, Durrer D (1980): Flow of 'injury' current and patterns of excitation during early ventricular arrhythmias in acute regional myocardial ischemia in isolated porcine and canine hearts. *Circ. Res.* 47: 151–65.

Kerber RE (1990): External direct current defibrillation and cardioversion. In *Cardiac Electrophysiology,* ed. DP Zipes, J Jalife, pp. 954–9, W.B. Saunders, Philadelphia.

Kubota H, Yamaguchi M, Yamamoto I (1993): Development of magnetic defibrillator—Distribution of eddy-currents by stimulating coils. *J. Jpn. Biomagn. Bioelectromagn. Soc.* 6: 78–81.

Mines GR (1913): On dynamic equilibrium in the heart. *J. Physiol. (Lond.)* 46: 349–82.

Mouchawar GA, Bourland JD, Nyenhuis JA, Geddes LA, Foster KS, Jones JT, Graber GP (1992): Closed-chest cardiac stimulation with a pulsed magnetic field. *Med. & Biol. Eng. & Comput.* 30:(2) 162–8.

Plonsey R, Barr RC, Witkowski FX (1991): One-dimensional model of cardiac defibrillation. *Med. & Biol. Eng. & Comput.* 29:(5) 465–9.

Spach MS, Dolber PC (1985): The relation between discontinuous propagation in anisotropic cardiac muscle and the 'vulnerable period' of reentry. In *Cardiac Electrophysiology and Arrhythmias,* ed. DP Zipes, J Jalife, pp. 241–52, Grune and Stratton, Orlando.

Witkowski FX, Penkoske PA, Plonsey R (1990): Mechanism of cardiac defibrillation in open-chest dogs with unipolar DC-coupled simultaneous activation and shock potential recordings. *Circulation* 82:(1) 244–60.

VIII

Measurement of the Intrinsic Electric Properties of Biological Tissues

The third subdivision of bioelectromagnetism discusses the measurement of intrinsic electric and magnetic properties of biological tissue. Part VIII briefly discusses, for example, the measurement of tissue impedance and of the electrodermal response.

The measurement of tissue impedance was first applied to impedance plethysmography. The most successful application of this technique, however, is impedance cardiography, which can be used for the noninvasive measurement of the stroke volume. Impedance plethysmography has also other applications— for example, measurement of the amount of fluid in the pleural cavities or detection of thromboses in the veins of the legs. Impedance plethysmography has also been used successfully in detecting the gastric activity in small babies.

A new application of the impedance technique is impedance tomography, an attempt to image the electric conductivity of the body. Unlike x-ray tomography (CT scanning) and nuclear magnetic resonance imaging (NMRI), impedance tomography has not been very successful clinically. The reason for this is that the resolution of impedance measurements, even in two dimensions where most work has been performed, has been poor.

The electrodermal response has wide applications in psychophysiology. On this subject there is a large body of literature. For the sake of completenes of this book, the electrodermal response is briefly discussed.

Part VIII could have included a discussion of applications where magnetic properties of the tissue are measured: for example, magnetic susceptibility plethysmography and nuclear magnetic resonance imaging (NMRI). These are, however, not included to avoid an increase of the number of pages. It should also be noted that the first of these two techniques is not in clinical use, and the second, which involves the magnetic properties of the tissue on a nuclear level, is essentially outside the scope of this book. Because NMRI has been succesfully applied in clinical use there is also a very large literature on this subject elsewhere.

25

Impedance Plethysmography

25.1 INTRODUCTION

Impedance plethysmography is a method of determining changing tissue volumes in the body, based on the measurement of electric impedance at the body surface. This chapter presents the bioelectric basis of impedance plethysmography with emphasis on impedance cardiography—that is, determination of cardiac stroke volume. The first publications concerning this method date back to the 1930s and 1940s (Atzler and Lehmann, 1931; Rosa, 1940; Holzer, Polzer, and Marko, 1946; Nyboer et al., 1940; Nyboer, Bango, and Nims, 1943; Nyboer, 1950). The method reached clinical value about 20 years ago based on the research work by Kinnen, Kubicek, et al. (Kinnen et al., 1964a,b,c; Kubicek et al., 1966; Kubicek, Patterson, and Witsoe, 1970). A related method, *integral rheography*, for measuring the cardiac output was developed by Tiščenko and co-workers (1973). This method has, however, hardly been used outside the (former) Soviet Union.

Determination of the cardiac stroke volume is an area in which accurate, easily applied, noninvasive methods are needed. Impedance cardiography is easy to apply, noninvasive, and also cheap; however, it has serious methodological limitations, which are discussed below. We also provide a brief overview of other applications of impedance plethysmography.

The magnetic method corresponding to electric impedance plethysmography is called *magnetic susceptibility plethysmography*. This method may be used for monitoring blood volume changes in the thorax. Most living tissues are diamagnetic since water is their major constituent. If a strong magnetic field is applied to the region of the thorax, the movements of the heart, blood, and chest wall during the heart cycle cause variations in magnetic flux. Thus it is possible to monitor these variations with a SQUID magnetometer during the heart cycle (Wikswo, 1975; Maniewski et al., 1988). Currently, magnetic susceptibility plethysmography does not have clinical applications and, therefore, this method is not discussed in detail in this book.

25.2 BIOELECTRIC BASIS OF IMPEDANCE PLETHYSMOGRAPHY

25.2.1 Relationship Between the Principles of Impedance Measurement and Bioelectric Signal Measurement

As discussed in Chapter 1 and illustrated in Figure 1.3, the measurement of tissue impedance is closely connected to other parts of this book. This is so because the sensitivity distribution of the impedance measurement may be determined with the aid of lead field theory. Through the lead field theoretic approach we may conclude that any change in the conductivity of a region produces in the impedance signal a change which is proportional to the amount of current flowing in that region. (To be accurate, a change in the conductivity changes the distribution of the introduced current in the volume conductor as well. This is, of course, also true in any lead field analysis in the measurement of bioelectric and biomagnetic sources.)

Otto H. Schmitt first suggested that the concept of lead field could be used in connection with impedance plethysmography. David Geselowitz (1971) mathematically proved this relationship between the measured impedance changes and the changes in conductivity within a volume conductor. John Lehr (1972) later presented another proof of this relationship. In the following we give the result of Geselowitz using the terminology and sign convention of this book. (Note that Geselowitz (1971) defined the lead fields as the electric fields per reciprocal current and we define them as the current fields per unit reciprocal current. These are, of course, directly related by Ohm's law.)

$$\Delta Z = \int_v \frac{1}{\Delta \sigma} \bar{J}_{LE}(t_0) \cdot \bar{J}_{LI}(t_1) \, dv \quad (25.1)$$

where

ΔZ = impedance change [Ω/m^3]
t_0, t_1 = time instants
$\Delta \sigma$ = conductivity change between the two
      time instants [S/m = $1/\Omega \cdot$ m]
$\bar{J}_{LE}$ = lead field of the voltage measurement
      electrodes for unit reciprocal current
      [$1/m^2$]
$\bar{J}_{LI}$ = lead field of the current feeding
      electrodes for unit current [$1/m^2$]
v = volume [m^3]

In Equation 25.1, the region v consists of an inhomogeneous volume conductor whose conductivity (as a function of position) at time t_0 is $\sigma(t_0)$. At t_1, this has changed to $\sigma(t_1)$, and it is this change $\sigma(t_1) - \sigma(t_0) = \Delta\sigma$ which is responsible for the measured impedance change ΔZ. Thus Equation 25.1 describes how the changes in volume conductor conductivity are converted into the impedance change evaluated

from a measured voltage (at the voltage electrode pair) divided by applied current (at the current electrode pair). Note that the 4-electrode impedance method underlies Equation 25.1.

A special case of Equation 25.1 is one where we consider $\sigma(t_1) = \epsilon\sigma(t_0)$, where ϵ is very small:

$$Z = \int_v \frac{1}{\sigma} \bar{J}_{LE} \cdot \bar{J}_{LI} dv \quad (25.2)$$

where all variables are evaluated at t_0. Equation 25.2 describes how the macroscopic resistivity Z (impedance per unit volume) is derived from the spatial distribution of conductivity σ weighted by the dot product of the lead fields of the current and voltage electrodes. Note the similarity between Equation 25.2 and the fundamental equation of the lead field theory, Equation 11.30 (or 11.52), which describes the electric signal in the lead produced by a volume source formed by a distribution of the impressed current $\bar{J}^i$. In these equations the corresponding variables are the measured signals: V_{LE} and Z (= measured voltage per applied current), the distributions of sensitivity: $\bar{J}_{LE}$ in both of them, as well as the source distributions: $\bar{J}^i$ and $\bar{J}_{LI}$.

If the introduction of the current is done with the same electrodes as the voltage measurement is made, the sensitivity distribution, that is the lead field $\bar{J}_{LE}$ is the same as the distribution of the applied current $\bar{J}_{LI}$. This technique is, however, seldom used because of the artifact due to the electrode impedance. If the current-feeding electrodes are different from those of the voltage measurement electrodes, the sensitivity distribution is the dot product of the lead fields of the voltage electrodes $\bar{J}_{LE}$ and the current electrodes $\bar{J}_{LI}$. Thus, any previous discussion in this book on the electric and magnetic lead fields in general (Chapters 11 and 12), in the head (Chapters 13 and 14) or in the thorax (Chapters 15–18 and 20) may readily be applied to impedance plethysmography. Just as in the study of electrocardiography, one can design electrode systems for impedance measurement to give special emphasis to particular regions (the aorta, the ventricles, etc.). One can even have situations where the dot product is negative in a particular region so that if the conductivity increases in that region, the impedance Z will also increase. Some examples can be found in Plonsey and Collin (1977) and Penney (1986).

While Equation 25.1 is a suitable theoretical basis for impedance plethysmography, we are still left with considerable uncertainty how σ varies throughout the heart and torso or in what way the circulation modifies the thorax structure and conductivity as a function of time throughout the cardiac cycle. Further research is required to develop a physiologically adequate circulation model. Note, however, that Equation 25.1 may be more readily applied over a longer time frame ($t_1 - t_0$) to, say, the growth of a localized tumor in the thorax (other regions remaining the same).

25.2.2 Tissue Impedance

The physical quantity measured in impedance plethysmography (and imaged in impedance tomography) is tissue impedance. (The impedance of various tissues was discussed in Section 7.4.) From Table 7.3 it can be seen that the resistivity of body organs varies about 100-fold from about 1.6 Ωm in blood to about 170 Ωm in bone. Within the soft tissues the variability is about 10-fold, with about 20 Ωm in the lung and in fat.

In measuring bioelectric sources the reactive component of tissue impedance is not important because the frequency range is under 1 kHz. Actually, in Section 7.2.4 it was shown that it can be omitted with the assumption of quasistationarity. In impedance plethysmography (and tomography) the frequency dependence of tissue impedance is a factor which can be utilized for increasing the selectivity of the system. Because the impedance of different tissues has different reactive components, the impedance may be measured with applied currents at different frequencies (Lozano, Rosell, and Pallás-Areny, 1990). The frequencies may be selected so that the separation of certain tissues is maximized. With appropriate filtering the measurement may be done simultaneously with different frequencies in order to save measurement time.

A useful method for illustrating the behavior of tissue impedance as a function of frequency is the Cole-Cole plot (Cole and Cole, 1941). In this presentation, real component R is plotted versus imaginary component X in the complex series impedance ($R + jX$) with the frequency as a parameter. Figure 25.1B shows the Cole-Cole plot of a three-element impedance with a single time constant, as shown in Figure

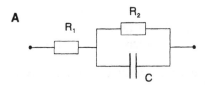

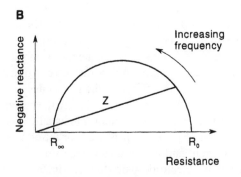

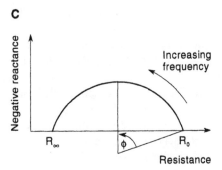

Fig. 25.1 (A) Three-element model of tissue impedance exhibiting a single time constant. (B) Cole-Cole plot for impedance with a single time constant. (C) The depressed Cole-Cole plot.

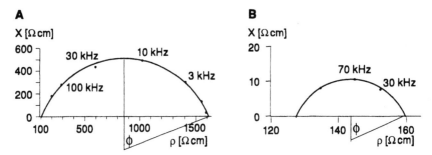

Fig. 25.2 Cole-Cole plots for (A) transverse and (B) longitudinal impedances of skeletal muscle.(Redrawn from Epstein and Foster, 1983.)

25.1A. The Cole-Cole plot obeys the following equation:

$$Z_f = R_\infty + \frac{R_0 - R_\infty}{1 + j\omega\tau}$$

$$= R_\infty + \frac{R_0 - R_\infty}{1 + \omega^2\tau^2} - j\omega\tau\frac{R_0 - R_\infty}{1 + \omega^2\tau^2}$$ (25.3)

where

Z_f = impedance (as a function of frequency f)
R_0 = resistance at $f = 0$
R_∞ = resistance at $f = \infty$
τ = time constant (R_2C)

The Cole-Cole plot is a semicircle with radius $(R_0 - R_\infty)/2$ which intercepts the real axis at R_0 and R_∞, a conclusion that can be verified by noting that the real (Re) and imaginary (Im) parts of Equation 25.3 satisfy

$$\left(Re - \frac{R_0 + R_\infty}{2}\right)^2 + Im^2 = \left(\frac{R_0 - R_\infty}{4}\right)^2$$ (25.4)

The right-hand side of Equation 25.4 is a constant where one recognizes the equation to be that of a circle whose center is at Im = 0, Re = $(R_0 + R_\infty)/2$ with a radius of $(R_0 - R_\infty)/2$, as stated. In the three-element circuit of Figure 25.1A, $R_0 = R_1 + R_2$, $R_\infty = R_1$, and $\tau = R_2C$.

In practice, the center of the semicircle is not necessarily on the real axis, but is located beneath it. The equation representing practical measurements may be described by Equation 25.4 (Schwan and Kay, 1957):

$$Z_f = R_\infty + \frac{R_0 - R_\infty}{1 + j\omega\tau^{(1-\alpha)}}$$ (25.5)

In the corresponding Cole-Cole plot, shown in Figure 25.1C, the depression angle is $\phi = (1 - \alpha)\pi/2$. Figure 25.2 shows the depression of the semicircle in the Cole-Cole plots for the transverse and longitudinal impedances of skeletal muscle as measured by Epstein and Foster (1983).

The reactive component of human blood has been studied, for example, by Tanaka et al. (1970) and Zhao (1992). The reactive component of tissue impedance seems to have an important role in impedance plethysmography, as will be discussed later in this chapter in connection with determining body composition.

25.3 IMPEDANCE CARDIOGRAPHY

25.3.1 Measurement of the Impedance of the Thorax

The impedance measurement is made by introducing an electric current in the frequency range of 20–100 kHz into the volume conductor and measuring the corresponding voltage. The ratio of voltage to current gives impedance Z. Usually the DC value is eliminated and only the impedance variation ΔZ is further examined. To eliminate the effect of the electrodes, separate electrode pairs for introducing the current and for measuring the voltage are usually used; the outer electrode pair is used for introducing the current and the voltage is measured across the inner electrode pair (though, in fact, any electrode pair may be chosen for current and for voltage).

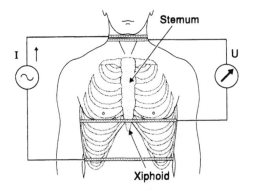

Fig. 25.3 Placement of the band electrodes in the measurement of the thorax impedance.

The impedance of the thorax is measured longitudinally by four band electrodes, shown in Figure 25.3. In the physical arrangement of the outer pair, one electrode is placed around the abdomen and the other around the upper part of the neck. For the inner electrode pair, one electrode is placed around the thorax at the level of the joint between the *xiphoid* and the *sternum*, called the *xiphisternal joint*, and the other around the lower part of the neck. In recent studies of impedance cardiography, the band electrodes are often replaced with normal ECG electrodes.

Figure 25.4 presents a typical thorax impedance curve (Z), its first time derivative (*dZ/dt*), and the simultaneous electrocardiogram (ECG), and phonocardiogram (PCG) curves. The impedance curve is usually shown so that a decrease in impedance results in an increase in the y-axis magnitude. This sign convention describes the changing admittance; for example, a decreasing impedance could arise from an increasing amount of low impedance blood in the thorax. The polarity of the first derivative curve is consistent with the impedance curve.

25.3.2 Simplified Model of the Impedance of the Thorax

In a very simple model, the impedance of the thorax can be considered to be divided into two

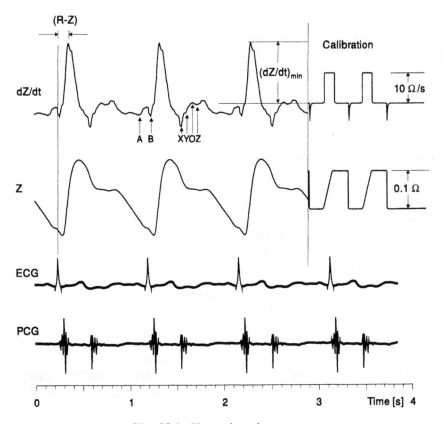

Fig. 25.4 Thorax impedance curve.

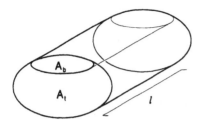

Fig. 25.5 Simplified cylindrical model of the average thorax containing a uniform blood and tissue compartment for determining the net torso impedance.

parts: the impedance of both tissue and fluids, as illustrated in Figure 25.5. If the patient does not breathe, all components forming the impedance of the thorax are constant, except the amount and distribution of blood.

The amount of blood in the thorax changes as a function of the heart cycle. During systole, the right ventricle ejects an amount of blood into the lungs which equals the stroke volume. Subsequently, blood flows from the lungs to the left atrium. The effect of these changes in the distribution of blood in the thorax as a function of the heart cycle can be determined by measuring the impedance changes of the thorax. The problem is to determine cardiac stroke volume as a function of changes in thoracic impedance.

25.3.3 Determining Changes in Blood Volume in the Thorax

To relate blood volume changes to impedance changes, we use the simplified model of the thorax, described in Figure 25.5. We designate the cross sections of blood and tissue and their longitudinal impedances by A_b, A_t, Z_b, and Z_t, respectively. The total longitudinal impedance of the model is

$$Z = \frac{Z_b Z_t}{Z_b + Z_t} \qquad (25.6)$$

where

Z = longitudinal impedance of the model
Z_b = impedance of the blood volume
Z_t = impedance of the tissue volume

The relationship between the impedance change of the thorax and the impedance change of the blood volume is found by differentiating Equation 25.6 with respect to Z_b:

$$dZ = \frac{Z^2}{Z_b^2} dZ_b \qquad (25.7)$$

The impedance of the blood volume with blood resistivity ρ_b based on the cylindrical geometry of Figure 25.5, is:

$$Z_b = \frac{\rho_b l}{A_b} \qquad (25.8)$$

where

ρ_b = blood resistivity
A_b = cross section of the blood area
l = length of the thorax model

The relationship between changes in blood volume v_b and the blood impedance is found by solving for the blood volume in Equation 25.8 and differentiating:

$$dv_b = d(lA_b) = - \frac{\rho_b l^2}{Z_b^2} dZ_b \qquad (25.9)$$

where

v_b = blood volume

We finally derive the dependence of the change in blood volume on the change in thoracic impedance by solving for dZ_b in Equation 25.7 and substituting it into Equation 25.9:

$$dv_b = - \frac{\rho_b l^2}{Z^2} dZ \qquad (25.10)$$

25.3.4 Determining the Stroke Volume

When determining stroke volume from thoracic impedance changes, Kubicek and colleagues (1966) and Kubicek (1968) made some assumptions concerning the relationship between stroke volume and net change in the thorax blood volume as evaluated in Equation 25.10. These assumptions are highly simplified and may be unreliable.

As was mentioned earlier, during systole, the right ventricle ejects a volume of blood into the lungs. At the same time blood flows away from the lungs to the left atrium. The stroke volume can thus be determined from the impedance curve by extrapolating to the impedance (ΔZ), that would result if no blood were to flow out of the lungs during systole. (The underlying assumption is that ΔZ is determined mainly by changes in lung conductivity.)

In this extrapolation, it is assumed that if no blood were to flow away from the thorax during systole, the thorax impedance would continuously decrease during systole at a rate equal to the maximum rate of decrease of Z. Thus, ΔZ can be approximated graphically by drawing a tangent to the impedance curve at the point of its maximum rate of decrease, as illustrated in Figure 25.6. Then, the difference between the impedance values of the tangent line at the beginning and at the end of the ejection time is ΔZ.

The value of ΔZ is easy to determine with the help of the first derivative curve of the thoracic impedance signal. According to the definition of the derivative:

$$\frac{\Delta Z}{\Delta t} = f'(Z) \qquad (25.11)$$

Assuming that Δt equals the ejection time t_e, ΔZ can be determined from equation

$$\Delta Z = f'(Z) \cdot t_e \qquad (25.12)$$

With the above assumptions, the impedance change ΔZ can be determined by multiplying the ejection time by the minimum value of the first derivative of the impedance curve (that is, the maximum slope magnitude; the reader must remember that the slope is negative).

Finally, the formula for determining the stroke volume is obtained by substituting Equation 25.12 into Equation 25.10, which gives:

$$SV = \rho_b \frac{l^2}{Z^2} \left| \frac{dZ}{dt} \right|_{min} \cdot t_e \qquad \textbf{(25.13)}$$

where

SV = stroke volume [ml]
ρ_b = resistivity of the blood [$\Omega \cdot$ cm]
l = mean distance between the inner electrodes [cm]
Z = mean impedance of the thorax [Ω]
$\left| \dfrac{dZ}{dt} \right|_{min}$ = absolute value of the maximum deviation of the first derivative signal during systole [Ω/s]
t_e = ejection time [s]

The ejection time can be determined from the first-derivative impedance curve with the help of the phonocardiogram or carotid pulse. Then, the impedance curve itself is used only for control purposes (e.g., checking the breathing).

The resistivity of the blood is of the order of 160 Ωcm. Its value depends on hematocrit, as discussed in Section 7.4.1.

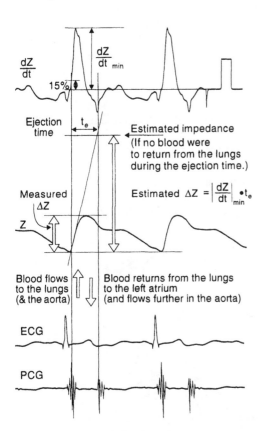

Fig. 25.6 Determination of the impedance change corresponding to the stroke volume.

25.3.5 Discussion of the Stroke Volume Calculation Method

The method described above, developed by Kinnen and Kubicek, is widely used to estimate stroke volume from impedance recordings. We discuss later efforts to identify the source or sources of the measured changes in impedance. It will be seen that such research implicates changes in blood volume in the vena cava, atria, ventricles, aorta, thoracic musculature, and lungs. Obviously, the two-compartment model, above, is a gross simplification. Furthermore, the assumed cylindrical geometry is also a highly simplified approximation. And, finally, the change of blood conductivity with change in velocity has been entirely neglected in this model.

25.4   ORIGIN OF IMPEDANCE SIGNAL IN IMPEDANCE CARDIOGRAPHY

25.4.1   Model Studies

Kinnen et al. (1964c) constructed a cylindrical thorax model to investigate the origin of the impedance signal (see Fig. 25.7). The inner cylinder represents the blood volume of the heart and the primary arteriovenous system of the thorax. The medium outside the inner cylinder represented the lungs. In this model, the computed resistance for the inner cylinder was 495 Ω and for the interspace 32 Ω. These values indicated that most of the current flux would tend to travel through the model's lungs so that the origin of the impedance signal should be based primarily on the right ventricle. This is consistent with observations in patients with septal defects (Lababidi et al., 1971). In these patients the cardiac output, measured by im-

pedance plethysmography, correlates well with the blood flow in the pulmonary circulation.

Sakamoto et al. (1979) constructed an anatomically more realistic model in which changes in vena cava, heart, lungs, aorta, and torso shape were investigated (see Fig. 25.8). The model permits an examination of the effect of conductivity changes of component structures on the measured impedance. The weakness in this work is that one does not know what quantitative changes in conductivity are brought about as a result of real or simulated blood circulation. Sakamoto et al. (1979) also did studies with dogs and humans where they measured the isopotential lines on the surface of the thorax.

25.4.2   Animal and Human Studies

Compared to the model studies, some practical experiments performed on animals gave different results concerning the origin of the signal. Baker, Hill, and Pale (1974) cite an experiment performed on a calf in which the natural heart was replaced by an implanted prosthesis containing artificial right and left ventricles. In this experiment the ventricles were operated either simultaneously or separately. The contribution of the left ventricle to the impedance signal was 62% of the total signal whereas that from the right ventricle was 38%.

Witsoe and Kottke (1967) conducted experiments with dogs, using venous occlusion achieved by an inflated ball. In these experi-

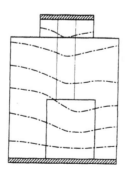
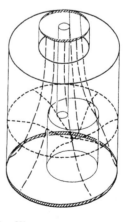

Fig. 25.7   Thorax model by Kinnen.

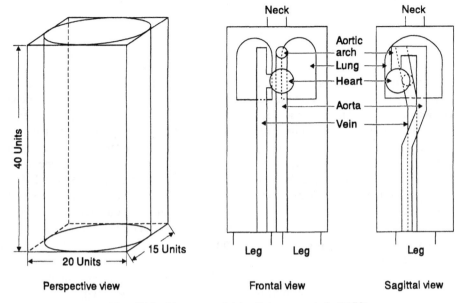

Fig. 25.8 Thorax model by Sakamoto et al. (1979).

ments the origin of the impedance signal was found to be contributed totally by the left ventricle. (This is also seen in humans.) Stroke volume measurements with impedance plethysmography on patients with aortic valve insufficiency give values that are too high.

Penney (1986) summarized a number of studies and estimated, on the base of these observations, the contributions to the impedance signal shown in Table 25.1.

Mohapatra (1981) conducted a critical analysis of a number of hypotheses concerning the origin of the cardiac impedance signal. He concluded that it was due to cardiac hemodynamics only. Furthermore, the signal reflects both a change in the blood velocity as well as change in blood volume. The changing speed of ejection has its primary effect on the systolic behavior of ΔZ whereas the changing volume (mainly

of the atria and great veins) affects the diastolic portion of the impedance curve.

These facts point out that the weakest feature of impedance plethysmography is that the source of the signal is not accurately known. Additional critical comments may be found in Mohapatra (1988).

25.4.3 Determining the Systolic Time Intervals from the Impedance Signal

Lababidi et al. (1970) carefully studied the timing of each significant notch in the first derivative curve of the thoracic impedance signal and assigned them to certain events in the heart cycle. According to their study, the relationship is as shown in Table 25.2 (see also Fig. 25.3).

Table 25.1 Origin of the impedance signal in impedance cardiography

Contributing organ	Contribution
Vena cava and right atrium	+20%
Right ventricle	−30%
Pulmonary artery and lungs	+60%
Pulmonary vein and left atrium	+20%
Left ventricle	−30%
Aorta and thoracic musculature	+60%

Source: Penney (1986)

Table 25.2 Timing of various notches in the first derivative impedance signal in impedance cardiography.

Event in the cardiac cycle	Notch
Atrial contraction	A
Closure of tricuspid valve	B
Closure of aortic valve	X
Closure of pulmonic valve	Y
Opening snap of mitral valve	O
Third heart sound	Z

Source: Lababidi et al. (1970)

The first-derivative impedance curve can be used with some accuracy in timing various events in the cardiac cycle. The ejection time can be determined as the time between where the dZ/dt curve crosses the zero line after the B point, and the X point. However, in general, the determination of ejection time from the dZ/dt curve is more complicated. Thus, the need of the phonocardiogram in determining the ejection time depends on the quality and clarity of the dZ/dt curve. Though the timing of the various notches of the dZ/dt curve is well known, the origins of the main deflections are not well understood.

25.4.4 The Effect of the Electrodes

In impedance plethysmography, the current is fed from a constant current generator to the thorax by an electrode pair, and the voltage generated by this current is measured by another electrode pair. With a well-designed constant current generator the current in the thorax can be maintained constant despite electrode skin resistance changes. The mean impedance of the thorax is about 20 Ω. Consequently, the source impedance for the detected voltage is very low. If the voltmeter circuit is designed to have a high input impedance, the contact resistance can be neglected. In commercially manufactured equipment, the impedance is about 100 $k\Omega$, in comparison to which the effects of contact impedance changes lie within an acceptable level (Kubicek, 1968).

Hill, Jaensen, and Fling (1967) have introduced a critical comment concerning the effect of the contact impedance on the signal: they claim that the entire signal is an electrode artifact. Based on the preceding arguments and the experiments concerning the origin of the signal (Lababidi et al., 1971; Baker, Hill, and Pale, 1974) these claims can be ignored.

The effect of changes in the mean thoracic impedance has also been investigated (Hill and Lowe, 1973). Placement of a defibrillator back electrode under the back of a supine patient changed the mean impedance recorded by the instrument by up to 20%, but did not have any significant influence on the stroke volume value determined by the instrument, because of a simultaneous change in $(dZ/dt)_{min}$, which compensated for the change in Z. This is easily seen by noting that stroke volume is proportional to Z^{-2}, whereas dZ is proportional to Z^2. Slight displacement of the detector electrodes changes the measured mean impedance and first derivative signal, but their effect on the computed stroke volume is compensated by the changed value of the mean distance of the electrodes. This is also easy to prove using the previous theory. It is also interesting to note that the signals remain unchanged when one half of the lower detector electrode is removed (Hill and Lowe, 1973). This implies that the electrode is situated on an equipotential surface, thus supporting the assumption of cylindrical symmetry.

25.4.5 Accuracy of the Impedance Cardiography

Today, more than one hundred publications exist on the accuracy of impedance cardiography. Lamberts, Visser, and Ziljstra (1984) have made an extensive review of 76 studies. In this chapter we discuss some representative studies where the accuracy of impedance cardiography has been evaluated. These can be divided into two main categories. In the first category the effect of the hematocrit on the blood resistivity is ignored and a constant value is used in the calculations for the resistivity of blood, usually 150 Ωcm. In the second category, the value of the blood resistivity is first determined for each subject.

Experiments Where the Blood Resistivity Is Constant

Kinnen and co-workers (1964b) determined the stroke volume from the equation

$$SV = \frac{\Delta Z}{Z} v_{tx} \qquad (25.13)$$

where

ΔZ = change of the impedance of the thorax
Z = mean value of the impedance of the thorax
v_{tx} = volume of the thorax between the inner electrode pair

They used the Fick principle as a reference for evaluating stroke volume. (The Fick principle determines the cardiac output from the oxygen consumption and the oxygen contents of the atrial and venous bloods.) In a study of six subjects at various exercise levels, the correlation between the impedance and Fick cardiac outputs was $r = .962$, with an estimated standard error of 12% of the average value of the cardiac output.

Harley and Greenfield (1968) performed two series of experiments with simultaneous dye dilution and impedance techniques. They estimated ΔZ from the impedance curve itself, instead of using the first-derivative technique. In the first experiment, 13 healthy male subjects were examined before and after an intravenous infusion of isoproterenol. The mean indicator dilution cardiac output was 6.3 ℓ/min before and 9.5 ℓ/min after infusion. The ratios of the cardiac outputs measured with impedance plethysmography and indicator dilution were 1.34 and 1.23, respectively. This difference ($p > .2$) was not significant. The second experiment included 24 patients with heart disease, including aortic and mitral insufficiencies. A correlation coefficient of $r = .26$ was obtained for this data. The poor correlation was caused in those cases with aortic and mitral insufficiency.

Bache, Harley, and Greenfield (1969) performed an experiment with eight patients with various types of heart disease excluding valvular insufficiencies. As a reference they used the pressure gradient technique. Individual correlation coefficients ranged from .58 to .96 with an overall correlation coefficient as low as .28.

Baker et al. (1971) compared the impedance and radioisotope dilution values of cardiac output for 17 normal male subjects before and after exercise. The regression function for this data was $CO_Z = 0.80 \cdot CO_I + 4.3$ with a correlation coefficient $r = .58$. The comparison between the paired values before and after exercise showed better correlation for the impedance technique. Baker examined another group of 10 normal male subjects by both impedance and dye techniques. In 21 measurements the regression function was $CO_Z = 1.06 \cdot CO_D + 0.52$, with correlation coefficient $r = .68$. In addition to this set of data, the impedance cardiac output was determined by using individual resistivity values determined from the hematocrit. The relation between resistivity and Hct was, however, not mentioned.

In this case, the regression function was CO_Z = $0.96 \cdot CO_D + 0.56$ with correlation coefficient $r = .66$. A set of measurements was performed also on 11 dogs using electromagnetic flowmeters and the impedance technique. A comparison of 214 paired data points was made with intravenous injections of epinephrine, norepinephrine, acetylcholine, and isoproterenol. Values of the correlation coefficients from each animal ranged from .58 to .98 with a mean value of .92. The first two experiments of this paper are also presented in Judy et al. (1969).

Experiments with Individual Resistivity Values

Lababidi et al. (1971) studied 95 children with various types of congenital heart disease using dye dilution and Fick principles as reference methods. In 20 subjects, paired impedance-dye dilution values had an average absolute difference of 6.6% ranging from -12% to $+13\%$ with a standard deviation of 0.259 ℓ/min/m^2. Paired impedance-cardiac output values had an absolute difference of 3.1%, ranging from -15% to $+3.2\%$ with a standard deviation of 0.192 ℓ/min/m^2. The F-test showed the reproducibility of both methods to be similar: $F = 1.82$ and $p > .05$. For 53 sequential determinations of impedance cardiac output and dye dilution, the absolute mean difference was -1.8%, $t = 1.19$ and $p > .05$. When determining, sequentially, the relationship between Fick and dye dilution principles, 37 of 39 points fell within 20% limits. The absolute mean difference was 8.3%, and the algebraic mean difference was $+3.4\%$. The correlation between impedance and Fick cardiac outputs was $r = .97$. These studies were performed with patients without intracardiac shunts or valvular insufficiencies.

A comparison of impedance cardiac output to Fick systemic cardiac output in patients with left to right shunts showed the correlation to be poor: $r = .21$. However, a comparison of the impedance cardiac output to the Fick pulmonary blood flow in these cases gave a correlation of $r = .96$ (see Fig. 25.9).

Baker, Hill, and Pale (1974) compared impedance and dye dilution cardiac outputs in three dogs and got a correlation of $r = .879$.

Malmivuo (1974) compared impedance and Fick methods in 18 patients without valvular incompetencies, but with one subject having a

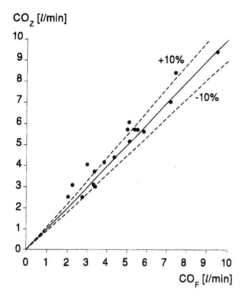

Fig. 25.9 Comparison of the impedance and Fick methods in determining the pulmonary blood flow.

ers the correlation coefficient r, then between Fick and dye dilution $.95 < r < .999$; Fick and thermodilution $.70 < r < .99$; Fick to carbon dioxide breathing, $r = .94$; dye to thermodilution, $.68 < r < .99$.

25.5   OTHER APPLICATIONS OF IMPEDANCE PLETHYSMOGRAPHY

25.5.1   Peripheral Blood Flow

Impedance plethysmography is also a convenient method for conducting measurements of blood volume changes in applications other than cardiac stroke volume. The peripheral circulation can be studied by using an inflated cuff for blocking the venous flow and monitoring the blood volume increase in the limb. In such studies, Equation 25.9 is readily applicable (van de Water et al., 1971). Yamamoto, Yamamoto, and Öberg (1991, 1992) have made technical and theoretical studies of the impedance plethysmography technique for measuring the blood flow in human limbs.

Concerning the accuracy of impedance plethysmography in determining peripheral blood flow, there are much fewer data available as few detailed experiments have been published. Van de Water et al. (1971) reported on a series of measurements in a hind limb of a dog using an electromagnetic flowmeter as a reference method. A correlation of $r = .962$ was obtained, using a constant value for the resistivity of the blood.

left to right shunt. For this special subject a comparison was made to pulmonary blood flow. The regression function was $CO_Z = 0.97 \cdot CO_F + 0.45$ yielding a correlation coefficient of $r = .97$ (see Fig. 25.8).

Malmivuo, Orko, and Luomanmäki (1975) compared impedance and Fick methods in 11 patients with atrial fibrillation and without intracardiac shunts or valvular insufficiencies. The regression function was $CO_Z = 1.05 \cdot CO_F + 0.1$, with a correlation coefficient of $r = .96$.

25.5.2   Cerebral Blood Flow

There are also applications where impedance plethysmography was used in an attempt to monitor cerebral blood flow. In these experiments one should be extremely careful in electrode placement to ensure that the impedance signal comes mainly from the intracranial region. As can be seen from the discussion in Section 13.4, even in the case where the bipolar leads in the inhomogeneous concentric spherical head model are located at opposite sides of the model, more than one third of the lead field current flows outside the skull. By moving the

Other Studies

Additional studies of the correlation between impedance methods and cardiac output reference techniques are summarized in Penney (1986). The results are generally similar to those described above. From these studies one can conclude that impedance cardiography is satisfactory for the determination of relative cardiac output for most normals. Under conditions of hypoxia, drugs, ventilatory maneuvers, and so on, the correlation may become poor.

In evaluating the significance of a particular correlation coefficient between impedance and reference methods, Penney points out that the reference methods themselves are not completely consistent. For example, if one consid-

electrodes closer to each other, the relative amount of current outside the skull increases rapidly.

From this it is easy to deduce that if the impedance measurement is made with electrodes placed on one side of the head only or if, when using circular band electrodes, the electrodes are relatively close to each other, the major part of the signal comes from the blood flow in the scalp, not from that in the brain area. This shading effect of the skull does not show up as clearly in the EEG-measurement, because no bioelectric sources exist outside the skull (Malmivuo, 1992).

25.5.3 Intrathoracic Fluid Volume

Impedance plethysmography technique can also be used for monitoring intrathoracic fluids other than blood. The fluid in the pleural cavity has a considerable effect on the mean impedance of the thorax. Equation 25.9 can again be used to monitor the pleural fluid changes in the thorax (van de Water et al. 1971).

Van de Water et al. (1971) infused 400 cm^3 of saline in 25 cm^3 increments into a thoracic cavity of a dog weighing 15 kg. The regression formula between the infused saline volume and the thoracic impedance was $Z = 0.02281$ cm^3 $+ 46.944$ with a correlation coefficient of $r = .988$. They reported also one case when 900 cm^3 of pleural fluid was removed from a patient in 50 cm^3 increments. The regression formula in this case was $Z = 0.0024$ cm^3 $+ 17.57$, with a correlation coefficient of $r = .965$.

25.5.4 Determination of Body Composition

Bioelectric impedance may be used in determining the body composition. In this procedure the impedance is measured between one arm and one leg by feeding a current less than 1 mA rms at 50 kHz frequency. The determination of the body composition is based on measurement of the resistive and reactive components of the body impedance (Baumgartner, Chunlea, and Roche, 1988). With this method it is possible to estimate several parameters of the body composition such as total body water,

fat free mass, body cell mass, and caloric consumption (Kushner and Shoeller, 1986; Lukaski et al., 1985). De Vries et al. (1989) have applied this technique for determining intracellular and extracellular fluid volumes during hemodialysis.

25.5.5 Other Applications

There have been some attempts to use the impedance technique to monitor cardiac contractility. Siegel et al. (1970), in an experiment with dogs, quantified myocardial contractility and the first-derivative thoracic impedance signal. Myocardial contractility and vascular tone was altered by the use of norepinephrine, isoproterenol, and methoxamine. They measured the time from the peak of the ECG R wave to the peak first derivative of the isovolumic portion of the ventricular contraction (dp/dt_{min}) and to the inflection point in the first derivative of impedance (dZ/dt). From these curves they obtained a correlation of $r = .88$. This application has, however, not yet reached wide acceptance.

25.6 DISCUSSION

The reliability of impedance plethysmography has been the focus of much controversy. This is easy to understand if one considers the earlier publications concerning the accuracy of the method. In the experiments reviewed in the previous section, where a simplified form of the formula for determining stroke volume was used or the individual variation of the resistivity of the blood was ignored, the accuracy of impedance plethysmography was relatively poor. These experiments have also included patients with heart diseases not appropriate for the method. The reliability of the method in the experiments performed with more detailed knowledge concerning the application of impedance plethysmography seems to be considerably higher.

The method undoubtedly has some disadvantages. These include the errors caused by aortic valve insufficiency, severe mitral valve insufficiency, and shunts in the circulation in, for example, septal defects or tetralogy of Fallot. The method does not give any indication of the presence of these pathologies, and they must therefore be diagnosed by other means. The method is also difficult to apply to patients with atrial fibrillation.

On the other hand, impedance plethysmography is noninvasive and harmless. The accuracy of the method in careful examinations in patients, excluding the previously mentioned groups, gives promising results. The accuracy in determining the absolute value of cardiac output seems to be of the same order as the accuracy of the dilution methods. The accuracy in determining changes in cardiac output seems to be still higher.

As noted in the previous section, extreme care should be followed in applying impedance plethysmography to measuring the blood flow in the brain area to ensure that the recorded signal really originates mostly from the intracranial region.

REFERENCES

Atzler E, Lehmann G (1931–1932): Über ein Neues Verfahren zur Darstellung der Herztätigkeit (Dielektrographie). *Arbeitsphysiol.* 6: 636–80.

Bache RJ, Harley A, Greenfield JC (1969): Evaluation of thoracic impedance plethysmography as an indicator of stroke volume in man. *Am. J. Med. Sci.* 258:(8) 100–13.

Baker LE, Hill DW, Pale TD (1974): Comparison of several pulse-pressure techniques for monitoring stroke volume. *Med. Biol. Eng.* 12:(1) 81–8.

Baker LE, Judy WV, Geddes LE, Langley FM, Hill DW (1971): The measurement of cardiac output by means of electric impedance. *Cardiovasc. Res. Cent. Bull.* 9:(4) 135–45.

Baumgartner RN, Chunlea WG, Roche AF (1988): Bioelectric impedance phase angle and body composition. *Am. J. Clin. Nutr.* 48: 16–23.

Cole KS, Cole RH (1941): Dispersion and absorption in dielectrics. *J. Chem. Physics* 9: 341–51.

Epstein BR, Foster KR (1983): Anisotropy as a dielectric property of skeletal muscle. *Med. & Biol. Eng. & Comput.* 21:(1) 51–5.

Geselowitz DB (1971): An application of electrocardiographic lead theory to impedance plethysmography. *IEEE Trans. Biomed. Eng.* BME 18:(1) 38–41.

Harley A, Greenfield JC (1968): Determination of cardiac output in man by means of impedance plethysmography. *Aerospace Med.* 39:(3) 248–52.

Hill DW, Lowe HJ (1973): The use of the electrical impedance technique for the monitoring of cardiac output and limb blood flow during anesthesia. *Med. Biol. Eng.* 11:(5) 534–45.

Hill RV, Jaensen JC, Fling JL (1967): Electrical impedance plethysmography: A critical analysis. *J. Appl. Physiol.* 22:(1) 161–8.

Holzer W, Polzer K, Marko A (1946): *RKG. Rheography. A Method of Circulation's Investigation and Diagnosis in Circular Motion*, Wilhelm Maudrich, Vienna. (English transl.)

Judy WV, Langley FM, McCowen KD, Stinnet DM, Baker LE, Johnson PC (1969): Comparative evaluation of the thoracic impedance and isotope dilution methods for measuring cardiac output. *Aerospace Med.* 40: 532–6.

Kinnen E, Kubicek WG, Hill DW, Turton G (1964a): Thoracic cage impedance measurements: Impedance plethysmographic determination of cardiac output (A comparative study). *U.S. Air Force School of Aerospace Medicine, Brooks Air Force Base, Texas* SAM-TDR-64:(15) 8.

Kinnen E, Kubicek WG, Hill DW, Turton G (1964b): Thoracic cage impedance measurements: impedance plethysmographic determination of cardiac output (An interpretative study). *U.S. Air Force School of Aerospace Medicine, Brooks Air Force Base, Texas* SAM-TDR-64:(23) 12.

Kinnen E, Kubicek WG, Hill DW, Turton G (1964c): Thoracic cage impedance measurements, tissue resistivity in vivo and transthoracic impedance at 100 kc. *U.S. Air Force School of Aerospace Medicine, Brooks Air Force Base, Texas* SAM-TDR-64:(5) 14.

Kubicek WG (1968): *Minnesota Impedance Cardiograph Model 303. Instruction Manual*, 4 pp. Univ. of Minnesota Press, Minneapolis.

Kubicek WG, Karnegis JN, Patterson RP, Witsoe DA, Mattson RH (1966): Development and evaluation of an impedance cardiac output system. *Aerospace Med.* 37:(12) 1208–12.

Kubicek WG, Patterson RP, Witsoe DA (1970): Impedance cardiography as a non-invasive method for monitoring cardiac function and other parameters of the cardiovascular system. *Ann. N.Y. Acad. Sci.* 170: 724–32.

Kushner RF, Shoeller DA (1986): Estimation of total body water by bioelectrical impedance analysis. *Am. J. Clin. Nutr.* 44:(Sept.) 417–24.

Lababidi Z, Ehmke DA, Durnin RE, Leaverton PE, Lauer RM (1970): The first derivative thoracic impedance cardiogram. *Circulation* 41:(4) 651–8.

Lababidi Z, Ehmke DA, Durnin RE, Leaverton PE, Lauer RM (1971): Evaluation of impedance cardiac output in children. *Pediatr.* 47:(5) 870–9.

Lamberts R, Visser KR, Zijlstra WG (1984): *Impedance Cadiography*, 160 pp. Van Gorcum, Assen, The Netherlands.

Lehr J (1972): A vector derivation useful in impedance plethysmographic field calculations. *IEEE Trans. Biomed. Eng.* BME-19:(2) 156–7.

Lozano A, Rosell J, Pallás-Areny R (1990): Two-frequency impedance plethysmograph: real and imaginary parts. *Med. & Biol. Eng. & Comput.* 28:(1) 38–42.

Lukaski HC, Johnson PE, Bolonchuk WW, Lykken GI (1985): Assessment of fat-free mass using bioelectrical impedance measurement of the human body. *Am. J. Clin. Nutr.* 41:(April) 810–7.

Malmivuo JA (1974): *Impedance Plethysmography*, Helsinki University Central Hospital, I Medical Clinic, Helsinki. (Report)

Malmivuo JA (1992): Distribution of electric current in inhomogeneous volume conductors. In *Proceedings of the 8th Internat. Conference on Electrical Bio-Impedance*, ed. T Lahtinen, pp. 18–20, University of Kuopio, Center for Training and Development, Kuopio, Finland.

Malmivuo JA, Orko R, Luomanmäki K (1975): Validity of impedance cardiography in measuring cardiac output in patients with atrial fibrillation. In *Proceedings of the III Nordic Meeting on Medical and Biological Engineering*, ed. A Uusitalo, N Saranummi, pp. 58.1–3, Finnish Society for Medical and Biological Engineering, Tampere, Finland.

Maniewski R, Katila T, Poutanen T, Siltanen P, Varpula T, Wikswo JP (1988): Magnetic measurement of cardiac mechanical activity. *IEEE Trans. Biomed. Eng.* BME-35:(9) 662–70.

Mohapatra SN (1981): *Noninvasive Cardiovascular Monitoring of Electrical Impedance Technique*, Pitman, London.

Mohapatra SN (1988): Impedance cardiography. In *Encyclopedia of Medical Devices and Instruments*, ed. JG Webster, pp. 1622–32, John Wiley & Sons, New York.

Nyboer J (1950): Plethysmography. Impedance. In *Medical Physics*, Vol. 2, ed. O Glasser, pp. 736–43, Year Book Pub., Chicago.

Nyboer J, Bango S, Barnett A, Halsey RH (1940): Radiocardiograms: Electrical impedance changes of the heart in relation to electrocardiograms and heart sounds. *J. Clin. Invest.* 19: 773. (Abstract).

Nyboer J, Bango S, Nims LF (1943): The impedance plethysmograph and electrical volume recorder. *CAM Report, OSPR* : 149.

Penney BC (1986): Theory and cardiac applications of electrical impedance measurements. *CRC Crit. Rev. Bioeng.* 13: 227–81.

Plonsey R, Collin R (1977): Electrode guarding in electrical impedance measurements of physiological systems—A critique. *Med. & Biol. Eng. & Comput.* 15: 519–27.

Rosa L (1940): Diagnostische Anwendung des Kurzwellenfeldes in der Herz und Kreislaufpathologie (Radiokardiographie). *Z. Kreislaufforsch.* 32: 118–35.

Sakamoto K, Muto K, Kanai H, Iizuka M (1979): Problems of impedance cardiography. *Med. & Biol. Eng. & Comput.* 17:(6) 697–709.

Schwan HP, Kay CF (1957): Capacitive properties of body tissues. *Circ. Res.* 5:(4) 439–43.

Siegel JH, Fabian M, Lankau C, Levine M, Cole A, Nahmad M (1970): Clinical and experimental use of thoracic impedance plethysmography in quantifying myocardial contractility. *Surgery* 67: 907–17.

Tanaka K, Kanai H, Nakayama K, Ono N (1970): The impedance of blood: The effects of red cell orientation and its application. *Jpn. J. Med. Eng.* 8: 436–43.

Ti%s%cenko MI, Smirnov AD, Danilov LN, Aleksandrov AL (1973): Characteristics and clinical use of integral rheography. A new method of measuring the stroke volume. *Kardiologiia* 13: 54–62.

de Vries PMJM, Meijer JH, Vlaanderen K, Visser V, Donker AJM, Schneider H (1989): Measurement of transcellular fluid shift during haemodialysis. *Med. & Biol. Eng. & Comput.* 27:(March) 152–8.

van de Water JM, Dmochowski JR, Dove GB, Couch NP (1971): Evaluation of an impedance flowmeter in arterial surgery. *Surgery* 70:(6) 954–61.

van de Water JM, Philips PA, Thouin LG, Watanabe LS, Lappen RS (1971): Bioelectric impedance. New developments and clinical application. *Arch. Surg.* 102:(6) 541–7.

Wikswo JP (1975): Non-invasive magnetic measurement of the electrical and mechanical activity of the heart. *Stanford University, Stanford*, Thesis, pp. 304. (Ph.D. thesis)

Witsoe DA, Kottke FJ (1967): The origin of cardiogenic changes in thoracic electrical impedance (del Z). *Fed. Proc.* 26: 595. (Abstract No 1890).

Yamamoto Y, Yamamoto T, Öberg PÅ (1991): Impedance plethysmography in human limbs. Part 1. On electrodes and electrode geometry. *Med. & Biol. Eng. & Comput.* 29: 419–24.

Yamamoto Y, Yamamoto T, Öberg PÅ (1992): Impedance plethysmography for blood flow measurements in human limbs. Part 2. Influence of limb cross-sectional area. *Med. & Biol. Eng. & Comput.* 30:(Sept.) 518–24.

Zhao T (1992): Electrical capacitance of human blood. In *Proc. Of the 8th Internat. Conf. Of Electrical Bioimpedance*, 1st ed. Vol. 1, ed. T Lahtinen, pp. 185–7, University of Kuopio, Kuopio, Finland.

26

Impedance Tomography

26.1 INTRODUCTION

In the previous chapter, in which impedance plethysmography was discussed, the impedance signal was one single signal detected between a single pair of electrodes. Thus it represented the average impedance of the region between those electrodes, weighted by the dot product between the lead field of the measurement electrodes and the current feeding electrodes (see Equation 25.2).

The spatial resolution of the impedance measurement may be enhanced by using an array of electrodes around the volume conductor of interest. Electric current may be fed consecutively through different available electrode pairs and the corresponding voltage measured consecutively by all remaining electrode pairs. In this way it is possible, by using certain reconstruction algorithms, to create an image of the impedance of different regions of the volume conductor. This imaging method is called *impedance imaging*. Because the image is usually constructed in two dimensions from a slice of the volume conductor, the method is also called *impedance tomography* and *ECCT* (electric current computed tomography). Thus impedance tomography is an imaging method which may be used to complement *x-ray tomography* (computer tomography, CT), *ultra-*

sound imaging, positron emission tomography (PET), and others. The reader may find more information about the modern medical imaging methods from such references as Krestel (1990), Webb (1992), and Wells (1982).

In creating an image, it is desirable to limit the region which is involved and to know the geometry of this region. In general, this is known accurately only if the energy signal proceeds linearly. This condition is satisfied for x-rays and for nuclear radiation. It is also true in ordinary photography with the addition that the light rays bend in the lens in an accurately known way. If the radiating energy proceeds along an unknown path, or if it proceeds from the source to the target via several paths (i.e., through a large volume), it is not possible to create an accurate image. As examples of this in photography (or vision), one may mention the halo around the sun or the mirage.

In impedance tomography the fundamental problem in the image reconstruction is that, in a general case, the electric current cannot be forced to flow linearly (or even along a known path) in an inhomogeneous volume conductor. Since there are no sources within the volume conductor (the sources all lie on the bounding surface in the form of applied currents) then the potential field, Φ, must satisfy $\nabla \cdot (\sigma \nabla \Phi) = 0$ and only a limited class of functions can satisfy this. When σ is a constant then Φ satisfies Laplace's equation and, thus, even fewer functional forms are available (such as Legendre polynomials, etc.). As was shown in Section 11.6.9, it is possible to create a linear current field in a *homogeneous* volume conductor of arbitrary shape. In the sense of impedance tomography such a volume conductor is, however, of minor interest, because its image would be 50% gray (i.e., uniform) throughout.

The accuracy of these images is not, however, limited by the size of the electrodes, as it is by the size of the focus of the x-ray tube and the detector in computer tomography. In impedance imaging, the image is blurred because in an inhomogeneous volume conductor the path of the electric current is not linear and in the general case it is not known accurately.

It should be noted that, though the basic purpose of impedance tomography is to reconstruct an impedance image from a slice of three-dimensional body area, it may also be used for a more accurate monitoring of some physiological parameter. Woo et al. (1992) presented an example of this kind of instrumentation for a more reliable infant apnea monitor. With the impedance tomography technique it is possible to concentrate the collection of impedance data more accurately to the lung area and thus to avoid the artifacts caused by the chest-wall movements.

In this chapter we briefly review some fundamental questions in impedance tomography. The reader may obtain more information from such excellent sources as Brown and Barber (1992), Hames (1990), and Webster (1990).

26.2 IMPEDANCE MEASUREMENT METHODS

The electric impedance may be measured either traditionally by pure electric methods or by electromagnetic methods. The traditional electric methods are discussed first.

26.2.1 Electric Measurement of the Impedance

As in impedance plethysmography, also in impedance tomography the current is fed and the voltage is measured through different pairs of electrodes to avoid the error due to the contact impedance. We note, however, the assertion of Cheng et al. (1990) that, in spite of the problem of skin impedance, to obtain the greatest sensitivity to changes in the resistivity of the body, voltages from current carrying electrodes should also be included. In the following we describe some of the measurement methods that are used.

Neighboring Method

Brown and Segar (1987) suggested a method whereby the current is applied through neighboring electrodes and the voltage is measured successively from all other adjacent electrode pairs. Figure 26.1 illustrates the application of this method for a cylindrical volume conductor with 16 equally spaced electrodes.

The current is first applied through electrodes 1 and 2 (Fig. 26.1A). The current density is, of course, highest between these electrodes, decreasing rapidly as a function of distance. The voltage is measured successively with electrode pairs 3–4, 4–5, . . . , 15–16. From these 13 voltage measurements the first four measurements are illustrated in Figure 26.1A. All these 13 measurements are independent. Each of them is assumed to represent the impedance between the equipotential lines intersecting the measurement electrodes. This is indicated with shading for the voltage measurement between electrodes 6 and 7.

The next set of 13 voltage measurements is obtained by feeding the current through electrodes 2 and 3, as shown in Figure 26.1B. For a 16-electrode system, $16 \times 13 = 208$ voltage measurements are obtained. Because of reciprocity, those measurements in which the current electrodes and voltage electrodes are interchanged yield identical measurement results. Therefore, only 104 measurements are independent. In the neighboring method, the measured voltage is at a maximum with adjacent electrode pairs. With opposite electrode pairs, the voltage is only about 2.5% of that.

Cross Method

A more uniform current distribution is obtained when the current is injected between a pair of more distant electrodes. Hua, Webster, and

A

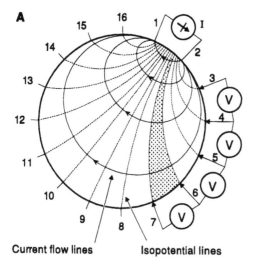

Current flow lines   Isopotential lines

B

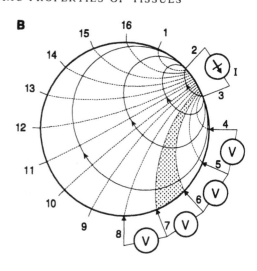

Fig. 26.1 Neighboring method of impedance data collection illustrated for a cylindrical volume conductor and 16 equally spaced electrodes. (A) The first four voltage measurements for the set of 13 measurements are shown. (B) Another set of 13 measurements is obtained by changing the current feeding electrodes.

Tompkins (1987) suggested such a method called the *cross method* (see Fig. 26.2).

In the cross method, adjacent electrodes—for instance 16 and 1, as shown in Figure 26.2A—are first selected for current and voltage reference electrodes, respectively. The other current electrode, electrode number 2 is first used. The voltage is measured successively for all other 13 electrodes with the aforementioned electrode 1 as a reference. (The first four voltage measurements are again shown in Fig. 26.2A.) The current is then applied through electrode 4 and the voltage is again measured successively for all other 13 electrodes with electrode 1 as a reference, as shown in Figure 26.2B. One repeats this procedure using electrodes 6, 8, . . . , 14; the entire procedure thus includes 7 × 13 = 91 measurements.

The measurement sequence is then repeated using electrodes 3 and 2 as current and voltage reference electrodes, respectively (see Fig. 26.2C). Applying current first to electrode 5, one then measures the voltage successively for all other 13 electrodes with electrode 2 as a reference. One repeats this procedure again by applying current to electrode 7 (see Fig. 26.2D). Applying current successively to electrodes 9,

11, . . . , 1 and measuring the voltage for all other 13 electrodes with the aforementioned electrode 2 as a reference, one makes 91 measurements. From these 182 measurements only 104 are independent. The cross method does not have as good a sensitivity in the periphery as does the neighboring method, but has better sensitivity over the entire region.

Opposite Method

Another alternative for the impedance measurement is the *opposite method*, illustrated in Figure 26.3 (Hua, Webster, and Tompkins, 1987). In this method current is injected through two diametrically opposed electrodes (electrodes 16 and 8 in Fig. 26.3A). The electrode adjacent to the current-injecting electrode is used as the voltage reference. Voltage is measured from all other electrodes except from the current electrodes, yielding 13 voltage measurements (the first four of these measurements are again shown).

The next set of 13 voltage measurements is obtained by selecting electrodes 1 and 9 for current electrodes (Figure 26.3B). When 16 electrodes are used, the opposite method yields 8 × 13 = 104 data points. The current distri-

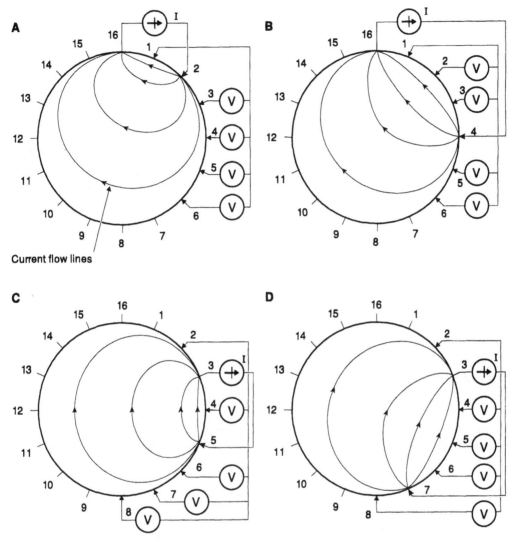

Fig. 26.2 Cross method of impedance data collection. The four different steps of this procedure are illustrated in A through D.

bution in this method is more uniform and, therefore, has a good sensitivity.

Adaptive Method

In the aforementioned methods, current has been injected with a pair of electrodes and voltage has been measured similarly. In the *adaptive method*, proposed by Gisser, Isaacson, and Newell (1987), current is injected through all electrodes (see Fig. 26.4A). Because current flows through all electrodes simultaneously, as many independent current generators are

needed as are electrodes used. The electrodes can feed a current from -5 to $+5$ mA, allowing different current distributions. Homogeneous current distribution may be obtained only in a homogeneous volume conductor, as discussed in Section 11.6.9. If the volume conductor is cylindrical with circular cross section, the injected current must be proportional to $\cos \theta$ to obtain a homogeneous current distribution.

The voltages are measured with respect to a single grounded electrode. When one is using

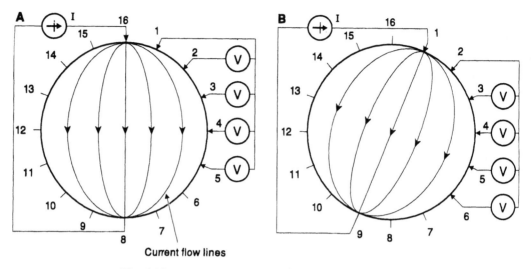

Fig. 26.3 Opposite method of impedance data collection.

16 electrodes, the number of voltage measurements for a certain current distribution is 15. The desired current distribution is then rotated one electrode increment (22.5° for a 16-electrode system; see Fig. 26.4B). Thus 8 different current distributions are obtained, yielding 8 × 15 = 120 independent voltage measurements.

26.2.2 Electromagnetic Measurement of the Electric Impedance

Earlier in this chapter, as well as in the previous chapter discussing impedance plethysmogra-

phy, the electric impedance of the tissue was measured by feeding an electric current to the volume conductor formed by the body and by measuring the generated electric potential difference (i.e., voltage). As discussed in Appendix B, Maxwell's equations tie the time-varying electric and magnetic fields together so that when there is an electric field, there is also a magnetic field and vice versa. As was mentioned in the Introduction in Section 1.2.1, this electromagnetic connection may be applied to the measurement of the electric impedance of the tissue.

In the electromagnetic measurement of the

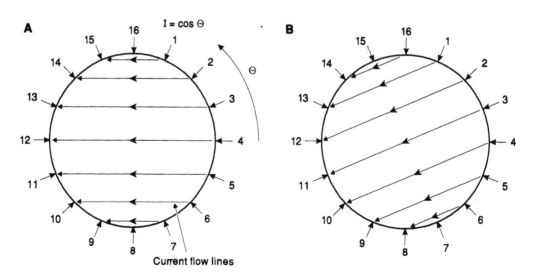

Fig. 26.4 Adaptive method of impedance data collection.

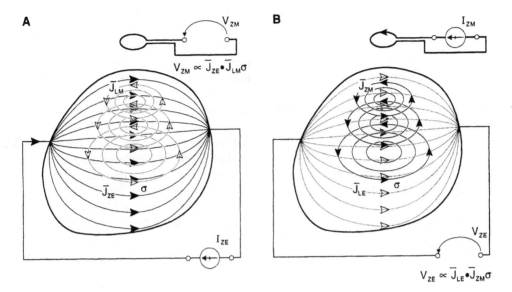

Fig. 26.5 Electromagnetic method of impedance data collection. (A) Electric current is fed through electrodes, and the current distribution is detected with a magnetometer. (B) Electric current is induced with a coil, and the induced voltage is measured with electrodes.

electric impedance, as in pure electric measurement, the sensitivity distribution of the measurement is similarly proportional to the dot product between the electric current field in the volume conductor and the lead field of the voltage measurement. This holds true irrespective of whether or not the electric current in the volume conductor is generated through direct application of electric currents or is induced by a time-varying magnetic field, and whether the detector is a magnetometer or a voltmeter, respectively. In Figure 1.2B these principles of electromagnetic measurement of electric impedance were introduced briefly; they are presented in more detail below.

One way to utilize the electromagnetic connection in the electric impedance measurement is to feed the electric current to the volume conductor by means of electrodes on its surface, but instead of detecting the generated voltage with another pair of electrodes, the induced magnetic field is detected with a magnetometer. In this method the electric current distribution is irrotational (zero curl). As discussed in Chapter 12, the lead field of the magnetometer is tangentially oriented. The back-projection for impedance imaging can be made by first determining the electric current distribution in the volume conductor from the magnetic field mea-

surements and thereafter the impedance distribution. Figure 26.5A illustrates this principle. Impedance images obtained with this method have not been published. Ahlfors and Ilmoniemi (1992) have published the electric current field *change* caused by an insulating cylinder placed in a saltwater tank, as measured with a 24-channel SQUID magnetometer.

The electromagnetic connection may also be used the other way around in the measurement of the electric impedance of the volume conductor. Due to the electromagnetic connection, the electric current may also be induced to the volume conductor by a time-varying magnetic field generated by a coil or a set of coils around the volume conductor (Purvis, Tozer, and Freeston, 1990). This gives an opportunity to create different kinds of current distributions compared to the feeding of electric current through electrodes. In this case the electric current field is solenoidal (zero divergence). This principle of measuring the electric impedance is illustrated in Figure 26.5B. Healey, Tozer, and Freeston (1992) published impedance images measured from a three-dimensional phantom. They used three equally spaced coils around a cylindrical phantom and measured the potentials by 16 equally spaced surface electrodes.

Note that because the sensitivity distribution of the electromagnetic measurement of the electric impedance is proportional to the dot product of the electric current field and the detector lead field, in both of these configurations, owing to the principle of reciprocity, the sensitivity distribution is the same, provided that similar coil and electrode structures are used.

26.3   IMAGE RECONSTRUCTION

From the collected data, the image of the distribution of the electric impedance may be constructed by use of certain reconstruction algo-

rithms. These algorithms are discussed in more detail in Webster (1990) and are not repeated here. The best obtained accuracy of the image reconstruction is at present about 5% of the dimension of the volume conductor in phantom tests and about 10% in vivo measurements at the thorax. An ultimate achievable resolution of 1.5% has been reported by Barber and Brown (1984). As regards the skull, the impedance method is not applicable because of the skulls very high resistivity. The distinguishability in impedance imaging is theoretically discussed in Cheney and Isaacson (1992).

An example of the reconstructed image is presented in Figure 26.6 (Woo, 1990). In this experiment, the impedance image was deter-

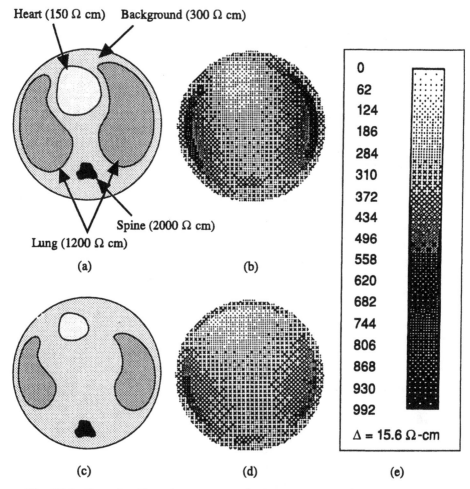

Fig. 26.6   Example of impedance tomography image reconstruction in phantom. (a) and (c) True images of the physical phantom modeling the human thorax. (b) and (d) Reconstructed images of (a) and (c), respectively. (e) Scale of resistivity images.

mined for two different phantoms that resembled the cross section of the human thorax. The phantoms were constructed by mixing agar powder and NaCl with boiling water. Figure 26.6a and c shows the true images of the two phantoms. The reconstructed impedance images of these phantoms are shown in b and d, respectively. Figure 26.6e illustrates the scale for the resistivity image.

As a nonionizing and inexpensive method, electric impedance tomography is an interesting addendum to the various medical imaging methods. Though the image resolution of in-vivo studies is continuously increasing, it will theoretically remain lower than that of x-ray and ultrasound. This low resolution will certainly limit its application to that of monitoring, rather than to accurate anatomical imaging applications.

Healey TJ, Tozer RC, Freeston IL (1992): Impedance imaging of 3D objects using magnetically induced currents. In *Proc. 14th Annual Int. Conf. IEEE Eng. in Med. and Biol. Society, Paris,* Vol. 14, ed. JP Morucci, R Plonsey, JL Coatrieux, S Laxminarayan, pp. 1719–20, IEEE, New York, N.Y.

Hua P, Webster JG, Tompkins WJ (1987): Effect of the measurement method on noise handling and image quality of EIT imaging. In *Proc. Ninth Int. Conf. IEEE Eng. in Med. and Biol. Society,* Vol. 2, pp. 1429–30, IEEE, New York, N.Y.

Purvis WR, Tozer RC, Freeston IL (1990): Impedance imaging using induced current. In *Proc. 12th Annual Int. Conf. IEEE Eng. in Med. and Biol. Society,* Vol. 1, pp. 114–5, IEEE, New York, N.Y.

Woo EJ (1990): Finite element method and reconstruction algorithms in electrical impedance tomography. *Dept. of Electrical and Computer Eng., Univ. of Wisconsin, Madison,* (Ph.D. thesis)

Woo EJ, Hua P, Webster JG, Tompkins WJ (1992): Measuring lung resistivity using electrical impedance tomography. *IEEE Trans. Biomed. Eng.* BME-39:(7) 756–60.

REFERENCES

Ahlfors S, Ilmoniemi R (1992): Magnetic imaging of conductivity. In *Proc. 14th Annual Int. Conf. IEEE Eng. in Med. and Biol. Society, Paris,* Vol. 14, ed. JP Morucci, R Plonsey, JL Coatrieux, S Laxminarayan, pp. 1717–8, IEEE, Piscatway, N.J.

Barber DC, Brown BH (1984): Applied potential tomography. *J. Phys. E.: Sci. Instrum.* 17: 723–33.

Brown BH, Segar AD (1987): The Sheffield data collection system. *Clin. Phys. Physiol. Measurement* 8(Suppl. A): 91–7.

Cheney M, Isaacson D (1992): Distinguishability in impedance imaging. *IEEE Trans. Biomed. Eng.* BME-39:(8) 852–60.

Cheng KS, Simske SJ, Isaacson D, Newell JC, Gisser DG (1990): Errors due to measuring voltage on current-carrying electrodes in electric current computed tomography. *IEEE Trans. Biomed. Eng.* BME-37:(60) 60–5.

Gisser DG, Isaacson D, Newell JC (1987): Current topics in impedance imaging. *Clin. Phys. Physiol. Measurement* 8(Suppl. A): 39–46.

REFERENCES, BOOKS

Brown BH, Barber DC (eds.) (1992): *Electrical Impedance Tomography,* 207 pp. The Institute of Physical Sciences in Medicine, York. (Clinical Physics and Physiological Measurement, Vol. 13, Suppl. A.)

Hames TK (ed.) (1990): *Proc. Meeting on Electrical Impedance Tomography, Copenhagen, 14th–16th July 1990,* 284 pp. European Community Concerted Action on Electrical Impedance Tomography, Brussels.

Krestel E (ed.) (1990): *Imaging Systems for Medical Diagnostics,* 636 pp. Siemens Aktiengesellschaft, Berlin and Munich.

Webb S (ed.) (1992): *The Physics of Medical Imaging,* 2nd ed., 633 pp. IOP Publishing Ltd, Bristol.

Webster JG (ed.) (1990): *Electrical Impedance Tomography,* 223 pp. Adam Hilger, Bristol and New York.

Wells PNT (ed.) (1982): *Scientific Basis of Medical Imaging,* 284 pp. Churchill Livingstone, New York.

27

The Electrodermal Response

27.1 INTRODUCTION

In previous chapters we described the need to take into account the interaction of the skin with electrodes whose purpose it was to record the surface potential noninvasively or to introduce stimulating currents. The skin and its properties were usually seen in these examples as providing certain difficulties to be understood and counteracted. In this chapter the sphere of interest is the *skin response* itself.

Interest in the conductance between skin electrodes, usually placed at the palmar surface, arose because of the involvement of the sweat glands in this measurement. Since sweat gland activity, in turn, is controlled by sympathetic nerve activity, this measurement has been considered as an ideal way to monitor the autonomic nervous system. In this chapter we describe what is currently understood to underlie the *electrodermal response* (EDR) to sympathetic stimulation. The source of the material for this chapter comes mainly from the summary papers of Fowles (1974, 1986) and Venables and Christie (1980) which are suggested as the first recourse of the reader seeking further information.

In the earlier chapters of this book such topics have been chosen that illustrate the fundamental principles of this discipline. In this chapter we

discover that the basis for the EDR is not well understood and much remains to be discovered to explain the phenomena in basic physiological and biophysical terms. In spite of this shortcoming EDR is nevertheless widely used. Since it is a topic in bioelectricity it deserves attention precisely because of the need for further study. Clearly, here is a bioelectromagnetic application where a valid quantitative model would have an immediate and salutary effect on its use in research and in clinical applications.

27.2 PHYSIOLOGY OF THE SKIN

The interpretation of skin conductance and/or skin potential requires some understanding about the structure of tissues at and beneath the skin surface. Figure 27.1 shows the main features of the skin. The most superficial layer is called the *epidermis* and consists of the *stratum corneum*, the *stratum lucidum* (seen only on "frictional surfaces"), the *granular layer*, the *prickle cell layer*, and the *basal* or *germinating layer*. The surface of the corneum (i.e., surface of the skin) is composed of dead cells, while at its base one finds healthy, living cells. Between these two sites there are transitional cells. This layer is also called the *horny layer*. Blood

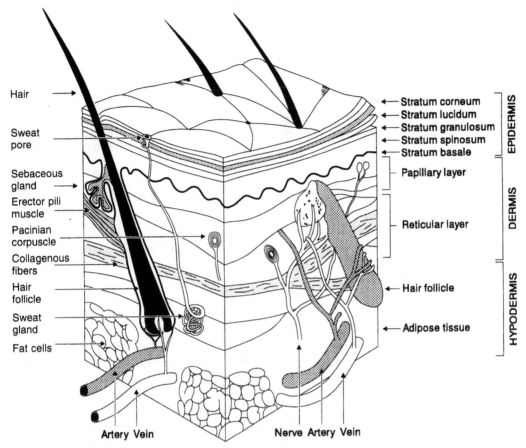

Fig. 27.1 Section of smooth skin taken from the sole of the foot. Blood vessels have been injected. (Redrawn from Ebling, Eady, and Leigh, 1992.)

vessels are found in the *dermis* whereas the eccrine sweat gland secretory cells are found at the boundary between the dermis and the *paniculus adiposus*, also referred to as *hypodermis* and *superficial fascia*. The excretory duct of the eccrine sweat glands consists of a simple tube made up of a single or double layer of epithelial cells; this ascends to and opens on the surface of the skin. It is undulating in the dermis but then follows a spiral and inverted conical path through the epidermis to terminate in a pore on the skin surface. Cholinergic stimulation via fibers from the sympathetic nervous system constitutes the major influence on the production of sweat by these eccrine glands.

From an examination of Figure 27.1 one can appreciate that the epidermis ordinarily has a high electric resistance due to the thick layer of dead cells with thickened keratin mem-

branes. This aspect is not surprising, since the function of skin is to provide a barrier and protection against abrasion, mechanical assaults, and so on. The entire epidermis (with the exception of the desquamating cells) constitutes the *barrier layer*), a permeability barrier to flow. Experiments show its behavior to be that of a passive membrane.

However, the corneum is penetrated by the aforementioned sweat ducts from underlying cells; as these ducts fill, a relatively good conductor (sweat can be considered the equivalent of a 0.3% NaCl salt solution and, hence, a weak electrolyte) emerges, and many low-resistance parallel pathways result. A further increase in conductance results from the hydration of the corneum due to the flow of sweat across the duct walls (a process that is facilitated by the corkscrew duct pathway and the extremely hydrophilic nature of the corneum). As a consequence the effective skin conductance can vary greatly, depending on present and past eccrine activity. The aforementioned behavior is particularly great in the palmar and plantar regions because, while the epidermis is very thick, at the same time the eccrine glands are unusually dense. It should be noted that the loading of ducts with sweat can be taking place before any (observable) release of sweat from the skin surface and/or noticeable diffusion into the corneum.

We have noted that the main function of the skin is to protect the body from the environment. One aspect of this is to prevent the loss of water by the body. However, at the same time, the evaporation of water as a means of regulating body temperature must be facilitated. These requirements appear to be carried out by the stratum corneum as a barrier layer that prevents the loss of water to the outside except through the sweat glands, whose activity can be controlled. This in turn is mediated by the autonomic (sympathetic) nervous system. Measurement of the output of the sweat glands, which EDR is thought to do, provides a simple gauge of the level and extent of sympathetic activity. This is the simple and basic concept underlying EDR and its application to psychophysiology.

27.3   ELECTRODERMAL MEASURES

That the electrodermal response is associated with sweat gland activity is well established. Convincing evidence arises from experiments in which a direct correlation is seen between EDR and stimulated sweat gland activity. Furthermore, when sweat gland activity is abolished, then there is an absence of EDR signals (Fowles, 1986).

There are two major measures of the electrodermal response. The first, involving the measurement of resistance or conductance between two electrodes placed in the palmar region, was originally suggested by Féré (1888). It is possible also to detect voltages between these electrodes; these potential waveforms appear to be similar to the passive resistance changes,

Table 27.1 Abbreviations used to distinguish the type of electrodermal measurements

Abbreviation	Significance
EDA	Electrodermal Activity
EDL	Electrodermal Level
EDR	Electrodermal Response
SCL	Skin Conductance Level
SCR	Skin Conductance Response
SRL	Skin Resistance Level
SRR	Skin Resistance Response
SPL	Skin Potential Level
SPR	Skin Potential Response

though its interpretation is less well understood. This measurement was pioneered by Tarchanoff (1889). The first type of measurement is referred to as *exosomatic*, since the current on which the measurement is based is introduced from the outside. The second type, which is less commonly used, is called *endosomatic*, since the source of voltage is internal. Researchers also distinguish whether the measurement is of the (tonic) background level (L), or the time-varying (phasic) response (R) type. These simple ideas have led to a number of specific measures, each described by a three-letter abbreviation. These are listed in Table 27.1.

Older terminology no longer in use, such as the *galvanic skin response*, has not been included in the table. The resistance and conductance measurements are reciprocals, of course; however, one or the other might turn out to be linearly related to the stimuli under study and be somewhat more useful as a result.

27.4   MEASUREMENT SITES AND CHARACTERISTIC SIGNALS

As discussed above, EDA is best measured at palmar sites. Suggested locations for electrode placement are given in Figure 27.2. In general, the electrodes used are of the Ag/AgCl type which are recessed from the skin and require the use of a suitable electrode paste. Since this is a reversible type of electrode, polarization and bias potentials are minimized. This is obviously of importance since such contributions

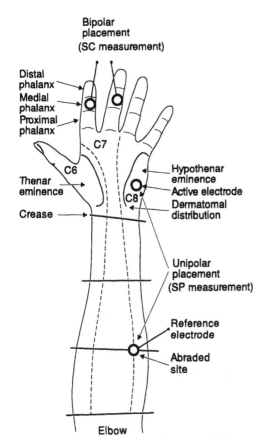

Fig. 27.2 Suggested electrode sites on the palm for the measurement of skin resistance and skin potentials. (Redrawn from Venables and Christie, 1980.)

introduce artifact in the SP and SC determinations. There is also a half-cell potential under each electrode, but if these are similar and overlie identical chloride concentrations their effects are equal and cancel. For this reason an electrode paste with NaCl at the concentration of sweat (approximately 0.3% NaCl) is to be preferred.

As described in Figure 27.2, the reference site should be abraded, a procedure that may possibly remove the corneum and introduce much reduced contact resistance. The site itself, on the forearm, is selected to be a neutral (nonactive) location so that only good contact is required. Although the removal of the corneum at the active site would interfere with the examination of the system there, no such requirement needs to be imposed at the reference site, since it should be nonactive.

Shown in Figure 27.3 are signals characteristic of SCR and SPR waveforms. Those identified as having *slow recovery*, shown in Figure 27.3A, have a duration of around 40 s, with phasic amplitudes of around 2 μS for conductance and 10–20 mV for potential. Since the amplitude values depend on electrode area in a nonlinear way, these values cannot be readily normalized and, consequently, are difficult to compare with others. Data collected by Venables and Christie (1980) give a mean SCL of 0.3 μS and SCR of 0.52 μS in a study of a particular population (N = 500–600). *Rapid-recovery* SCRs and SPRs are shown in Figure 27.3B.

The electronics associated with measurement of EDR is fairly simple. For exosomatic conditions either a constant current or a constant voltage source is used. As illustrated by Venables and Christie (1980), the circuit in either case consists of a battery with voltage E_B connected to the skin through a series resistance R_A; the circuit is completed by the skin resistance R_s. Constant current conditions can be implemented by letting R_A be very large. (In the example given, E_B = 100 V; R_A = 10 MΩ; and, even for high values of skin resistance (i.e., $R_s \approx 250$ kΩ, corresponding to 4 μS), the current differs from a nominal 10.0 μA by under 2.5%. For constant-voltage conditions R_A is small compared to R_s, so the voltage across R_s is the fixed battery voltage. In the constant-current case, the skin voltage $V_s(t)$ is measured and

$$SC(t) = \frac{E_b}{R_A V_s(t)} \qquad (27.1)$$

For constant-voltage conditions the voltage V_A is measured across the series resistance. Then

$$SR(t) = \frac{E_b R_A}{V_A} \qquad (27.2)$$

Present-day practice utilizes a battery voltage E_b of 0.5 V, whereas constant current and constant voltage are better obtained electronically.

For endosomatic measurements the skin potential is desired, and the optimum condition is where the input resistance of the amplifier is very high compared to the skin resistance. The use of an operational amplifier is called for. Additional requirements are evident from

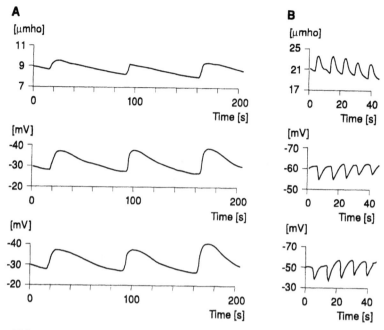

Fig. 27.3 (A) Upper trace is a slow-recovery SCR, whereas middle and lower are monophasic negative SPRs. (B) The upper trace is a rapid-recovery SCR, whereas the middle and lower traces are positive monophasic SPRs. (Redrawn from Fowles, 1974.)

the sample waveforms in Figure 27.3; in general, an input voltage in the range of $+10$ to -70 mV at a bandwidth of from DC to a few Hz. Geddes and Baker (1989) suggest 0–5Hz for tonic measurements, with 0.03–5Hz being adequate for phasic measurements. Recommendations for electrodermal measurements were drawn up by a committee selected by the editor of *Psychophysiology* and published by that journal (Fowles et al., 1981). The paper by MacPherson, MacNeil, and Marble (1976) on measurement devices may also be useful.

27.5 THEORY OF EDR

A comprehensive model underlying EDR has been developed by Fowles (1974) and appears essentially unchanged in Fowles (1986); its principle is given here in Figure 27.4. This model is useful only in a qualitative sense since there is no quantitative data either to support the circuit or to provide an evaluation of any of its elements. The top of the figure represents the surface of the skin, whereas the bottom represents the interface between the hypoder-

mis and the dermis. The active electrode is at the top (skin surface), whereas the reference electrode is considered to be at the bottom (hypodermis).

R_1 and R_2 represent the resistance to current flow through the sweat ducts located in the epidermis and dermis, respectively. These are major current flow pathways when these ducts contain sweat, and their resistance decreases as the ducts fill. Such filling starts in the dermis and continues into the epidermis.

E_1 and R_4 represent access to the ducts through the duct wall in the dermis, whereas E_2 and R_3 describe the same pathway, but in the epidermis. Transduct potentials E_1 and E_2 arise as a result of unequal ionic concentrations across the duct as well as selective ionic permeabilities (as discussed in Chapter 3). This potential is affected by the production of sweat, particularly if, as is thought, the buildup of hydrostatic pressure results in depolarization of the ductal membranes. Such depolarization results in increased permeability to ion flow; this is manifested in the model by decreased values of R_3 and R_4. In particular, this is regarded as an important mechanism to explain rapid-

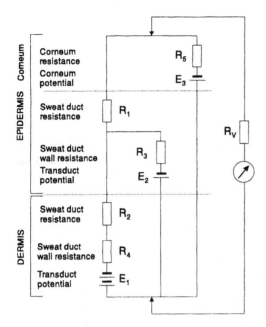

Fig. 27.4 A simplified equivalent circuit describing the electrodermal system. Components are identified in the text. (From Fowles, 1986.)

recovery signals (since the restoration of normal permeability is equally fast). The potentials of E_1 and E_2 are normally lumen-negative.

The resistance R_5 is that of the corneum, whereas E_3 is its potential (treating this region as the site of liquid junction potentials). The phenomenon of hydration of the corneum, resulting from the diffusion of sweat from the sweat ducts into the normally dry and absorbant corneum, leads to a reduction in the value of R_5.

The predicted outcome of an experiment depends on (among others) the size of the response to a stimulus and the prior sweat gland condition. For an SCR determination Fowles (1986) states that the potentials can be ignored (these appear to be relatively small factors). If one assumes initial resting conditions, then a sweat response consists of sweat rising in the ducts, and correspondingly R_2 slowly diminishes. The response latency is associated with the time required for this to take place. If the response is a small one and R_1 and R_5 are not affected, then the SCR may not show any change. For a larger response, although sweat still remains within the ducts, it now extends also into the corneum and hence reduces R_1 as

well as R_2. If it is large enough, then flow across the duct wall will take place, causing hydration of the corneum and a decrease in R_5. With a very large sweat response (or if a moderate response takes place after the ducts are already partly filled), then the response also includes the triggering of the epidermal duct membrane due to associated hydrostatic pressure buildup, and a consequent reduction of R_3.

For SP recordings Figure 27.4 can also serve as a guide on the possible outcome of the response to a stimulus. The measured potential is thought to represent, mainly, that across the epidermis—namely E_3 minus the voltage drop in R_5. Factors that are considered include the reabsorption of sodium across the duct walls by active transport which generates large lumen-negative potentials. Their effect on the measured potentials depends on the relative values of R_1, R_2, and R_4 (with low values enhancing surface measurement of E_1, and low R_5 values diminishing this measurement (Edelberg, 1968)). With modest responses when the corneum is relatively unhydrated, the increased lumen-negative duct potential and decrease in R_2 and possibly R_1 act to produce a monophasic negative SPR. Large responses that trigger the membrane response and a large and rapid decrease in R_3 result in a decrease in the measured negative potential and possibly a positive component if the ducts are already filled.

The reader can appreciate that the model is not a quantitative one and, hence, cannot be appealed to as a source of information regarding the outcome of an experiment except in very qualitative terms. One needs to examine to what extent a lumped-parameter circuit can represent the actual distributed system. Possibly such a circuit is justifiable; perhaps additional layers are needed. Most importantly, each circuit element needs to be described biophysically and quantitatively. Presumably this will require isolation of different parts of the system and also appropriate in vitro experiments. In the meantime, EDA appears to be useful as an empirical tool for registering the level of sympathetic activity in a psychophysiological experiment.

One problem in the use of EDR should be mentioned. When skin conductance responses are used to evaluate an immediate outcome to a specific stimulus, it can be difficult to distinguish the stimulus specific response from the spontaneous SCR activity. To deal with this problem, investigators use a response window of 1–5 s following the stimulus, during which a signal will be accepted. If one assumes a spontaneous SCR rate of 7.5/min, the reduction in a confounding spontaneous SCR is 50%. A narrower window has been suggested to discriminate further against the unwanted signal.

27.6 APPLICATIONS

The applications of EDR lie in the area of psychophysiology and relate to studies in which a quantitative measure of sympathetic activity is desired. Fowles (1986) states:

The stimuli that elicit these [EDA] responses are so ubiquitous that it has proved difficult to offer a conceptualization of the features common to these stimuli. There is no doubt, however, that the response often occurs to stimuli that depend for their efficacy on their physiological significance as opposed to their physical intensity.

One measure of the extent of interest in EDR is the references to papers that list EDR as a keyword. In the SCI's *Citation Index* for 1991, one finds approximately 25 such references (i.e., publications). The importance attached to such measurements includes the statement in one recent paper that palmar sweat is one of the most salient symptoms of an anxiety state and, for some, the single most noticeable bodily reaction. But such applications lie outside the scope of this book, and we shall not pursue this topic further. The interested reader may wish to consult issues of the journal *Psychophysiology* for many of the current research papers.

REFERENCES

Ebling FJG, Eady RAJ, Leigh IM (1992): Anatomy and organization of the human skin. In *Textbook of Dermatology,* 5th ed., ed. RH Champion, JL Burton, FJG Ebling, 3160 pp. Blackwell, London.

Edelberg R (1968): Biopotentials from the skin surface: The hydration effect. *Ann. N.Y. Acad. Sci.* 148: 252–62.

Féré C (1888): Note sur les modifications de la résistance électrique sous l'influence des excitations sensorielles et des émotions. *C. R. Soc. Biol. (Paris)* 5: 217–9.

Fowles DC (1974): Mechanisms of electrodermal activity. In *Methods in Physiological Psychology. Bioelectric Recording Techniques,* C ed. Vol. 1, ed. RF Thompson, MM Patterson, pp. 231–71, Academic Press, New York.

Fowles DC, Christie MJ, Edelberg R, Grings WW, Lykken DT, Venables PH (1981): Committee report: Publication recommendations for electrodermal measurements. *Psychophysiol.* 18: 232–9.

Fowles DC (1986): The eccrine system and electrodermal activity. In *Psychophysiology,* ed. MGH Coles, E Donchin, SW Porges, pp. 51–96, Guilford Press, New York.

Geddes LA, Baker LE (1989): *Principles of Applied Biomedical Instrumentation,* 3rd ed., John Wiley, New York, N.Y.

MacPherson RD, MacNeil G, Marble AE (1976): Integrated circuit measurement of skin conductance. *Behav. Res. Methods Instrum.* 8: 361–4.

Tarchanoff J (1889): Décharges électriques dans la peau de l'homme sous l'influence de l'excitation des organes des sens et de différentes formes d'activité psychique. *C. R. Soc. Biol. (Paris)* 41: 447–51.

Venables PH, Christie MJ (1980): Electrodermal activity. In *Techniques in Psychophysiology,* ed. I Martin, PH Venables, pp. 2–67, John Wiley, New York.

IX

Other Bioelectromagnetic Phenomena

The main source of bioelectric signals are those produced by excitable tissues—that is, nerve and muscle cells. There are, however, other spontaneous bioelectric signals. An important example is the *electro-oculogram* (EOG), which is discussed in this section. The EOG is not produced by an excitable tissue but by the static electric polarization of the eye. Through the movement of the eye it produces electric potential changes that can be measured around the eye. This phenomenon may, of course, also be detected magnetically. The EOG and its subdivision, the *electronystagmogram* (ENG) have wide clinical applications. These do not, however, fall directly within the scope of this book, and only the mechanism behind the generation of the EOG-signal and its measurement principle are discussed here.

There are excitable tissues in the eye and these produce bioelectric signals of the type discussed throughout the earlier chapters of the book. These include the *electroretinogram* (ERG), which is the electric response of the retina to light. Visual information proceeds from the retina to the central nervous system along the optic nerve. Since these bioelectric signals involve an excitable (nervous) tissue, they could, on the basis of their mechanism, have been included in Part IV (Neurological bioelectromagnetism). They are discussed here, however, in connection with other bioelectric signals originating in the eye.

28

The Electric Signals Originating in the Eye

28.1 INTRODUCTION

The eye is a seat of a steady electric potential field that is quite unrelated to light stimulation. In fact, this field may be detected with the eye in total darkness and/or with the eyes closed. It can be described as a fixed dipole with positive pole at the cornea and negative pole at the retina. The magnitude of this *corneoretinal potential* is in the range 0.4–1.0 mV. It is not generated by excitable tissue but, rather, is attributed to the higher metabolic rate in the retina. The polarity of this potential difference in the eyes of invertebrates is opposite to that of vertebrates. This potential difference and the rotation of the eye are the basis for a signal measured at a pair of periorbital surface electrodes. The signal is known as the *electro-oculogram*, (EOG). It is useful in the study of eye movement. A particular application of the EOG is in the measurement of *nystagmus*, which denotes small movements of the eye. The resulting signal is called an *electronystagmogram*. It depends both on the *visual system* and the *vestibular system* and provides useful clinical information concerning each. Some details concerning the EOG as it relates to eye movement, including nystagmus, is contained in the following sections.

The lens of the eye brings the illuminated external scene to a focus at the retina. The retina is the site of cells that are sensitive to the incident light energy; as with other peripheral nerve cells, they generate receptor potentials. The collective behavior of the entire retina is a bioelectric generator, which sets up a field in the surrounding volume conductor. This potential field is normally measured between an electrode on the cornea (contact-lens type) and a reference electrode on the forehead. The recorded signal is known as the *electroretinogram* (ERG). It may be examined both for basic science studies and for clinical diagnostic purposes. Though the electroretinogram is produced by the activity of excitable nervous tissue, and should therefore be discussed in Part IV, it is discussed in this chapter in connection with the electro-oculogram to follow the anatomical division of bioelectromagnetism. It is, of course, more practical to discuss all electric signals originating in the eye after the anatomy and physiology of this organ are presented.

28.2 ANATOMY AND PHYSIOLOGY OF THE EYE AND ITS NEURAL PATHWAYS

28.2.1 Major Components of the Eye

The eye and its major components are shown in Figure 28.1. Light enters the front of the eye

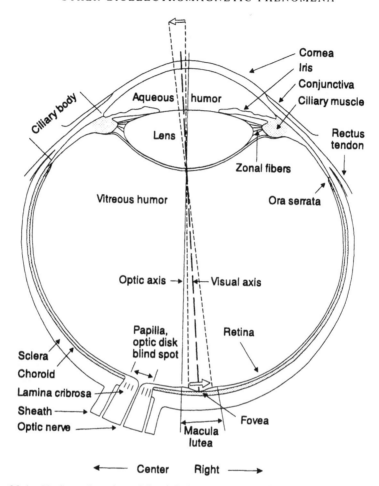

Fig. 28.1 Horizontal section of the right human eye seen from above. The anteroposterior diameter averages 24 mm.

at the *cornea*. Behind the cornea exists a transparent fluid called the *aqueous humor*. Its main function is to make up for the absence of vasculature in the cornea and lens by providing nutrients and oxygen. The aqueous also is responsible for generating a pressure of 20–25 mmHg, which inflates the eye against the relatively inelastic boundaries provided by the *sclera* and *choroid*. This ensures an appropriate geometrical configuration for the formation of clear images by the optical pathway. The lens is located behind the aqueous humor. Its shape and refractive index are controlled by the *ciliary muscles*. The lens completes the focusing of the light, begun at the cornea, on the *retina*. Between the lens and the retina is the vitreous chamber, which is filled with gel-like transparent material known as the *vitreous humor*.

The center of the visual image is focused on the retina to the *fovea*, where visual accuracy is the highest. The retina contains photosensitive cells and several layers of neural cells. This combination generates action pulses relative to the visual image which passes out of the eye to the brain on the optic nerve (Rodieck, 1973).

28.2.2 The Retina

A drawing of the major elements of the retinal cellular structure is shown in Figure 28.2. In this figure, light enters from the top and passes through the neural structure to the *photoreceptors*, which are the *rods* and *cones*. Just behind the rods and cones is the *retinal pigment epithelium* (RPE). Its major function is to supply the

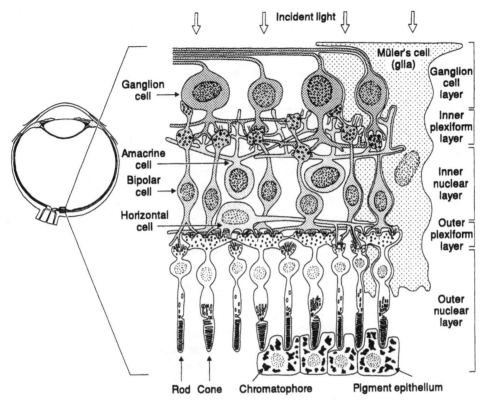

Fig. 28.2 The retinal cellular structure.

metabolic needs (as well as other supportive functions) of the photoreceptors. The rods respond to dim light, whereas the cones contribute to vision in bright light and in color. This area is the site of visual excitation (Charles, 1979).

The initial step in the translation of light information from a spot of light into an electric signal propagating to the visual cortex takes place in the photoreceptors in a process known as *transduction*. This consists of the *cis-trans isomerization* of the *carotenoid chromophore*, which leads to a transient change in the membrane potential of the cell. The result consists of a graded response, seen as a hyperpolarization of the photoreceptor, and an electrotonic current linking the outer and inner segments. A photoreceptor is capable of transducing the energy of a single photon (about 4×10^{-12} erg) into a pulsed reduction of axial current of about 1 pA lasting about 1 s with an energy equivalent of 2×10^{-7} erg (Levick and Dvorak, 1986). Thus, a photoreceptor serves as a photomultiplier with an energy gain of some

10^5 times. The combined volume conductor signal from all photoreceptors contributes what is known as a *late receptor potential* (LRP).

The photoreceptors synapse with a *horizontal cell* and *bipolar cell* in what is known as the *triad*. The signal transmitted via the horizontal cell results in the inhibition of neighboring receptor cells (lateral inhibition) and, hence, an enhancement in contrast. The bipolar cell responds electrotonically with either a hyperpolarization or depolarization. The bipolar cells synapse with *ganglion cells*. This synaptic connection, however, is modulated by the *amacrine cells*. These cells provide negative feedback and thus allow regulation of the sensitivity of transmission from the bipolar to ganglion cells to suitable levels, depending on the immediate past light levels. At the ganglion cell the prior (slow) graded signals are converted into an action pulse that can now be conveyed by nerve conduction to the brain. The magnitude of the slow potential is used by the ganglion cell to establish the firing rate, a process sometimes described as converting from amplitude modulation to pulse-frequency modulation.

The region of the retinal pigment epithelium and the posterior portion of the photoreceptors (rods and cones) is called the *outer nuclear layer*. The region of contact of the photoreceptors with the bipolar cells is known as the *outer plexiform layer* (OPL). The main function of the OPL appears to be signal processing. Since there are 100×10^6 rods and 6×10^6 cones but only 1×10^6 ganglion cells, a marked convergence must take place in the course of signal processing. The bipolar and amacrine cells form the *inner nuclear layer*. The region of contact of the bipolar and amacrine cells with the ganglion cells is known as the *inner plexiform layer* (IPL). The amacrine cells play a role similar to the horizontal cells in the OPL, except that the amacrine cells act in the temporal domain whereas the horizontal cells affect the spatial domain.

28.3 ELECTRO-OCULOGRAM

28.3.1 Introduction

Emil du Bois-Reymond (1848) observed that the cornea of the eye is electrically positive relative to the back of the eye. Since this potential was not affected by the presence or absence of light, it was thought of as a resting potential. In fact, as we discuss in a subsequent section, it is not constant but slowly varying and is the basis for the *electro-oculogram* (EOG).

This source behaves as if it were a single dipole oriented from the retina to the cornea. Such corneoretinal potentials are well established and are in the range of 0.4–1.0 mV. Eye movements thus produce a moving (rotating) dipole source and, accordingly, signals that are a measure of the movement may be obtained. The chief application of the EOG is in the measurement of eye movement.

Figure 28.3 illustrates the measurement of horizontal eye movements by the placement of a pair of electrodes at the outside of the left and right eye (outer canthi). With the eye at rest the electrodes are effectively at the same

potential and no voltage is recorded. The rotation of the eye to the right results in a difference of potential, with the electrode in the direction of movement (i.e., the right canthus) becoming positive relative to the second electrode. (Ideally the difference in potential should be proportional to the sine of the angle.) The opposite effect results from a rotation to the left, as illustrated. The calibration of the signal may be achieved by having the patient look consecutively at two different fixation points located a known angle apart and recording the concomitant EOGs. Typical achievable accuracy is $\pm 2°$, and maximum rotation is $\pm 70°$; however, linearity becomes progressively worse for angles beyond 30° (Young and Sheena, 1988). Typical signal magnitudes range from 5–20 μV/°.

Electro-oculography has both advantages and disadvantages over other methods for determining eye movement. The most important disadvantages relate to the fact that the corneoretinal potential is not fixed but has been found to vary diurnally, and to be affected by light, fatigue, and other qualities. Consequently, there is a need for frequent calibration and recalibration. Additional difficulties arise owing to muscle artifacts and the basic nonlinearity of the method (Carpenter, 1988). The advantages of this technique include recording with minimal interference with subject activities and minimal discomfort. Furthermore, it is a method where recordings may be made in total darkness and/or with the eyes closed. Today the recording of the EOG is a routinely applied diagnostic method in investigating the human oculomotor system. The application of digital computers has considerably increased the diagnostic power of this method (Rahko et al., 1980). In the following, we discuss in greater detail the two subdivisions of electro-oculography—the *saccadic response* and *nystagmography*.

28.3.2 Saccadic Response

Saccadic movements describe quick jumps of the eye from one fixation point to another. The speed may be 20–700°/s. *Smooth* movements are slow, broad rotations of the eye that enable it to maintain fixation on an object moving with respect to the head. The angular motion is in

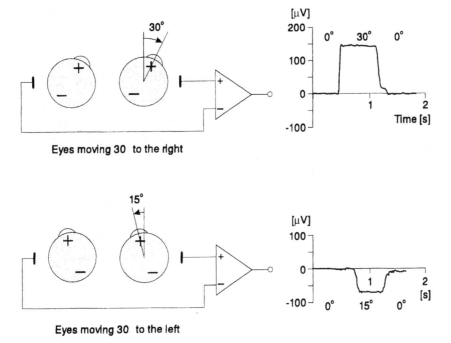

Fig. 28.3 An illustration of the electro-oculogram (EOG) signal generated by horizontal movement of the eyes. The polarity of the signal is positive at the electrode to which the eye is moving.

the range of 1–30°/s. The adjective *pursuit* is added if only the eye is moving, and *compensatory* if the eye motion is elicited by body and/or head movement. The aforementioned eye movements are normally *conjugate* that is, involve parallel motion of the right and left eye. In fact, this is assumed in the instrumentation shown in Figure 28.3; were this not the case, separate electrode pairs on the sides of each eye would become necessary.

A normal saccadic response to a rapidly moving target is described in Figure 28.4. The stimulus movement is described here as a step, and eye movement speeds of 700°/s are not uncommon. The object of the oculomotor system in a saccade is to rapidly move the sight to a new visual object in a way that minimizes the transfer time.

The parameters commonly employed in the analysis of saccadic performance are the maximum angular velocity, amplitude, duration, and latency. The trajectory and velocity of saccades cannot voluntarily be altered. Typical values of these parameters are 400°/s for the maximum

velocity, 20° for the amplitude, 80 ms for the duration, and 200 ms for the latency.

When following a target moving in stepwise jumps, the eyes normally accelerate rapidly, reaching the maximum velocity about midway to the target. When making large saccades (≥25°), the eyes reach the maximum velocity earlier, and then have a prolonged deceleration. The movement of the eyes usually undershoots the target and requires another small saccade to reach it. Overshooting of the target is uncommon in normal subjects. Normally the duration and amplitude are approximately linearly correlated to each other. Several factors such as fatigue, diseases, drugs, and alcohol influence saccades as well as other eye movements.

28.3.3 Nystagmography

Nystagmography refers to the behavior of the visual control system when both vestibular (balance) and visual stimuli exist. *Nystagmoid* movement is applied to a general class of unstable eye movements, and includes both smooth

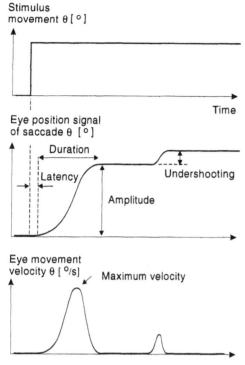

Fig. 28.4 An illustration of the eye movement response to a step stimulus (i.e., a spot of light whose horizontal position instantaneously shifts). After a latency the eye rapidly moves toward the new position, undershoots, and moves a second time. The movements are illustrative of *saccades,* and the parameters include latency, amplitude, velocity, duration, overshooting, and undershooting.

and saccadic contributions. Based on the origin of the nystagmoid movement, it is possible to separate it into *vestibular* and *optokinetic* nystagmus. Despite their different physiological origin, these signals do not differ largely from each other.

Vestibular Nystagmus

Nystagmography is a useful tool in the clinical investigation of the vestibular system (Stockwell, 1988). The vestibular system senses head motion from the signals generated by receptors located in the labyrinths of the inner ear. Under normal conditions the oculomotor system uses vestibular input to move the eyes to compensate for head and body motion. This can occur with saccadic and/or pursuit motion (Fig. 28.5A).

If the vestibular system is damaged then the signals sent to the oculomotor system will be in error and the confusion experienced by the patient results in dizziness. Conversely, for a patient who complains of dizziness, an examination of the eye movements arising from vestibular stimuli can help identify whether, in fact, the dizziness is due to vestibular damage.

Inappropriate compensatory eye movements can easily be recognized by the trained clinician. Such an examination must be made in the absence of visual fixation (since the latter suppresses vestibular eye movements) and is usually carried out in darkness or with the patient's eyes closed. Consequently, monitoring eye movement by EOG is the method of choice.

Optokinetic Nystagmus

Another example of nystagmoid movement is where the subject is stationary but the target is in rapid motion. The oculomotor system endeavors to keep the image of the target focused at the retinal fovea. When the target can no longer be tracked, a saccadic reflex returns the eye to a new target. The movements of the eye describe a sawtooth pattern, such as shown in Figure 28.5B. This is described as *optokinetic nystagmus*. This may also be provoked in the laboratory by rotating a cylinder with dark stripes on a light background in front of a person's eyes.

28.4 ELECTRORETINOGRAM

28.4.1 Introduction

F. Holmgren (1865) showed that an additional time-varying potential was elicited by a brief flash of light, and that it had a repeatable waveform. This result was also obtained, independently, by Dewar and McKendrick (1873). This signal is the *electroretinogram* (ERG), a typical example of which is shown in Figure 28.6. It is clinically recorded with a specially constructed contact lens that carries a chlorided silver wire. The electrode, which may include a cup that is filled with saline, is placed on the cornea. The reference electrode is usually placed on the forehead, temple, or earlobe. The

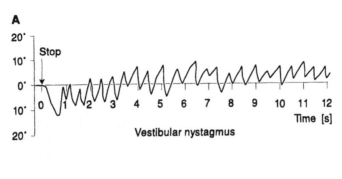

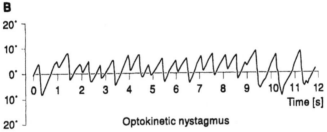

Fig. 28.5 (A) An illustrative record of saccades arising from vestibular nystagmus. (B) An illustrative record of saccades arising from optokinetic nystagmus.

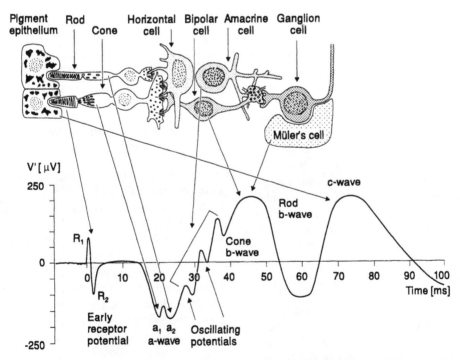

Fig. 28.6 The cells of the retina and their response to a spot light flash. The photoreceptors are the rods and cones in which a negative receptor potential is elicited. This drives the bipolar cell to become either depolarized or hyperpolarized. The amacrine cell has a negative feedback effect. The ganglion cell fires an action pulse so that the resulting spike train is proportional to the light stimulus level.

amplitude depends on the stimulating and physiological conditions, but ranges in the tenths of a millivolt.

The sources of the ERG arise in various layers of the retina, discussed above. These sources are therefore distributed and lie in a volume conductor that includes the eye, orbit, and, to an extent, the entire head. The recording electrodes are at the surface of this region. For the ERG one can identify the progressively changing layer from which different portions of the waveform arise, initiated by a brief light flash stimulus to the photoreceptors.

The earliest signal is generated by the initial changes in the photopigment molecules of the photoreceptors due to the action of the light. This usually gives rise to a positive R_1 deflection followed by a negative R_2 deflection, together making up the *early receptor potential* (ERP). This is followed, after around 2 ms, by the late receptor potential (LRP) mentioned earlier, which (combined with the remainder of the ERP) forms the main constituent of the *a-wave*, a corneo-negative waveform (see Figure 28.6). Both rods and cones contribute to the a-wave; however, with appropriate stimuli these may be separated. For example, a dim blue flash to the dark-adapted eye results in a rod ERG, whereas a bright red flash to a light-adapted eye results in a cone ERG.

The second maxima, which is corneo-positive, is the *b-wave*. To explain its origin we need to note that in the inner retinal layers there are *Müller's cells*. These cells are glial cells and have no synaptic connection to the retinal cells. The transmembrane potential of Müller's cells depends on its potassium Nernst potential, which is influenced by changes in the extracellular potassium. The latter is increased by the release of potassium when the photoreceptors are stimulated. In addition, the ganglion cell action pulse is associated with a potassium efflux. (The aforementioned electrophysiological events follow that described in Chapters 3 and 4.) The consequence of these events is to bring about a Müller's cell response. And it is the latter that is the source of the b-wave. Müller's cells can contribute to a b-wave from either cone or rod receptors separately.

The c-*wave* is positive like the b-wave, but otherwise is considerably slower. It is generated by the retinal pigment epithelium (RPE) as a consequence of interaction with the rods.

The *oscillatory potentials* shown in Figure 28.6 are small amplitude waves that appear in the light-adapted b-wave. Although they are known to be generated in the inner retinal layer and require a bright stimulus, the significance of each wave is unknown. Some additional details are found in the paper by Charles (1979).

In retrospect, the sources that are responsible for the ERG and that lie within and behind the retina, are entirely electrotonic. They constitute a specific example of the *receptor* and *generator* potentials described and discussed in Chapter 5. This contrasts with the sources of the ECG in that the latter, which arise from cardiac muscle cells, are generated entirely from action pulses. Nevertheless, as described in Chapters 8 and 9, a double-layer source is established in a cell membrane whenever there is spatial variation in transmembrane potential. Such spatial variation can result from a propagating action pulse and also from a spreading electrotonic potential. In both cases currents are generated in the surrounding volume conductor and the associated potential field may be sampled with surface electrodes that register the EOG and ERG. An examination of the ERG volume conductor is given below.

28.4.2 Volume Conductor Influence on the ERG

We have described the sources of the ERG lying in the retina (or the RPE) and being measured by a corneal and (say) temple electrode. To model this system requires a description of the volume conductor that links the source with its field. A first effort in this direction is the axially symmetric three-dimensional model of Doslak, Plonsey, and Thomas (1980) described in Figure 28.7. Because of the assumed axial symmetry, the model can be treated as two-dimensional—a large simplification in the calculation of numerical solutions. In this model, the following inhomogeneities were identified:

1. The aqueous humor and vitreous body were assumed to constitute a single region of uni-

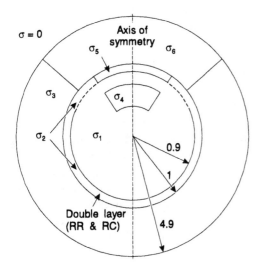

Fig. 28.7 The two-dimensional model depicting the ERG source and volume conductor inhomogeneities. The retina and R-membrane impedance are represented together by double layer and RR and RC, respectively. The other parameters correspond to the conductivities and are listed in Table 28.1.

form conductivity since, in fact, they have nearly the same conductivity (σ_1).

2. The sclera (σ_2).
3. The extraocular region was considered to have a uniform conductivity, much the same as simplified models of the ECG consider the torso uniform (σ_3).
4. The lens (σ_4).
5. The cornea (σ_5).

6. The air in front of the eye, which has a conductivity of zero (σ_6).
7. The model includes the R-membrane, which lies at the same radius as the retina and continues to the cornea. This membrane was treated as a distribution of parallel RC elements (RR, RC).
8. The retina itself was assumed to be the location of a uniform double layer source, considered to extend over a hemisphere.

Since quasistatic conditions apply, temporal changes in source strength can be ignored; these may be added later through superposition. Values of the aforementioned parameters are given in Table 28.1.

In the model described by Figure 28.7 we seek the potential Φ that satisfies

$$\nabla^2\Phi = 0 \qquad (28.1)$$

namely, Laplace's equation subject to the following boundary conditions: At all passive interfaces between regions of different conductivity the normal component of current density is continuous and the electric potential is continuous. For the retinal double layer, the normal component of current density is continuous, but the potential is discontinuous across this source by a value equal to the double layer strength (expressed in volts). Finally, for the R-membrane, the current density is also continuous, but there is a discontinuity in potential; this is given by the product of membrane impedance

Table 28.1 Normalized values of volume conductor parameters of the model of the eye

Parameter	Structure	Value in model	Dimension
σ_1	Aqueous & Vitreous	1.0	57·[S/cm]
σ_2	Sclera	.01 15	57·[S/cm]
σ_3	Extraocular	.005 06	57·[S/cm]
σ_4	Lens	.08 3	57·[S/cm]
σ_5	Cornea	.03 86	57·[S/cm]
σ_6	Air	0.0	57·[S/cm]
RR	R-membrane resistiv.	1.67 . . . 6.25	$\frac{1}{57}$ [Ωcm^2]
RC	$1/(2\pi Cs)$	27.8 . . . 58.8	
RXC	Capacitive reactance	RC/frequency	

Note: C is the R-membrane capacitance. Division of σ_i by 57 gives conductivity in [S/cm]. Multiplication of RR, RC, and RXC by 57 gives resistivity in [Ωcm^2].

Source: Doslak, Plonsey, and Thomas (1980)

(Ωcm^2) and the normal component of current density. Doslak, Plonsey, and Thomas (1980) solved this by locating a system of nodal points over the entire region and then using the method of finite differences and overrelaxation. Mathematical details are contained in Doslak, Plonsey, and Thomas (1982). The model was used by Doslak and Hsu (1984) to study the effect of blood in the vitreous humor on the ERG magnitude. They were able to establish that little effect on ERG magnitude could be expected from this condition.

28.4.3 Ragnar Granit's Contribution

Hermann von Helmholtz (1867) developed the theory of color vision on the basis of the ideas of English scientist Thomas Young (1802). He proposed that the human ability to discriminate a spectrum of colors is based on three different kinds of receptors which are sensitive to different wavelengths of light—red, green, and violet. The perception of other colors would arise from the combined stimulation of these elements.

Ragnar Granit's first experiments in color vision, performed in 1937, employed the electroretinogram (ERG) to confirm the extent of spectral differentiation. Using the microelectrode, which he developed in 1939, he studied color vision further and established the spectral sensitivities of the three types of cone cells: blue, green, and red. These results he confirmed in a later study on color vision (Granit, 1955). Ragnar Granit shared the 1967 Nobel Prize with H. Keffer Hartline and George Wald "for their discoveries concerning the primary physiological and chemical visual processes in the eye."

A seminal study of the ERG was conducted by Ragnar Granit (1955). He recognized the distributed nature of the sources and designed experiments to block different parts in an effort to identify the major elements contributing to the waveform. He deduced the presence of three main components, namely P_I, P_{II}, and P_{III}. P_I is a slowly developing positive potential and is associated with the c-wave. P_{II} is also positive but develops more rapidly and is chiefly responsible for the b-wave. P_{III} is the negative component; its initial phase develops rapidly and is associated with the onset of the a-wave. The total ERG is found by superposition (summing) of $P_I + P_{II} + P_{III}$.

A seminal study of recordings from different retinal layers and individual retinal cells was later made also by Torsten Wiesel and K.T. Brown (1961). Torsten Nils Wiesel (Swedish, 1924–) shared the 1981 Nobel Prize with David Hunter Hubel "for discoveries concerning information processing in the visual system."

The scientific works of Ragnar Granit are well summarized in Granit (1955). It includes also a large list of references to his works in vision and in other fields of bioelectromagnetism and neurophysiology.

REFERENCES

du Bois-Reymond EH (1848): *Untersuchungen Ueber Thierische Elektricität*, Vol. 1, 56+743 pp. G Reimer, Berlin.

Carpenter RHS (1988): *Movements of the Eyes*, 2nd ed., 593 pp. Pion, London.

Charles S (1979): Electrical signals of the retinal microcircuitry. In *Physiology of the Human Eye and Visual System,* ed. RE Records, pp. 319–27, Harper & Row, Hagerstown.

Clark JW (1978): The electroretinogram. In *Medical Instrumentation,* ed. JG Webster, pp. 177–84, Houghton Mifflin, Boston.

Dewar J, McKendrick JG (1873): On the physiological action of light. *Proc. R. Soc. (Edinburgh)* 8: 179–82.

Doslak MJ (1988): Electroretinography. In *Encyclopedia of Medical Devices and Instrumentation,* Vol. 2, ed. JG Webster, pp. 1168–80, John Wiley, New York.

Doslak MJ, Hsu P-C (1984): Application of a bioelectric field model of the ERG to the effect of vitreous haemorrhage. *Med. & Biol. Eng. & Comput.* 22: 552–7.

Doslak MJ, Plonsey R, Thomas CW (1980): The effects of variations of the conducting media inhomogeneities on the electroretinogram. *IEEE Trans. Biomed. Eng.* BME-27: 88–94.

Doslak MJ, Plonsey R, Thomas CW (1982): Numerical solution of the bioelectric field. *Med. & Biol. Eng. & Comput.* 19: 149–56.

Granit R (1955): *Receptors and Sensory Perception,* 369 pp. Yale University Press, New Haven.

Holmgren F (1865): Method att objectivera effecten af ljusintryck på retina. *Uppsala Läk. För. Förh.* 1: 184–98.

Levick WR, Dvorak DR (1986): The retina—From molecules to networks. *Trends Neurosci.* 9: 181–5.

Oster PJ, Stern JA (1980): Electro-oculography. In *Techniques in Psychophysiology,* ed. I Martin, PH Venables, pp. 276–97, John Wiley, New York.

Rahko T, Karma P, Torikka T, Malmivuo JA (1980): Microprocessor-based four-channel electronystagmography system. *Med. & Biol. Eng. & Comput.* 18:(1) 104–8.

Rodieck RW (1973): *The Vertebrate Retina,* 1044 pp. Freeman, San Francisco.

Stockwell CW (1988): Nystagmography. In *Encyclopedia of Medical Devices and Instrumentation,* Vol. 3, ed. JG Webster, pp. 2090–4, John Wiley, New York.

Wiesel TN, Brown KT (1961): Localization of origins of electroretinogram components by intraretinal recording in the intact cat eye. *J. Physiol. (Lond.)* 158: 257–80.

Young LR, Sheena D (1975): Eye movement measurement techniques. *Amer. Physiologist* 30: 315–30. (Reprinted in: *Encyclopedia of Medical Devices and Instrumentation,* Webster, JG, ed., J. Wiley & Sons, New York, vol. 2., pp. 1259–1269, 1988).

Young LR, Sheena D (1988): Eye-movement measurement techniques. In *Encyclopedia of Medical Devices and Instrumentation,* ed. JG Webster, pp. 1259–69, John Wiley, New York.

FURTHER READING

Berthoz A, Melvill Jones G (1985): Adaptive mechanisms in gaze control. In *Reviews of Oculomotor Research,* Vol. 1, ed. DA Robinson, H Collewjin, p. 386, Elsevier, Amsterdam.

Büttner-Ennever JA (1989): Neuroanatomy of the oculomotor system. In *Reviews of Oculomotor Research,* Vol. 2, ed. DA Robinson, H Collewjin, p. 478, Elsevier, Amsterdam.

Kowler E (1990): Eye movements and their role in visual and cognitive processes. In *Reviews of Oculomotor Research,* Vol. 4, ed. DA Robinson, H Collewjin, p. 496, Elsevier, Amsterdam.

Wurtz RH, Goldberg ME (1989): The neurobiology of saccadic eye movements. In *Reviews of Oculomotor Research,* Vol. 3, ed. DA Robinson, H Collewjin, Elsevier, Amsterdam.

APPENDIX A

Consistent System of Rectangular and Spherical Coordinates for Electrocardiology and Magnetocardiology

A.1 INTRODUCTION

Detailed analysis of the electric and magnetic fields produced by the human heart requires a convenient and mathematically consistent coordinate system. Several different rectangular and spherical coordinate systems are being used in clinical electrocardiography, but none fulfill these requirements. In clinical electrocardiology the right-handed rectangular coordinate system standardized in 1967 by the American Heart Association (AHA; American Heart Association, 1967) has been most frequently used. However, this coordinate system is a result of historical development and is not necessarily the rational choice from all possible alternatives.

The basis for the AHA coordinate system arises from the basic research performed by Willem Einthoven. Einthoven defined the positive x axis as oriented from the right to the left side of the patient (which actually means from left to right when viewed from an observer, as traditionally defined in physics). Because the electric heart vector is typically directed to the left, back, and down, Einthoven chose the y axis to point down so that the main deflection of the QRS complex is positive. Einthoven investigated the ECG signal only in the frontal plane and therefore did not need the z coordinate.

When constructing his vectorcardiographic system, Frank decided to accept the x and y directions defined by Einthoven and defined the z coordinate to point to the back in order to have a right-handed coordinate system. This coordinate system is the one standardized by AHA.

The coordinate system of AHA includes the following shortcomings:

1. Relative to the natural observation planes of the patient (i.e., the frontal plane observed from the front, the sagittal plane observed from left, and the transverse plane observed from above), only the sagittal plane is observed from the positive side.
2. The spherical coordinate system, fixed to this coordinate system with the generally accepted axes, results in an unfamiliar orientation.

Additionally, Einthoven's attempt to obtain a positive deflection of the electric y signal results in a negative deflection in the magnetic signal.

For these reasons Malmivuo developed a consistent coordinate system for electrocardiology, which avoids the aforementioned drawbacks (Malmivuo, 1976; Malmivuo et al., 1977).

A.2 REQUIREMENTS FOR A CONSISTENT SYSTEM OF RECTANGULAR COORDINATES

The rectangular coordinate system should fulfill the following requirements:

1. The rectangular coordinate system should be right-handed to be consistent with conventions in the physical sciences and to permit straightforward application of the standard equations used in vector analysis and electromagnetism.
2. The three coordinate planes are the xy, yz, and zx planes.
3. Each plane is viewed from positive side.
4. Angles in the xy, yz, and zx planes are measured in the positive direction (counterclockwise) from the x, y, and z axes, respectively, with a range from either $0°$ to $360°$ or $0°$ to $\pm180°$, with negative angles being measured in a clockwise direction from the axis.

5. The four quadrants in each coordinate plane are specified in a positive, counterclockwise, sequence:

$$
\begin{array}{ll}
\text{I:} & 0° \text{ to } 90° \\
\text{II:} & 90° \text{ to } 180° \\
\text{III:} & 180° \text{ to } 270° \\
\text{IV:} & 270° \text{ to } 360°
\end{array}
$$

A.3 ALIGNMENT OF THE COORDINATE SYSTEM WITH THE BODY

The origin of the coordinate system should be in the geometric center of the heart. The orientation of the coordinate system with respect to the body is of little mathematical consequence but of great practical importance.

It is convenient to align the rectangular coordinate axes with the body axes (i.e., sagittal, transverse, and longitudinal axes). This means that the coordinate planes correspond to the

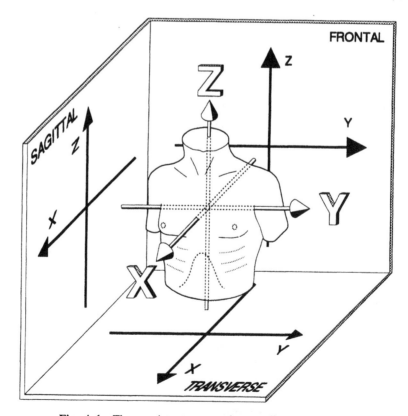

Fig. A.1 The consistent rectangular coordinate system.

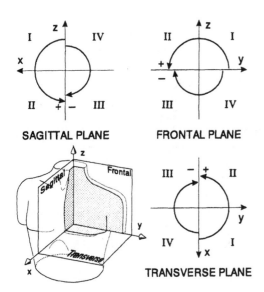

SAGITTAL PLANE

FRONTAL PLANE

TRANSVERSE PLANE

Fig. A.2 Display of the three standard projections in the consistent rectangular coordinate system. The arcs indicate the positive and negative deviation of the angles in each coordinate plane.

frontal, left sagittal, and transverse planes. In order that the planes be viewed from their positive side and that these views be the same as those used in clinical vector electrocardiography, the positive directions of the *x*, *y*, and *z* axes are chosen to be *anterior*, *left*, and *superior*, respectively. The consistent rectangular

coordinate system is illustrated in Figure A.1. The three coordinate planes including their four quadrants and the convention for measuring the angles are illustrated in Figure A.2.

Note that selection of the positive directions of the axes in the above order provides the most practical orientation for the *illustrative spherical coordinates* (see Fig. A.3B).

A.4 CONSISTENT SPHERICAL COORDINATE SYSTEMS

There are two spherical coordinate systems which are consistent with the rectangular coordinate system:

A.4.1 Mathematically Consistent Spherical Polar Coordinate System

For mathematical calculations the following spherical polar coordinate system which fulfills the definition of the Laplace equation (Morse and Feshbach, 1953, p. 658; Smythe, 1968, p. 52) is defined:

$$r = \sqrt{x^2 + y^2 + z^2}$$
$$\cos\theta = \frac{z}{\sqrt{x^2 + y^2 + z^2}} \qquad (A.1)$$
$$\tan\phi = \frac{y}{x}$$

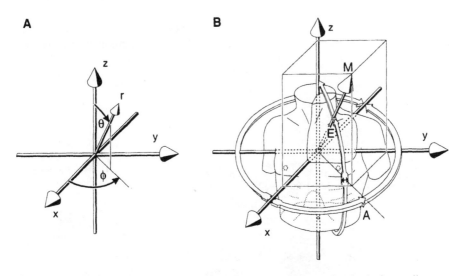

Fig. A.3 Relationship between the consistent rectangular and spherical coordinate systems. (A) Mathematically consistent spherical polar coordinate system. (B) Illustrative spherical coordinate system.

The radius vector is described by the symbol *r*. The angles θ and φ are called *colatitude* and *longitude,* respectively. The angle θ is also called *polar* angle because it is an angle dimensioned from the pole (i.e., *z* axis). These requirements for rectangular and spherical polar coordinates are based on existing mathematical conventions. This mathematically consistent coordinate system is illustrated in Figure A.3A.

A.4.2 Illustrative Spherical Coordinate System

If the behavior of the electric or the magnetic heart vector is displayed in the mathematically consistent spherical polar coordinate system, the direction of increasing values on the vertical axis is inconveniently downward. Therefore to avoid this deficiency it is preferable to use the same spherical coordinate system which is familiar in the geographical projection of the Earth. This coordinate system differs from the mathematically consistent coordinate system in that instead of the colatitude angle, the *latitude* angle is used. The latter is measured from the *xy* plane. In this coordinate system the spherical coordinates are related to the rectangular coordinates by the following equations:

$$M = \sqrt{x^2 + y^2 + z^2}$$
$$\sin E = \frac{z}{\sqrt{x^2 + y^2 + z^2}} \qquad (A.2)$$
$$\tan A = \frac{y}{x}$$

In the illustrative spherical coordinate system, the vector magnitude is represented by the symbol *M* (being the same as the radius vector *r* in the spherical polar coordinate system). The angles *E* and *A* are called the *elevation* and *azimuth,* respectively. This coordinate system is illustrated in Figure A.3B. (Note, that when the elevation and azimuth angles are those used in connection with the AHA coordinate system, they are represented by symbols *V* and *H* and they differ from those of the consistent system introduced in this chapter.)

The elevation and azimuth angles correspond exactly to the *latitude* and *longitude* angles, respectively, used in geography. Therefore, ordinary (and familiar) geographic map projection techniques can be immediately applied to maps of electric potential and magnetic field over the entire torso surface, as described in Figure A.4.

A.5 COMPARISON OF THE CONSISTENT COORDINATE SYSTEM AND THE AHA SYSTEM

The consistent coordinate system differs from that recommended by the American Heart Association (1967), and the conversion of the respective coordinate axes is as shown in Table A.1.

In the rectangular coordinates, the *x* and *z* coordinates in the consistent system have op-

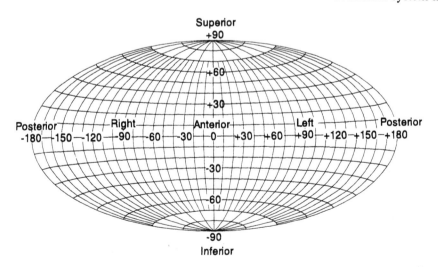

Fig. A.4 Display of the torso surface in the illustrative spherical coordinate system.

Table A.1 Conversion of the coordinate axes and angles between the consistent coordinate system and the AHA coordinate system

Consistent coordinate system	AHA coordinate system
x	$-z$
y	$+x$
z	$-y$
E	$-V$
A	$H+90°$
M	M

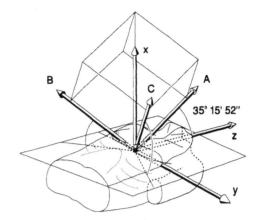

Fig. A.5 The directional relationship between the ABC coordinates and the xyz coordinates.

posite polarity to those in the AHA system. However, the consistent system and the AHA system have *identical vector loop displays.*

In the spherical coordinates, the elevation angles (E and V) are the same in both systems except for different polarity. The azimuth angles (A and H) have the same polarity in both systems, but because of the different reference axis the values in the consistent system differ by 90° from the values in the AHA system. The vector magnitude M is, of course, the same in both systems. (Note that in the existing literature one may find other definitions for the elevation and azimuth angles than those of the AHA.)

A.6 RECTANGULAR ABC COORDINATES

In addition to the XYZ coordinate system in magnetocardiography, another right-handed coordinate system is needed that is oriented more symmetrically in relation to the frontal plane (Malmivuo, 1976). The three axes of this coordinate system are selected to be the three edges of a cube whose diagonal is parallel to the x axis. This system is called the ABC coordinate system. Figure A.5 shows the orientation of these axes in relation to the x, y, and z axes. The ABC axes form an angle of 35° 15′ 52″ with the yz plane, and the angle between their projections on this plane is 120°. The projection of the A axis is parallel to the z axis.

The components of a vector in the ABC coordinate system may be transformed to the XYZ coordinate system with the following linear transformation (Equation A.3):

The components of a vector in the XYZ coordinate system may be transformed to the ABC coordinate system with the following linear transformation (Equation A.4):

$$
\begin{vmatrix} x \\ y \\ z \end{vmatrix} = \begin{vmatrix} \dfrac{1}{\sqrt{3}} & \dfrac{1}{\sqrt{3}} & \dfrac{1}{\sqrt{3}} \\ 0 & \dfrac{-1}{\sqrt{2}} & \dfrac{1}{\sqrt{2}} \\ \dfrac{2}{\sqrt{3}} & \dfrac{-1}{\sqrt{6}} & \dfrac{-1}{\sqrt{6}} \end{vmatrix} \begin{vmatrix} A \\ B \\ C \end{vmatrix} \quad \text{(A.3)}
$$

$$
\begin{vmatrix} A \\ B \\ C \end{vmatrix} = \begin{vmatrix} \dfrac{1}{\sqrt{3}} & 0 & \dfrac{\sqrt{2}}{\sqrt{3}} \\ \dfrac{1}{\sqrt{3}} & \dfrac{-1}{\sqrt{2}} & \dfrac{-1}{\sqrt{6}} \\ \dfrac{1}{\sqrt{3}} & \dfrac{1}{\sqrt{2}} & \dfrac{-1}{\sqrt{6}} \end{vmatrix} \begin{vmatrix} x \\ y \\ z \end{vmatrix} \quad \text{(A.4)}
$$

REFERENCES

American Heart Association (1967): Recommendations for standardization of leads and of specifications for instruments in electrocardiography and vectorcardiography. *Circulation* 35: 583–7. (Report of Committee on Electrocardiography).

Frank E (1956): An accurate, clinically practical system for spatial vectorcardiography. *Circulation* 13:(5) 737–49.

Malmivuo JA (1976): On the detection of the magnetic heart vector—An application of the reciprocity theorem. *Helsinki Univ. Tech.*, Acta Polytechn. Scand., El. Eng. Series. Vol. 39., pp. 112. (Dr. tech. thesis)

Malmivuo JA, Wikswo JP, Barry WH, Harrison DC, Fairbank WM (1977): Consistent system of rectangular and spherical coordinates for electrocardiography and magnetocardiography. *Med. & Biol. Eng. & Comput.* 15:(4) 413–5.

Morse PM, Feshbach H (1953): *Methods of Theoretical Physics. Part I,* 997 pp. McGraw-Hill, New York.

Smythe WR (1968): *Static and Dynamic Electricity,* 3rd ed., 623 pp. McGraw-Hill, New York.

APPENDIX B

Application of Maxwell's Equations in Bioelectromagnetism

B.1 INTRODUCTION

The behavior of time-varying and static electric and magnetic fields are governed by Maxwell's equations formulated by James Clerk Maxwell (1865, 1873). These equations simply summarize the mathematical consequences of the classical experiments of Faraday, Ampère, Coulomb, Maxwell, and others.

Maxwell's equations can be found in general texts on electromagnetic theory. However, they are essentially applicable to electromagnetic fields in free space (i.e., radiation fields). Where conducting and/or magnetic media are involved, then, although the equations continue to be valid, current sources can arise in other ways than specified under free space conditions. These modifications must be introduced through a consideration of the particular nature of current sources appropriate for the problem at hand.

Our goal here, after introducing Maxwell's equations in the form valid for free space conditions, is to specialize them so that they correctly describe conditions that arise in bioelectromagnetism. Following this, our goal is to simplify the equations where possible, based on practical electrophysiological considerations.

B.2 MAXWELL'S EQUATIONS UNDER FREE SPACE CONDITIONS

PRECONDITIONS:

Sources and Fields: *Time-varying $\bar{J}$, ρ, $\bar{E}$, $\bar{H}$*

Conductor: *Infinite, homogeneous free space*
$\sigma = 0$, $\mu = \mu_0$, $\epsilon = \epsilon_0$

Maxwell's equations are usually written in differential (and vector) form for free space conditions as follows, where for simplicity a harmonic time variation is assumed:

$$\nabla \times \bar{E} = -j\omega\mu_0\bar{H} \tag{B.1}$$

$$\nabla \times \bar{H} = j\omega\epsilon_0\bar{E} + \bar{J} \tag{B.2}$$

$$\nabla \cdot \bar{D} = \rho \tag{B.3}$$

$$\nabla \cdot \bar{J} = -j\omega\rho \tag{B.4}$$

$$\nabla \cdot \bar{B} = 0 \tag{B.5}$$

Equation B.1 is a statement of *Faraday's law* that a time-varying magnetic field $\bar{H}$ induces an electric field $\bar{E}$.

Equation B.2 is a statement of *Ampère's law* that the line integral of magnetic field $\bar{H}$ around a closed loop equals the total current through the loop. The current is described as a displacement current $j\omega\epsilon_0\bar{E}$ plus source

455

currents $\bar{J}$ arising from the actual convection of charge in a vacuum.

Equation B.3 arises from *Coulomb's law* and relates the electric displacement $\bar{D}$ to the sources that generate it, namely the charge density ρ.

Equation B.4 is a statement of the *conservation of charge*, namely that its outflow from any closed region (evaluated from $\nabla \cdot \bar{J}$) can arise only if the charge contained is depleted.

Equation B.5 recognizes that *no magnetic charges exist*, and hence the magnetic induction $\bar{B}$, must be solenoidal.

B.3 MAXWELL'S EQUATIONS FOR FINITE CONDUCTING MEDIA

PRECONDITIONS:

Sources and Fields: *Static or quasistatic emf, $\bar{J}^i$, $\bar{E}$, $\bar{H}$*

Conductor: *Finite, inhomogeneous*
$\sigma = \sigma(x,y,z)$, $\mu = \mu_0$, $\epsilon = \epsilon_0$

Our interest lies in describing electric and magnetic fields within and outside electrophysiological preparations. Electrophysiological preparations are isolated regions (lying in air) that involve excitable tissue surrounded by a conducting medium (*volume conductor*). The conductivity σ of the volume conductor, in general, is a function of position $[\sigma(x,y,z)]$; that is, it is assumed to be inhomogeneous. Its magnetic permeability μ is normally assumed to be that of free space (μ_0), and, except for a membrane region the dielectric permittivity also has the free space value (ϵ_0).

If we consider for the moment a static condition, then we find that Equation B.1 requires that $\nabla \times \bar{E} = 0$. This means that $\bar{E}$ must be conservative, a condition that is appropriate for electric fields arising from static charges in free space (i.e., electrostatics). But in our conducting medium, currents can flow only if there are nonconservative sources present. So we must assume the existence of electromotive forces emf. Thus for conducting media, Equation B.1 must be modified to the form of Equation B.6.

By the same reasoning, we must also recognize the presence of *impressed* (applied) current fields, which we designate $\bar{J}^i$; these must be included on the right side of Equation B.7, which corresponds to Equation B.2 as applied to conducting media. Such sources may be essentially time-invariant as with an electrochemical battery that supplies an essentially steady current flow to a volume conductor. They may also be *quasistatic*, as exemplified by activated (excitable) tissue; in this case, time-varying nonconservative current sources result which, in turn, drive currents throughout the surrounding volume conductor.

In a conducting medium there cannot be a convection current such as was envisaged by the parameter $\bar{J}$ in Equation B.2, and it is therefore omitted from Equation B.7. The convection current is meant to describe the flow of charges in a vacuum such as occurs in high-power amplifier tubes. (For the same reason, Equation B.4 is not valid in conducting media.) In the consideration of applied magnetic fields, one can treat the applied current flowing in a physical coil by idealizing it as a free-space current, and hence accounting for it with the $\bar{J}$ on the right side of Equation B.2. Since this current is essentially solenoidal, there is no associated charge density. In this formalism the means whereby $\bar{J}$ is established need not be considered explicitly.

Because of the electric conductivity σ of the volume conductor we need to include in the right side of Equation B.7 the conduction current $\sigma\bar{E}$, in addition to the existing displacement current $j\omega\epsilon\bar{E}$.

Another modification comes from the recognition that a volume charge density ρ cannot exist within a conducting medium (though surface charges can accumulate at the interface between regions of different conductivity— essentially equivalent to the charges that lie on the plates of a capacitor). Therefore, Equation B.3 is not applicable in conducting media.

With these considerations, Maxwell's equations may now be rewritten for finite conducting media as

$$\nabla \times \bar{E} = -j\omega\mu_0\bar{H} + \text{emf} \qquad (\text{B.6})$$

$$\nabla \times \bar{H} = (\sigma + j\omega\epsilon_0)\bar{E} + \bar{J}^i \qquad (\text{B.7})$$

$$\nabla \cdot \overline{E} = - \frac{\nabla \cdot \overline{J}^i}{\sigma + j\omega\epsilon_0} \qquad (B.8)$$

$$\nabla \cdot \overline{B} = 0 \qquad (B.9)$$

In this set of equations, we obtain Equation B.8 by taking the divergence of both sides of Equation B.7 and noting that the divergence of the curl of any vector function is identically zero ($\nabla \cdot \nabla \times \overline{H} \equiv 0$).

B.4 SIMPLIFICATION OF MAXWELL'S EQUATIONS IN PHYSIOLOGICAL PREPARATIONS

PRECONDITIONS:

Sources and Fields: *Quasistatic ($\omega < 1000$ Hz) emf, $\overline{J}^i$, $\overline{E}$, $\overline{H}$*

Conductor: *Limited finite ($r < 1$ m) inhomogeneous resistive ($\omega\epsilon/\sigma < 0.15$) $= \mu_0$, $\epsilon = \epsilon_0$*

Physiological preparations of electrophysiological interest have several characteristics on which can be based certain simplifications of the general Maxwell's equations. We have already mentioned that we expect the permittivity ϵ and permeability μ in the volume conductor to be those of free space (ϵ_0, μ_0). Three other conditions will be introduced here.

B.4.1 Frequency Limit

The power density spectra of signals of biological origin have been measured. These have been found to vary depending on the nature of the source (e.g., nerve, muscle, etc.). The highest frequencies are seen in electrocardiography. Here the bandwidth for clinical instruments normally lies under 100 Hz, though the very highest quality requires an upper frequency of 200–500 Hz. In research it is usually assumed to be under 1000 Hz, and we shall consider this the nominal upper frequency limit. Barr and Spach (1977) have shown that for intramural cardiac potentials frequencies as high as 10 kHz may need to be included for faithful signal reproduction. When one considers that the action pulse rise time is on the order of 1ms, then signals due to such sources ought to have little energy beyond 1 kHz. Relative to the entire frequency spectrum to which Maxwell's equations have been applied, this is indeed a low-frequency range. The resulting simplifications are described in the next section.

B.4.2 Size Limitation

Except for the very special case where one is studying, say, the ECG of a whale, the size of the volume conductor can be expected to lie within a sphere of radius of 1 m. Such a sphere would accommodate almost all intact human bodies, and certainly typical in vitro preparations under study in the laboratory. A consequence, to be discussed in the next section, is that the "retarded" potentials of general interest do not arise.

B.4.3 Volume Conductor Impedance

The volume conductor normally contains several discrete elements such as nerve, muscle, connective tissue, vascular tissue, skin, and other organs. For many cases, the conducting properties can be described by a conductivity $\sigma(x,y,z)$ obtained by averaging over a small but multicellular region. Since such a macroscopic region contains lipid cellular membranes the permittivity may depart from its free-space value. The values of both σ and ϵ entering Equations B.7 and B.8 will depend on the particular tissue characteristics and on frequency. By making macroscopic measurements, Schwan and Kay (1957) determined that $\omega\epsilon/\sigma$ for the frequency range 10 Hz $< f <$ 1000 Hz is under 0.15. But in many cases it is possible to treat all membranes specifically. In this case it is the remaining intracellular and interstitial space that constitutes the volume conductor; and, since the lipids are absent, the medium will behave resistively over the entire frequency spectrum of interest. In either case it is reasonable to ignore the displacement current $j\omega\epsilon_0\overline{E}$ within the volume conductor in Equations B.7 and B.8. (One should always, of course, include the capacitive membrane current when considering components of the total membrane current.) Consequently, these equations can be simplified to Equations B.10 and B.11, respectively.

Thus Maxwell's equations for physiological applications have the form:

$$\nabla \times \bar{E} = -j\omega\mu_0\bar{H} + \text{emf} \qquad (B.6)$$

$$\nabla \times \bar{H} = \sigma\bar{E} + \bar{J}^i \qquad (B.10)$$

$$\nabla \cdot \bar{E} = -\frac{\nabla \cdot \bar{J}^i}{\sigma} \qquad (B.11)$$

$$\nabla \cdot \bar{B} = 0 \qquad (B.9)$$

B.5 MAGNETIC VECTOR POTENTIAL AND ELECTRIC SCALAR POTENTIAL IN THE REGION OUTSIDE THE SOURCES

PRECONDITIONS:

Source: *Quasistatic $\bar{J}^i$ (ω < 1000 Hz)*

Conductor: *Limited finite (r < 1 m) region outside the sources inhomogeneous resistive ($\omega\epsilon/\sigma$ < 0.15)*

$\mu = \mu_0$, $\epsilon = \epsilon_0$

In this section we derive from Maxwell's equations the equations for magnetic vector potential $\bar{A}$ and electric scalar potential Φ in physiological applications, Equations B.19 and B.21, respectively.

Since the divergence of $\bar{B}$ is identically zero (Equation B.9), the magnetic field may be derived from the curl of an arbitrary vector field $\bar{A}$, which is called the *magnetic vector potential*. This fulfills the requirement stated in Equation B.9 because the divergence of the curl of any vector field is necessarily zero. Consequently,

$$\bar{B} = \nabla \times \bar{A} \qquad (B.12)$$

Since $\bar{B} = \mu_0\bar{H}$, we can substitute Equation B.12 into Equation B.6. We consider only the volume conductor region external to the membranes where the emf's are zero (note that the emfs are explicitly included *within* the membrane in the form of Nernst potential batteries), and we consequently obtain

$$\nabla \times (\bar{E} + j\omega\bar{A}) = 0 \qquad (B.13)$$

Now, when the curl of a vector field is zero, that vector field can be derived as the (negative) gradient of an arbitrary scalar potential field (which we designate with the symbol Φ and which denotes the *electric scalar potential*). This assignment is valid because the curl of the gradient of any scalar field equals zero. Thus Equation B.13 further simplifies to

$$\bar{E} + j\omega\bar{A} = -\nabla\Phi \qquad (B.14)$$

According to the *Helmholtz theorem*, a vector field is uniquely specified by both its divergence and curl (Plonsey and Collin, 1961). Since only the curl of the vector field $\bar{A}$ has been specified so far (in Equation B.12), we may now choose

$$\nabla \cdot \bar{A} = -\sigma\mu_0\Phi \qquad (B.15)$$

This particular choice eliminates Φ from the differential equation for $\bar{A}$ (Equation B.17). That is, it has the desirable effect of uncoupling the magnetic vector potential $\bar{A}$ from the electric scalar potential Φ. Such a consideration was originally suggested by Lorentz when dealing with the free-space form of Maxwell's equations. Lorentz introduced an equation similar to Equation B.15 known as the *Lorentz condition*, which is that

$$\nabla \cdot \bar{A} = -j\omega\epsilon\mu\Phi \qquad (B.16)$$

We have modified this expression since we have eliminated in Equations B.10 and B.11 the displacement current $j\omega\epsilon\bar{E}$ in favor of a conduction current $\sigma\bar{E}$. This amounts to replacing $j\omega\epsilon$ by σ in the classical Lorentz condition (Equation B.16), resulting in Equation B.15. The Lorentz condition can also be shown to have another important property, namely that it ensures the satisfaction of the continuity condition.

Now, if we substitute Equations B.12, B.14, and B.15 into Equation B.10, keeping in mind that $\bar{H} = \bar{B}/\mu_0$, and if we use the vector identity that

$$\nabla \times \nabla \times \bar{A} \equiv \nabla\nabla \cdot \bar{A} - \nabla^2\bar{A} \quad (B.17)$$

we obtain

$$\nabla^2\bar{A} - j\omega\mu_0\sigma\bar{A} = -\mu_0\bar{J}^i \qquad (B.18)$$

Just as emf's were eliminated by confining attention to the region external to the excitable cell membranes, so too could one eliminate the nonconservative current $\bar{J}^i$ in Equation B.10. In this case all equations describe conditions in the passive extracellular and intracellular spaces; the effect of sources within the membranes then enters solely through boundary conditions at and across the membranes. On the other hand, it is useful to retain $\bar{J}^i$ as a distributed source function in Equation B.10. While it is actually confined to cell membranes ensuring the aforementioned boundary conditions, it may be simplified (averaged) and regarded as an equivalent source that is uniformly distributed throughout the "source volume." For field points outside the source region which are at a distance that is large compared to cellular dimensions (over which averaging of $\bar{J}^i$ occurs) the generated field approaches the correct value.

Equation B.18 is known as the *vector Helmholtz equation*, for which solutions in integral form are well known in classical electricity and magnetism (Plonsey and Collin, 1961). Adapting such a solution to our specific equation gives

$$\bar{A} = \frac{\mu_0}{4\pi} \int \frac{\bar{J}^i e^{-kr} e^{jkr}}{r} \, dV \qquad (B.19)$$

where

$$k = \sqrt{\omega\mu_0\sigma/2} \; [1/m]$$
$$r = (x,y,z,x',y',z')$$
$$= \sqrt{(x-x')^2 + (y-y')^2 + (z-z')^2}$$

Note that r is the radial distance from a source element $dV(x,y,z)$ (unprimed coordinates) to the field point $P(x',y',z')$ (primed coordinates), and is thus a function of both the unprimed and primed coordinates.

To evaluate an upper bound to the magnitude of kr in the exponential terms in Equation B.19 we choose:

$$r_{max} = 100 \text{ cm}$$
$$\omega = 2\pi \times 1000 \text{ 1/s}$$
$$\mu_0 = 4\pi \times 10^{-9} \text{ H/cm}$$
$$\sigma = 0.004 \text{ S/cm}$$

Then

$$kr_{max} = .04$$

Since $e^{-.04} = .96$, these exponential terms can be ignored and we get a simplification for Equa-

tion B.19, giving the magnetic vector potential under electrophysiological conditions:

$$\bar{A} = \frac{\mu_0}{4\pi} \int \frac{\bar{J}^i}{r} \, dV \qquad (B.20)$$

The electric scalar potential Φ may be found from $\bar{A}$ by using Equation B.15 with Equation B.20. In doing so, we note that Equation B.20 involves an integration over the source coordinates (x,y,z) while Equation B.15 involves operations at the field coordinates (x',y',z'). Consequently, we get

$$\Phi = \frac{1}{4\pi\sigma} \int \bar{J}^i \cdot \nabla' \left(\frac{1}{r}\right) dV \qquad (B.21)$$

where ∇' operates only on the field coordinates, which is why $\bar{J}^i$ is not affected. Since $\nabla'(1/r) = -\nabla(1/r)$, we finally get for the electric scalar potential:

$$\Phi = \frac{1}{4\pi\sigma} \int \bar{J}^i \cdot \nabla \left(\frac{1}{r}\right) dV \qquad (B.22)$$

Equation B.22 is identical to static field expressions for the electric field, where $\bar{J}^i$ is interpreted as a volume dipole density source function. This equation corresponds exactly to Equation 7–5. Although a staticlike equation applies, $\bar{J}^i$ is actually time-varying, and consequently, so must Φ be time-varying synchronously. We call this situation a *quasistatic* one.

When the source arises electrically (including that due to cellular excitation), a magnetic field is necessarily set up by the resulting current flow. The latter gives rise to a vector potential $\bar{A}$, which in turn contributes to the resulting electric field $\bar{E}$ through the term $j\omega\bar{A}$ in Equation B.14. However, under the conditions specified, $|\omega\bar{A}|$ is negligible compared to the term $|\nabla\Phi|$ as discussed in Plonsey and Heppner (1967). Under these conditions we are left with the scalar potential term alone, and Equation B.14 simplifies to

$$\bar{E} = -\nabla\Phi \qquad (B.23)$$

which also corresponds to a static formulation. It should be kept in mind that Equation B.23 is not exact, but only a good approximation. It corresponds to the quasistatic condition where the electric field resembles that arising under static conditions. Under truly static conditions the electric and magnetic fields are completely independent. Under quasistatic conditions, while the fields satisfy static equations, a low frequency time variation may be superimposed (justified by the low frequency conditions discussed earlier), in which case the magnetic field effects, although extant, can normally be ignored.

Note that in this case, where the sources are exclusively bioelectric and the simplification of Equation B.23 is valid, Equation B.11 leads to Equation 7.2 ($\bar{J} = \bar{J}^i - \sigma \nabla \Phi$).

B.6 STIMULATION WITH ELECTRIC AND MAGNETIC FIELDS

B.6.1 Stimulation with Electric Field

PRECONDITIONS:

Source: *Steady-state electric field $\bar{E}$*

Conductor: *Uniform fiber in volume conductor*

The above comments notwithstanding, we are also interested in a situation where excitable tissue is stimulated solely with an applied magnetic field. In this case the vector potential $\bar{A}$ is large and cannot be ignored. In fact, to ignore $\bar{A}$ under these circumstances is to drop the underlying forcing function, which would leave an absurd result of no field, either electric or magnetic.

We have shown in Chapter 3 that for a single uniform fiber under steady-state conditions a homogeneous partial differential equation (Equation 3.46) arises:

$$\frac{\partial^2 V_m}{\partial x^2} - \frac{V_m}{\lambda^2} = 0 \qquad (B.24)$$

where

V_m = transmembrane potential

λ = space constant, characteristic of the physical and electric properties of the fiber

x = coordinate along the direction of the fiber

For a point source at the origin we have also essentially shown, in Chapter 3, that the solution to Equation B.24 is (Equation 3.49)

$$V'(x) = V_m(0)e^{-x/\lambda} \qquad (B.25)$$

where

$V'(x)$ = deviation of the membrane voltage from the resting voltage

In this equation

$$V_m(0) = \frac{r_i \lambda I_0}{2} \qquad (B.26)$$

where

$V_m(0)$ = transmembrane potential at the origin

I_0 = applied intracellular point current

r_i = intracellular axial resistance per unit length

We remark, here, that for a more general applied scalar potential field, Φ_e, Equation B.24 becomes

$$\frac{\partial^2 V_m}{\partial x^2} - \frac{V_m}{\lambda^2} = -\frac{\partial^2 \Phi_e/\partial x^2}{\lambda^2} \qquad (B.27)$$

One can recognize in this equation that the second derivative of the applied potential field along the fiber is the forcing function (in fact, it has been called the "activating function"), whereas the dependent variable, V_m, is the membrane response to the stimulation. Using Equation B.23, one can write Equation B.24 as

$$\frac{\partial^2 V_m}{\partial x^2} - \frac{V_m}{\lambda^2} = \frac{\partial \bar{E}/\partial x}{\lambda^2} \qquad (B.28)$$

where $\bar{E}$ is the applied electric field.

B.6.2 Stimulation with Magnetic Field

PRECONDITIONS:

Source: *Time-varying magnetic field $\bar{B}$*

Conductor: *Uniform fiber in volume conductor*

Electric stimulation may be produced by applying a time-varying magnetic field $\bar{B}$ to the tissue. As given in Equation B.12, this magnetic field is defined as the curl of a vector potential $\bar{A}$. Now the stimulus is introduced solely through a magnetic field that induces an electric field $\bar{E}$. Equation B.27 is still completely valid except that the applied field $\bar{E}$ is found from Equation B.14, namely where $\bar{E} = -j\omega\bar{A}$.

The determination of the vector field $\bar{A}$ from a physical coil is found, basically, from Equation B.20 (which corresponds to Equation

12.33). This relationship has also been worked out and published for many other coil configurations.

We also note that since the differential equations B.24, B.27, and B.28 are linear, and the solution given in Equation B.25 is essentially the response to a (spatial) unit impulse at the origin (set $I_0 = \delta(x)$), then linear systems theory describes the solution to Equation B.27, (or B.28), as

$$V_m(x) = V'(x' - x) \otimes - \left(r_m \frac{\partial^2 \Phi_e/\partial x'^2}{\lambda^2} \right) \quad \text{(B.29)}$$

where $\otimes$ denotes convolution. (The added factor of r_m is required in order to convert the right side of Equation B.29 into a current density.) The convolution operation can be performed by taking the inverse Fourier transform of the product of the Fourier transform of V' and the Fourier transform of the second derivative of Φ_e. Such operations are readily carried out using the fast Fourier transform (FFT).

B.7 SIMPLIFIED MAXWELL'S EQUATIONS IN PHYSIOLOGICAL PREPARATIONS IN THE REGION OUTSIDE THE SOURCES

PRECONDITIONS:

Sources and Fields: *Quasistatic (ω < 1000 Hz)* $\bar{J}^i, \bar{E}, \bar{H}$

Conductor: *Limited finite (r < 1 m) region outside the sources inhomogeneous resistive ($\omega\epsilon/\sigma$ < 0.15)*

$\mu = \mu_0, \epsilon = \epsilon_0$

We finally collect the Maxwell's equations in their simplest form. These equations are valid under quasistatic electrophysiological conditions outside the region of bioelectric sources:

$$\bar{E} = -\nabla\Phi \quad \text{(B.23)}$$

$$\nabla \times \bar{H} = \sigma\bar{E} + \bar{J}^i \quad \text{(B.10)}$$

$$\nabla \cdot \bar{E} = -\frac{\nabla \cdot \bar{J}^i}{\sigma} \quad \text{(B.11)}$$

$$\nabla \cdot \bar{B} = 0 \quad \text{(B.9)}$$

REFERENCES

Barr RC, Spach MS (1977): Sampling rates required for digital recording of intracellular and extracellular cardiac potentials. *Circulation* 55: 40–8.

Maxwell J (1865): A dynamical theory of the electromagnetic field. *Phil. Trans. R. Soc. (Lond.)* 155: 459–512.

Maxwell J (1873): *Treatise on Electricity and Magnetism*, Vol. 2, Oxford. (Reprint by Dover, New York, 1954.)

Plonsey R, Collin R (1961): *Principles and Applications of Electromagnetic Fields*, 554 pp. McGraw-Hill, New York.

Plonsey R, Heppner DB (1967): Considerations of quasistationarity in electrophysiological systems. *Bull. Math. Biophys.* 29:(4) 657–64.

Schwan HP, Kay CF (1957): The conductivity of living tissue. *Ann. N.Y. Acad. Sci.* 65: 1007.

Name Index

Subject Index

Printed in the USA
CPSIA information can be obtained
at www.ICGtesting.com
CBHW081957040924
13927CB00031B/599